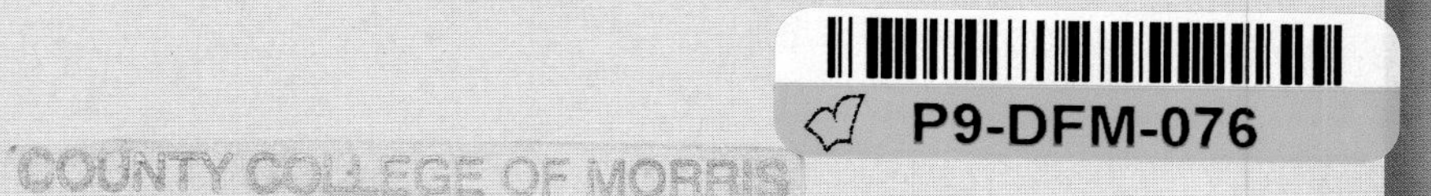

Electronic Health Records

third edition

Byron R. Hamilton

CEO, Med-Soft National Training Institution—Colorado, BA, MA

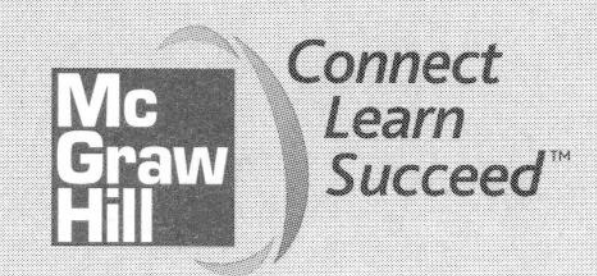

The McGraw·Hill Companies

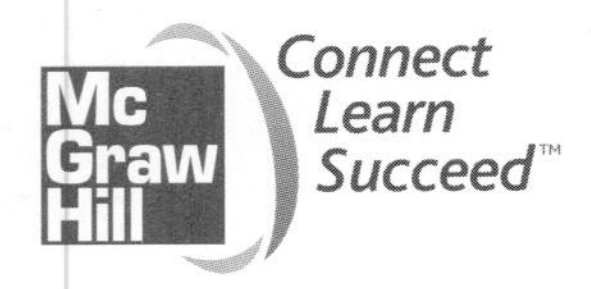

ELECTRONIC HEALTH RECORDS, THIRD EDITION

Published by McGraw-Hill, a business unit of The McGraw-Hill Companies, Inc., 1221 Avenue of the Americas, New York, NY, 10020.

Some ancillaries, including electronic and print components, may not be available to customers outside the United States.

This book is printed on acid-free paper.

5 6 7 8 9 0 RMN/RMN 1 0 9 8 7 6 5 4

ISBN 978-0-07-340214-7
MHID 0-07-340214-1

Senior Vice President, Products & Markets: *Kurt L. Strand*
Vice President, General Manager, Products & Markets: *Martin J. Lange*
Vice President, Content Production & Technology Services: *Kimberly Meriwether David*
Managing Director: *Michael S. Ledbetter*
Senior Brand Manager: *Natalie J. Ruffatto*
Managing Development Editor: *Michelle L. Flomenhoft*
Development Editor: *Raisa Priebe Kreek*
Executive Marketing Manager: *Roxan Kinsey*
Digital Development Editor: *Katherine Ward*
Project Manager: *Kathryn D. Wright*
Buyer: *Susan Culbertson*
Senior Designer: *Srdjan Savanovic*
Cover Designer: *George Kokkonas*
Interior Designer: *PV Design*
Cover Image: © *Katya Triling | Dreamstime.com*
Senior Content Licensing Specialist: *Keri Johnson*
Media Project Manager: *Brent dela Cruz*
Media Project Manager: *Cathy L. Tepper*
Typeface: *10.5/12.5 Palatino*
Compositor: *Aptara®, Inc.*
Printer: *R. R. Donnelley*

Library of Congress Cataloging-in-Publication Data

Hamilton, Byron, 1958–
Electronic health records / Byron R. Hamilton.—3rd ed.
p. ; cm.
Includes bibliographical references and index.
ISBN 978-0-07-340214-7 (alk. paper)—ISBN 0-07-340214-1 (alk. paper)
1. Medical records—Data processing. I. Title.
[DNLM: 1. Electronic Health Records—Problems and Exercises. WX 18.2]
R864.H32 2013
610.285—dc23

2012013845

www.mhhe.com

about the author

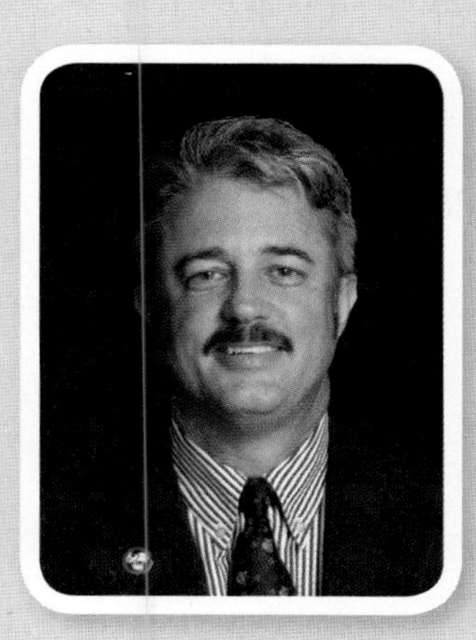

Byron R. Hamilton received a BA in Education from the College of Advanced Education in Australia, and taught for several years in both private and public institutions. He earned an MA in Biblical Literature in Springfield, MO, and has taught EHR as part of the Continuing Education Department at Ozark Technical Community College in Springfield, Missouri.

In 1997, Byron and his wife, Leesa, established *MedTech Medical Management Systems,* a medical billing and consulting company for both practice management software and electronic medical records. For the following decade they were involved with medical billing, supervision of healthcare information management, medical software consultation, and training. Byron has been involved with electronic health record systems from the inception of the industry.

In 2004, he launched *Med-Soft National Training Institute,* (MNTI), a software training group conducting on-site and online training on medical software, including Medisoft™ PMS and SpringCharts™ EHR, both nationally and internationally. He has written the product training manuals for several PMS and EHR programs and has authored numerous articles for professional magazines. MNTI also provides strategies for healthcare organizations in the selection, implementation and project management of electronic health records.

In 2010, Hamilton co-authored *Nursing Documentation Using Electronic Health Records,* a textbook focused on educating nursing students in the skills of documenting patient care electronically. Byron is a national speaker at career college workshops, business college associations, and medical professional groups.

brief contents

table of contents

Preface

Health information technology continues to expand rapidly across the entire spectrum of the medical community. Affordability of computer technology and medical software continues to exert a major influence on physicians to adopt electronic health records (EHRs). Additionally, the availability and reliability of wireless computer networks, the public concern for patient safety, and the affordability of health information technology have contributed to the federal government's involvement in setting technical standards and timetables for the implementation of EHRs. The remarkable surge of interest in EHRs is leading to further development in comprehensive clinical decision support, which will continue to enhance computerized knowledge management systems and create even more robust EHRs. Through the EHR, patients have become the beneficiary of improved medical care, greater safety, and increased control over medical records, enabling them to make important contributions to their healthcare.

Because of the changes in the way that health records are kept, healthcare professionals must have exposure to and hands-on experience with electronic documentation. Specialization of informatics that now manages and processes medical data has created the urgent need for professionals with the ability to chart clerical skills, clinical skills, and patient care in an EHR system.

What You Can Expect In *Electronic Health Records*, Third Edition

- **The ONC-certified™ SpringCharts® premium EHR program is available with each text at no additional cost.** Students learn EHR documentation through this industry-standard software. It combines the right mix of rich functionality and intuitive ease of use to enable rapid and complete clinical and clerical documentation.
- An abundance of **screen captures and menu icons** from SpringCharts EHR software provide step-by-step instructions for easy reference and application.
- **HITECH Meaningful Use** standards have been detailed in tables and strategically placed throughout the text relevant to the discussion on EHR features and functionality, linking EHR software skills to the meaningful use of EHR.
- A **Certificate of Training** is available on McGraw-Hill's Online Learning Center (OLC) at **www.mhhe.com/hamiltonehr3e** for each student completing the course.

Organization of *Electronic Health Records*, 3e

The first two chapters of *Electronic Health Records* introduce the concepts and history of EHR software, including meaningful use. Chapter 3 orients you in the SpringCharts software. Chapters 4–10 emphasize different aspects of SpringCharts, from the basic patient's chart to labs, tests, codes, and templates. Chapters 11–12 give you a chance to apply the skills you have learned.

What's New in the Third Edition of *EHR?*

- *Electronic Health Records, third edition,* uses SpringCharts EHR version 2011, an upgrade of two major releases since the previous edition of *EHR*. SpringCharts V2011 is ONC-certified for ambulatory EHR criteria to qualify eligible professionals (EPs) who participate in the Medicare and Medicaid programs for financial incentive payments under the Health Information Technology for Economic and Clinical Health (HITECH) Act.
- International Classification of Diseases, 10th Revision (ICD-10) is discussed and provides an opportunity to practice creating and documenting ICD-10 codes in an EHR.
- History of EHR standards have been expanded to discuss the many private and government-sponsored organizations involved in the spread and education of EHRs, such as the Beacon Community Cooperative Agreement Program, the Health Information Technology Extension Program, Regional Extension Centers, and the national Health Information Technology Research Center (HITRC).
- Under the provisions of the American Recovery and Reinvestment Act of 2009, the ONC has established 15 mandatory EHR criteria that eligible healthcare professionals will use to demonstrate meaningful use (MU) of an EHR system in order to

qualify for robust financial incentives. These 15 criteria are a focal point of this text, along with an additional 5 standards that physicians must choose from a menu of 10 measures to demonstrate MU.

- Each chapter in the third edition of *Electronic Health Records* has:
  - o Updated Learning Outcomes linked directly to each section of the chapter.
  - o Updated Key Terms.
  - o Updated exercises using ONC-Certified SpringCharts 2011.
  - o Updated Concept Checkup questions at the end of each section.
  - o An end-of-chapter tabular summary correlated with the learning outcomes.
  - o Updated end-of-chapter matching and multiple-choice review questions.
  - o New Applying Your Knowledge critical-thinking exercises in the end-of-chapter review.

Chapter by Chapter

- **Chapter 1 The Electronic Health Record**
  - o New table showing how workflow in an office using EHR compares to workflow in an office using paper charts
  - o New Section 1.8 on potential developments in the future of the EHR
  - o Updated sections on government involvement with implementation and regulation of EHRs
- **Chapter 2 Standards and Features of Electronic Health Records**
  - o Updated section on EHR standards, including ONC and new certification bodies
  - o New section on meaningful use and EHR
  - o Updated discussion of EHR privacy and security
  - o New Section 2.5 on EHR competencies
- **Chapter 3 Introduction and Setup**
  - o New table linking MU criteria to EHR functionality
- **Chapter 4 The Clinic Administration**
  - o Existing Exercise 4.1 separated into 8 smaller exercises
  - o Existing Exercise 4.2 separated into 13 smaller exercises
- **Chapter 5 The Patient Chart**
  - o Reorganization of material by features rather than software menu items
  - o Six new tables linking mandated MU requirements to EHR features
- **Chapter 6 The Office Visit**
  - o Reorganization of material by features rather than software menu items
  - o New chapter organization for greater clarity
  - o Three new tables linking mandated MU requirements to EHR features
- **Chapter 7 Clinical Tools**
  - o Three new tables linking mandated MU requirements to EHR features
- **Chapter 8 Creating Templates**
  - o Removed IT material on exporting and importing
  - o New table linking mandated MU requirements to EHR feature
- **Chapter 9 Tests, Procedures, and Codes**
  - o New discussion and focus on ICD-10 codes
  - o New Exercise 9.8 about use of ICD-10 codes in EHR
  - o Three new tables linking mandated MU requirements to EHR features
- **Chapter 10 Productivity Center and Utilities**
  - o Removed IT material
  - o Two new tables linking mandated MU requirements to EHR features
- **Chapter 11 Applying Your Knowledge**
  - o New Introduction
  - o Reference from each exercise to text material where the underlying skill was added
  - o New Exercise 11.13 (printing the face sheet)
- **Chapter 12 EHR Practicum**
  - o New chapter title to reflect practical application in this chapter
  - o Reference from each exercise to text material where the underlying skill was introduced

(Information about the book's pedagogical elements appears in the Walkthrough starting on page xviii.)

To the Instructor

McGraw-Hill knows how much effort it takes to prepare for a new course. Through focus groups, symposia, reviews, and conversations with instructors like you, we have gathered information about what materials you need to facilitate successful courses. We are committed to providing you with high-quality, accurate instructor support.

You can rely on the following materials to help you and your students work through the material in the book, all of which are available on the book's website, **www.mhhe.com/hamiltonehr3e** (instructors can request a password through their sales representative):

Supplement	Features
Instructor's Manual (organized by Learning Outcomes)	Sample Syllabi and Lesson Plans Answer Keys for Concept Checkups and Chapter Review Documentation of Steps and Screenshots for SpringCharts Exercises
PowerPoint Presentations (organized by Learning Outcomes)	Key Terms Key Concepts Teaching Notes
Electronic Testbank	EZ Test Online (computerized) Word Version Questions are tagged with: • Learning Outcome • Level of Difficulty • Level of Bloom's Taxonomy • Feedback
Tools to Plan Course	Correlations of the Learning Outcomes to Accrediting Bodies such as CAHIIM, ABHES, CAAHEP, NHA, and SCANS Sample Syllabi and Lesson Plans Certificate of Completion Asset Map—details on the supplements for each chapter, as well as information on the content available through *Connect Plus*

Additional practice is available at McGraw-Hill's *Connect Plus. Connect Plus* uses the latest technology and learning techniques to better connect professors to their students, and students to the information and customized resources they need to master a subject. It includes a variety of digital learning tools that enable instructors to easily customize courses and allow students to master content and succeed in the course.

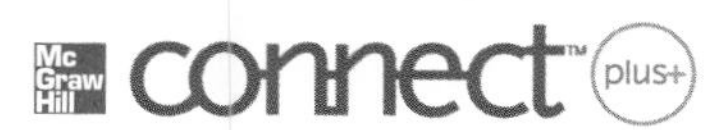

The *Connect Plus* course for *Electronic Health Records*, 3rd edition, contains all of the Concept Checkups and Chapter Review exercises, as well as some interactive exercises for each chapter. All of these exercises are tagged with the following in *Connect Plus*:

- *Learning Outcome*
- *Level of Difficulty*
- *Level of Bloom's Taxonomy*
- *Correct Response Feedback*
- *Estimated Length of Time to Complete Exercise*

In addition, all of the Learning Outcomes are correlated to the key accrediting bodies—including CAHIIM, ABHES, and CAAHEP—for instructors at **www.mhhe.com/hamiltonehr3e.**

Need help? Contact McGraw-Hill's Customer Experience Group (CXG). Visit the CXG website at www.mhhe.com/support. Browse our FAQs (Frequently Asked Questions) and product documentation, and/or contact a CXG representative. CXG is available Sunday through Friday.

To the Student

Downloading SpringCharts EHR

SpringCharts EHR is an electronic medical records software suite based on the latest industry-standard Java technology. It requires a very modest network system for installation:

- PC: A 2.8 GHz, or faster, processor.
- Mac: Core 2 Duo, 64-bit, or faster, processor.
- 500 MB available disk space (after loading Java Runtime Environment).
- 4 GB of memory.
- A computer running one of the following operating systems: Windows XP or above, or MacOS Snow Leopard (10.5) or above.

SpringCharts is available in two different system configurations: Single Computer and Network Option.

(Students, please check with your instructor about which version you need.) For the Single Computer option, SpringCharts can be installed either on a computer or on a flash drive for greater portability. Before installing SpringCharts, ensure Java Runtime Environment (JRE) 1.6.0 is installed on your computer; if it is not, you will need to install JRE before installing SpringCharts. Directions for checking if JRE is installed on your computer are available in the *McGraw-Hill Guide to Success with SpringCharts,* which is located on the McGraw-Hill Online Learning Center (OLC) at **www.mhhe.com/hamiltonehr3e.**

Before you can begin working on the exercises in *Electronic Health Records,* you will need to access and download both the SpringCharts EHR software and the *EHR Material* folder located at **www.mhhe.com/hamiltonehr3e.** The *EHR Material* folder contains images, documents, and files to give you authentic scenarios for importing EHR documentation throughout the course. For instructions on how to download the SpringCharts EHR program and the *EHR Material* folder, please refer to the *McGraw-Hill Guide to Success with SpringCharts,* which is located at **www.mhhe.com/hamiltonehr3e.**

Once you have installed JRE, SpringCharts, and the *EHR Material* folder, follow the instructions in the *McGraw-Hill Guide to Success with SpringCharts* to launch SpringCharts and complete the exercises in Chapters 3–12 as directed by your instructor.

Need help? Contact McGraw-Hill's Customer Experience Group (CXG). Visit the CXG website at www.mhhe.com/support. Browse our FAQs (Frequently Asked Questions) and product documentation, or contact a CXG representative. CXG is available Sunday through Friday.

acknowledgments

Suggestions have been received from faculty and students throughout the country. We rely on this vital feedback with all of our books. Each person who has offered comments and suggestions has our thanks.

The efforts of many people are needed to develop and improve a product. Among these people are the reviewers and consultants who point out areas of concern, cite areas of strength, and make recommendations for change. In this regard, the following instructors provided feedback that was enormously helpful in preparing the third edition of *Electronic Health Records*.

Workshops

In 2011 and 2012, McGraw-Hill conducted over a dozen health professions workshops, providing an opportunity for more than 600 faculty members to gain continuing education credits as well as to provide feedback on our products.

Book Reviews

A panel of instructors shared feedback on the second edition of *Electronic Health Records* in preparation for development of the third edition.

Joey L. Brown, MA, NRCMA
Great Lakes Institute of Technology

Georganne Copeland, BA, M Ed
Centralia College

Brian Dickens, MBA, RMA, CHI
Keiser Career College, Southeastern Institute

Cynthia Greiner Holmes, MAM

Marsha Lalley, BS, MS
Minneapolis Community and Technical College

Rhonda Lazette, BS, CMA (AAMA), CPC
Stautzenberger College

Yeva Madden, RHIA
South Hills School of Business and Technology

Heather Marti, CPC, CMA, PCT
Carrington College

Karen McAbee, CMA (AAMA), CPC
Miami-Jacobs Career College

Laura Melenedez, BS, RMA, RT BMO
Keiser Career College

Cheryl A. Miller, MBA/HCM
Westmoreland County Community College

Carey Lee Mortensen, CMA
Southern Careers Institute

Julie Lindstrom Myhre, BS, CMT
Century Community and Technical College

Karen M. Phelps, MBA/HM, RT, CPC, NCICS
Everest College Phoenix

Noreen Semanski, LPN, ASB, CHI
McCann School of Business & Technology

Many instructors participated in manuscript reviews throughout the development of the book.

Pamela Christianson, CMA, CPhT, BS
Montana State University

Ruth E. Dearborn, MBA-HCM, CCS, CCS-P
University of Alaska

Dawn Eitel, BAS, CMA (AAMA)
Kirkwood Community College

Rhonda Epps, CMA (AAMA), RMA, AS
National College of Business and Technology

Howard Gunning, MS Ed, CMA (AAMA)
Southwestern Illinois College

Elizabeth Hoffman, MA Ed, CMA (AAMA), CPT, (ASPT)
Baker College of Clinton Township

Christine Jerson, RHIA
Lakeland Community College

Rhonda Johns, MS, CMA (AAMA)
Baker College

Marsha Lalley, BS, MS
Minneapolis Community and Technical College

Jorge Lopez
San Antonio College

Amie Mayhall, MBA, CCA
Olney Central College

Nancy G. Measell, BS, CMA (AAMA)
Ivy Tech Community College

Cindy Minor, Ed M, MS, BS, CPS
John A. Logan College

Gwendolyn Parker, BBA, CBS
College of the Mainland

Nina Pustylnik, MBA, DHA/DBA, RMA
Keiser Career College

Arthur Reynolds, MA, MHA, JD
University of Maryland University College Graduate School

Kamala S. Robinson, MS
Northeast Community College

Stacey Spilka, CEHRS

Cindy Thompson, RN, RMA
Davenport University

Marianne Van Deursen, MS Ed, CMA (AAMA)
Warren County Community College

Kathy Vitale, CPC, CEHRS
Branford Hall Career Institute

Becky Voelker, CMA (AAMA), MBA
Baker College

Ethel B. Ware, CPC, CPC-I
West Tennessee Business College

Katherine Webb, BS Ed, RHIT
Ozarks Technical Community College

Ron Winston, BA
San Juan College

Technical Edit/Accuracy Panel

A panel of instructors completed a technical edit and review of all content and exercises in the book page proofs to verify their accuracy.

Pamela Christianson, CMA, CPhT, BS
Montana State University

Amy Ensign, CMA (AAMA), RMA (AMT)
Baker College of Clinton Township

Elizabeth Hoffman, MA Ed, CMA (AAMA), CPT, (ASPT)
Baker College of Clinton Township

Christine Jerson, RHIA
Lakeland Community College

Rhonda Johns, MS, CMA (AAMA)
Baker College

Laura Michelsen, MS, RHIA
Joliet Junior College

Michael Newsham, BA
Harris School of Business

Barbara Parker, CPC, CCS-P, CMA (AAMA)
Olympic College

Kamala S. Robinson, MS
Northeast Community College

Kathy Vitale, CPC, CEHRS
Branford Hall Career Institute

Digital Resources

Many instructors provided feedback to shape the development of digital resources for *EHR 3e* within Connect Plus.

Pamela Christianson, CMA, CPhT, BS
Montana State University

Rhonda Epps, CMA (AAMA), RMA, AS
National College of Business and Technology

Elizabeth Hoffman, MA Ed, CMA (AAMA), CPT, (ASPT)
Baker College of Clinton Township

Christine Jerson, RHIA
Lakeland Community College

Rhonda Johns, MS, CMA (AAMA)
Baker College

Cindy Minor, Ed M, MS, BS, CPS
John A. Logan College

Gwendolyn Parker, BBA, CBS
College of the Mainland

Nina Pustylnik, MBA, DHA/DBA, RMA
Keiser Career College

Arthur Reynolds, MA, MHA, JD
University of Maryland University College Graduate School

Kamala S. Robinson, MS
Northeast Community College

Ethel B. Ware, CPC, CPC-I
West Tennessee Business College

Katherine Webb, BS Ed, RHIT
Ozarks Technical Community College

Kathy Vitale, CPC, CEHRS
Branford Hall Career Institute

Special thanks are due to the following instructors for their help creating and reviewing activities for this edition of *Electronic Health Records:*

Christine Jerson, RHIA
Lakeland Community College

Rhonda Johns, MS, CMA (AAMA)
Baker College

Acknowledgments from the Author

Electronic Health Records is dedicated to my wife Leesa. Leesa and I were enrolled in full-time studies when a revision of the EHR text became necessary. Because of the current dynamics of the EHR industry and establishment of mandates by the federal government regulating standards, certification, and qualifying deployment of the EHR, it soon became obvious to me that what I had envisioned as a revision of the text would have to be a rewrite. It was necessary for me to take a 12-month sabbatical from our educational pursuits to dedicate my time to the creation of this third edition. Leesa agreed, and selflessly continued on without me. I'm appreciative of her understanding and support.

Electronic Health Records is also dedicated to my son Jeremie, who spent countless hours beside me in the office working the exercises, concept checkups, and review questions while he listened to my easy-listening '60s and '70s music. Thank God we enjoy the same genre!

Thanks to all the individuals at McGraw-Hill whose tireless efforts have moved this project through to its final publication. I especially want to thank the McGraw-Hill editorial team—Michael S. Ledbetter, Natalie J. Ruffatto, and Michelle L. Flomenhoft—for their encouragement and support throughout this process. A special thanks to Raisa Priebe Kreek, my developmental editor, who kept a firm grip on the helm, cracked the whip, and always kept a smile on her face.

I also want to thank other McGraw Hill staff who provided invaluable assistance, including project manager Kathryn Wright, executive marketing manager Roxan Kinsey, digital development editor Katherine Ward, buyer Sue Culbertson, senior designer Srdjan Savanovic, senior content licensing specialist Keri Johnson, and media project managers Brent dela Cruz and Cathy Tepper. Without them, this book would not have been possible.

My appreciation is also expressed to Nancy Peterson. As a freelance editor with years of experience in higher-education publishing and her experience as a healthcare professional, Nancy's understanding of the industry has been invaluable in shaping this text.

My indebtedness is extended to Jack B. Smyth, who had the foresight in 2007 as president and CEO of Spring Medical Systems Inc. to support incorporating a full-featured, popular electronic health record software into the college environment. With Jack's backing and his keen understanding of the growth of the EHR industry, the medical student has a unique opportunity to receive hands-on training on industry-standard electronic medical records at no additional cost. Thus, students are taken from a sterile, abstract educational setting to a dynamic, realistic learning environment. This hands-on experience will successfully equip each student with the knowledge and confidence necessary to contribute to the electronic health records in the medical office.

Byron R. Hamilton

walkthrough

Chapter Openers

Every chapter opens with Learning Outcomes, Key Terms, and a What You Need to Know section that prepares the student for the chapter they are about to read.

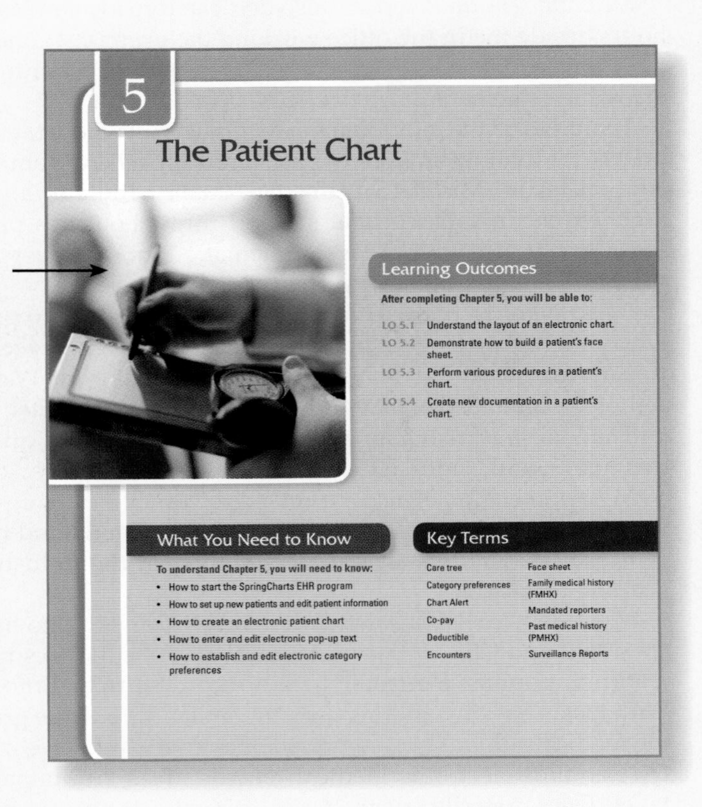

5

The Patient Chart

Learning Outcomes

After completing Chapter 5, you will be able to:

LO 5.1 Understand the layout of an electronic chart.

LO 5.2 Demonstrate how to build a patient's face sheet.

LO 5.3 Perform various procedures in a patient's chart.

LO 5.4 Create new documentation in a patient's chart.

What You Need to Know

To understand Chapter 5, you will need to know:

- How to start the SpringCharts EHR program
- How to set up new patients and edit patient information
- How to create an electronic patient chart
- How to enter and edit electronic pop-up text
- How to establish and edit electronic category preferences

Key Terms

Care tree
Category preferences
Chart Alert
Co-pay
Deductible
Encounters
Face sheet
Family medical history (FMHX)
Mandated reporters
Past medical history (PMHX)
Surveillance Reports

Learning Outcomes Tags

Each section heading, Concept Checkup box, practice exercise, and review question is tied directly to the chapter's learning outcomes. This tagging allows instructors to move students from general theory to application in a step-by-step, logical manner through a variety of activities and exercises tied to the learning outcomes of the chapter.

5.1 Overview of the Patient Chart

In EHR systems, electronic charts can be accessed from many different places in the program. In SpringCharts, the electronic chart can be accessed from the *Practice View* screen in several different ways by clicking on:

- The patient's name in the *Appointment Schedule* and selecting the [Get Chart] button
- The patient's name in the *Patient Tracker* and selecting the [Get Chart] button
- A *ToDo* item associated with a patient
- A message associated with a patient and selecting the [Get Chart] button
- The *Open a Patient's Chart* icon on the speed Toolbar (Figure 5.1)
- The *Actions* menu and then selecting *Open a Chart*
- The *Recent Charts* menu

Focal Points and Tips

Focal Points appear throughout the text as marginal inserts, spotlighting critical data necessary to master the skills being learned. HIPAA/HITECH Tips emphasize legal compliance and protection of patient privacy. SpringCharts Tips highlight quick tips and shortcuts for easy navigation in the EHR program.

Focal Point

Past Medical History (PMHX)

The PMHX section of the face sheet includes information about the patient's past healthcare history, such as major illnesses, previous surgeries, injuries, and operations relevant to the medical practice.

HIPAA/HITECH Tip

A patient's authorization to release PHI is not needed when the purpose is for treatment, payment, or operations (TPO). However, because state laws vary, many practices will ask patients to sign releases.

SpringCharts Tip

The *eRx* icon on the far right of the toolbar is only seen when the medical clinic has activated the e-prescribing feature of SpringCharts EHR.

Key Term Definitions

Key Term definitions appear in the margin every time a new Key Term is introduced for quick and easy reference.

Surveillance Reports
These reports provide information to the federal Centers for Disease Control and Prevention to enable effective monitoring of rates and distribution of disease, detection of outbreaks, monitoring of interventions, and prediction of emerging hazards.

Concept Checkups

Concept Checkups appear after each Learning Outcome, emphasizing the topics and skills that were just covered.

Concept Checkup 5.1

A. An electronic chart created through computer automation in the medical clinic is the repository for what information?

B. Name three ways in which a user can access the patient's chart in the Spring-Charts program.

C. Can the same patient's chart be opened by multiple users at the same time?

D. Where would a user set up preference lists that are used in the social history, past medical history, and family medical history sections of the face sheet?

E. What information is stored in the care tree?

Chapter Review

Each chapter ends with a review including Using Terminology, Checking Your Understanding, and Applying Your Understanding questions to reinforce the learning outcomes that were presented in the chapter.

chapter 5 review

Name ______ Instructor ______ Class ______ Date ______

Using Terminology

Match the terms on the left with the definitions on the right.

____ 1. **LO 5.1** Care tree
____ 2. **LO 5.1** Category preferences
____ 3. **LO 5.2** Chart Alert
____ 4. **LO 5.1** Electronic chart
____ 5. **LO 5.1** Encounters
____ 6. **LO 5.3** Deductible
____ 7. LO

A. Information generated in an EHR that is provided to the Centers for Disease Control and Prevention, enabling effective monitoring of rates and distribution of disease.
B. The portion a medical insurance policyholder pays for each medical office visit or a specific type of medical service covered under the health insurance policy.
C. The portion of a patient's chart that displays the patient's demographics, medical history, and healthcare information.
D. The portion of the patient's chart that lists progress notes, tests,

Checking Your Understanding

Choose the best answer and circle the corresponding letter.

10. **LO 5.1** SpringCharts EHR provides practitioners a unique electronic view of the patient's chart similar to a:
    a) Practice management system
    b) Paper chart layout
    c) Patient's intake sheet
    d) Physician's order form

11. **LO 5.1** All of the preset categories in the care tree:
    a) Cannot be altered or edited
    b) Can be altered and edited
    c) Can be customized to the clinic's needs
    d) Mat

13. **LO 5.1** Three areas of the face sheet cannot be altered or edited. Select the one that *can* be altered.
    a) Prescription history
    b) Diagnosis history
    c) Problem list
    d) Procedure history

14. **LO 5.3** Before creating new documentation or activities for a patient, the patient's chart must be:
    a) Opened
    b) Closed
    c) In the *Recent Charts* list

Applying Your Knowledge

Use your critical-thinking skills to answer the following questions.

26. **LO 5.2** While in the waiting room, a new patient fills out the following information on the intake form: *Lipitor 10mg, Wellbutrin XL 300mg, Glyburide 2.5 mg.* Where will this information be placed in the chart?

27. **LO 5.3** Why is it important that a patient's past immunizations be added to the patient's electronic chart?

28. **LO 5.4** When a user is saving a copy of the patient's excuse note in the chart, why is it unnecessary to select a care tree category to save it to?

A Commitment to Accuracy

You have a right to expect an accurate textbook, and McGraw-Hill invests considerable time and effort to make sure that we deliver one. Listed below are the many steps we take to make sure this happens.

Our Accuracy Verification Process

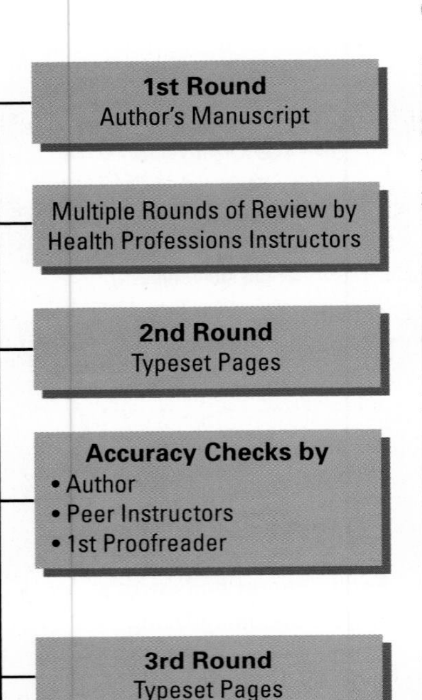

First Round—Development Reviews

STEP 1: Numerous **health professions instructors** review the draft manuscript and report on any errors they may find. The author makes these corrections in his final manuscript.

Second Round—Page Proofs

STEP 2: Once the manuscript has been typeset, the **author** checks his manuscript against the page proofs to ensure all illustrations, graphs, examples, and exercises have been correctly laid out on the pages.

STEP 3: An outside panel of **peer instructors** completes a review of content in the page proofs to verify its accuracy. The author adds these corrections to his review of the page proofs.

STEP 4: A **proofreader** adds a triple layer of accuracy assurance in pages by looking for errors; then a confirming, corrected round of page proofs is produced.

Third Round—Confirming Page Proofs

STEP 5: The **author** reviews the confirming round of page proofs to make certain any previous corrections were properly made and to look for any errors he might have missed on the first round.

STEP 6: The **project manager,** who has overseen the book from the beginning, performs **another proofread** to make sure no new errors have been introduced during the production process.

Final Round—Printer's Proofs

STEP 7: The **project manager** performs a **final proofread** of the book during the printing process, providing a final accuracy review. In concert with the main text, all supplements undergo a proofreading and technical editing stage to ensure their accuracy.

Results

What results is a textbook as accurate and error-free as is humanly possible. Our authors and publishing staff are confident the many layers of quality assurance have produced books that are leaders in the industry for their integrity and correctness. *Please view the Acknowledgments section for more details on the many people involved in this process.*

1

The Electronic Health Record

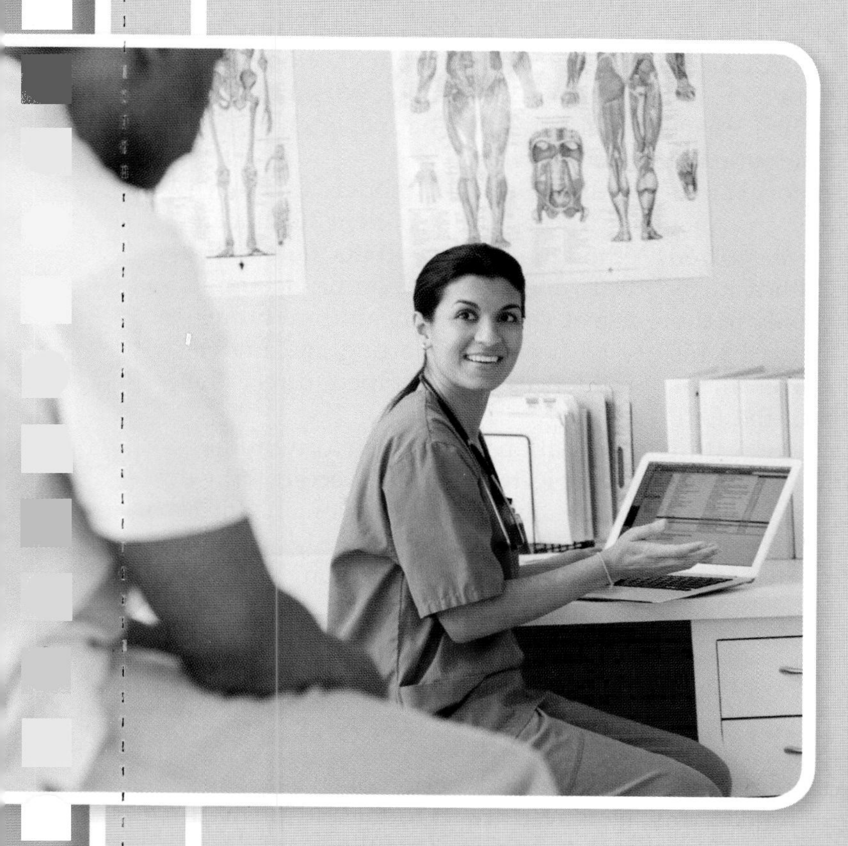

Learning Outcomes

After completing Chapter 1, you will be able to:

LO 1.1 Define the concept of an electronic health record (EHR).

LO 1.2 Explain key events in the history of EHRs.

LO 1.3 Distinguish between the terms commonly used to refer to EHRs.

LO 1.4 Describe the government's involvement in EHRs.

LO 1.5 Differentiate between medical office processes that use a paper chart and an EHR.

LO 1.6 Summarize the major barriers and benefits of using an EHR.

LO 1.7 Describe potential developments in the future of the EHR.

Key Terms

- Ambulatory
- American Recovery and Reinvestment Act (ARRA)
- Best practice guidelines
- Centers for Medicare and Medicaid Services (CMS)
- Electronic health record (EHR)
- Electronic medical record (EMR)
- E-prescribing
- Health information exchange (HIE)
- Health information technology (HIT)
- Health Information Technology for Economic and Clinical Health (HITECH) Act
- Inpatient
- Interoperability
- Medicare Improvements for Patients and Providers Act of 2008 (MIPPA)
- Medicare Part A
- Medicare Part B
- Office of the National Coordinator for Health Information Technology (ONC)
- Outpatient
- Patient portal
- Personal digital assistant (PDA)
- Personal health record (PHR)
- Point of care
- Practice management system (PMS)
- Return on investment (ROI)

What You Need to Know

To understand Chapter 1, you will need to know:

- The concept of a patient's chart in a medical office

Introduction

Electronic health record (EHR)
An electronic health record is the most commonly accepted term for software with a full range of functionalities to store, access, and use patient healthcare information.

What is an **electronic health record (EHR)**? An EHR system is a computerized, organized collection of individual patients' healthcare information in a digital format. An EHR system can store, share, and transmit electronic data between healthcare facilities. This chapter will introduce you to the concept of the EHR and describe the three different models of EHR systems used around the world. EHR programs have revolutionized the way healthcare processes are conducted in medical facilities. Everything from checking in a patient, to searching a patient's chart for wellness screenings, to submitting data for research reports can be managed efficiently now that paper charts are not the focal point for storing patient health information.

Multiple terms are used to explain the different EHR models that have developed as the technology and methods for capturing patient healthcare information electronically have evolved. Although primitive EHRs were introduced in large medical facilities in the 1960s, the proliferation of electronic health records has occurred only in more recent years. As a healthcare professional, it is important to know the history of electronic charting and understand what private and governmental influences have helped direct the development and adoption of the EHR.

The EHR is now a permanent feature in the national healthcare community. Although the future is difficult to forecast, the electronic health record industry is heading in exciting directions both nationally and internationally. Electronic exchange systems are currently being designed that will give healthcare providers instant access to patient healthcare information from many sources in real time and enable the compilation of population disease tracking and intervention.

1.1 Overview of the Electronic Health Record

Electronic health record programs have evolved over a period of 60 years and have been referred to by various terms. However, the concept and purpose of electronic charting has always remained the same. Healthcare philosophies, management, and organization differ from country to country based on types of governments and political values; these factors have influenced the development of electronic health records around the world. As a result, various models for storing, accessing, and using patient healthcare information have emerged.

The Concept

Inpatient
An **inpatient** is a person who is admitted to the hospital and stays overnight or for an indeterminate amount of time, usually several days or weeks.

Outpatient
An **outpatient** is a person who is not hospitalized for 24 hours or more but may visit a hospital, a medical clinic, or other healthcare facility for diagnosis or treatment.

EHR programs collect the health information of individual patients in a digital (i.e., computerized) format, as seen in Figure 1.1. The information gathered is typical of what would normally be assembled into a paper chart at an **inpatient** or **outpatient** healthcare facility (Figure 1.2): patient demographics; insurance information; personal and family healthcare history; allergies; ongoing medical problems; routine and current medications; physical examination notes; lab, imaging, and medical test results; and so on. Beyond being a computerized repository for medical information, EHR programs have the ability to interface with external healthcare computer programs. This ability enables healthcare professionals to:

- Electronically transmit and receive lab and medical orders and test results.

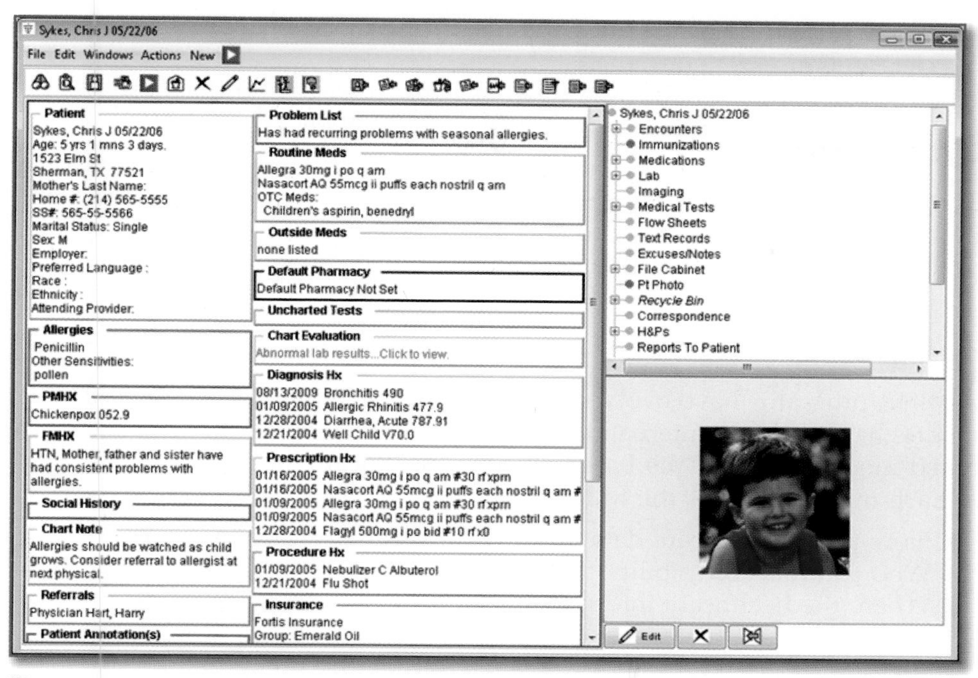

Figure 1.1 Example of the facesheet portion from a patient's electronic chart, as shown in SpringCharts EHR program.

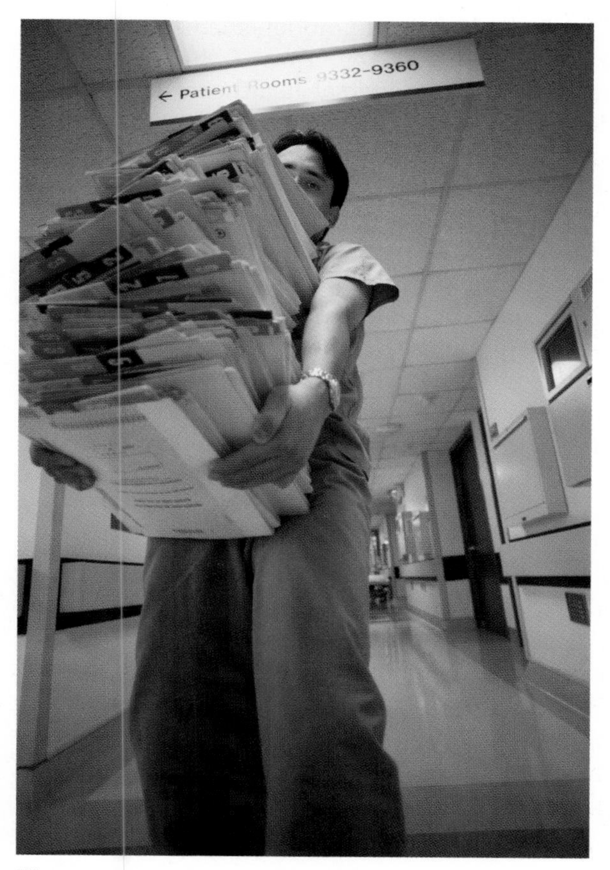

Figure 1.2 Examples of paper charts used to store patients' healthcare information.

Focal Point

EHR programs store computerized healthcare information on individual patients and interface with other electronic healthcare programs to transmit and receive orders, test results, and prescriptions and to produce healthcare reports.

Focal Point

Due to the varying healthcare systems used by countries around the world and the number of EHR vendors, EHR models have developed into three distinct models: distribution-based, facility-based, and Web-based.

- Automatically transmit prescriptions to pharmacies via an electronic clearinghouse.
- Produce comprehensive reports of specific diseases and diagnoses that can be transmitted to government healthcare agencies.

The purpose of EHRs is to provide a complete record of patient medical encounters in an electronic format that automates and streamlines the work-flow in healthcare settings, and to increase safety through "evidence-based decision support, quality management, and outcomes reporting."[1]

EHR Models

As EHR programs have evolved over the past several decades, three distinct models have emerged internationally: the distribution-based model, the facility-based model, and the Web-based personal healthcare model.

Each model specifies the following factors:

- How much healthcare data is stored in a patient's health record
- Who controls accessibility to this medical data
- Where the healthcare information is stored

Distribution-Based Model Universal healthcare is the concept of a government-organized healthcare system. Governments of countries with universal healthcare programs control both healthcare financing and health services. As such, these countries have developed and deployed EHR programs differently than countries operating under a private healthcare model, such as the United States.

Australia, for example, operates under a universal healthcare system and uses a distribution-based model. In this model, selected healthcare data is transmitted to a centralized electronic record.[2] Health*Connect* was a healthcare management strategy initiated by the Australian government to facilitate standards of electronic communication to all healthcare facilities that capture, store, and transmit electronic medical data so that vital health information could be securely exchanged among parties such as patients, physicians, pharmacies, and hospitals.[3] As a result, Health*Connect* provided business-grade broadband (high-speed) services to eligible healthcare organizations to support the transfer of healthcare data more accurately and securely between healthcare professionals. The patient's complete medical record is not transferred; rather, the data consists of information considered to be useful to other healthcare providers who are involved in the current and future care of the patient—information agreed upon by the patient and the provider. Once this data is transmitted to the Health*Connect* patient record, it is available to other healthcare providers and medical facilities.

Although private health facilities and private insurance exist in Australia, primary healthcare remains the responsibility of the Australian federal government. Estimates were that this centralized national EHR system would save the Australian government $300 million per year by reducing medical errors and duplication of effort.[4]

Facility-Based Model In the United States, healthcare facilities are largely privately owned and operated, rather than controlled by a centralized government agency. Therefore the focus has primarily been on the need to support a national health information infrastructure and establish benchmarks for data transfer and compatibility between multiple EHR programs. These technical aspects of EHR implementation have related to standardizing terminology, computer language, features, and reporting.[5] Various government and commercial organizations have been involved in establishing EHR standards and advancing certification programs to unify the many EHR vendors and their programs. At this stage of EHR development in the United States, the style is that of a facility-based model in which patient data resides in the electronic health information system at the healthcare facility or with a third-party hosting company. Wellness reports regarding generalized healthcare from a facility's patient data can be sent to centralized public health authorities, rather than shared individualized patient records being made available at a centralized government healthcare agency, as in the Australian model. Public health agencies analyze the wellness reports data, which is displayed by factors such as age, race, sex, how the disease is transmitted in the population, and the number of reported cases by state.[6]

Web-Based Personal Healthcare Model The third model for EHR development is the Web-based personal healthcare model, in which personal EHR accounts provide patients with secure Web space. Within that space, patients can accumulate their healthcare data and make it accessible online to providers that have the digital credentials to access the information. Large Internet companies like Yahoo!, Microsoft, and WebMD have launched secure healthcare **patient portals** that enable the general public to store and update their own medical records. Search engines at these sites allow patients to locate and manage health information related to their medical conditions. Patient-selected providers, such as physicians and pharmacists, can also update some of these Web-based systems. The Web-based model, however, is still in its infancy and tends to have limited functionality at this time. Advocates of the Web-based health record model anticipate a time when a greater percentage of the population will take advantage of Internet host sites, when healthcare facilities can receive data directly from medical monitoring devices, and when data can transfer directly from EHR systems to a patient's online medical record. The fact remains that a relatively small proportion of the population, perhaps 7 percent, have utilized the Web-based model, due to concerns about Internet security and identity fraud.[7]

Patient portals
Patient portals are online applications that are designed to allow patients access to and storage of some of their medical records and allow communication with their healthcare providers across the Internet. Some patient portals exist as stand-alone websites while others are integrated into the existing website of the healthcare provider.

Concept Checkup 1.1

A. EHRs are more than computerized repositories for medical information. They can also interface with other electronic healthcare devices. What three tasks does this enable EHRs to accomplish?

B. Describe each of the following EHR models:

1. Distribution-based model
2. Facility-based model
3. Web-based personal healthcare model

1.2 History of the Electronic Health Record

Focal Point

Improvement in the quality of patient medical care and safety has always been the catalyst for development of the electronic health record concept.

The concept of storing a patient's medical information electronically instead of on paper is not a new one. In the 1960s, as medical care became more complex, medical facilities realized that in certain situations the patient's complete health history needed to be accessible to make informed medical decisions. This need brought about the innovation of electronic storage of patients' healthcare information. Improvement of patient medical care was and continues to be the catalyst for the electronic health record.

The Mayo Clinic in Rochester, Minnesota; the University Hospital in Burlington, Vermont; and the Latter Day Saints Hospital in Salt Lake City, Utah, were some of the first medical facilities to use electronic health record systems. Their systems were developed in the early 1960s. Over the next two decades, more information and functionality were added to electronic health record systems to improve patient care. Drug dosages, side effects, allergies, and drug interactions became available electronically to doctors, enabling that information to be incorporated into electronic healthcare systems. Electronic diagnostic and treatment plans proliferated and were integrated into electronic health record systems, giving physicians additional information for medical decision making and patient care. More academic and research institutes developed their own computerized medical record systems as tools to track patient treatment. Overall, utilization and development of these computer models focused on increasing the quality of patient care.

Although large hospitals began developing electronic patient records as early as the 1960s, the earliest use of computers in the independent medical office began in the 1990s, to aid in the administration of insurance claims and financial accounting. Computer programs focused on fiscal management for processing insurance claims and patient statements are known as **practice management systems (PMSs)**. Small- to average-sized private medical practices, however, were slow to implement electronic health record programs due to the high cost of computer hardware and software, the huge task of data entry, and the resulting need to change office processes and procedures.

Practice management system (PMS)
A software program that manages, among other things, financial transactions, both charges and payments; the billing of insurance claims; and the issuing of patient statements.

The adoption of PMS programs in the mid-1990s did not accelerate in the private sector until government insurance agencies, such as Medicare and Medicaid, offered medical providers financial incentives to implement electronic PMS programs and levied penalties on them for noncompliance. Government insurance entities required medical providers to use electronic data transfer of claims to receive financial reimbursement for services rendered.

Focal Point

In recent years, government mandates for standardizing EHR features and government incentive programs for EHR adoption have accelerated the acquisition of EHR programs.

At the turn of the twenty-first century, as computer hardware and software costs became more affordable, personal computers more compact and portable, and wireless transfer of data more reliable, the feasibility of independent medical offices using electronic health records became a reality. In the early 2000s, EHR vendors began to proliferate, and healthcare providers could choose from an array of several hundred electronic health record programs offering a collection of different features. Because of a wide assortment of functionalities, lack of official industry standards, and absence of government regulations, healthcare providers lagged in acquiring and implementing electronic charting programs in the first decade of the century. However, by 2010, government mandates and funding spurred the standardization of features in the electronic records industry, introduced an EHR certification program, and offered major financial incentives to providers for purchasing and deploying EHR programs. Due to the federal government's involvement in the EHR industry, particularly the offering of financial incentives tied to the use of EHRs, we are witnessing

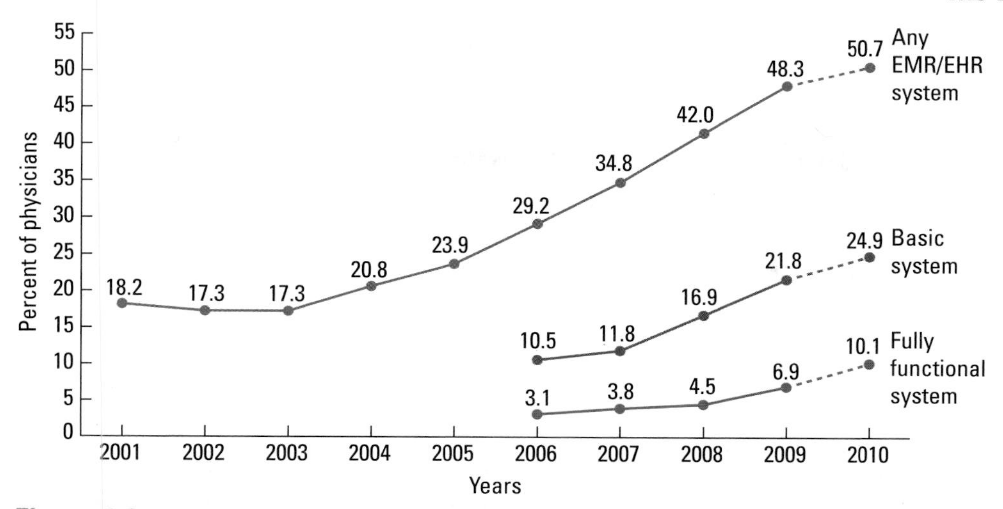

Figure 1.3 Percentage of independent physicians using EHRs.
Source: Hsiao et al, 2010.

a similar surge in medical offices acquiring electronic health record systems as we saw in the 1990s with the acquisition of PMS programs.

The electronic health record program is now here to stay. A nationwide healthcare infrastructure is quickly forming that will link medical facilities, pharmacies, laboratories, testing services, rural and urban health clinics, and healthcare providers to the secured patient chart. This infrastructure will also allow collection and analysis of U.S. population health data, based on patient healthcare surveillance reports that providers regularly transmit to the Centers for Disease Control and Prevention (CDC). A 2010 survey conducted by the CDC's National Center for Health Statistics (NCHS) indicates that 50.7 percent of the approximately 230,000 physician practices in the United States reported using some form of an EHR system. Between 2006 and 2010, the percentage of physicians who reported having electronic programs that met the criteria of a basic system increased by 14.4 percent (Figure 1.3).[8] With the government implementing incentive programs followed by possible financial penalties in 2016, industry experts predict that EHR use by office-based healthcare providers will reach 95 percent saturation within the next three years.

Concept Checkup 1.2

A. What is the reason for the initial and continuing development of electronic health records (EHRs)?

B. The earliest use of computers in the medical office was to utilize practice management systems. What is the PMS program designed to manage?

C. What has been the primary cause for the acceleration of the acquisition of both PMS and EHR programs?

1.3 EHR Terminology

An alphabet soup of terms and acronyms surrounds the evolution of electronic health records. These terms are somewhat flexible in meaning, depending on how government agencies and independent associations that influenced the development of EHRs have evolved and changed the way they use the terms.

Focal Point

Different terms used for electronically storing a patient's healthcare information reflect the evolution of the electronic health record and reveal distinctions in their purposes.

Although the following terms and acronyms and their definitions are supplied to help provide clarity, they are still sometimes used interchangeably to describe the concept of an electronic patient record.

Computer-Based Patient Record (CPR). This term was one of the first used to conceptualize the idea of an electronic patient record. A computer-based patient record is a lifetime patient record that includes all information from all specialties, including dentistry and psychiatry. The record is available to all providers nationally and potentially internationally. Because the CPR requires full **interoperability** among all electronic medical data, the goal was not realistic in the early development of the electronic record. In the 1990s there was an initiative to use the CPR; however, the concept evolved into less ambitious forms of centralized medical data.

Interoperability
Interoperability is the ability of a software program to accept, send, and communicate data from its database to and from multiple vendors' software programs.

Electronic Medical Record (EMR). This phrase was widely used as the terminology migrated away from computer-based patient record. As definitions became clearer, EMR began to be used for electronic medical software that did not contain high-end functionalities such as health maintenance and disease management, care alerts, patient Internet access, interconnectivity with providers outside the practice, and interoperability with external medical testing facilities.

Electronic medical record (EMR)
The term for medical software that lacks a full range of higher-end functionalities to store, access, and use patient medical information. EMRs are not interoperable.

Electronic Health Record (EHR). Currently, this term is the most commonly accepted and used phrase for the storage and access of patient medical information electronically. The EHR encompasses a full range of functionalities and information, including full patient records, laboratory data, radiology reports, automated evaluation and management coding, care alerts, evidence-based decision support, drug and allergy interaction checking, and health maintenance analysis. EHRs are now being certified by the U.S. Department of Health and Human Services (HHS). As such, they require the functionality to e-prescribe, transmit electronic reports to Medicare and Medicaid, and be interoperable with external medical facilities. In the future, EHRs may be required to transmit electronic patient medical data to other healthcare providers involved in a patient's healthcare. Standards for this functionality are being developed.

Continuity of Care Document (CCD) or Continuity of Care Record (CCR). The CCD/CCR is a healthcare provider–oriented record comprising a core set of data considered to be the most relevant summary of a patient's medical healthcare. The CCD/CCR would be considered a subset of the EHR. Typically it includes patient information, diagnoses, recent procedures, allergies, medications, and future treatment plans. Its primary use is to provide a snapshot of the pertinent clinical, demographic, and administrative data for a specific patient. The electronic CCD/CCR is designed to be vendor and technology neutral; that is, content is created in a common computer language and accessible by all EHRs and other electronic systems. Currently developing standards would enable the electronic CCD/CCR to be read, interpreted, and stored by any EHR software application.

Personal health record (PHR)
PHRs allow the patient access via the Internet to the medical office's website to store and update personal medical information. A PHR allows the patient to make inquiries of the healthcare provider regarding prescriptions, appointments, and other concerns.

Personal Health Record (PHR). PHRs allow patients to become interactive sources of health information and health management through an Internet-based connection to a medical practice website. Through a secure connection, patients can schedule appointments, receive reminders, request medication refills, access lab and radiology results, and ask questions about their health. Some PHRs enable patients to update family or social histories, read their medical records, and notify providers of incorrect or missing information.

Concept Checkup 1.3

Provide the definitions of the following acronyms:

A. CPR

B. CCD/CCR

C. PHR

1.4 Government Involvement in the EHR

Many organizations have promoted the EHR concept because of the benefits EHRs bring to healthcare. Recognizing these advantages, in 1991, the Institute of Medicine (IOM) called for implementing EHRs and eliminating paper-based patient records as early as 2001. In his 2004 State of the Union address, then-President George W. Bush stated, "By computerizing health records, we can avoid dangerous medical mistakes, reduce costs, and improve care."[9] President Bush created a subcabinet-level position within the Department of Health and Human Services (HHS) called the **Office of the National Coordinator for Health Information Technology (ONC)**. In April 2004, he outlined a plan "to ensure that most Americans have electronic health records within the next 10 years."[10] From that plan, government agencies have been able to promote the use of and overcome barriers to EHRs. Although the Bush administration empowered the HHS to promote EHRs, strong advocacy for electronic health records occurred mainly in the private sector.

In 2008, President Barack Obama echoed concerns over reducing costs, improving patient healthcare, and implementing an electronic infrastructure for national healthcare. The Obama administration promised to sponsor the adoption of EHRs through a sizable federal financial commitment as part of a broader economic stimulus package. In its economic recovery plan of 2009, the federal government outlined strategies to spend $19.2 billion to accelerate the use of computerized health records in physician's offices and inpatient settings over a period of five years. In his speech to Congress in February 2009, President Obama stated:

> Our recovery plan will invest in electronic health records and new technology that will reduce errors, bring down costs, ensure privacy, and save lives.[11]

Medicare Improvements for Patients and Providers Act of 2008

On July 15, 2008, Congress enacted the **Medicare Improvements for Patients and Providers Act of 2008 (MIPPA)**. The Act establishes Medicare reimbursement for providers, reduces racial and ethnic disparities among Medicare recipients, increases benefits to low-income beneficiaries, and places limits on certain rapidly growing Medicare supplemental insurance policies.[12] In addition to these important changes, MIPPA provided positive incentives for practitioners who used **e-prescribing**, a program that began in 2009 and continues

Focal Point

Because of the known benefits that EHRs bring to patient healthcare, many government agencies and private organizations promote the use of electronic medical records.

Office of the National Coordinator for Health Information Technology (ONC)
The ONC's purpose is to serve as a resource for the entire health system, support the adoption of HIT, and promote a nationwide health information exchange.

Medicare Improvements for Patients and Providers Act of 2008 (MIPPA)
Enacted by Congress in 2008, this 275-page piece of legislation blocked scheduled cuts in Medicare's payments to physicians and increased benefits to low-income beneficiaries and other vulnerable areas of the population.

E-prescribing
The use of computerized tools, usually embedded in an EHR program, to create and sign prescriptions for medicines, thereby replacing handwritten prescriptions. Electronic prescriptions are sent to pharmacies over the Internet via a clearinghouse.

practices in EHR adoption, meaningful use, and provider support for the 62 RECs across the country. RECs have been chosen from every geographic region of the United States to ensure adequate support for healthcare providers.

During 2011 and 2012, the goal of the Health Information Technology Extension Program was to provide outreach and support services to at least 100,000 priority primary care providers. Regional Extension Centers were mandated to:

- Provide training and support services to assist primary healthcare providers in adopting EHRs.
- Offer information and guidance to help with EHR implementation and achieving meaningful use to qualify for incentive payments.
- Give technical assistance as needed.

Concept Checkup 1.4

A. Provide the definitions for the following acronyms:

1. MIPPA
2. ARRA
3. CMS

B. What is the function of a Health Information Technology Regional Extension Center?

1.5 Healthcare Processes and the EHR

The introduction of EHRs into healthcare facilities over the past decade has revolutionized procedures and processes in medical offices. Because EHRs are patient focused, all healthcare personnel—both clerical and clinical, from the front office to the back office—use EHR functionality to perform their duties. Although some medical offices are using a combination of paper charts and electronic storage of some medical data, no paper charts exist in a fully electronically integrated medical facility; everything from a simple phone call, to documenting a procedure, to receiving lab results, to billing insurance claims occurs in the EHR. The most fundamental processes of tracking patient care and workflow have undergone major transformations from the paper chart environment to the introduction of the EHR, as outlined in Table 1.2.

After reviewing the workflow and processes shown in Table 1.2, one will see an obvious disadvantage of the paper chart is accessibility. With every patient encounter and handling of associated documents, the chart must be located, pulled, handled, and then refiled. This process takes an enormous amount of cumulative time and therefore expense. A significant amount of time is also spent waiting for documents to arrive and be processed and for the appropriate actions and communications to be taken.

Accessibility is not an issue with EHRs. The patient's chart is always available, even from a remote location via the Internet. Multiple providers and staff members can access the chart simultaneously. The information for accurate medical decision making is always available at the time of encountering the patient, and documentation is speedy and accurate. With the adoption of an EHR program, physicians have reported being able to see four to six additional patients a day or spend more counseling time with existing patients.[17]

Focal Point

Introduction of the EHR has answered the problem of chart accessibility, document processing, and the availability of accurate healthcare information at the time of patient encounter.

Table 1.2 Comparison of Paper Chart Environment with Electronic Chart Environment

Paper Chart Environment	Electronic Chart Environment
Patient Setup	
Scheduling an Appointment: The patient calls the medical office to schedule an appointment.	The patient accesses the Internet from home and logs on to the clinic's website. The patient enters a patient portal and requests an appointment date on the online calendar.
Preparing Charts and Verifying Insurance Coverage: At the medical clinic, paper charts are located and pulled the night before and organized by provider and appointment time slots. A staff member calls the insurance company of each patient and verifies insurance eligibility over the phone.	No charts need to be located, pulled, or organized. Electronic charts are available immediately in the EHR. The night prior to the appointment, the medical office computer automatically interfaces with insurance companies across the country to verify eligibility for patients scheduled the following day. An eligibility report is available the following day.
Checking in the Patient: The patient arrives at the medical office and verifies personal demographics and insurance information.	An existing patient verifies and updates personal demographics and insurance information via the patient portal on the clinic's website prior to arriving for an appointment. Front-office personnel check the patient in on the electronic schedule upon arrival and enter the patient's name into a patient tracking module.
Verifying Patient's Identification: For new patients, photocopies of the patient's ID and insurance card are made and placed in the paper chart.	A digital photo is taken of the patient using a digital camera or webcam and stored in the EHR. The patient's insurance card is placed in a device that scans both sides of the card and stores the image in the patient's chart.
Collecting Patient Healthcare Information: A clipboard with forms to complete is given to the patient so that personal healthcare history, family medical history, problem list, and routine medications can be updated and documented.	A new patient is escorted to a private area of the waiting room and instructed how to use the patient kiosk, a computer on which the patient will complete an electronic-guided questionnaire regarding personal and family healthcare history, problem list, routine medications, and so on.
Signing Official Forms: New patients sign a privacy notice and medical release authorization. All forms are placed in the paper chart.	Patient signs his or her digital signature on an electronic pad after reading the privacy notice and medical release authorization. The digital signature is stored in the patient's EHR.
Initial Clinical Encounter	
Recording Vital Signs and Chief Complaint: When front-office personnel communicate that the patient is ready and a clinical staff member calls the patient from the waiting room, the patient's chief complaint and vital signs are recorded and placed in the front of the paper chart. The patient is escorted to an open exam room.	Front-office personnel change patient status to "ready" in the patient tracking program. A clinical staff member observes this change on the computer, calls the patient, and escorts him or her to the nurse station. The patient's chief complaint and vital signs are transmitted wirelessly from the measuring devices directly into the patient's EHR. Body mass index is calculated automatically. The patient is escorted to an open exam room.
Reviewing Patient's Healthcare Information: A clinician reviews the patient's completed healthcare questionnaire and makes additional handwritten notations based on input from the patient.	A clinician reviews the patient's healthcare information, which was entered by the patient at the kiosk in the waiting room or via the electronic patient portal on the clinic's website. Modifications can be keyed in by the clinician based on input from the patient.
Checking Status of Wellness Screenings: The patient is asked if he/she is up-to-date on screening tests and other procedures. The clinician flips through the patient's chart looking for diagnoses and other indicators that may help flag the need for any wellness screenings or tests.	The clinician clicks a button in the EHR to conduct a chart evaluation. A window is displayed immediately, indicating whether the patient is behind in specific wellness screenings. The clinician talks with the patient about when and how to take care of necessary screenings and indicates the patient's response in the electronic chart note.

(continued)

Concept Checkup 1.5

A. What has been revolutionized over the past decade by the introduction of electronic medical records into healthcare facilities?

B. Briefly describe the process of ordering a prescription in a paper chart environment.

C. Briefly describe the process of ordering a prescription in an electronic chart environment.

D. What is the major disadvantage to using the paper chart?

Focal Point

The establishment of an EHR certification program, a financial incentive program, and Regional Extension Centers by the ONC largely addressed healthcare providers' concerns regarding barriers to the implementation of EHR programs.

Focal Point

A lack of feature uniformity and affordability, and change to clinical processes were some of the barriers to the adoption of ambulatory EHRs in the 1990s.

Return on investment (ROI)
This measure, expressed as a percentage, is the amount earned from a company's total purchase or investment, calculated by dividing the total capital into earnings or financial benefits.

Point of care
Point of care is the time and place the healthcare provider gives the patient medical care.

Ambulatory
This term means the ability to walk or to move from one place to another. In the medical sense it is used to distinguish walking patients from bedridden ones, as in those in inpatient hospitals or skilled nursing facilities.

1.6 Barriers and Benefits of the EHR

Barriers to the EHR

Although electronic health records bring tremendous benefits to patient care and to healthcare providers, use of EHRs instead of paper charts did not become widespread among independent physicians during the 1990s, despite that PMS programs were in wide use. Certainly, healthcare providers were motivated to improve patient care and utilize the availability of medical data, but they were hesitant to begin using this tool. The lack of EHR implementation until recent years may have been due to:

- Lack of standards
- Unknown costs and return on investment
- Difficulties operating EHR systems
- Significant changes in clinical/clerical processes
- Lack of trust and safety

Lack of Standards In the early 2000s, the content within EHR systems was not uniform and therefore did not allow for compatibility or interoperability. Various EHR programs offered different features, and the exchange of data was not possible. The issue of feature uniformity was not completely addressed until 2010 by the ONC.

Unknown Costs and Return on Investment Healthcare providers found it difficult to accurately calculate costs and **return on investment (ROI)** with the use of an EHR. The full cost of an EHR includes the software purchase price, additional computer hardware, and implementation, including staff training, system customization, ongoing technical support, system maintenance, and future program upgrades. However, when the federal government established a financial incentive program in 2009, providers' concerns regarding cost and estimating ROI substantially decreased.

Difficulties Operating EHR Systems Another barrier to the adoption of EHRs was practitioners' perception that data entry would be more time-consuming than handwriting. Learning where the information should be entered or accessed seemed complicated, and computers were not always accessible at the **point of care**. Some providers had trouble judging whether long-term benefits would outweigh perceived short-term operation difficulties until system warnings, medical alerts, and reporting features were developed in the **ambulatory** EHR in more recent years.

Significant Changes in Clinical/Clerical Processes Although an EHR can be customized for specific medical practices, there is always some process change required by the provider and medical staff. An EHR may bring a more rigid structure to office workflow and processes, and adapting to new standards of operation for entering and locating information can be difficult initially. Once again, practitioners needed to be educated on the real and tangible benefits of the EHR to overcome the barrier of unwanted process changes. The ONC established the Regional Extension Centers in 2010 principally to address the issues of EHR education, implementation, and support among primary care providers.

Lack of Trust and Safety The concern about the security of medical records stored electronically instead of on paper was common in the early stages of EHR deployment. Healthcare providers were often concerned that the electronic medical record could be inappropriately accessed or shared without their consent or knowledge. Providers needed to be assured that medical records were safely stored for future access and protected. The HITECH Act of 2009 established stringent security requirements for all EHR programs that sought ONC certification, thus eliminating providers' apprehension regarding safety and unauthorized accessibility.

Benefits of the EHR

Entry into the twenty-first century witnessed an upsurge in electronic social networking, instant communication, and demand for the immediate availability of information. Because of our mobile society, patients are more likely to change doctors or to be seen by a number of practitioners, which makes the efficient transfer of medical records a necessity. Access to personal medical information across the Internet has become a need, not only for healthcare providers, but also for patients. The need to share examination assessments and test results has also accelerated EHR adoption in more recent years. Industry analysts have identified major benefits motivating physicians toward clinical automation, including:

- Enhanced accessibility to clinical information
- Improved patient safety
- Enhanced quality of patient care
- Greater efficiency and savings

Focal Point

Many barriers to the adoption of ambulatory EHRs have been addressed in recent years, causing the implementation of EHRs to rapidly increase in the small- to medium-sized medical practice groups.

Enhanced Accessibility to Clinical Information EHRs provide enhanced accessibility of clinical information to healthcare providers. Access to a patient's healthcare information is no longer limited to the location of the paper chart, but is available at the point of care. Healthcare providers can easily retrieve information, such as past health history, family health history, and immunization records. Up-to-date data, including test results, routine and current medications, and allergy information, is crucial for informed decision making. For example, in the outpatient setting, if a patient calls with an issue concerning a current medication, the healthcare provider can instantly access the patient's medication information on the EHR (even if the provider is not in the office), make an informed decision, create a prescription, and document the consultation rapidly with a few mouse clicks or the tap of a stylus pen on a portable touch-screen computer. In addition, information regarding drug interactions with current and routine medications, dosage information for the prescription being created, and instant alerts with allergy warnings are all accessible within the EHR.

In contrast, in a paper chart environment, information such as drug interaction is not present. In addition, the provider may not have access to the paper chart, making the process more complicated, time-consuming, and error-prone. In the inpatient setting, nurses and other staff have immediate access to information collected in the past, such as allergies and past health history, and need only identify and document changes.

Focal Point

Immediate access to all patient medical information promotes informed medical decisions. Automated medical alerts and less reliance on handwriting promote patient safety.

Improved Patient Safety The EHR contributes to patient safety in several ways. For example, illegible handwriting is recognized as the source of many medical errors. EHR use eliminates the challenge of reading handwritten notes, orders, and prescriptions. Patient information is clear and legible. Reports and letters to other specialists and patients are comprehensive, professional, and easy to create, promoting safe patient transfers and continuity of care. Because information is readily accessible in the EHR, important data is not misplaced, which is possible with paper charts.

EHRs also contribute to patient safety through various alert systems, particularly related to medications and allergies. Alerts appear when a medication order is not within normal prescribing parameters, and EHRs can signal drug interactions and food–drug interactions. Allergy alerts indicate when a contraindicated medication is ordered, preventing a possible allergic or hypersensitivity reaction. National attention to patient safety is driving the healthcare industry toward drastically reducing errors through the use of e-prescription and electronic provider orders.

Enhanced Quality of Patient Care As healthcare becomes more complex, healthcare providers rely increasingly on evidence-based practice guidelines to support their practice. Through incorporation in the EHR, these guidelines are readily available to healthcare professionals to assist in their decisions, promote adherence, and ensure quality care for patients. Clinical decision support systems such as this allow healthcare professionals to easily access guidelines and correlate them with a patient's past health history, family history, gender, age, and allergies. Electronic reminders are available for routine screening and treatments, such as mammograms and immunizations, and may be individualized based on patient needs. For example, although a reminder for a routine colonoscopy may be set to appear for all patients older than 50 years, an EHR can also identify that a patient who is younger than 50, but has a family history of colon cancer, needs to have a colonoscopy screening. These evidence-based treatment protocols and electronic recommendations for diagnostic tests help prevent oversight by the practitioner and ensure optimal care for patients.

In addition to health promotion guidelines, over 2,000 best practice guidelines have been developed by reputable healthcare organizations to guide the diagnosis and treatment of many illnesses. The Illinois State Medical Society states:

> Practice guidelines, based on "evidence-based medicine," often are very complex, with what is best for a patient with a particular condition depending on a variety of factors, including the patient's history, the patient's family's history, other conditions of the patient and patient medications, and the availability of different modes of treatment in a community. No physician is able to keep up with all the latest practices and apply them to the particular conditions of each of his or her patients.[18]

The EHR provides a mechanism to ensure that patients receive the most current standard of care, consistently. Kaiser Permanente of Ohio achieved improvement in compliance with guidelines after implementing an automated health record system and adding reminders at the point of care:[19]

- Stratification (staging) for patients with diabetes mellitus and asthma increased to 76 percent in 26 months and 65 percent in 29 months, respectively. In addition, referrals to podiatry for medium- and high-risk diabetics increased from 14 percent to 66 percent in 12 months.
- Percentage of patients older than 64 years of age who were offered an influenza vaccination during a primary care visit increased from 56 percent to 69 percent in 36 months.

EHRs also improve the quality of patient care by providing information to patients concerning their diagnosis and the planned treatments. Office staff can easily access these instructions in the EHR and print or e-mail them to the patient, giving the patient a resource to help manage an illness or prepare for a diagnostic procedure. The EHR reports and records the distribution of treatment plans and the instructions for procedural preparation and posttreatment care for the patient. As a result, patient care is enhanced and healthcare providers may be safeguarded against liabilities.

Another mechanism to promote quality care is the proficient handling of drug recalls. Reports generated through an EHR identify which patients are currently taking specific medications. When a drug recall is issued, form letters can be rapidly generated, alerting patients to the recall and requesting follow-up with their healthcare provider. The alternative process in a paper chart environment is time-consuming and error-prone.

EHRs reduce the repetition of lab tests and other diagnostic studies through messages that inform the practitioner that a diagnostic procedure has already been ordered. Diagnostic test information is clearly displayed and readily accessed. Lost or delayed test and/or lab results are not common with EHR programs, resulting in a more expeditious diagnosis and treatment plan for the patient and increased patient satisfaction.

Greater Efficiency and Savings Greater efficiency and financial savings are major motivations for increased use of an EHR. These time and cost savings occur through eliminating redundant diagnostic testing and paper charts and decreasing storage and retrieval costs. One study cites that "a chart pull costs $20 . . . Their electronic chart solution reduced electronic chart pulls to less than $1 apiece."[20]

The use of simple electronic messaging systems built into an EHR enable faster communication between staff members. Communication to the healthcare provider concerning diagnoses, drug refills, pre-authorizations for treatments, and general patient concerns is expedited and simplified. Electronic communication among staff regarding referrals, telephone call documentation, and letters to patients and other professionals are accelerated, and documentation is automatically saved in the patient's record.

Use of EHRs also results in significant time saving for clinicians through streamlined job processes. Studies by Dassenko and Slowinski reported a reduction in clinician intake time from 35 minutes to 20 minutes for initial office visits and from 35 minutes to 15 minutes for return visits at the University of Wisconsin Hospital and Clinics. The elimination of repeatedly collecting and entering information and the addition of the enhanced display of the patient's history, vital signs, weight, and health problems attributed to greater efficiency and time savings.[21]

EHRs expedite and facilitate reporting to public health organizations as well. The simplification of this process for both ambulatory and inpatient settings is another example of time savings that translates into cost savings. Records are easily accessed and patient data sorted by diagnoses, treatments, or care plans and then sent to the appropriate agencies. EHR programs use the Internet to transmit healthcare information, so to ensure security, the data is encrypted, and only the receiver(s) has the unique deciphering "key," built into the receiving software, to decode the transmission, returning it to its readable state.

When healthcare providers complete documentation in an EHR, the need for transcription services is often eliminated. This efficiency has generated an estimated savings of $300 to $1,000 or more per month per practitioner. In one six-provider practice, transcription took 150 hours per week. After implementing an EHR, that time was decreased by one-third, and the turnaround time for transcription went from 7 days to 1 day. The time and money savings enabled the practice to add two additional providers.[22]

In the independent medical practice setting, EHR coding programs give healthcare providers confidence and support for accurately coding the level of patient encounters. Often, under-coding occurs by healthcare providers. However, with an EHR, more accurate level-of-care coding is automated and based on documentation from the review of systems and examination notes within the office visit assessment. In addition, some malpractice insurance carriers give discounts to insured providers that use an EHR program due to more thorough documentation and improved patient care.

The Illinois State Medical Society reported the following details on the ROI of a Chicago-area hospital that implemented an EHR costing over $40 million:

> The hospital estimates that it will save $10 million annually. The new system is substantially enhancing patient care. The turnaround time for obtaining test results has fallen significantly, with mammograms now taking a day compared to up to three weeks, and cardiographics reports dropping from as long as 10 days to one day. Entire categories of medication errors and potential errors have been eliminated, including transcription errors, errors due to misunderstood abbreviations and mix-ups due to look-alike drug names. In addition, delayed administration of patient medications has decreased 70 percent while omitted administration of medications has dropped 20 percent across the organization due to the electronic medication administration records and system tools that alert nurses of new patient orders and of overdue medications.[23]

Focal Point

The availability of care plans and practice guidelines increases the accuracy of patient care. Rapid documentation and accurate coding have reduced costs and increased reimbursement as a result of EHR implementation.

Concept Checkup 1.6

A. List four perceived benefits of implementing an EHR program.

B. What has made the transfer of medical records a necessity in our society?

1.7 The Future of the Electronic Health Record

As in any industry, future developments for specific products are difficult to predict; however, we do know the EHR is here to stay and has revolutionized all aspects of the medical community. Few American industries have witnessed such a massive overhaul as that currently observed in healthcare information systems. This overhaul is due mainly to the enormous financial stimulus provided by the federal government to encourage the development of a national electronic healthcare infrastructure.

The National Health Information Network (NHIN) is an ambitious, key component of the federal government's goal to digitize patients' health records and create a sophisticated network accessible by hospitals, insurers, doctors, pharmacies, and other medical stakeholders nationwide. It is designed to provide a common platform for health information exchange over the Internet. Agencies known as Health Information Exchange Organizations (HIOs) are currently developing HIE networks at the local, state, regional, and national levels; however, federal and state regulations regarding HIEs and HIT are still being defined. In January 2011, $16 million was made available to states through the ONC's new Challenge Grants program. The program provides state funding to encourage breakthrough HIE innovations that can then be leveraged widely to support nationwide HIE and interoperability. Once developed, the NHIN will be in place. Because EHRs are central to creating a nationwide, interoperable HIT network, the federal government is investing billions of dollars through the HITECH Act to encourage the rapid deployment of EHR programs.

Focal Point

The National Health Information Network (NHIN) is a set of standards, services, and policies that enable secure health information exchange over the Internet. Its purpose is to create a sophisticated network of healthcare information accessible by hospitals, insurers, doctors, pharmacies, and other medical stakeholders nationwide.

Technology is also advancing rapidly. Handheld computers were introduced to the general public only a few years ago, and now a large percentage of the population is using complex personal digital devices. The mobility now afforded by **personal digital assistants (PDAs)** and smartphones, the expansion of wireless networks from local regions and departments to systemwide corporations, and the development of high-speed Internet access will allow an enormous amount of information to be instantly available at the point of care. Practitioners and medical staff will see vast growth in accessible databases and data repositories, enabling the collection, searching through, and analyzing of large amounts of healthcare data, as well as instant support of medical decision making.

Personal digital assistant (PDA)
The term *PDA* was first used in 1992 by Apple Computer CEO John Sculley. These handheld mobile devices function as a personal information manager.

Interestingly, the computer-based patient record (CPR), which initially inspired the EHR, is coming back into focus. The lack of interoperability and standards that once plagued the electronic healthcare industry has now been removed, so a computerized lifetime patient record that includes all information from all specialties, available across a secured Internet, is now foreseeable. A virtual nationwide (potentially worldwide) medical information system will evolve, in which practitioners can view and process healthcare resources through interactive information systems beyond the confines of their own clinics and facilities. Clinical data will no longer reside exclusively in a physician's office but be available to the patient, medical personnel, and third-party entities wherever the Internet is available.

Scientists who study genomes and map human DNA sequencing that links disease to genetics are having a powerful impact on the medical industry, which will affect the EHR. In the future, federal agencies may require gene testing prior to issuing prescriptions and administering procedures. The clinician will trigger analysis reports from enormous information systems of DNA sequence data that will potentially interact with hundreds of drugs and procedures and create medical decision-making proposals.

The use of EHR programs, particularly in small- to medium-sized practices, is expanding rapidly. Nearly 90 percent of office-based physicians practice within groups of five or fewer practitioners.[24] The explosive growth of EHR implementation in this segment of the medical community has generated a great need for both clerical and clinical support staff who have professional training in and exposure to EHRs. Concerns about the transition from traditional paper charts to EHRs are now being overcome. The official certification of EHR vendors and their software in recent years has addressed more fully many of the expressed concerns about EHRs. Although medical practices' motivations vary from wanting to simply "become paperless" to improving patient care, they are quickly recognizing the EHR is an effective tool for enhancing patient care.

Concept Checkup 1.7

A. Define the concept of a PDA.

B. What is the goal of the National Health Information Network (NHIN)?

chapter 1 summary

Learning Outcome	Key Concepts/Examples
1.1 Define the concept of an electronic health record (EHR). **Pages 2–5**	An EHR is the collection of health information of individual patients that is stored in a digital format. An EHR can interface with external healthcare computer programs, enabling them to electronically transmit and receive test results, data on prescription medications, and comprehensive reports to government healthcare agencies. EHR programs can be grouped into three distinct models that are used internationally: • The distribution-based model transmits selected healthcare data to a centralized electronic record. • The facility-based model stores patient data on the health information system at a particular healthcare facility or with a third-party hosting company. • The Web-based model provides secure Web space in which patients can accumulate their healthcare data and make it available to providers.
1.2 Explain key events in the history of EHRs. **Pages 6–7**	The initial creation and use of the computerized patient record occurred in large hospitals during the 1960s. Databases and functionality were added to EHRs in order to improve patient care during the 1970s and 1980s. Computers and practice management system (PMS) programs were used in independent medical offices for insurance claims and financial accounting in the 1990s. By 2010, government mandates and funding had spurred the standardization of EHR features, introduced an EHR certification program, and offered major financial incentives to providers for the purchase and implementation of EHR programs.
1.3 Distinguish between the terms commonly used to refer to EHRs. **Pages 7–9**	CPR—Computer-Based Patient Record EMR—Electronic Medical Record EHR—Electronic Health Record CCD/CCR—Continuity of Care Document/Continuity of Care Record PHR—Personal Health Record
1.4 Describe the government's involvement in EHRs. **Pages 9–12**	In 2004, the Bush administration created a subcabinet-level position called the Office of the National Coordinator for Health Information Technology at the Department of Health and Human Services to promote the use of and overcome barriers to the EHR. In 2008, MIPPA provided financial incentives for practitioners who used e-prescribing beginning in 2009 through 2013. In 2009, the Obama administration introduced an economic recovery plan to accelerate the use of computerized health records in physician's offices and inpatient settings over a period of five years. In 2009, ARRA provided $19.2 billion through the HITECH Act to aid in the development of a healthcare infrastructure and assist individual providers adopt and use health information technology. In 2010, the Beacon Community Cooperative Agreement Program provided funding through the HITECH Act to 17 selected communities to encourage the development of EHR adoption and health information exchange (HIE) systems. In 2010, the Health Information Technology Extension Program provided funding through the HITECH Act to establish nationwide Regional Extension Centers (RECs) and a national Health Information Technology Research Center (HITRC). • RECs support and serve primary healthcare clinicians to assist them in becoming proficient and meaningful users of EHRs. • HITRC gathers information on effective practices in EHR adoption, meaningful use, and provider support for the 62 RECs across the country.

Learning Outcome	Key Concepts/Examples
1.5 Differentiate between medical office processes that use a paper chart and an EHR. **Pages 12–16**	Processes that change with the implementation of an EHR: • Scheduling an appointment • Preparing charts and verifying insurance coverage • Checking in the patient • Verifying patient's identification • Collecting patient healthcare information • Signing official forms • Recording vital signs and the chief complaint • Reviewing patient's healthcare information • Checking status of wellness screenings • Readying patient for physician examination • Reviewing clinician's notes • Documenting physical examination • Ordering in-house tests • Processing prescriptions • Completing physician's note • Ordering outside tests • Completing the superbill • Distributing patient education material • Checking out the patient • Entering billing data • Processing lab and medical test results • Sending healthcare records to other physicians
1.6 Summarize the major barriers and benefits of using an EHR. **Pages 16–20**	Even though they were motivated to improve patient care, healthcare providers have been hesitant to begin using EHRs because of: • Lack of standards for EHR systems • Unknown cost and return on investment • Difficulties operating EHR systems • Significant changes in clinic/clerical processes • Lack of trust and safety Some of the major benefits that are motivating providers toward clinical automation are: • Enhanced accessibility to clinical information • Improved patient safety • Enhanced quality of patient care • Greater efficiency and savings
1.7 Describe potential developments in the future of the EHR. **Pages 21–22**	The National Health Information Network (NHIN) will provide a common platform for HIE over the Internet to create a national network accessible by hospitals, insurers, doctors, pharmacies, and other healthcare stakeholders. Funding available through the Challenge Grants program will encourage breakthrough innovations for HIE systems and interoperability that will advance the rapid uptake of EHR programs. The PDA, wireless networks, and high-speed Internet access will allow an enormous amount of information to be instantly available at the point of care. Clinical data will no longer reside exclusively in a physician's office, but will be available to the patient, medical personnel, and third-party entities wherever the Internet is available to form the computer-based patient record (CPR).

chapter 1 review

Name ______________________ Instructor ______________ Class ______________ Date ______________

Using Terminology

Match the terms on the left with the definitions on the right.

_____ 1. **LO 1.1** EHR

_____ 2. **LO 1.3** Interoperability

_____ 3. **LO 1.4** Medicare Part B

_____ 4. **LO 1.7** PDA

_____ 5. **LO 1.1** Patient portals

_____ 6. **LO 1.4** HITECH Act

_____ 7. **LO 1.6** Ambulatory

_____ 8. **LO 1.4** E-prescribing

_____ 9. **LO 1.6** Point of care

_____ 10. **LO 1.2** PMS

A. A software program that manages financial transactions, both charges and payments; the billing of insurance claims; and the issuing of patient statements.

B. This legislation was initiated by Congress to stimulate and increase the use of electronic health records by independent physicians and hospitals over a five-year period.

C. The time and place at which a healthcare provider gives the patient medical care.

D. A handheld mobile device that functions as a personal information manager.

E. The capability of walking or the ability to move from one place to another. In a medical sense it is used to distinguish walking patients from patients who are bedridden, as in an inpatient hospital or skilled nursing facility.

F. The most commonly accepted and used term for storing and accessing patient healthcare information electronically.

G. The use of computerized tools, usually embedded in an EHR program, to create and sign prescriptions for medicines, thereby replacing handwritten prescriptions.

H. Part of the federally funded insurance program that covers medical providers' supervision, outpatient hospital care, diagnostic tests, and other ambulatory services.

I. Online applications that are designed to allow patients access to their medical records and allow communication with their healthcare providers across the Internet.

J. The ability of a software program to accept, send, or communicate data from its database to other software programs from multiple vendors.

Checking Your Understanding

Select the letter that best completes the statement or answers the question.

11. LO 1.6 EHR programs were not fully utilized until more recent years for all the following reasons *except:*

a) Lack of standards

b) Unknown cost and ROI

c) Difficulty in operating EHR programs

d) Lack of availability of computers

12. LO 1.4 The HITECH Act allocated $19.2 billion to aid in the development of a healthcare infrastructure and to assist the following entities in adopting and using health information technology:

a) Individual providers and hospitals

b) The government and patients

c) EHR vendors and EHR programs

d) Only primary healthcare providers

13. **LO 1.4** MIPPA was enacted in 2008 and is an acronym for:
    a) Medical Improvements for Patients and Professionals Act
    b) Medicare Improvements for Patients and Providers Act
    c) Medicaid Incentive Program for eligible Professionals Act
    d) Medicare/Medicaid Improvements for Providers and Professionals Act

14. **LO 1.1** As EHR programs have evolved internationally, three distinct models of electronic records have emerged. Which of the following is *not* a model of electronic health records?
    a) Distribution-based model
    b) Facility-based model
    c) International-based model
    d) Web-based personal healthcare model

15. **LO 1.5** Because EHRs are patient-focused, who utilize EHR functionality to perform their duties?
    a) All clerical and clinical staff
    b) Only physicians and patients
    c) Only physicians and billing personnel
    d) Only clinical staff

16. **LO 1.7** Which government-sponsored organization or program is responsible for providing EHR training and support services for primary healthcare providers?
    a) Beacon Community Program
    b) Health Information Technology Research Center
    c) Health Information Exchange
    d) Regional Extension Centers

17. **LO 1.6** Which of the following is *not* a benefit of EHR?
    a) Little or no training necessary
    b) Enhanced access to clinical information
    c) Improved patient safety
    d) Enhanced quality of patient care

18. **LO 1.6** Which of the following items is *not* a cost saving of using EHRs rather than paper-based charts?
    a) Storage and retrieval costs are often eliminated
    b) The need for medical assistants is often eliminated
    c) The need for a transcriptionist is often eliminated
    d) Redundant diagnostic testing is eliminated

19. **LO 1.2** Some of the earliest electronic health record programs were developed and utilized in:
    a) 1950 at the University of Utah
    b) The 1980s at the Mayo Clinic
    c) The 1960s at Medical Center Hospital of Vermont and the Mayo Clinic
    d) This information cannot be determined

20. **LO 1.3** Which acronym was one of the first terms used to conceptualize the idea of storing medical information electronically?
    a) EHR
    b) PHR
    c) CPR
    d) BYO

21. **LO 1.6** Ambulatory means:
    a) Return on investment
    b) Point of care
    c) The capability of walking or moving from one place to another
    d) Lack of EHR standards

22. **LO 1.6** With an EHR, healthcare practitioners provide better and more consistent care for patients because the information is:
    a) More accessible and better utilized with care plans and alerts
    b) Reviewed with the patient
    c) Stored offsite at a remote location
    d) Backed up electronically on a regular basis

23. **LO 1.4** The stimulus package of 2009 is officially known as:
    a) Centers for Medicare & Medicaid Services (CMS)
    b) American Recovery and Reinvestment Act (ARRA)
    c) Health Information Technology for Economic and Clinical Health (HITECH) Act
    d) Troubled Asset Relief Program (TARP)

24. **LO 1.4** ONC stands for:
    a) Office for National Committee on EHR Standards
    b) Office of the National Commission for Health Information Systems
    c) Office for New Codes and Technology
    d) Office of the National Coordinator for Health Information Technology

25. **LO 1.7** The future of the EHR anticipates:
   a) The majority of doctors retiring early because of high levels of technology
   b) Budget cuts eliminating chances for long-term or widespread use
   c) An enormous amount of Internet data available at the point of care
   d) Increased medical costs because of the purchase of expensive equipment

Applying Your Knowledge

Use your critical-thinking skills to answer the following questions.

26. **LO 1.4** You are employed in a primary care medical office that is in the process of selecting an EHR program. The physician knows you have received training in EHR features and functionality and asks for your input. The clinic is looking for guidance in selecting an EHR program and technical assistance in implementing the program. Which government service would you suggest the clinic contact and why?

27. **LO 1.5** Explain the differences between a paper and an EHR environment in the process of fulfilling a referring physician's request for a copy of a patient's chart.

28. **LO 1.6** You are assisting your office manager with implementing an EHR program in the medical office. Some staff members are not proficient with the use of computers and nervous about the established clinic processes that inevitably will change. They are also concerned about a decline in patient safety and care because of the use of computers. What would you say to help ease their anxieties?

2

Standards and Features of Electronic Health Records

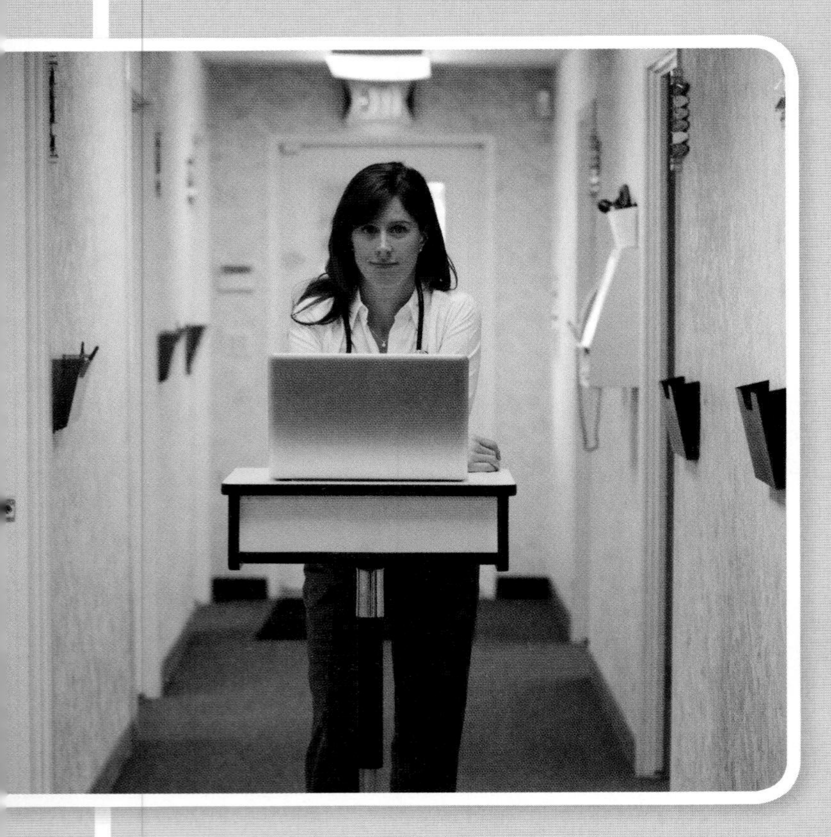

Learning Outcomes

After completing Chapter 2, you will be able to:

- LO 2.1 Identify major events in the development of standards for the EHR.
- LO 2.2 Describe meaningful use (MU) criteria, including specific EHR functions that meet MU requirements.
- LO 2.3 Describe key privacy and security issues related to EHRs.
- LO 2.4 Explain the basic technology used in EHR implementation.
- LO 2.5 List EHR competencies identified by the Competency Model Clearinghouse.

Key Terms

Application server provider (ASP)
Certification Commission for Health Information Technology (CCHIT)
Computer on wheels (COW)/ workstation on wheels (WOW)
Computerized provider order entry (CPOE)
Consolidated Health Informatics (CHI)
Current Procedural Terminology (CPT) codes
Drug formulary
Eligible professional (EP)
Encrypting
Health Insurance Portability and Accountability Act (HIPAA)
Health Level Seven (HL7)
Healthcare Common Procedure Coding System (HCPCS) codes
Institute of Medicine (IOM)
International Classification of Diseases (ICD) codes
Intranet
Local area network (LAN)
Meaningful use (MU)
National Committee on Vital and Health Statistics (NCVHS)
Protected health information (PHI)
Server
Structured data
Tablet
Telehealth services
Template
Test script
Wireless connectivity

What You Need to Know

To understand Chapter 2, you will need to know:

- The concept of a patient's chart in a medical office
- The history of the development of electronic health records

Introduction

National standards related to the features and functionality of practice management systems (PMS) and medical billing programs have been in place since the 1990s. Many of these standards were applied to electronic health record (EHR) programs as they evolved during that decade. Since then, various government agencies and commercial interests have been responsible for developing national standards for operability, privacy, and security for the health information technology (HIT) industry. These criteria will continue to be evaluated routinely to meet the everchanging benchmarks of functionality; EHR vendors and their products will have to enhance their standards of functionality and features on an ongoing basis.

The privacy and security issues surrounding healthcare records have been valid concerns from EHRs' inception. Congressional legislation has addressed these concerns in recent years. As EHRs have developed and been increasingly used in the medical industry, various independent healthcare organizations and government agencies have also advanced privacy and security guidelines for EHR features and functionality—everything from simple e-mail to issues of national security. This chapter will outline the history of standards regulating this technology, the main aspects of the current federal government's EHR certification program, and EHRs' key features.

2.1 History of EHR Standards

With the established premise that EHRs can improve the quality of healthcare, the U.S. government and other institutions have been promoting the use of EHRs since the year 2000. Although obstacles such as cost, organization, standards, functionality, and interoperability have slowed EHR implementation and progress, the work of private commercial entities, various national committees, and independent associations have aided the federal government's efforts, established standards, and served as stepping stones to facilitate wider EHR use.

Health Insurance Portability and Accountability Act (HIPAA)

The U.S. Congress passed the **Health Insurance Portability and Accountability Act (HIPAA)** in 1996 to establish standards for accountability and criteria for the protection and confidentiality of electronically transported health information. HIPAA standards, which initially regulated PMS programs, played an important role in EHR development early in this century by requiring participants in the healthcare industry to use standardized transactions and code sets and by extending the reach of HIPAA to protect medical information beyond the initial covered entity.

In early 2000, the **National Committee on Vital and Health Statistics (NCVHS)** proposed establishing national standards for effective and significant use of EHR technology and expansion of quality reporting to improve patient care. The committee has legislative responsibility for making recommendations related to HIPAA and a broader mandate for national health information policy.

Health Insurance Portability and Accountability Act (HIPAA)
Passed by Congress in 1996, this legal act enforces standards for electronic patient health, administrative, and financial data.

National Committee on Vital and Health Statistics (NCVHS)
Formed in 1949 and restructured following the passage of HIPAA, the NCVHS is an advocate for uniform health data sets, particularly for underrepresented populations. This advisory committee has responsibility for providing recommendations on health information policy and standards to the Department of Health and Human Services (HHS).

Consolidated Health Informatics (CHI)

In the last decade, several associations and government departments called for further action to promote and set baseline functionality for EHRs, which prompted the next significant step in EHR standards. In 2003, **Consolidated Health Informatics (CHI)**, an initiative of the U.S. Office of Management and Budget (OMB), released the first set of EHR standards. The goal was to make the approximately 20 federal agencies involved in healthcare and health-related missions interoperable, that is, to effectively enable them to share electronic information. Those agencies included the Department of Veterans Affairs, the Department of Health and Human Services, the Department of Defense, and the Social Security Administration. The standards included common clinical vocabularies and standard methods for transmitting health information. In May 2004, 20 standards became the benchmark for how the information would be coded or termed for use in exchanging data to and from EHR programs.

Consolidated Health Informatics (CHI)
This federal government initiative promotes the adoption of health information interoperability standards for health vocabulary and messaging.

Focal Point

EHR vendors voluntarily adopted 20 Consolidated Health Informatics standards, designed to promote interoperability among health information systems.

Although CHI standards were not legally required, vendors doing business with the federal government voluntarily adopted them. The federal government, as the largest purchaser of healthcare services, continues to use these standards to promote interoperability between EHR systems. A few notable adopted standards are:

Health Level Seven (HL7). HL7 is a computer messaging and vocabulary standard for demographic information, units of measure, immunizations, and clinical encounters for text-based reports. Practically, the computer communication standard is used for scheduling, orders, tests, admittances, discharges, and transfers for coordinated patient care. HL7 computer language enables clinical systems to communicate, or interface, with each other so all clinical software understands what is being sent and received. HL7 is currently the selected standard for interfacing clinical data in most institutions.

HL7
Health Level 7 is an international computer language by which various healthcare systems can communicate. HL7 is currently the selected standard for the interfacing of clinical data between software programs in most institutions.

The National Council on Prescription Drug Programs (NCPDP). The NCPDP creates and promotes standards for the transfer of data to and from retail pharmacy services. NCPDP standards are focused on prescription drug messages and the activities involved in billing pharmacy claims and services, rebates, pharmacy ID cards, and standardized business transactions among pharmacies and the professionals who prescribe medications.

The Institute of Electrical and Electronics Engineers 11073 Medical Device Communications standard. IEEE (pronounced *eye-triple-e*) is an international organization tasked with advancing technology related to electricity. This particular standard addresses the interoperability of medical devices. The standard sets electronic standards to allow for the connection of medical devices to information and computer systems, allowing healthcare providers to monitor information from such places as ICUs and **telehealth services**, specifically on Native American reservations.

Telehealth services
These services use electronic and communication technology to deliver medical information and services over large and small distances through a standard telephone line.

Systematized Nomenclature of Medicine Clinical Terms (SNOMED CT). SNOMED CT provides a common language that enables a consistent way of capturing, sharing, and aggregating health data across specialties and sites of care. It provides standard terminology for laboratory result contents, anatomy, diagnoses, medical problems, and nursing.

Institute of Medicine (IOM)

We have learned that the focus of CHI was primarily interoperability standards affecting health terminology and messaging. In addition to technical standards, in 2003 HHS asked the **Institute of Medicine (IOM)** to provide

Institute of Medicine (IOM)
This independent, nonprofit organization works outside the government to provide unbiased and authoritative medical advice to decision makers and the public.

guidance on key EHR system capabilities. The IOM's Committee on Data Standards for Patient Safety identified eight key capabilities, or functions, EHRs should include. Four of the notable functions are as follows:

Health Information and Patient Data. This standard addresses the mandate that an EHR must contain pertinent patient data so the healthcare provider can easily access all the necessary information to make sound clinical decisions. For example, it must contain the patient's past medical history, diagnoses, a written account of the patient's chief complaint(s), and the current healthcare history. Patient allergy and drug interaction information should be clear and accessible. Availability of past laboratory results prevent redundant or unnecessary tests from being performed. All patient information must be well displayed so the end user can easily access the needed information.

Results Management. This capability addresses the management of laboratory and radiology test results. Healthcare providers must be able to easily access computerized test results, via HL7 interfaces, when and where needed. Reduced lag time between the physician order and electronic data entry of those results allows providers to more quickly detect medical abnormalities and treatment, thus increasing both office efficiency and patient safety.

Order Entry/Management. The order entry function concerns computerizing orders for lab work, other medical tests, and prescriptions to improve the workflow processes as well as eliminate lost or ambiguous orders, handwriting discrepancies, order duplication, and superfluous paperwork.

Medical Decision Support. This recommended functionality focuses on drug prescribing and dosage, disease screening, diagnosis and treatment, and improvement of the quality of care. The following information must be accessible through the EHR: prescription details, drug interactions, allergies, dosing, diagnoses, disease and symptom management, disease outbreaks, and adverse reactions or events. Having this information available significantly improves healthcare and is a major reason for promoting EHR use.

Focal Point

The IOM developed guidelines for key capabilities/functions that should exist in a quality electronic health record program.

The Certification Commission for Health Information Technology (CCHIT)

The **Certification Commission for Health Information Technology (CCHIT)** was organized in July 2004 with support from the American Health Information Management Association (AHIMA), the Healthcare Information and Management Systems Society (HIMSS), and the National Alliance for Health Information Technology (NAHIT). These three organizations committed resources during the formation phase to create the independent, nonprofit, private-sector Certification Commission. At that time, 21 volunteer commissioners guided more than 100 work group members, who in turn were charged with the commission's development work.[2]

HHS awarded the commission a contract in 2005 to develop certification criteria standards, evaluate these standards, and create an inspection process for HIT. The commission's work addressed three specific HIT areas:

1. Ambulatory healthcare EHRs for office-based healthcare providers
2. Inpatient EHRs for hospitals and health systems
3. Network components through which EHRs interoperate and share information

Certification Commission for Health Information Technology (CCHIT)
The Certification Commission's mission was to accelerate the adoption of health information technology by creating an efficient, credible, and sustainable product certification program.[1]

From 2006 to 2009, the commission annually developed new EHR criteria and feature requirements. To be CCHIT-certified, EHR vendors paid to have their products inspected and then receive a three-year term of certification. Since 2009, the Office of the National Coordinator for Health Information Technology (ONC) has taken responsibility for developing and managing the EHR certification program.

The Certification Commission provided the official recognition and approval process that both the private sector and government agencies had requested. Such industry standards–based criteria for EHRs promoted confidence in their use. In the past, the lack of uniform requirements and standards was a considerable hurdle to extensive EHR adoption. This barrier was specifically addressed when HHS awarded the Certification Commission the contract, to promote the use of EHRs by primary care providers, hospitals, home health, and other organizations.

Focal Point

Both HIPAA legislation and the CCHIT have exerted major influence on EHR development, features, and standards.

Office of the National Coordinator for Health Information Technology (ONC)

In 2004, the ONC was established within the Office of the Secretary for HHS. Its purpose was to serve as a resource for the entire health system, support HIT adoption, and promote a nationwide health information exchange, with the goal of improving healthcare in the United States.[3]

The American National Standards Institute (ANSI) Healthcare Information Technology Standards Panel (HITSP) was created in 2005 as part of the ONC's efforts to promote interoperability in healthcare by harmonizing HIT standards. CCHIT evaluated these uniform EHR standards as part of its development of conformance criteria and **test scripts**. The first set of 300 proposed ambulatory EHR criteria was published in May 2006 and used as the benchmark for the first EHR certification program conducted by CCHIT.

Test script
A test script in software testing is a set of instructions that is performed on the system to ensure the system functions as expected.

Focal Point

Although the private-sector organization CCHIT began certifying EHR programs in 2006, the ONC established a government-based certification program in 2010 in which CCHIT participates as an ONC-ATCB.

However, the need to guarantee basic government standards, national implementation specifications, and EHR program functionality to the medical community spurred the ONC to launch its own two-year temporary certification program, which began in September 2010. Several HIT organizations countrywide were selected to test and certify both ambulatory and inpatient EHR programs. Each entity is known as an ONC-Authorized Testing and Certification Body (ONC-ATCB). CCHIT became one of the six sanctioned ONC-ATCBs. EHR vendors are required to submit their EHR products for testing and certification to one of the ONC-ATCBs. Products that were previously CCHIT certified must be resubmitted for ONC-ATCB certification. To qualify for incentive money provided through the 2009 Health Information Technology for Economic and Clinical Health (HITECH) Act, practitioners must use an EHR program that is ONC-ATCB certified.

With a national standards process in place, healthcare providers and patients can be confident that electronic health information technology products and systems are secure, maintain data confidentially, perform a set of specified functions, and can share medical information with other systems.

Concept Checkup 2.1

A. The government regulation known as HIPAA initially regulated PMS programs. What important role did HIPAA exert in the early development of EHRs?

B. By 2004, CHI had set 20 standards to regulate information exchange between federal healthcare agencies. What did these standards regulate?

C. With what was the IOM tasked by HHS in the early development of the EHR industry?

D. List three purposes of the ONC in relation to improving healthcare in the United States.

2.2 EHR Functionality

As we learned in Chapter 1, versions of EHR programs have been available to the healthcare industry since the 1960s. However, due to barriers such as high costs and lack of uniform features, medical facilities—particularly small- to medium-sized independent medical offices—have been reluctant to invest time and money in implementing an EHR system. In 2004, the federal government addressed the sluggish adoption rate of EHRs, establishing the ONC to spearhead HIT implementation by acting as a resource to the national healthcare system. In 2009, because the uptake of EHR programs remained slow-moving, the HITECH Act authorized the ONC to promote EHR adoption by means of a financial incentive program based on healthcare practitioners' ability to use EHR technology in a meaningful manner.

Focal Point

The ONC's purpose is to serve as a resource to the entire health system, to support the adoption of health information technology, and to promote a nationwide health information exchange, in order to improve healthcare in the United States.

Meaningful Use (MU)

The HITECH Act seeks to improve healthcare delivery in the United States. Through various provisions and regulations, the act authorized the ONC to establish a certification program that ensures a standard of features and functionality in both ambulatory and inpatient EHR programs. The act also provides financial incentives, assistance, online tools, and resources for providers to implement, use, and prove **meaningful use (MU)** of electronic health records. MU refers to demonstrably effective use of an EHR program, determined via tangible, ONC-established functionalities. For example, one way an ONC-certified EHR program must demonstrate MU is by allowing the user to record a patient's height and weight and then automatically calculating and recording the patient's body mass index.

The ONC sanctioned six Authorized Testing and Certification Bodies (ATCBs) in summer 2010 to certify EHR programs. EHR vendors submit their programs for testing against a set of ONC-established standards and features. Products that achieve certification are placed on the Certified HIT Product List (CHPL), which the ONC maintains. ATCB certification signifies to each **eligible professional (EP)** and hospitals that the EHR technology has the capabilities to meet MU goals and objectives. By demonstrating meaningfully use with an ONC-ATCB–certified EHR system, providers qualify for the Medicare or Medicaid EHR Incentive Programs, which offer substantial financial incentives for achieving health and efficiency goals. The criteria for meaningful use are staged in three steps, which began in 2011 and continue over the next four years.[4]

Meaningful use (MU)
Meaningful use is healthcare providers' use of certified EHR technology in ways that can be measured significantly in quality (e.g., e-prescribing) and in quantity (e.g., set percentage of patients). By demonstrating MU with an ONC-certified EHR program, providers then can receive stimulus money, as set up through the HITECH Act of 2009.

Eligible professional (EP)
To participate in the HITECH Act incentive program for meaningful use (MU) on an ONC-certified EHR program, an EP qualifying under Medicare must be a doctor of either medicine, osteopathy, dental surgery, dental medicine, podiatry, optometry, or chiropractic. Individuals qualifying under the Medicaid program must be a doctor of medicine or osteopathy, nurse practitioner, certified nurse-midwife, dentist, or qualifying physician assistant.

The American Recovery and Reinvestment Act (ARRA) specifies three main components of meaningful use:

1. The use of a certified EHR in a specified significant manner, such as e-prescribing.
2. The use of certified EHR technology for electronic exchange of health information to improve healthcare quality, such as transmitting lab results.
3. The use of certified EHR technology to submit clinical quality reports and other measures.

To qualify for meaningful use in 2011 and 2012, EPs or hospitals had to demonstrate the use of a core set of 15 features in an EHR program and the selection of 5 additional objectives from a menu set of 10 objectives specified by the ONC.[5] To qualify for an incentive payment in 2011, each EP was required to use a certified EHR program for 90 consecutive days and achieve the MU requirements specified for stage 1. In 2012, EPs had to demonstrate MU for each month of the calendar year.

As an example, 3 of the 15 core features required to demonstrate MU in 2011 and 2012 are outlined below, using screen shots from the SpringCharts EHR program. See Table 2.1 for a complete list of the 15 mandatory objectives and the 10 menu set objectives.

Core Measure 1. Record patient demographics in the patient data section of the patient's electronic chart. The following demographic fields must be recorded for more than 50 percent of patients during the MU

Table 2.1 Meaningful Use (MU) Criteria for Stage 1 of ONC Incentive Program

Core Objectives/Mandatory Functions

The following 15 Core Objectives were demonstrated by the EP in an ONC-certified EHR program in 2011 and 2012 to qualify for incentive payments:

1. Create computerized provider order entry (CPOE).
2. Generate and transmit permissible prescriptions electronically (eRx).
3. Report a total of six ambulatory clinical quality measures to CMS.
4. Implement one clinical decision support rule.
5. Provide patients with an electronic copy of their health information, upon request.
6. Provide clinical summaries for patient for each office visit.
7. Perform drug–drug and drug–allergy interaction checks.
8. Enable a user to electronically record, modify, and retrieve patient demographic data, including preferred language, gender, race, ethnicity, and date of birth.
9. Maintain an up-to-date problem list of current and active diagnoses based on ICD-9 or SNOMED CT
10. Maintain the patient's active medication list.
11. Maintain the patient's active medication allergy list.
12. Record and chart changes in patient's vital signs:
    - Height
    - Weight
    - Blood pressure

    Calculate and display BMI; and plot and display growth charts for children 2–20 years (including BMI).

Table 2.1 *(Concluded)*

13. Record smoking status for patients 13 years old or older.
14. Exchange key clinical information among providers of care and patient-authorized entities electronically.
15. Protect electronic health information created or maintained by the certified EHR technology through the implementation of appropriate technical capabilities.

Menu Set Objectives/Mandatory & Optional Functions

Five of the following objectives had to be selected and performed in an ONC-certified EHR program in 2011 and 2012 to qualify for incentive payments. Objective #9 or #10 must be one of the five selected objectives.

1. Perform drug-formulary checks.
2. Document clinical lab test results as structured data.
3. Generate lists of patients by specific conditions.
4. Send reminders to patients per patient preference for preventive/follow-up care.
5. Provide patients with timely electronic access to their health information.
6. Use certified EHR technology to identify patient-specific education resources and provide to patient.
7. Perform medication reconciliation.
8. Create summary of care record for each transition of care/referrals.
9. Submit electronic data to immunization registries/systems (public health objective).
10. Provide electronic surveillance data to public health agencies (public health objective).

Sources: CMS.gov. Centers for Medicare and Medicaid Services, February 24, 2011. https://www.cms.gov/EHRIncentive Programs/30_Meaningful_Use.asp. CMS.gov. "Eligible Professional Meaningful Use Table of Contents: Core and Menu Set Objectives." https://www.cms.gov/EHRIncentivePrograms/Downloads/EP-MU-TOC.pdf (accessed November 2011).

period: date of birth, gender/sex, preferred language, race, and ethnicity (Figure 2.1).

Core Measure 2. Demonstrate the ability to maintain an active medications list. The practitioner must have at least one medication entered into the routine medication list or indicate the patient is not on any medications, for more than 80 percent of patients during the MU testing period of 90 consecutive days in 2011 and for each month in 2012 (Figure 2.2).

Core Measure 3. A medical practice qualifying for incentive payments under the HITECH Act must demonstrate the ability to record and maintain a patient's smoking status for more than 50 percent of patients 13 years of age or older during the reporting period (Figure 2.3).

An example of 3 of the 5 measures that must be chosen from a menu set of 10 objectives are as follows:

Menu Measure 1. Demonstrate the ability to conduct **drug formulary** checks. A certified EHR program must use a formulary check system with access to at least one internal or external drug formulary for the entire reporting period. In the SpringCharts EHR system, this feature is available whenever the user is managing prescriptions or prescription refills, by clicking on the eRx icon (Figure 2.4). The program provides many real-time clinical support tools, including drug formularies and drug/allergy interaction checking, illustrated in Figure 2.5.

Drug formulary
A drug formulary is a database of approved medications in drug therapy categories that includes information on the preparation, safety, effectiveness, and cost of the medications.

New Patient

First Name*: Jose
MI: R
Last Name*: Gomez
Date of Birth*: 08/02/1958
Address: 3006 DeContez Crt. #205
City: Sherman
State: TX
Zip+: 77521
Sex+: Male Female
Marital Status: Married
Employer: Gospel Publishing House
EMail: jgomez@gph.org
SS#: 048-68-5412
Category:
Preferred Language: Spanish
Race: American Indian or Al...
Ethnicity: Hispanic or Latino

Home Phone: (214) 512-4897
Home Fax:
Work Phone: (214) 526-8888
Work Fax:
Pager:
Mobile Phone: (214) 789-6541
PMS ID:
Patient ID:
Mother's Last Name: N/A
Attending Provider ID:
Attending Provider:

Other Provider Details Add

Name	Role	Edit	Del
John O. Smith, M. D.	Physician	Edit	Del

* Required
\+ Required for eRx

Previous Updates Exempt Save Cancel Copy Patient

Figure 2.1 Required patient demographics for meaningful use.

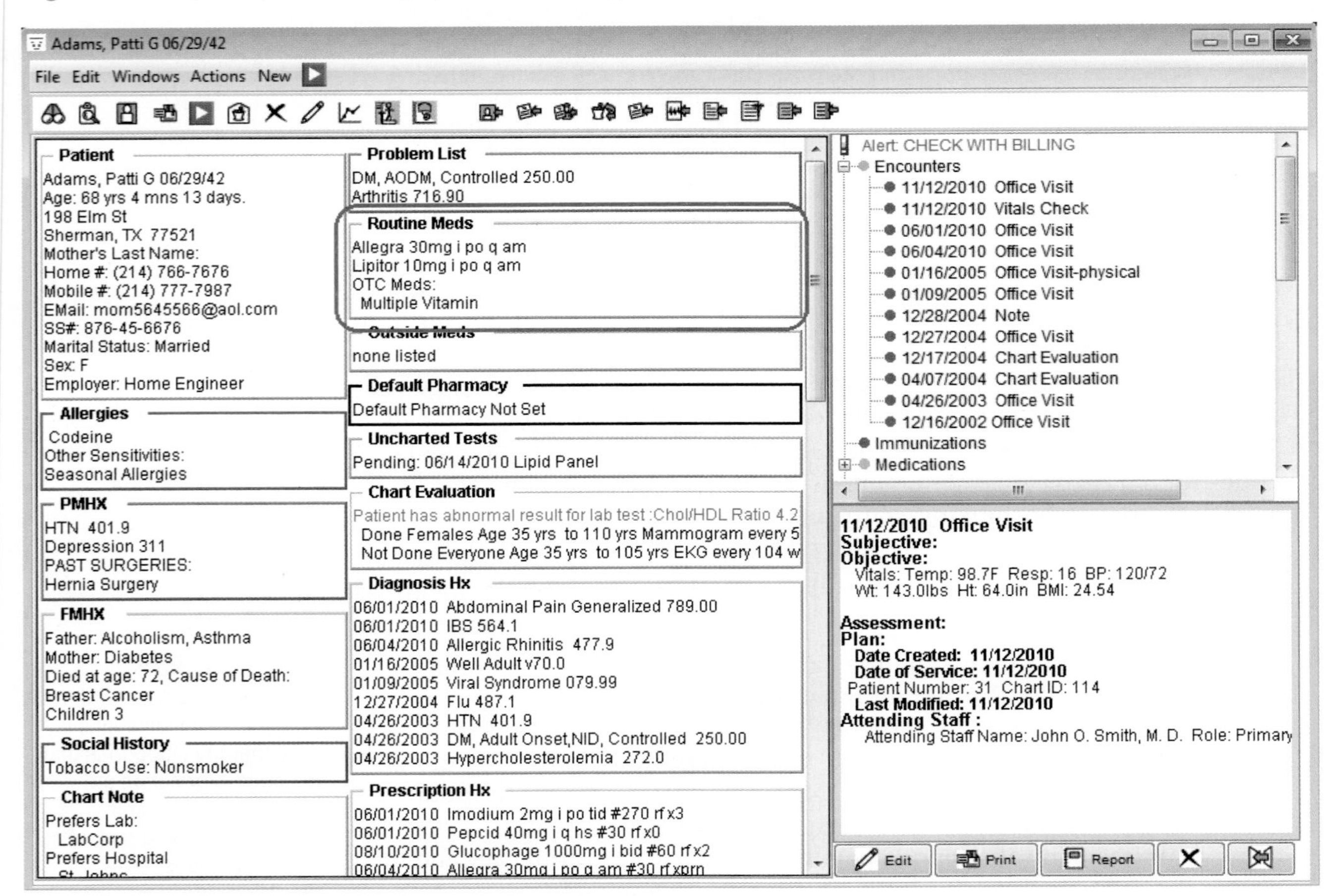
Adams, Patti G 06/29/42
File Edit Windows Actions New

Patient
Adams, Patti G 06/29/42
Age: 68 yrs 4 mns 13 days.
198 Elm St
Sherman, TX 77521
Mother's Last Name:
Home #: (214) 766-7676
Mobile #: (214) 777-7987
EMail: mom5645566@aol.com
SS#: 876-45-6676
Marital Status: Married
Sex: F
Employer: Home Engineer

Allergies
Codeine
Other Sensitivities:
Seasonal Allergies

PMHX
HTN 401.9
Depression 311
PAST SURGERIES:
Hernia Surgery

FMHX
Father: Alcoholism, Asthma
Mother: Diabetes
Died at age: 72, Cause of Death:
Breast Cancer
Children 3

Social History
Tobacco Use: Nonsmoker

Chart Note
Prefers Lab:
LabCorp
Prefers Hospital

Problem List
DM, AODM, Controlled 250.00
Arthritis 716.90

Routine Meds
Allegra 30mg i po q am
Lipitor 10mg i po q am
OTC Meds:
Multiple Vitamin

Outside Meds
none listed

Default Pharmacy
Default Pharmacy Not Set

Uncharted Tests
Pending: 06/14/2010 Lipid Panel

Chart Evaluation
Patient has abnormal result for lab test :Chol/HDL Ratio 4.2
Done Females Age 35 yrs to 110 yrs Mammogram every 5
Not Done Everyone Age 35 yrs to 105 yrs EKG every 104 w

Diagnosis Hx
06/01/2010 Abdominal Pain Generalized 789.00
06/01/2010 IBS 564.1
06/04/2010 Allergic Rhinitis 477.9
01/16/2005 Well Adult v70.0
01/09/2005 Viral Syndrome 079.99
12/27/2004 Flu 487.1
04/26/2003 HTN 401.9
04/26/2003 DM, Adult Onset,NID, Controlled 250.00
04/26/2003 Hypercholesterolemia 272.0

Prescription Hx
06/01/2010 Imodium 2mg i po tid #270 rf x3
06/01/2010 Pepcid 40mg i q hs #30 rf x0
08/10/2010 Glucophage 1000mg i bid #60 rf x2

Alert: CHECK WITH BILLING
Encounters
11/12/2010 Office Visit
11/12/2010 Vitals Check
06/01/2010 Office Visit
06/04/2010 Office Visit
01/16/2005 Office Visit-physical
01/09/2005 Office Visit
12/28/2004 Note
12/27/2004 Office Visit
12/17/2004 Chart Evaluation
04/07/2004 Chart Evaluation
04/26/2003 Office Visit
12/16/2002 Office Visit
Immunizations
Medications

11/12/2010 Office Visit
Subjective:
Objective:
Vitals: Temp: 98.7F Resp: 16 BP: 120/72
Wt: 143.0lbs Ht: 64.0in BMI: 24.54
Assessment:
Plan:
Date Created: 11/12/2010
Date of Service: 11/12/2010
Patient Number: 31 Chart ID: 114
Last Modified: 11/12/2010
Attending Staff :
Attending Staff Name: John O. Smith, M. D. Role: Primary

Edit Print Report

Figure 2.2 Routine medications on display in patient's electronic chart.

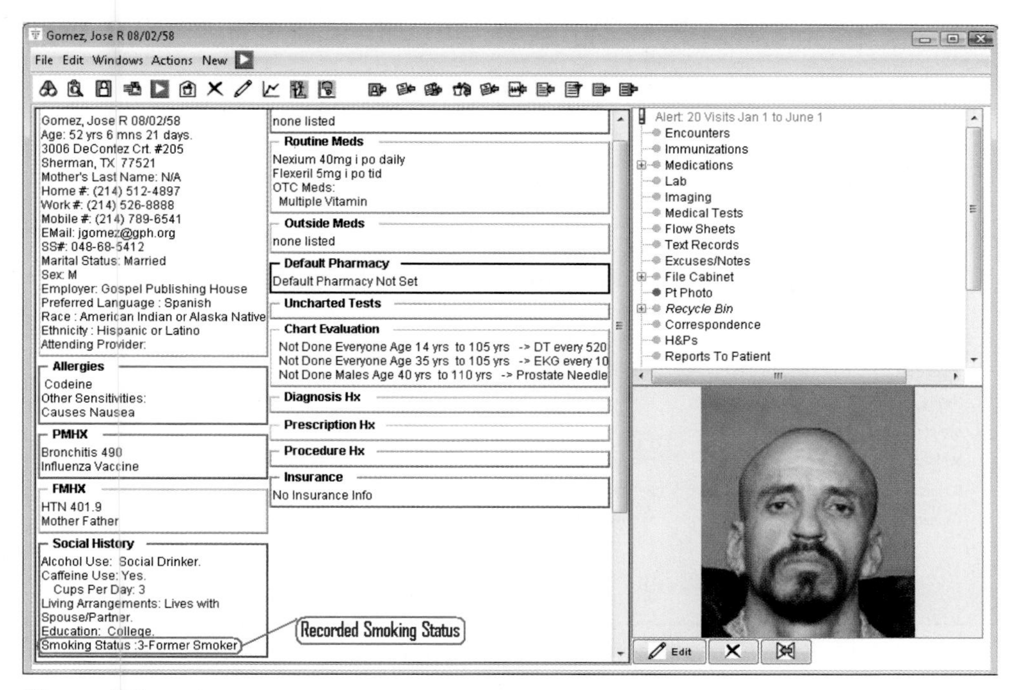

Figure 2.3 Patient's smoking status on display in electronic chart.

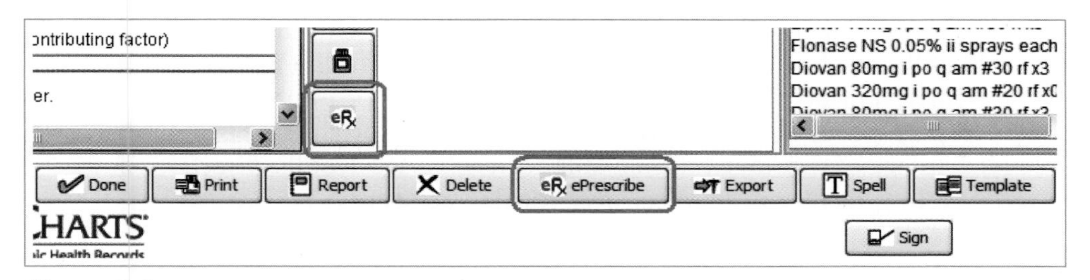

Figure 2.4 SpringScripts icon in the SpringCharts EHR program.

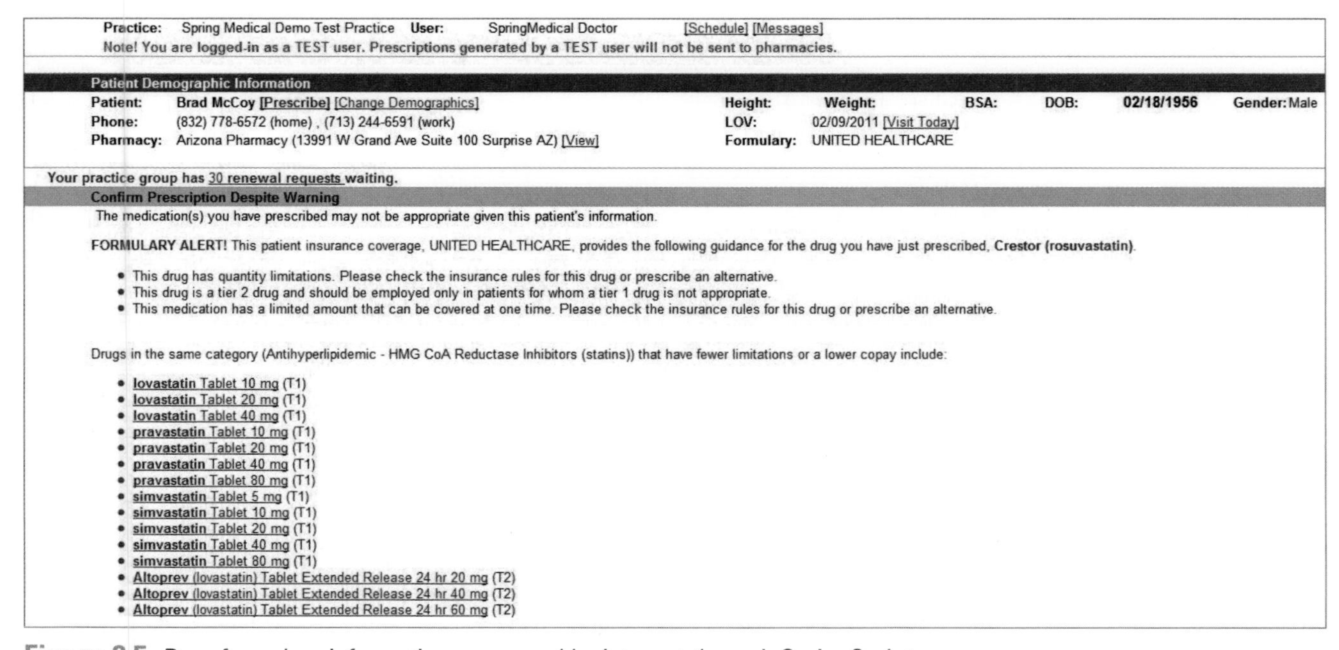

Figure 2.5 Drug formulary information, accessed by Internet through SpringScripts.

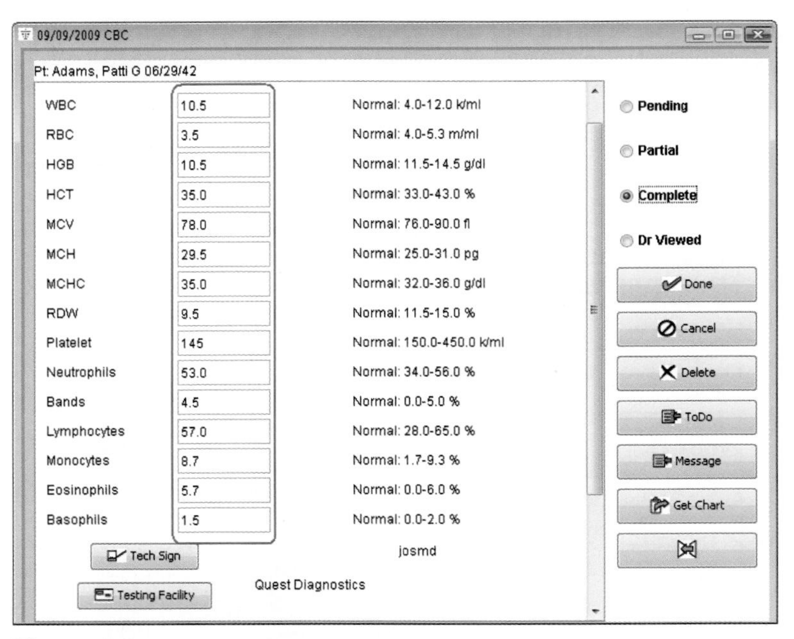

Figure 2.6 Manually entered lab results in an EHR program.

Structured data
Structured data is information that is organized in a coded manner so that it is identifiable, storable, retrievable, and analyzable in a computer system. Conversely, unstructured data is unidentifiable (e.g., free text).

Menu Measure 2. Each EP must demonstrate the ability to incorporate laboratory test results into a certified EHR as **structured data,** either manually or electronically. More than 40 percent of lab results during the reporting period should be in positive/negative or numeric format and incorporated as structured data (Figure 2.6). Through the SpringLabs HL7 interface, SpringCharts is able to receive lab results directly from the testing facility in an electronic format, as seen in Figure 2.7.

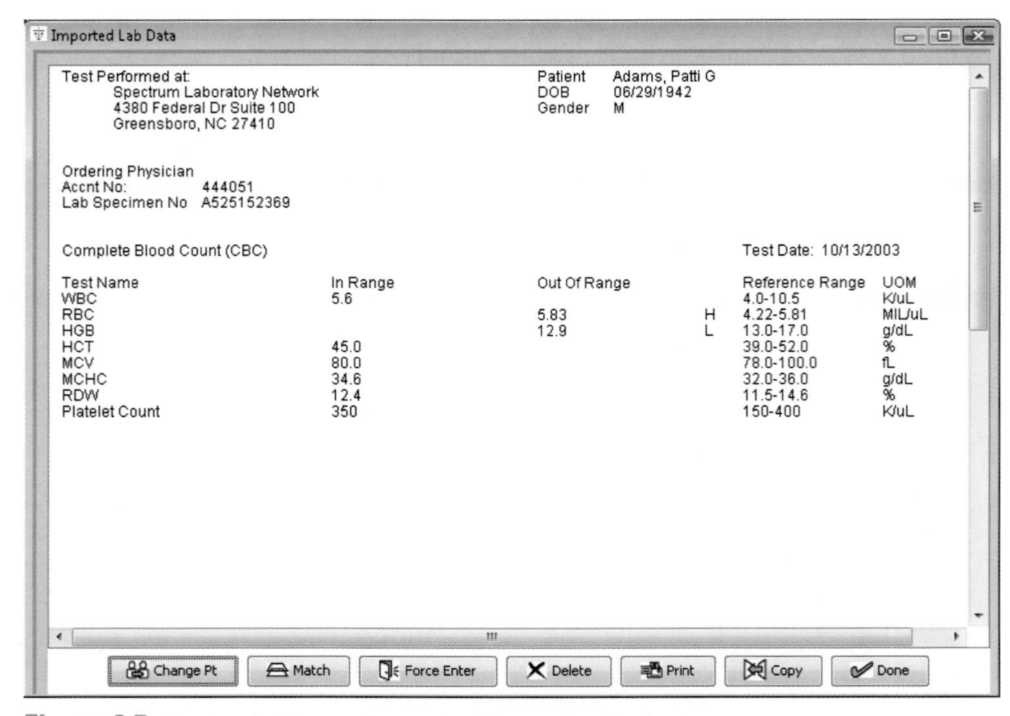

Figure 2.7 Electronic lab results received in a patient's chart.

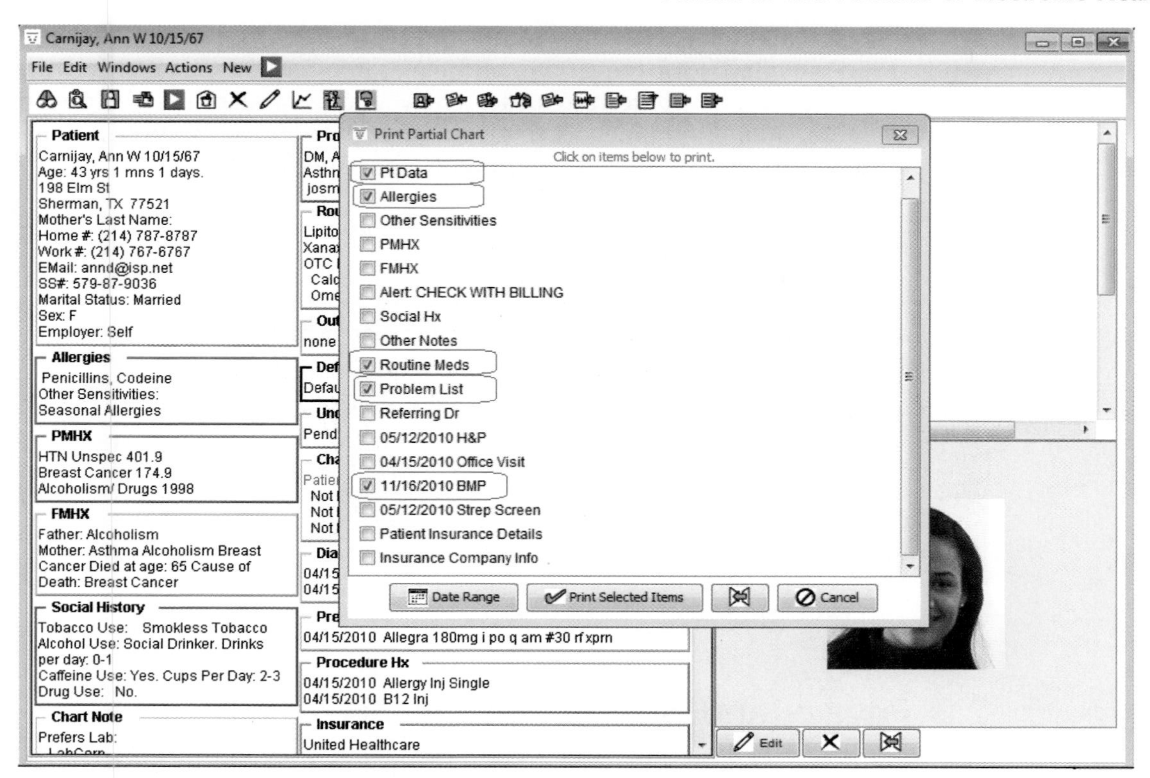

Figure 2.8 Selection of clinical data in patient's chart to create a summary of care record.

Menu Measure 3. During the 90-day reporting period of 2011 and the 12-month reporting period of 2012, EPs were required to demonstrate the ability to provide summary of care records from their certified EHR program for patients referred or transitioned to another provider, as illustrated in Figure 2.8. Clinical summaries from an EHR program must be provided for more than 50 percent of requesting patients.

Computerized Provider Order Entry (CPOE)

Computerized provider order entry (CPOE) is the means by which a physician or clinician electronically transmits instructions for a patient's treatment or the ordering of tests to a testing facility. These facilities may include pharmacies, laboratories, imaging centers, and other testing facilities responsible for fulfilling the order. CPOE is one of the core objectives that had to be met by hospitals and EPs to qualify for stage 1 MU in either 2011 or 2012.

Computerized provider order entry (CPOE)
The CPOE is the process of communicating a clinician's instructions for patient treatment over a computer network to departments within a hospital or testing facilities outside the patient setting.

The benefits of the CPOE function in EHRs include more expedient order completion, reduction in errors related to handwriting, and the opportunity to check for duplicate or incorrect tests. In the past, physicians have traditionally handwritten or verbally communicated orders for patient care. Manual order entry, nonstandard abbreviations, and poor legibility have led to errors and injuries to patients. Studies of CPOE indicate the medication prescription error rate can be reduced by 80 percent and other errors that can harm patients, by 55 percent.[6] ONC-ATCB certification requires that EHR programs have automatic alerts in their e-prescribing modules, warning practitioners of high medication dosages, dangerous drug combinations, and other potentially dangerous issues.

Despite the many years it has taken to create interoperability, develop national HIT standards for the CPOE, and overcome the resistance to change in clinical practices, computerized order entry is now a standard feature in certified EHRs, allowing clinicians to electronically order medications, imaging tests, lab work, nurse actions, diets, and other specialty requests.

Concept Checkup 2.2

A. What was the purpose of the EHR certification program that the HITECH Act authorized the ONC to establish?

B. Provide the term that each of these acronyms stands for.

1. MU
2. ATCB
3. CPOE

2.3 Privacy and Security of the EHR

Protected health information (PHI) Regulated under HIPAA, PHI includes any information (past, present, or future) about health status, provision of healthcare (including mental health), and payment for healthcare that can be linked to a specific individual.

Health information technology and the universal availability of the Internet have changed the way personal health information is collected, stored, and transmitted. Personal computers have replaced typewriters, e-mail and messaging have replaced memos and phone calls, and digital media have replaced the postal system. To ensure the security of **protected health information (PHI)** and protect doctor–patient confidentiality, all healthcare entities must safeguard computer systems and protect PHI from misuse. Computer hardware, EHR software, and healthcare data are at risk for damage and theft from events as simple as power surges, to computer viruses, to identification theft crimes via the Internet. Various government agencies and private healthcare entities have brought these concerns to Congress, which has passed laws to regulate security and privacy in the EHR industry.

USA PATRIOT Act and Homeland Security

The USA PATRIOT Act of 2001 (commonly known as the "Patriot Act") was signed into law in 2001 and stands for Uniting and Strengthening America by Providing Appropriate Tools Required to Intercept and Obstruct Terrorism. The act enhances the ability of law enforcement agencies to access and search e-mail communication, telephone, medical, financial, and other records, and eases restrictions on foreign intelligence gathering within the United States.[7] The Patriot Act is designed to deter and punish terrorist acts in the United States and world wide and improve law enforcement investigatory tools, including monitoring and collecting private information. The federal government may access medical records under the Patriot Act to protect against international and intelligence activities. In this case, a patient does not need to be notified of access or informed about specific sharing of healthcare information.

Although the Patriot Act allows for the disclosure of PHI in relationship to terrorism, HIPAA also provides for circumstances under which medical information may be disclosed for law enforcement purposes without explicitly requiring a warrant. These circumstances include:

- Law enforcement requests for information to identify or locate a suspect, fugitive, witness, or missing person
- Situations in which a crime was committed on the premises of the covered entity
- Medical emergencies connected with a crime

Issues related to national security and PHI can surface when considering acts of bioterrorism. EHR reporting capabilities enable practitioners and hospitals to track the spread of diseases and outbreaks of illness caused by contaminated foods and exposure to hazardous materials. Early determination of intentional and unintentional infections enables authorities to detect sources and contain their effects.

HIPAA and Privacy/Security

In April 2003, healthcare organizations became responsible for adherence to HIPAA regulations to protect the privacy of electronic protected health information (ePHI) in electronic health record programs. All healthcare members, covered entities (CEs), business associates (BAs), and computer systems became fully subject to all aspects of the HIPAA Security Final Rule, which gives greater control to patients over their care, provides patient education on privacy protection, ensures patient access to personal records, guarantees patient consent prior to release of medical information, and provides recourse if privacy violations occur.[8] Multiple and complex HIPAA regulations affect the patient's PHI and many areas of the healthcare industry. HIPAA's core regulations for the EHR industry address password management; unique user identification; access authorization; accounting of PHI disclosures; auditing abilities; code sets; data backup, storage, and security.

Focal Point

In 2003, new regulations added to the HIPAA Act provided protection for the privacy of certain individually identifiable health data, referred to as electronic protected health information (ePHI) in EHR programs.

HIPAA/HITECH Tip

Only covered entities and business associate organizations can be charged with HIPAA violations—not the employees of these organizations.

Password Management Policies and procedures are necessary for password management. EHRs must provide clinics with the ability to create, change, and safeguard passwords for the program. Password length formats of eight or more characters with a combination of alpha, numeric, and special characters are recommended, although not required. Default passwords must be eliminated, and a password expiration period of 90 to 120 days is recommended. Log-in attempts are monitored for auditing as well.

Unique User Identification Each EHR user must be assigned a unique name and/or number for identifying and tracking user activity within the EHR program. Modifications made to patients' demographic information and medical record are audited along with the user's log-in and log-out history.

Access Authorization Electronic PHI is protected by assigning access levels to identifiable health information strata. Users must be assigned an appropriate security access level based on the minimal data necessary to perform their jobs. Therefore, individuals with specific security levels are not able to access, modify, delete, or transmit certain information. For example, a receptionist may not be able to view lab results, and the EHR tracks who does view and modify the information. Also, an EHR should be able to limit user access based on the nature of an office visit; for example, access could be restricted the document cannot be altered after the digital signature has been affixed. Many certified EHR programs have these standards built into the software in order to achieve an entirely paperless medical chart with secure electronic signatures.

Concept Checkup 2.3

A. What does the acronym PHI stand for?

B. The Patriot Act allows the federal government to access medical records under what conditions?

C. Name the seven HIPAA regulations that affected the development of features within EHRs.

2.4 EHR Implementation and Technology

As computer technology continues to rapidly develop, EHR versatility increases. Access to patient information, health alerts, warnings, drug information, and disease management has become available at the point of care to healthcare providers in a more user-friendly form.

Modes of data entry in EHRs have also progressed. Traditionally, a keyboard was the only means of data entry. However, the need for convenience, efficiency, and speed has mandated other methods of input. Voice recognition systems adapt accurately to a person's voice and speech patterns so computer software inputs data as the operator speaks. Electronic handwriting recognition has also been enhanced and is now available to EHR operators. Although voice recognition and digital handwriting software have improved greatly in operation, these forms of data entry are not commonly used by healthcare providers because they require the user to repeat the same activity each time data is needed; that is, the activity of dictation and electronic handwriting have to be replicated with each occurrence of recording healthcare information. Although dictation of healthcare notes has been widely used in the past, concerns about the privacy of PHI, in terms of it being overheard or seen by unauthorized personnel outside the medical office, has always been an issue. EHR developers have now moved toward a template-based and pick list–based form of data entry.

The use of **templates,** or large bodies of preset text, reduces the need to constantly rekey data used multiple times. EHRs use templates to easily and quickly input data into a patient's record. For example, instead of retyping a routine referral letter that applies to many patients, healthcare providers can enter template data by tapping with a stylus pen on a touch screen or clicking a mouse at a computer terminal.

Touch screens are available on devices such as laptops and **tablets,** making the EHR portable. Traditionally, a stationary computer workstation in each exam room was cost-prohibitive for independent healthcare providers, and the lack of computer availability at the point of care resulted in delayed data entry. As a result, patient information was not readily available to other providers and healthcare staff. However, in recent years the increased use of laptops, **computers on wheels (COWs), workstations on wheels (WOWs),** and **wireless connectivity** has resulted in greater mobility and lower costs.

Focal Point

Modes of data entry into the EHR include keyboard, touch screen, voice recognition dictation, electronic handwriting recognition, templates, and pick lists.

Template
A template is an electronic file with a predesigned or set format and structure. It serves as a model for letters, faxes, and reports that need to be filled in to be completed.

Tablet
A tablet is a portable, handheld computer that allows users to document directly on the screen with a stylus pen or by touch.

Computer on wheels (COW)/workstation on wheels (WOW)
A computer is placed on a mobile desk or stand so it can be moved around an office, unit, or patient room.

Wireless connectivity
Wireless connectivity is the ability to make and maintain a connection between two or more points in a telecommunications system without using "hard" wires or cables. It allows for viewing of data between computer systems and transfer of data from one computer system to another, using electromagnetic waves.

Advances in electronic security and network reliability have also promoted EHR flexibility and mobility. A **local area network (LAN)** enables multiple computers to communicate with one another, typically using a main **server** for the database, and can be customized to a healthcare facility's needs. The LAN may consist of wired connections or use a wireless network (Figure 2.9). Wireless LANs enable healthcare providers to maintain full or open access to their EHR program from anywhere within the healthcare facility.

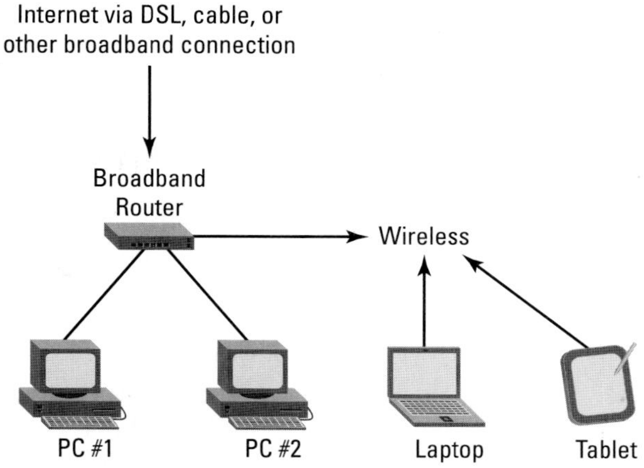

Figure 2.9 Hardwired and wireless LAN systems.

Internet and **intranet** technologies have increased the availability of healthcare databases that can be shared and accessed across large distances, giving healthcare providers access to EHRs from remote locations such as long-term care facilities, patients' homes, home offices, and hospitals. Access to these networks is restricted and data flowing on the network is encrypted for security. This configuration is ideal for home health nurses who need to access patient records stored on their healthcare agency's remote server. With the advent of portable wireless cards, data can be sent and received between a nurse's laptop and the network, providing access to the patient's record in real time via the Internet.

Another network option for healthcare facilities is the Web-based EHR offered by an **application server provider (ASP),** whereby the EHR is accessed via the Internet using high-speed (broadband) connections. In this model, the software is located on the computers of the EHR Web hosting company and is not housed on a computer server at the healthcare facility. The EHR hosting company is responsible for maintenance, updates, and backups. Some healthcare professionals' concerns about Web-based EHRs include EHR security, download and upload speeds of images and large files, and the reliability of Internet connectivity.[9]

Local area network (LAN)
A LAN is a wired and/or wireless connection of computers on a single campus or facility.

Server
A server is a main computer designed to provide services to clients, workstations, or desktop computers over a local area network or the Internet. Many network software programs have a server component and a workstation component.

Intranet
An intranet is a privately maintained computer network that provides secure accessibility to authorized people and enables sharing of software, databases, and files.

Application server provider (ASP)
An ASP enables access to an EHR via the Internet; the EHR software and database are housed and maintained by a separate company in a remote location.

Concept Checkup 2.4

A. Although there are many modes of data entry in EHRs, what two forms of data entry have emerged as the most common?

B. List two types of technologies that have increased the availability of medical databases and EHR access.

C. What does the term *ASP* mean?

2.5 Electronic Health Record Competencies

The Medical Assisting Education Review Board (MAERB) is a self-governing entity within the American Association of Medical Assistants Endowment. MAERB is responsible for medical assisting educational program reviews, accreditation recommendations, and the development and revision of the core curriculum for medical assistants as part of the Committees on Accreditation of the Commission on Accreditation of Allied Health Education Programs (CAAHEP). CAAHEP is a nonprofit allied health education organization that accredits entry-level, allied health education programs.

Learning Outcome	Key Concepts/Examples
2.3 Describe key privacy and security issues related to EHRs.—*Continued*	**HIPAA and Privacy/Security** In April 2003, healthcare organizations became responsible for adherence to HIPAA regulations to protect the privacy of patient health information in EHR programs. HIPAA's core regulations for the EHR industry are as follows: • Password management • Unique user identification • Access authorization • Accounting of PHI disclosures • Data backup, storage, and security • Auditing abilities • Code sets **Health Information Technology for Economic and Clinical Health (HITECH) Act** • This act authorized HIPAA's authority to include business associates of healthcare entities. • HIPAA's regulations and penalties were strengthened to cover these business associates. **Other Privacy Concerns** • E-mail • Electronic signatures
2.4 Explain the basic technology used in EHR implementation. **Pages 44–45**	Modes of EHR data entry include: • Keyboard • Voice recognition • Electronic handwriting • Templates • Touch screens and laptops • Computers on wheels (COWs) or workstations on wheels (WOWs) Types of network technologies include: • Local area network (LAN) • Servers and workstations • Wired connections and wireless connections • Internet and intranet • Application server providers (ASPs)
2.5 List EHR competencies identified by the Competency Model Clearinghouse. **Pages 45–46**	Due to the rapid increase in HIT in medical offices and the need for EHR-qualified clerical and clinical staff, competencies and core EHR curricula are currently being developed.

chapter 2 review

Name ______________ Instructor ______________ Class ______________ Date ______________

Using Terminology

Match the terms on the left with the definitions on the right.

_____ 1. **LO 2.3** CPT codes

_____ 2. **LO 2.4** ASP

_____ 3. **LO 2.2** Drug formulary

_____ 4. **LO 2.3** Encrypting

_____ 5. **LO 2.3** ICD codes

_____ 6. **LO 2.4** LAN

_____ 7. **LO 2.3** PHI

_____ 8. **LO 2.4** Tablet

_____ 9. **LO 2.1** Telehealth services

_____ 10. **LO 2.4** Wireless connectivity

A. Databases of approved medications in drug therapy categories that include information on the preparation, safety, effectiveness, and cost of medications.

B. The international standard diagnostic classification for all medical data concerning the incidence and prevalence of disease in large populations and for other health management purposes.

C. Five-digit codes developed by the AMA and adopted by insurance carriers and managed care companies as the means to identify common medical procedures.

D. Regulated under HIPAA, these records include any information (past, present, or future) about health status and provision of healthcare (including mental health) that can be linked to a specific individual.

E. A separate company in a remote location that enables access to an EHR via the Internet; the EHR software and database are housed at the remote location.

F. A portable, handheld computing device with the ability to document directly on the screen with a stylus pen or by touch.

G. The use of electronic and communication technology to deliver medical information and services over large and small distances through a standard telephone line.

H. A wired and/or wireless connection of computers on a single campus or facility.

I. The ability to make and maintain a mobile connection between two or more points in a telecommunications system.

J. When computer data is changed from its original form to be transmitted securely, so as to be unintelligible to unauthorized parties, and then changed back into its original form for use.

Checking Your Understanding

Choose the best answer and circle the corresponding letter.

11. LO 2.1 In 2003, the IOM identified eight key capabilities that should be included in an EHR program. Which of the following is *not* one of the key capabilities?

a) Health information and patient data
b) Order entry management
c) Insurance and patient billing
d) Medical decision support

12. LO 2.4 Which of the following is *not* a mode of data entry in the EHR?

a) Voice recognition software
b) Photocopying from a paper chart
c) Keyboard
d) Templates and pick lists

13. **LO 2.4** A privately maintained computer network that provides secure access to authorized people and enables sharing of software and files is an example of:
    a) Intranet technology
    b) Internet technology
    c) Laptop technology
    d) Certified technology

14. **LO 2.1** Which organization created standards so that approximately 20 government agencies could share healthcare and health-related information?
    a) HIPAA
    b) CHI
    c) AHIMA
    d) SNOMED CT

15. **LO 2.3** Password management and access authorization are two PHI regulations that fall under the governance of:
    a) The HITECH Act
    b) The PATRIOT Act
    c) ARRA
    d) HIPAA

16. **LO 2.1** The creation of the private-sector organization CCHIT in 2004 specifically addressed:
    a) EHR costs
    b) Security issues
    c) Lack of industry standards in EHRs
    d) The appropriation of government money

17. **LO 2.3** In 2009, the HITECH Act expanded HIPAA's security and privacy requirements to include:
    a) CNAs and MAs
    b) Business associates of covered entities
    c) International terrorists
    d) Computer hackers

18. **LO 2.4** In the context of health information technology, COW is an acronym for:
    a) Computer on Wheels
    b) Certified Office Workstation
    c) Certification of Wireless-Technology
    d) Cluster of Workstations

19. **LO 2.1** HIPAA is an acronym for:
    a) Health Information Portability and Accountability Act
    b) Health Information Problems and Answers Act
    c) Health Insurance Portability and Accountability Act
    d) Health Insurance Portability and Accessibility Act

20. **LO 2.2** In terms of the MU program, EP is an acronym for:
    a) Eligible professional
    b) Eligible physician
    c) Executive producer
    d) Exclusive protection

21. **LO 2.2** MU is part of the ONC's incentive program that seeks to determine if practitioners have achieved:
    a) Maintenance units with a certified EHR program
    b) Medical units with a certified EHR program
    c) Meaningful use with a certified EHR program
    d) Management and utilization with a certified EHR program

22. **LO 2.1** In 2010, the ONC launched a two-year temporary certification program to:
    a) Pay doctors and hospitals for purchasing EHR programs.
    b) Oversee the distribution of $19.2 billion of HITECH stimulus money.
    c) Guarantee basic standards and functionality in EHR programs.
    d) Buy back CCHIT-certified EHR programs.

23. **LO 2.3** The Patriot Act allows the federal government access to private medical records to:
    a) Oppose the ACLU.
    b) Create surveillance reports.
    c) Protect against international terrorists' activities.
    d) Protect PHI.

24. **LO 2.2** CPOE is a process of communicating a clinician's instructions over a computer network for:
    a) Computerized prescription order entry
    b) Electronic orders of patient tests, medications, and procedures
    c) Calibrated provider office EHR equipment
    d) The center for physician-owned EHR

25. **LO 2.5** Competency training and evaluation addresses a healthcare professional's ability to:
    a) Perform a certain job proficiently.
    b) Obtain a meaningful job in the medical industry.
    c) Achieve a superior-paying profession.
    d) Demonstrate advanced aptitude.

Applying Your Knowledge

Use your critical-thinking skills to answer the following questions.

26. **LO 2.1** The nonprofit, private organization known as CCHIT was established in 2004 for the purpose of accelerating the adoption of EHR programs by creating an EHR product certification program. The certification program increased industry confidence that uniform standards in EHR programs were being met. Why do you think the ONC needed to launch its own EHR certification program in 2010?

27. **LO 2.3** Why do you think there may be conflict between the legislation of the USA PATRIOT Act and the philosophy of certain private organizations whose purpose is to defend and preserve individual rights and liberties?

28. **LO 2.2** Why do you think eligible professionals (EPs) must implement and utilize an ONC-certified EHR program, rather than a non-certified program, to qualify for MU and obtain incentive money through the HITECH Act?

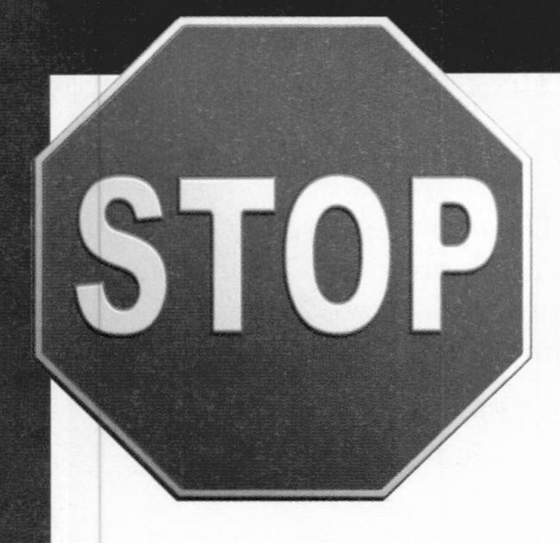

For the remainder of *Electronic Health Records,* you will work in the SpringCharts EHR program. Before you proceed, read these important tips! You need to make sure the EHR software and related files are loaded on your computer.

Step A. Is SpringCharts EHR Installed on My Computer?

SpringCharts has two different versions: the single-user version and the network version. You will be working on one or the other (if you are unsure, check with your instructor). The single-user version is downloaded from the *Electronic Health Records* Online Learning Center (OLC), **www.mhhe.com/hamiltonehr3e,** and then installed on your individual computer or onto a flash drive. The network version is sent directly to your school's IT department so it can be installed on multiple computers and shared across the network.

When either the single-user version or the network version of SpringCharts is installed, it places an icon on your desktop to provide easy access to the program (Figure S.1).

Figure S.1 SpringCharts desktop icon.

Check to see if you have this icon on your desktop. If it is not there, check with your instructor about downloading the software; you will need to follow the directions contained in the *Guide to Success with SpringCharts* at www.mhhe.com/hamiltonehr3e. You will not be able to complete the exercises in the rest of the chapters without the SpringCharts program.

Step B. Is the EHR Materials Folder Installed on My Computer?

You will need to import several files into your SpringCharts program to complete some exercises in this text. These files are contained in the folder titled *EHR Material* on the OLC (www.mhhe.com/hamiltonehr3e). Whether you are using the SpringCharts single-user version or network version, the folder should be downloaded to your desktop.

Check to see if you have the *EHR Material* on your desktop. If the folder is not on your desktop, please check with your instructor to ensure it has been downloaded. If it has not been downloaded and installed on your computer, please follow the instructions in the *Guide to Success with SpringCharts.*

Step C. How Do I Launch SpringCharts EHR?

When SpringCharts was installed on your computer or your flash drive, a shortcut icon to the SpringCharts program was placed on your desktop.

- Double-click on the SpringCharts icon to open the program. You *may* receive a Windows Security Alert screen (Figure S.2); it is designed to protect your computer system. Please click the [Unblock] button to continue. You only have to do this the first time you launch the SpringCharts EHR program.

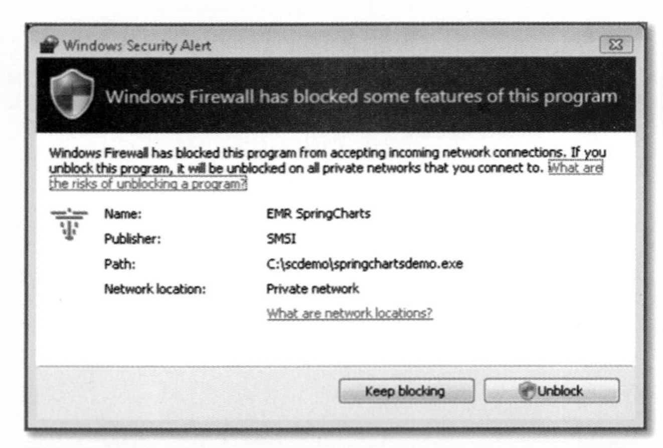

Figure S.2 Windows' firewall security activation window.

- A *Log On* window appears (Figure S.3). On the single-user version of SpringCharts the user name and password are hardcoded in, so you do not need to enter them. Select the [Log on] button to open the SpringCharts program. On the network version of SpringCharts the user name and password are *not* hardcoded in. You will need to request a log-in name and password from your instructor.

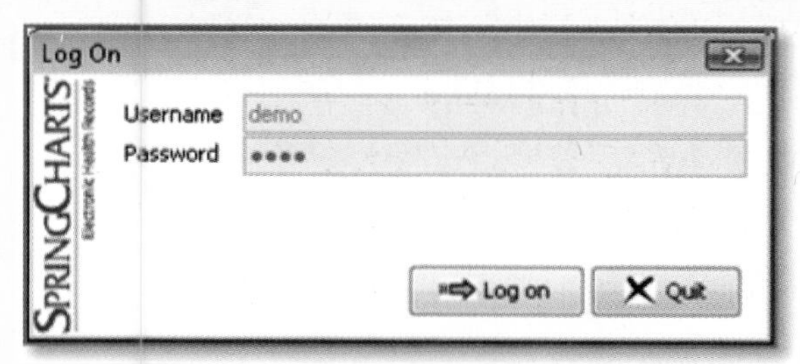

Figure S.3 SpringCharts *Log On* window.

- The single-user version of SpringCharts program opens and automatically places two patients on the *Office Calendar* and two patients in the *Patient Tracker* (Figure S.4). A small tutorial window displays in the center. This tutorial window appears every time you log in to this version of SpringCharts. Simply close this window by clicking on the red [X] in the upper right corner. The network version of SpringCharts does not automatically place patients on the schedule. You will be instructed how to add patients to the scheduler.

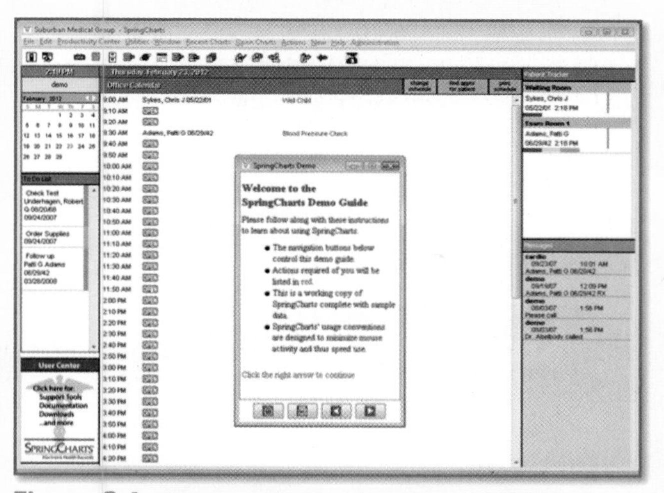

Figure S.4 Opening screen of SpringCharts EHR.

Congratulations! You have successfully launched SpringCharts EHR.

Check to be sure you have the correct version of SpringCharts. This may not be the first time your school has used the SpringCharts program. It is worthwhile to ensure you have accessed the correct version of SpringCharts.

- In the opening screen of SpringCharts, click on the *Help* menu and select the *About SpringCharts* option (Figure S.5).

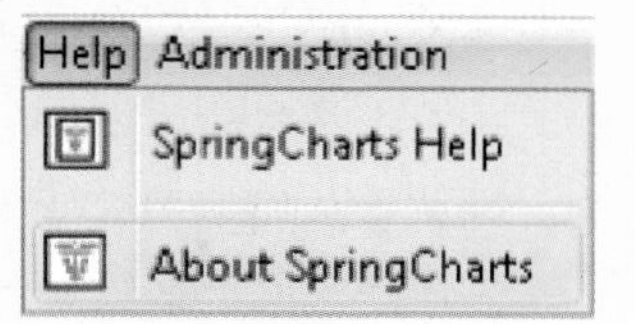

Figure S.5 Accessing *About SpringCharts.*

- In the *Program Information* window you can find the version of SpringCharts you have launched (Figure S.6). The correct version for this text is *2011 R 1.0.10*. If your screen displays a different version number, contact your instructor. You need the correct version to complete the exercises.

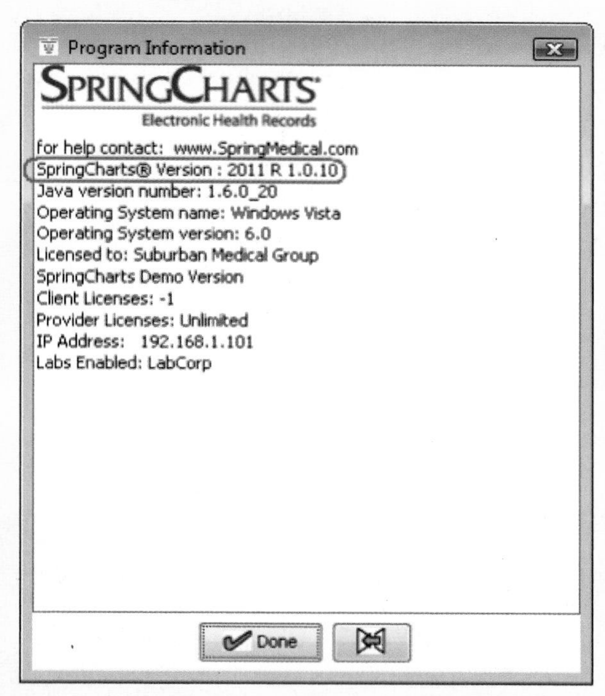

Figure S.6 *Program Information* window.

- Close the *Program Information* window by clicking the [Done] button. Close SpringCharts by clicking the *File* menu and selecting the *Quit* submenu. Answer *Yes* to the enquiry *Shut down SpringCharts?* Click the [No] button in the *Backup Recommended* window if you are using the single-user version of the program.

Congratulations! You are ready to begin your SpringCharts EHR adventure.

3

Introduction and Setup

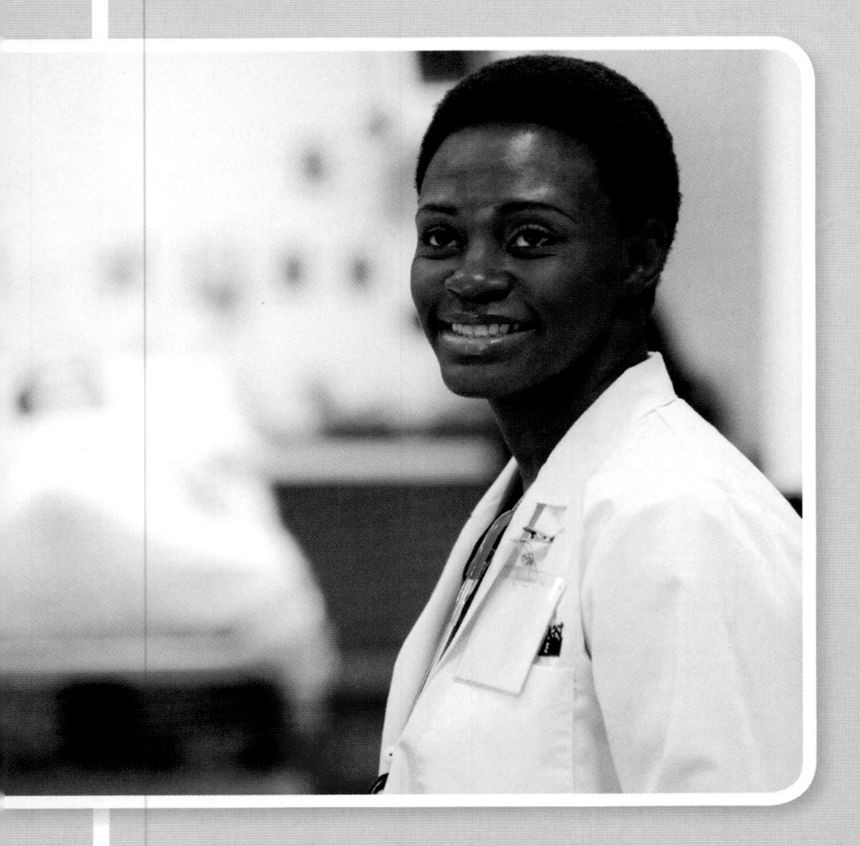

Learning Outcomes

After completing Chapter 3, you will be able to:

LO 3.1 Provide a brief history of SpringCharts EHR software and list three clinical and three administrative tools that it offers.

LO 3.2 Set up user preferences.

LO 3.3 Set up, edit, and print addresses in the physician, employee, pharmacy, and testing facility categories.

LO 3.4 Set up new patients, edit patient information, and export patient lists.

LO 3.5 Set up new insurance companies and edit existing insurance company information.

What You Need to Know

To understand Chapter 3, you will need to know:

- The concepts and processes of using paper charts and EHRs
- The development history of the EHR
- The standards history governing the functionality and use of EHRs
- How to download, install, and log on to SpringCharts EHR

Key Terms

Attending physician
Demographics
End-to-end solution
Graphical user interface (GUI)
Imperial units
Metric units
Office Visit (OV)
Primary insurance
Secondary insurance
User preferences

Introduction

This textbook teaches the knowledge and skills necessary to achieve EHR competency using SpringCharts EHR software. Although the specific layouts, access, and storage methods vary among different EHRs, the overall key functions and capabilities of ONC-certified EHR programs are the same. Beginning with this chapter, you will apply the theoretical knowledge learned in the first two chapters of the text to hands-on exercises covering a wide range of EHR features. The skills you'll develop by doing so will allow you to successfully enter the healthcare community with a comprehensive working knowledge and experience of EHRs.

3.1 The Story of SpringCharts EHR Software and Its Features

The ONC-ATCB certified SpringCharts EHR software was selected as the training tool for this textbook because of its ease of use, rich features, and ability to be customized to suit a wide range of medical specialties. SpringCharts is an international program used by more than 1,000 physicians in more than 65 different healthcare specialties. Although we have chosen SpringCharts as the tool to teach EHR functionality and skills, the text goes beyond a simple guide of the SpringCharts system; it provides education in both fundamental and advanced EHR features, moving from simple to complex skill sets. Mastery of these skills will allow students to transfer knowledge and experience from one EHR system to another.

Development of SpringCharts

SpringCharts EHR software was designed by practicing physicians and technology executives whose goal was to introduce easy-to-use, functional technology to practitioners who remained dependent on paper charting systems and traditional clinical workflow processes. The program is largely focused on streamlining communications and documentation, while improving workflow in both the administrative and clinical practice areas. SpringCharts EHR was developed and implemented over a period of 12 years to provide physicians, clinicians, and clerical staff with a powerful and intuitive software solution for both the healthcare and administrative sides of an office. The program manages all *nonfinancial* activities of a medical practice. It electronically links with practice management software (PMS) systems to create an **end-to-end solution** for medical offices that combines medical records and financial management of claims and statements.

End-to-end solution
This software industry term suggests that the vendor of an application program can provide all the hardware and software components to meet the client's requirement and that no other supplier need be involved.

SpringCharts provides instant access to more than 90 percent of the program's key functions through three main screens: the *Practice View*, *Patient Chart* and *Office Visit* screens, seen in Figures 3.1, 3.2, and 3.3, respectively. From these three windows, practitioners and clinical and clerical staff can perform charting and office procedures with flexibility, efficiency, and accuracy. Table 3.1 provides a sample list of functions that can be performed in these three windows.

SpringCharts EHR makes available one-click links to many powerful medical, pharmaceutical, and utility websites that provide integrated access to databases and services such as drug formularies (i.e., listings of pharmaceutical substances and formulas for making medicinal preparations), dosage information, patient education instructions, and the electronic reception of lab results.

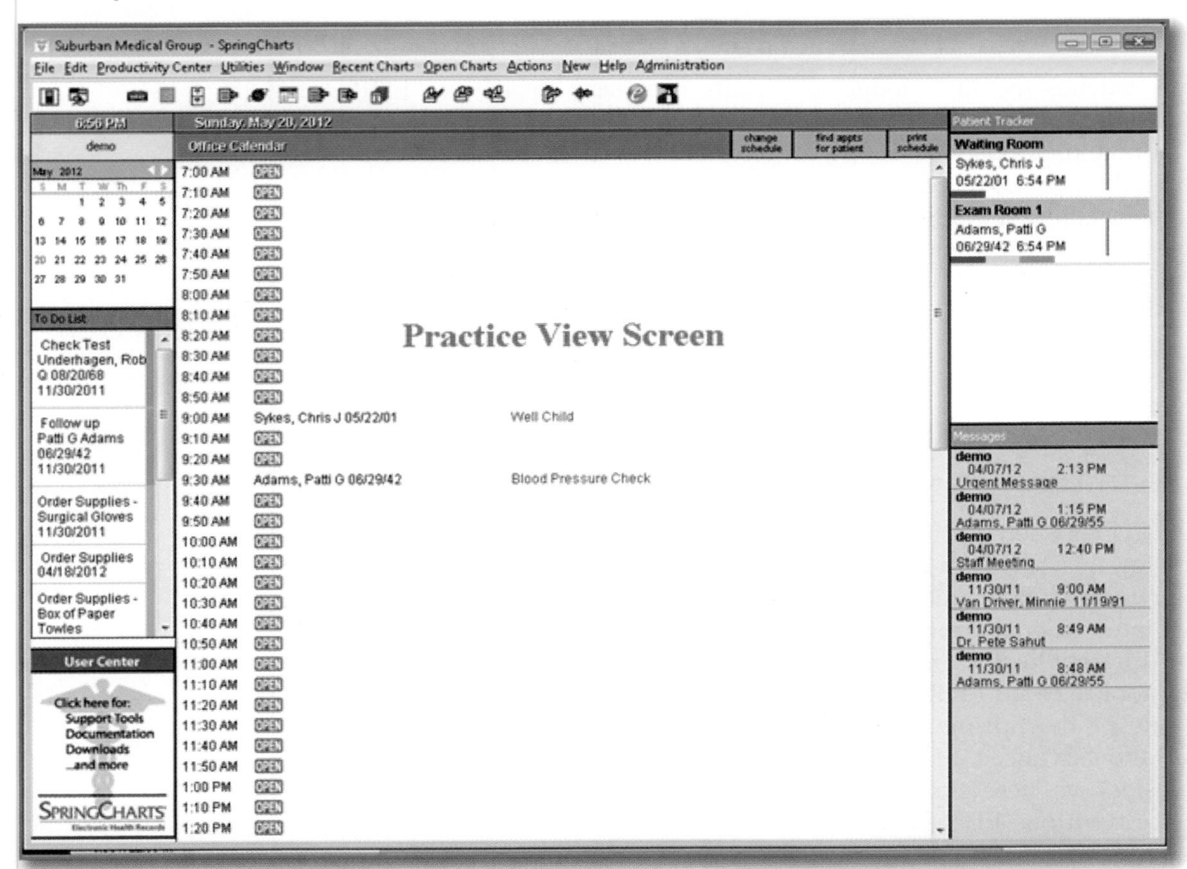

Figure 3.1 *Practice View* window.

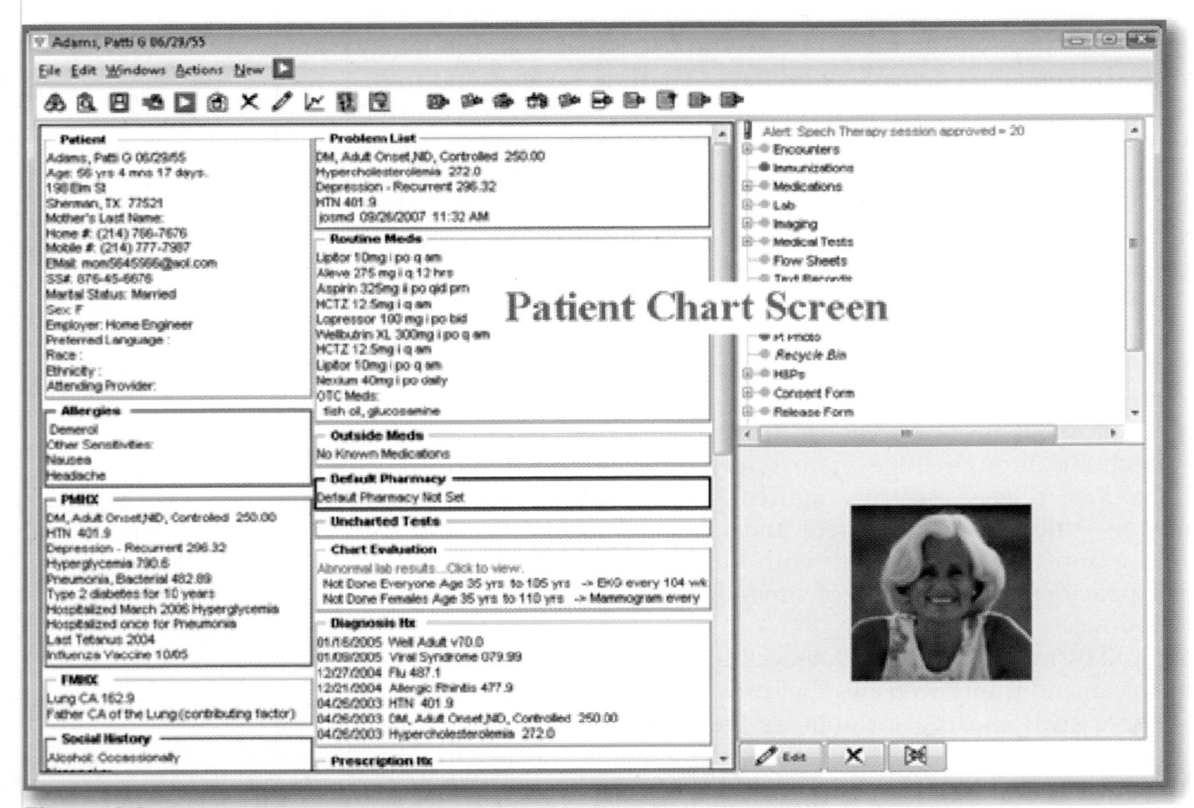

Figure 3.2 *Patient Chart* window.

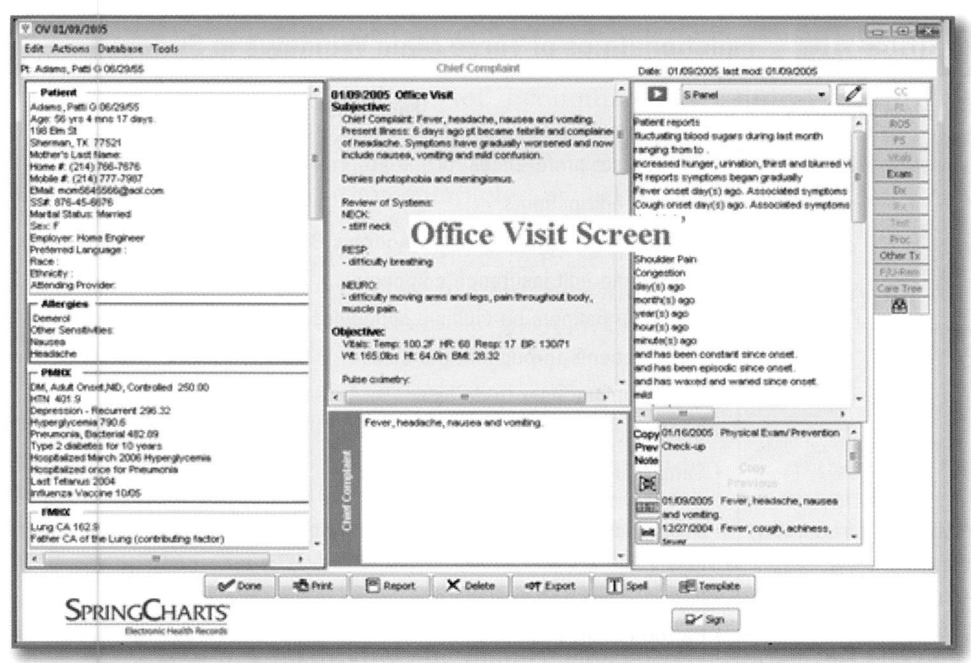

Figure 3.3 *Office Visit* window.

Clinical Tools

Among many other features, SpringCharts combines clinical tools to enhance patient care, including:

- Template-based office visit notes
- A chart evaluation manager for proactive patient healthcare maintenance
- An evaluation and management (E&M) coder for automatic and accurate E&M coding
- Plan-of-care practice guidelines
- Real-time e-prescribing
- Drug and allergy interaction alerts

Administrative Tools

SpringCharts's clerical tools are designed to speed and streamline office communication and documentation, including:

- Integrated patient tracking
- Integrated e-mail
- Messaging
- Reminders
- Employee time clock
- Electronic bulletin board
- Template-based letters and order forms

Certification and Meaningful Use Criteria

In 2007, SpringCharts was certified by the Certification Commission for Health Information Technology (CCHIT) for ambulatory EHRs. The

User preferences
User preferences are choices a user makes in software programs to preset elements—such as default practice name, physician name, and schedule—to be displayed when that user logs in to the program.

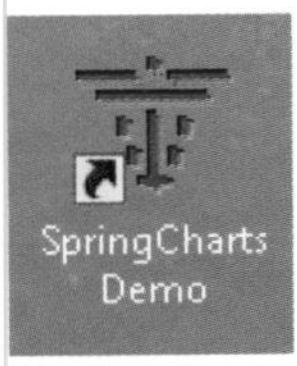

SpringCharts desktop icon

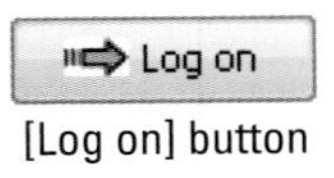

[Log on] button

Graphical user interface (GUI)
A GUI is a software program screen that can display icons, subwindows, text fields, and menus designed to standardize and simplify use of the computer program, by allowing a user to type in fields and use a mouse to manipulate text and images.

SpringCharts Tip

Activating the SpringCharts icon on the desktop is the only time you will need to double-click while using SpringCharts. Once you open the program, all functions are activated by a single mouse click.

SpringCharts Tip

Typically, a user will enter his or her unique user name and password in the *Log On* window. However, in the single-user version of SpringCharts, the user name and password are already embedded or fixed.

3.2 User Preferences

SpringCharts enables the user to set up **user preferences**, which determine the default **graphical user interface** (GUI—pronounced *goo-eee*) for several key areas in the program, specific to each user. Once these preferences are selected, SpringCharts adjusts these features for the specific user at each log-in to the program. The following steps will guide you through launching SpringCharts EHR and follow along as we discuss the features of an ONC-certified EHR program. (If you have not yet downloaded the EHR program, please follow the directions on pages xiii–xiv in the preface of this text.)

1. Double-click on the SpringCharts icon on your desktop (shown in margin).
2. When the *Log On* window displays, click on the [Log on] button (shown in margin). SpringCharts will launch and you will see a smaller demo tutorial screen.
3. You can close out of the *SpringCharts Demo* tutorial window by clicking on the [X] button in the upper right corner, as seen in Figure 3.4.

The SpringCharts program has three main work screens: *Practice View, Patient Chart,* and *Office Visit* windows. When you launch the EHR program, you will arrive at the *Practice View* screen (Figure 3.5).

Preferences 1

To set user preferences, access the main menu at the top of the screen and select *File > Preferences > User Preferences*. The *Set User Preferences* window will appear (Figure 3.6). At this point, you are working within the *Preferences 1* tab.

In the *Set User Preferences* window, users can set up the following default names and other program elements by simply clicking on the appropriate choice in the drop-down menu or on the appropriate radio button.

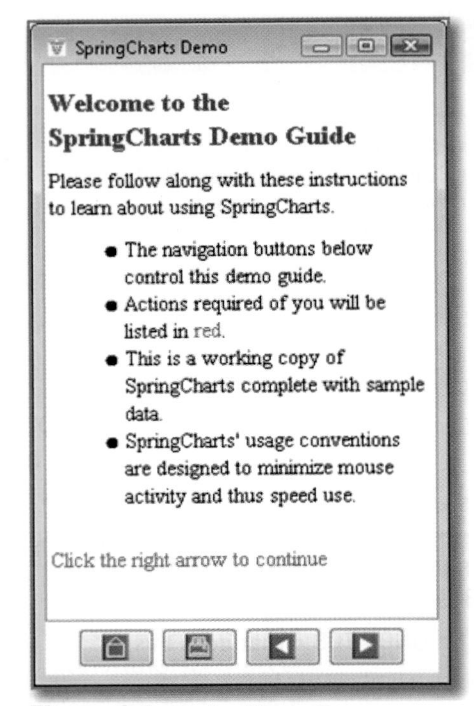

Figure 3.4 *SpringCharts Demo* tutorial window.

Your Provider. The selection in this field will determine the doctor's name that will appear as the default name on reports and letters the user sends from the EHR program. The list of doctors' names is based on the providers who are set up as doctors in the administration panel of the SpringCharts server when a medical office adopts and customizes the program. Remember, you are in a "user preference" area of the EHR program. The choices a user makes in the section will only affect how the program functions for that particular user.

Your Practice. The practice name selected here will be the default name that will appear on the letterhead of all correspondence, reports, orders, notes, and prescriptions this user sends from the system. Although

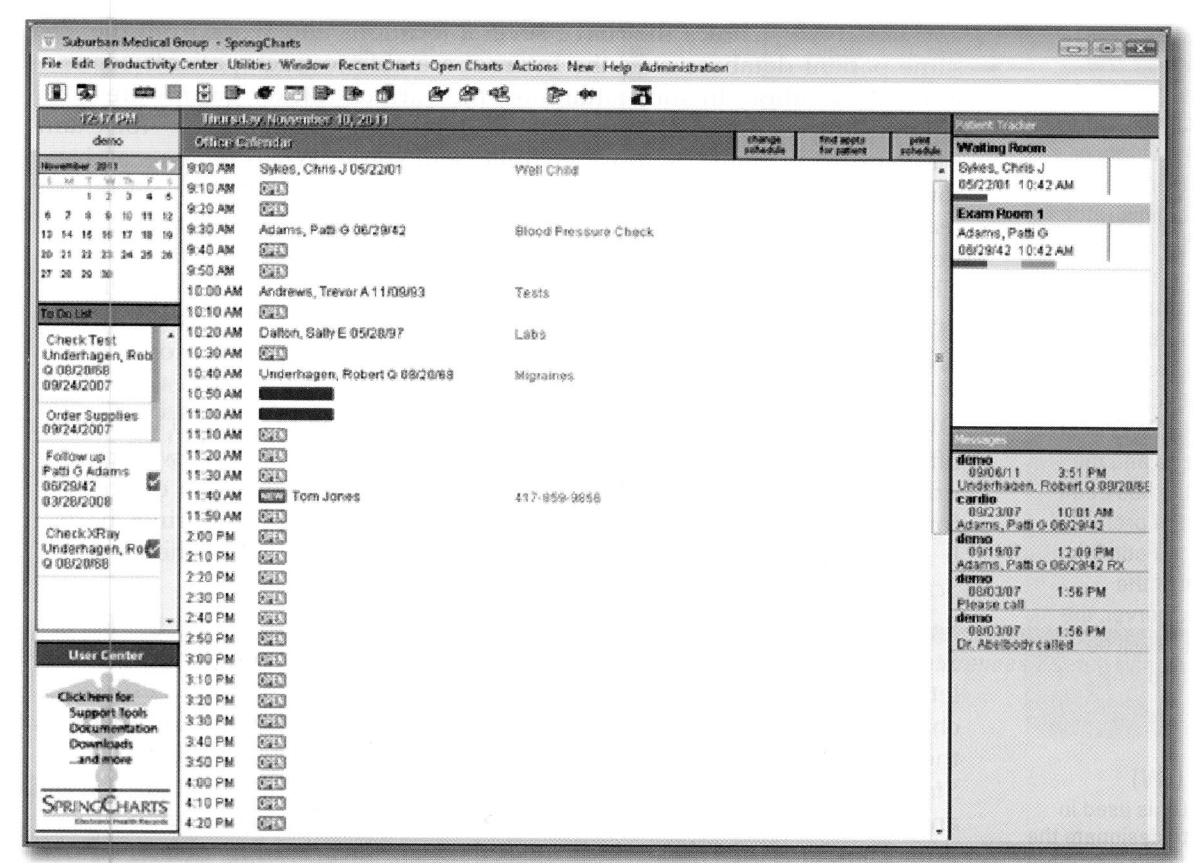

Figure 3.5 Typical *Practice View* screen after log-in.

the provider and practice names are selected here as the default, they can be changed within the program at the time various letters and reports are created. A clinic may have several practice sites in various locations, all accessing the same SpringCharts database via the Internet. This setup allows each practice unlimited access to any patient medical record regardless of location. The ability to select a specific practice name means each user will have the appropriate letterhead for his or her location. The practices' names and addresses are set up in the administration panel of the SpringCharts server.

Appt Schedule. Appointment schedules can be set up in SpringCharts for several different providers and therapy resources within the practice (for example, several providers' schedules and an in-house physical therapist's schedule). Here, users will use the drop-down menu to select which schedule they want to see by default as their main appointment screen. Although one schedule will be viewed on the main screen, the other schedules also can be viewed within SpringCharts.

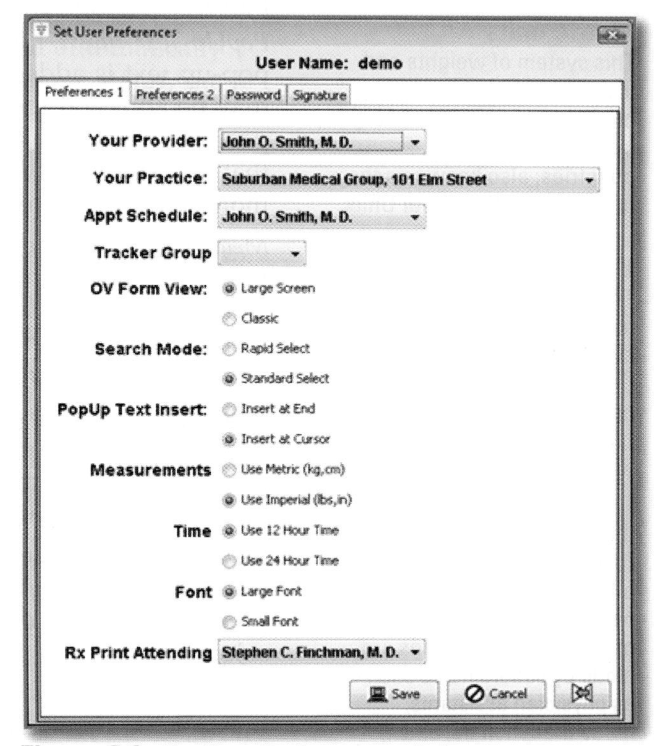

Figure 3.6 *Set User Preferences* window.

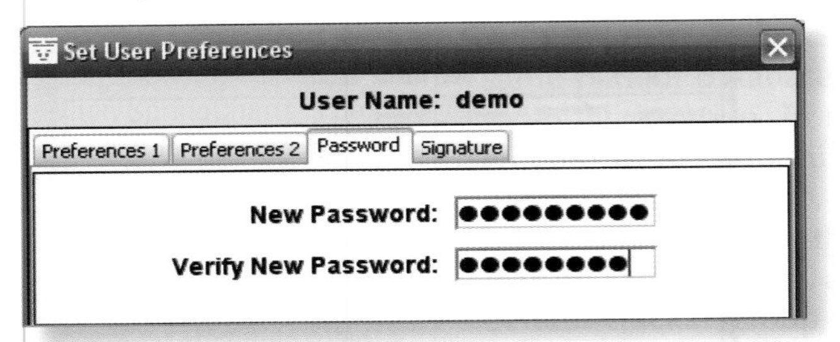

Figure 3.9 *Password* change tab.

the screen so that the office visit note is not covered by his or her hand, whereas a left-handed user will likely prefer these panels on the left. Once the preference has been chosen, the user clicks on the [Save] button.

Password

The third tab at the top of the *Set User Preferences* window is the *Password* tab (Figure 3.9).

When a medical office or other entity adopts SpringCharts EHR, user passwords are initially created on the SpringCharts server when the user profile is set up. After that, users may change their passwords in this window. The user would simply add a new password, verify it by retyping it, and click the [Change Password] button.

When SpringCharts EHR is initially installed at an office, the server administrator chooses between the *Low Security* and *High Security* options. Passwords may be changed as often as needed when *Low Security* has been selected. When *High Security* has been enabled on the server, the program enforces rigorous password rules, including requiring users to reset passwords every 2 months. Some of the security elements of password management include:

- Encrypted passwords that are obscured from the user's view
- Automatic password reset every 60 days; users are prohibited from logging on until the password is changed
- Password length of 8 to 16 characters
- Case-sensitive passwords
- Password guidelines that require at least one number, one character, and one special character (!@#$%&*)
- Strikeout password protection: users get a preset number of attempts before the program closes; the number of allowed unsuccessful attempts to log in is set on the SpringCharts server
- All user log-ins and log-outs are recorded in the audit manager

Signature

The fourth tab at the top of the *Set User Preferences* window is the *Signature* tab. Here, SpringCharts allows importing of the user's digital signature, which can then be used in various places throughout the program to stamp the user's real signature on letters, reports, prescriptions, and so on. There are three options available to set up a signature:

1. Create a handwritten signature, scan the image, and save it on the computer. Select the [Import] button (Figure 3.10) from the *Signature* tab to navigate to the file and import it into the *Signature* window.

Import
Export
Save
Clear
Enter Digital Signature for demo. Signature size is 2.3 " x 3/4"

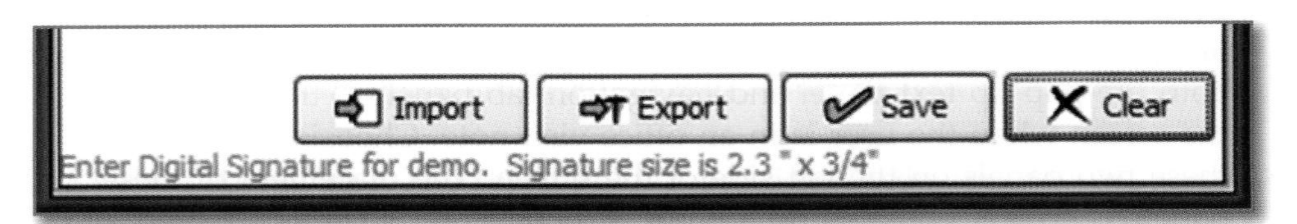

Figure 3.10 Digital signature [Import] button.

2. Using the stylus pen on a tablet or iPad, create the digital signature directly in the signature field at the top of the *Signature* window.
3. Create a signature in the field by signing an electronic signature pad connected to the computer via the USB port.

After the signature has been imported or otherwise placed in SpringCharts, the user selects the [Save] button, also seen in Figure 3.10. To save all the preferences, the user returns to the *Preferences 1* tab and saves all changes to the *Set User Preferences* window by clicking on the [Save] button.

If you have had SpringCharts open while going through the preceding material, the following steps will guide you through logging out of the EHR program:

1. Click the Log Off speed icon to log out of the program (shown in margin).
2. Answer [Yes] to confirm that you are exiting.
3. Click the [Quit] button in the *Log On* window, then the [Yes] button to confirm you are quitting the program.

SpringCharts Tip

Shortcut:

Log Off SpringCharts

The first speed icon located on the Toolbar enables the user to speedily log out of the EHR program without having to go through the drop-down menus.

Concept Checkup 3.2

A. Which two options in the *Set User Preferences* window does the user select that will be defaulted onto reports and letters?

B. What is the purpose of selecting a provider in the *Rx Print Attending* field?

C. When the *High Security* feature is activated, how often are users required to change their passwords?

Exercise 3.1 Setting Your User Preferences

1. Double-click on the SpringCharts icon on your desktop.
2. When the *Log On* window displays, click on the [Log on] button.
3. Close out of the small central *SpringCharts Demo* tutorial window by clicking on the [X] in the upper right corner.
4. Clink on the *Edit User Preferences* speed icon on the Toolbar (shown in margin). At this point, you are in the *Preferences 1* tab of the *Set User Preferences* window. Based on the items shown in Figure 3.6, set your preferences for the following:
   - Your Provider
   - Your Practice
   - Appt Schedule
   - Tracker Group
   - OV Form View
   - Search Mode
   - PopUp Text Insert
   - Measurements
   - Time
   - Font
   - Rx Print Attending

Note: Only change preferences under the *Preferences 1* tab. Do not change information under the *Preferences 2, Password,* or *Signature* tabs.

5. Click the [Save] button.

SpringCharts Tip

Shortcut:

Edit User Preferences

The second speed icon on the Toolbar enables the user to access the user preferences setup window without having to go through the drop-down menu items.

SpringCharts Tip

Patients are not added to the address book in SpringCharts because they have their own database, which is accessed via the *New Patient* window under the *New* menu of the *Practice View* screen.

SpringCharts Tip

The EHR program will default to the city, state, and area code of the healthcare practice when supplying information for these same fields in the address window.

SpringCharts Tip

When entering a company name that has multiple locations in the *Company* field, users need to add some defining information (such as location) in that same field (e.g., "Pharmacy Walgreens—Republic Road." This extra information helps distinguish the different companies in the *Address* search window (Figure 3.13).

3.3 Address Data Setup

In this section, you will learn how to add new addresses to the program and edit addresses that exist in the electronic Address Book.

New Address

New addresses are added to SpringCharts through the *New* menu option in the main *Practice View* window. Name and addresses of entities such as pharmacies, testing facilities, referring physicians, and vendors can be entered in the *New Address* window that appears (Figure 3.11). The address book can be accessed from various locations throughout SpringCharts.

Two fields must be completed to successfully add a new address to the database: 1) *Last Name* or *Company*, and, 2) the *Category* fields (shown in red font). Without these two items, the system will not allow the user to save the new entry. If users are adding information for a "nonperson," such as a company, data entry can begin on the *Company* line rather than the *First Name* field. If recording information for an individual, a user must at least complete the *Last Name* field; the *Company* field then is optional. The required *Category* field displays a drop-down list of preset options. This list of categories is set up on SpringCharts server by an administrator in the *Category Preferences* feature under the *Addresses* tab (Figure 3.12). By assigning a category to each address entry, SpringCharts can display groups of specific addresses throughout the program. For example, in the *Pending Tests* area of the program under the main *Edit* menu, the [Testing Facility] button will only display those facilities that have been assigned the classification of *TestingFacility* in the address setup window. Both the *Category* and *Specialty* fields in the *New Address* window are populated from lists set up on the SpringCharts server. If an additional item is needed on these lists, the administrator can add these line entries on the SpringCharts server in the

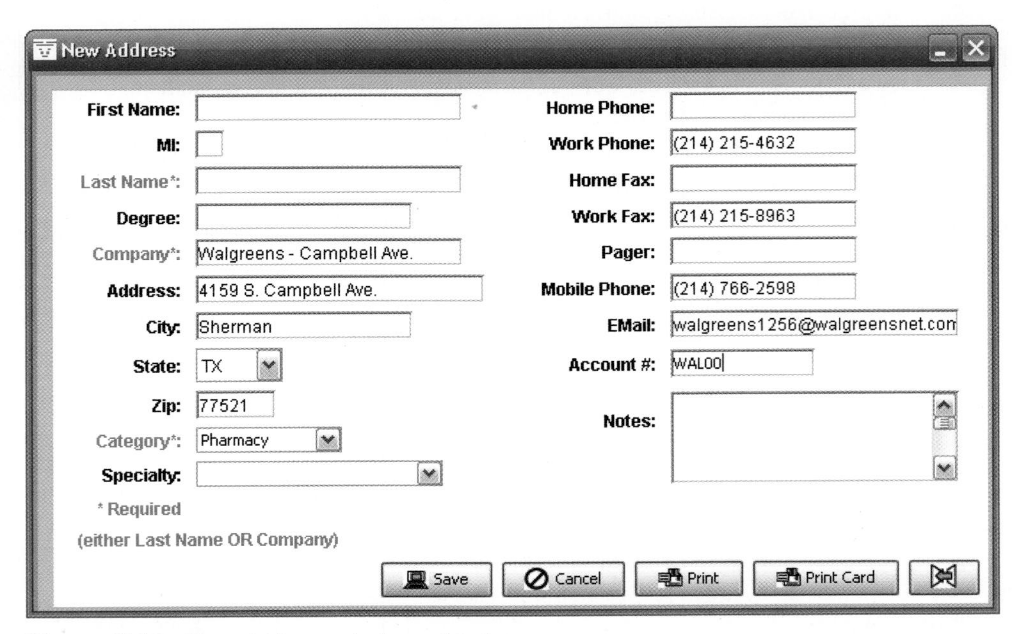

Figure 3.11 *New Address* window with data.

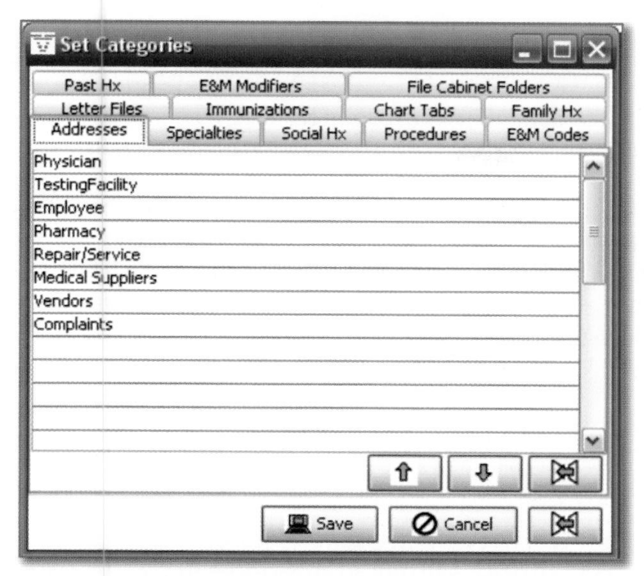

Figure 3.12 The *Addresses* tab of the *Set Categories* window on the SpringCharts server (also note the *Specialties* tab).

Category Preferences feature. The *Specialty* field is optional and is only used when adding a provider to the address book. (On a single-user program the server setup items are found under the *Administration* menu on the main screen).

If an e-mail address is included in the new address profile in the *EMail* field, SpringCharts is able to access it through the integrated e-mail feature when sending out messages, letters, and reports from within the program. The *EMail to Who?* window (Figure 3.14) appears when a user clicks on the e-mail function located in various places throughout SpringCharts.

SpringCharts Tip

Referring providers and consultants are added into the address book, but not the providers within the clinic. In-house physicians are set up on the SpringCharts server as "Providers" on the SpringCharts server administration screen.

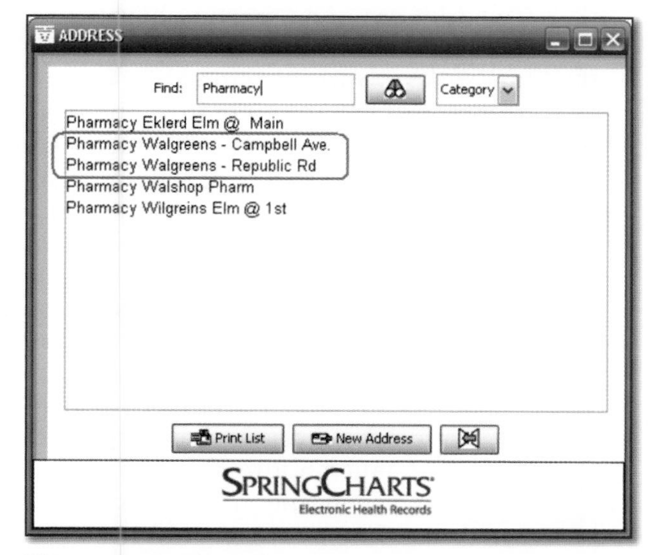

Figure 3.13 *Address* search window for the pharmacy category.

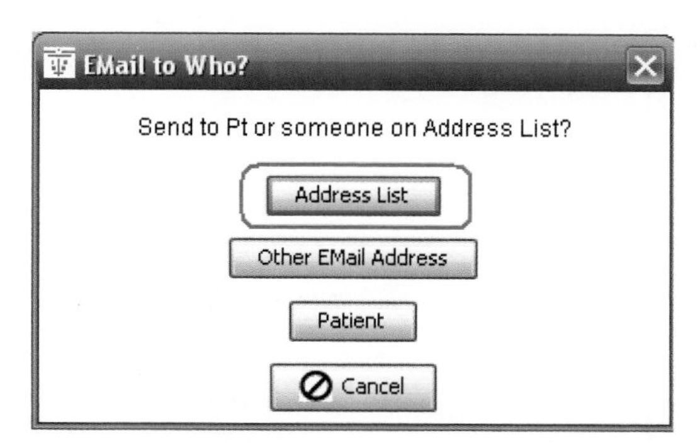

Figure 3.14 *EMail to Who?* window within SpringCharts.

SpringCharts Tip

Tab Key and Punctuation
The [Tab] key is used throughout the SpringCharts program to move from field to field in the data windows, rather than the [Enter] key. The program operates with an automatic capitalization feature when entering new entries into the database. For example, if you type in only lowercase letters, the program will capitalize the first letter of each new word. It also is not necessary to punctuate within Social Security and telephone numbers—SpringCharts will do that after you exit the field (using the [Tab] key). For example, if you type a patient's Social Security number and telephone number without the dashes and parentheses, the EHR program will automatically add them when you tab to a new line. These features aid in data entry speed.

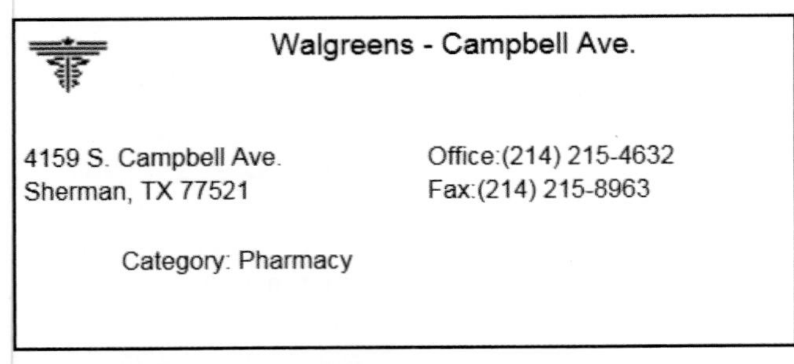

Figure 3.15 Business card-sized information created from using [Print Card] option in *New Address* window.

The [Print] button at the bottom of the *New Address* window will print the details of the address window. The [Print Card] option will allow the user to print or fax the address information to a business card-sized image measuring approximately 1.75 × 4 inches (Figure 3.15). This option can be useful when a patient needs an address and telephone number for a referral physician, facility, or pharmacy.

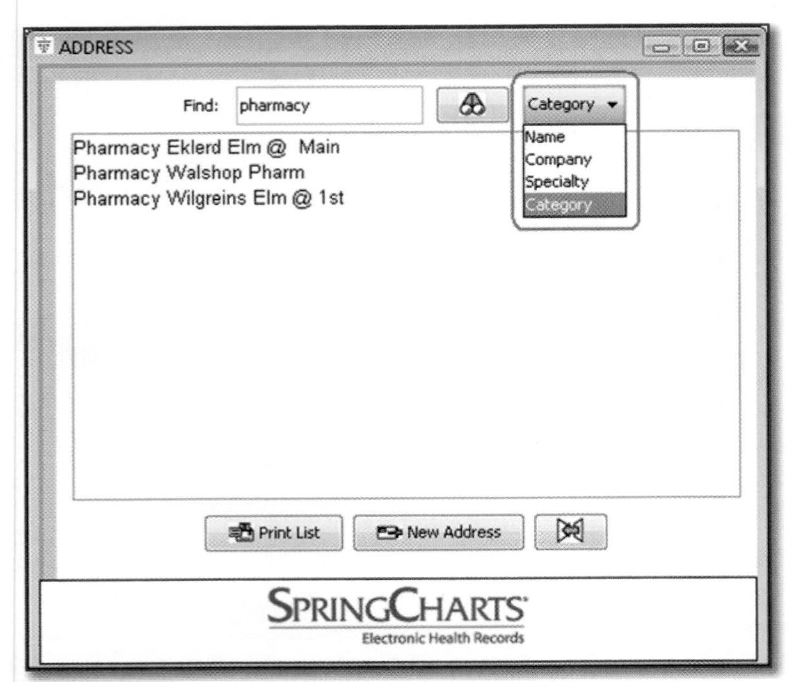

Figure 3.16 *Address* window under the *Productivity Center* menu, where addresses can be edited.

Editing Addresses

The *Address Book* feature located in the *Productivity Center* menu on the main screen is used to store, edit, and search for addresses of supporting businesses, such as pharmacies, testing facilities, therapists, and outside physicians. Within the *Address* window, the *Find* field is used to search for entries by name, company, specialty (Figure 3.16), or category determined from the drop-down menu to the right. (This list of search criteria cannot be amended.) The user enters the first few letters of the name, company, specialty, or category in the *Find* field, and then activates the *Search* icon. A list of addresses matching the search criteria is then displayed, and the detailed address information is provided when the user clicks on a name. At that point, the address can then be edited. A new address can also be added in the *Address* window by selecting the [New Address] button.

Concept Checkup 3.3

A. Are patients added into SpringCharts through the Address Book? Explain why or why not.

B. Name the two required fields when setting up an address entry.

C. Where are the *category* and *specialty* lists used in the address book set up?

Exercise 3.2 Adding New Addresses—Physician

1. Access the *New* menu at the top of the main screen and select *New Address.*
2. Enter the name and demographics of your personal primary care physician (PCP) or general practitioner (GP). (If you do not have a PCP or GP, you may make up the information.)
3. In the *Category* field, select *Physician* from the drop-down menu.
4. Choose the appropriate medical specialty from the drop-down menu in the *Specialty* field.
5. Complete the remaining fields except *Account #*, and leave *Notes* blank. (Again, you may make up any information, such as telephone numbers, that you do not have.)
6. Save the information by clicking on the [Save] button.

SpringCharts Tip

The *Specialty* field is only completed for a practitioner being set up in the Address Book. It is not necessary for any other type of address.

Exercise 3.3 Adding New Addresses—Employee

1. Access the *New* menu at the top of the main screen and select *New Address.*
2. Enter your name and demographics.
3. In the *Category* field, select *Employee* from the drop-down menu. (You do not need to complete the *Company* or *Specialty* fields when creating an address file for an individual.)
4. Complete all of the appropriate remaining fields except *Account #*, and leave *Notes* blank.
5. Save the information by clicking on the [Save] button.

SpringCharts Tip

Although SpringCharts users are set up as *Users* in the administration panel of SpringCharts server, they also need to be entered into the *Address Book* as employees in order to capture their addresses and other demographic information.

Exercise 3.4 Adding New Addresses—Pharmacy

1. Access the *New* menu at the top of the main screen and select *New Address.*
2. Set up a pharmacy of your choice, starting with entering information in the *Company* field. (You do not need to complete the *Last Name* information.)
3. Select *Pharmacy* in the *Category* field.
4. Complete all the appropriate remaining fields except *Account #*, and leave *Notes* blank. (Remember the *Specialty* field is only used to designate the medical *specialty* when setting up a provider.)
5. Save the information by clicking on the [Save] button.

Exercise 3.5 Adding New Addresses—Testing Facility

1. Access the *New* menu at the top of the main screen and select *New Address*.
2. Set up the following testing facility name: *MRI of the Ozarks, 103 E. Battlefield St., Springfield, MO 65807.* (As with the pharmacy, you do not need to complete the name information or choose a *Specialty*.
3. Select *TestingFacility* in the *Category* field.
4. Complete the remaining fields except *Account #,* and leave *Notes* blank. (You may make up information, such as telephone numbers.)
5. Save the information by clicking on the [Save] button.

SpringCharts Tip

Shortcut:

Open Address Book

The third-from-the-left speed icon located on the SpringCharts Toolbar enables users to open the address book, where nonpatient addresses can be added and edited.

Exercise 3.6 Editing an Address

1. Click on the *Open Address Book* speed icon on the Toolbar (shown in margin).
2. In the *Address* window, click on the down arrow in the classification box in the upper right and select *Category*.
3. In the *Find* field type *pharm* and click on the *Search* icon (shown in margin).
4. Click on the *Wilgreins Elm* pharmacy, which will open the address details for editing.
5. Click in the *Work Fax* field and add the following fax number: 2146765435. Tab off the line and allow the program to punctuate automatically.
6. Click the [Save] button and close the *Address Book* window by clicking on the [X] in the upper right corner.

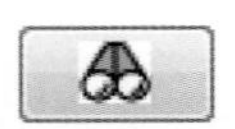

Search icon

Exercise 3.7 Printing Addresses

1. Access the *Productivity Center* menu at the top of the main screen and select the *Address Book* (Figure 3.17).
2. Locate each of your new addresses (physician, employee, pharmacy, and testing facility) by selecting the appropriate option (*Name, Company, Specialty,* or *Category*) in the drop-down menu and then entering the type of category or the name in the *Find* field. (Figure 3.18 shows an example).
3. In each category, click on the new address entry you added to open the address details.
4. Print out each of your addresses by selecting the [Print Card] button (shown in margin), choosing the printer, and then clicking [OK]. Samples of printed address cards appear in Figure 3.19. (Because you provided your own information for some of the exercise above, the information will not be the same on the sample cards illustration).
5. Close the *Address* window by clicking the red [X] in the upper right corner.
6. Write your name on each page and submit them to your instructor.

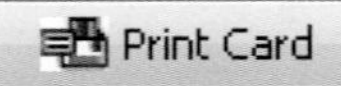

[Print Card] button

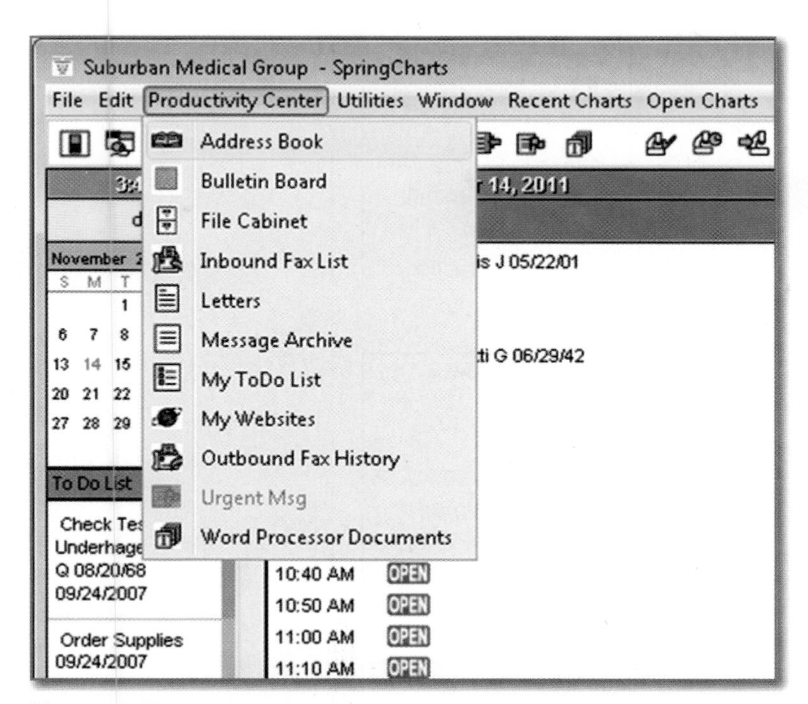

Figure 3.17 *Productivity Center > Address Book* menu.

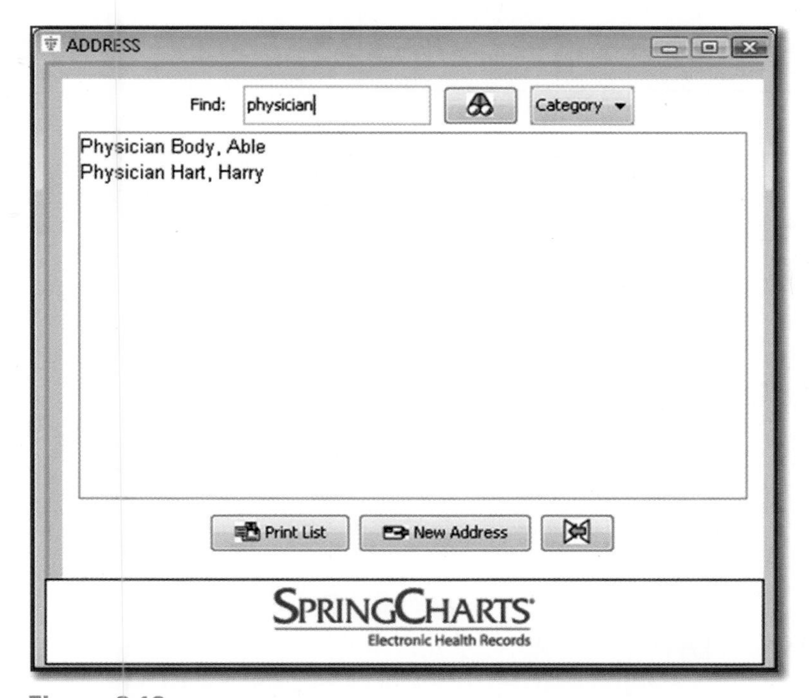

Figure 3.18 Searching for a physician in the address book.

Clarke, Jason M.D	
123 Main St.	Office:(417) 239-0856
Springfield, MO 65807	Fax:(214) 456-7890
Category: Physician Specialty: Family Practice	

Burnich, Steve M.A.	
	Office:(214) 567-8765
Sherman, TX 77521	Fax:(214) 123-9876
Category: Employee	

PharmWorld	
345 Davis Dr	Office:(214) 567-8765
Sherman, TX 77521	Fax:(214) 234-5678
Category: Pharmacy	

MRI Of The Ozarks	
103 E. Battlefield St.	Office:(214) 567-9087
Springfield, MO 65807	Fax:(214) 342-7896
Category: TestingFacility	

Figure 3.19 Samples of printed address cards.

3.4 Patient Data Setup

In this section, you will learn how to set up new patients in the SpringCharts EHR and edit their information.

You will recall from earlier in this book that the Office of the National Coordinator for Health Information Technology (ONC) is a position within the U.S. Department of Health and Human Services (HHS). Beginning in fall 2010, the ONC required EHR programs to meet a comprehensive set of criteria in order to attain certification. Certain healthcare providers who qualify as eligible professionals (EPs) must use an ONC-certified EHR program and demonstrate meaningful use (MU) to qualify for incentive payments through

Table 3.3 Meaningful Use Core Measure

Essential Patient Demographics	
Stage 1 Objective	**Measure**
Mandated to record the following patient demographics (sex, race, ethnicity, date of birth, and preferred language).	More than 50 percent of patients' demographic data recorded as structured data.

Notes:

- A unique patient can only be counted once during the reporting period for MU even though the patient may actually be seen by the EP more than one time during the same time period.
- Preferred language is understood to be the language that the patient prefers to communicate in.
- EPs are not required to communicate with the patient in the patient's preferred language in order to qualify for MU.
- A patient may decline to provide all or part of the demographic information. A notation made by a clinician indicating the refusal counts as an entry for the purposes of meeting this measure's requirements.
- Patients who do not know their ethnicity are treated the same way as patients who decline to provide race or ethnicity; notation is made in the patient's chart, and the entry is counted toward MU qualifications.

Demographics
Demographics are the statistical data of a person or population. They are typically comprised of address, phone numbers, gender, age, marital status, employment, and education. However, demographics can be very broad to include disabilities, mobility, home ownership, income, and personal preferences.

CMS. The specific measure for the *Essential Patient Demographics* requires the patient's sex, race, ethnicity, date of birth, and preferred language be recorded in an EHR (Table 3.3). More than 50 percent of an EP's patients had to have this data recorded, for the EP to qualify for stimulus money in the 2011 and 2012 reporting period.

New Patient

The *New Patient* feature is used to create an electronic chart for a new patient. Front-office users will access the *New* menu option at the top of the main *Practice View* window and click on the *New Patient* submenu. An empty *New Patient* window will appear (Figure 3.20).

Fields with labels in red are required to be completed to successfully save patient data and create a chart. Fields labeled in yellow are required for the e-prescribing function; if these are not completed, SpringCharts will be unable to transmit an electronic prescription to a clearinghouse.

A patient's chart can be created rapidly by recording only the patient's first and last name and date of birth. In a front-office clerical environment, this basic information can be obtained from the patient over the phone. The patient's electronic file can then be created and the patient added to the schedule. On the scheduled appointment day, the remaining information can be added after the patient completes the Intake Forms.

The *Category* field allows the user to assign a category to the patient, for example, *Nursing Home Patient, Obstetrics, Gynecology, Disabled,* and so on. The clinic will define the list of categories based on its medical specialty. The items in the *Category* drop-down menu can be added and modified in the *Patient Categories* section on the SpringCharts server in a network environment and under the *Administration* menu on a single-user version of SpringCharts. Grouping patients into categories allows staff to search and print information about selected groups of patients.

SpringCharts Tip
In the *New Patient* window, you can enter a patient's date of birth using the *mmddyyyy* format (without punctuation) in the *Date of Birth* field. Punctuation will be inserted automatically after you tab off the field. Another method of entering the date of birth is to click the pop-up calendar icon to the right of the field.

SpringCharts Tip
It is critical to record the patient's Social Security number in the *SS#* field. A duplicate patient alert is triggered as a warning message in SpringCharts when the Social Security number matches that in another patient's record.

Table 3.4 Edit Patient Functions

Function Button	Action
[New]	Create a new patient record
[Save]	Save the updated patient information
[Get Chart]	Open a patient's chart
[Track Patient]	Place a patient into the *Patient Tracker*
[Previous Updates]	Check to see which user updated the patient's information and what material was updated
[Exempt]	Identify a patient as exempt from database searches
[Delete]	Delete a patient from being viewed in the database
[Archive]	Remove a patient from the active list and move him or her to an archived patient list
[Undelete]	View a list of deleted patients and "undelete" a patient back into the active database
[Import]	Manually import a patient record from an interfaced PMS program
[Export]	Export an individual patient's data or export the entire patient database

As shown in Figure 3.22, the entire list of patients can be viewed by clicking the [Search] button without entering any data in the *Search* field. Users may need to export the database of patients to convert the list to a spreadsheet for further analysis. To export a list of patients, the administrator would select the [Export] button at the bottom right corner of the window, as seen in Figure 3.23, and choose either *Export Item* or *Export List* to export a specific highlighted patient or the entire database of patients, respectively.

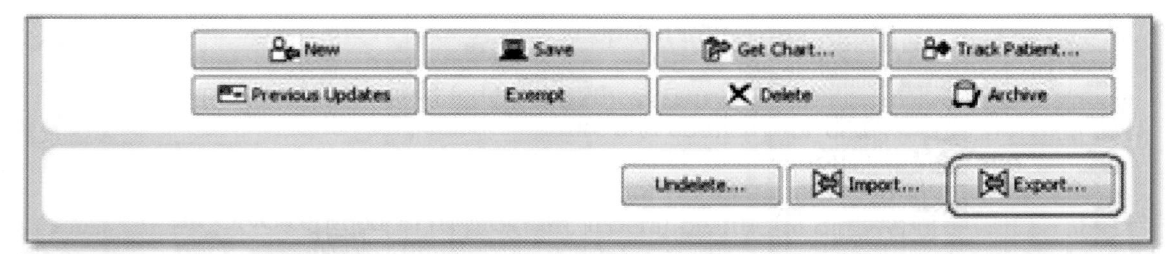

Figure 3.23 Export button in *Edit Patient* window.

Concept Checkup 3.4

A. New patients can be added into SpringCharts through which windows? Select all that apply.

1. *Address Book* **2.** *New Patient* **3.** *Edit Patient* **4.** *Edit Address Book*

B. Why are the race and ethnicity lists coded in SpringCharts's database?

C. To keep a selected patient out of the regular search function of the program, which button would be selected in the *Edit Patient* window?

1. [Get Chart] **2.** [Track Patient] **3.** [Exempt] **4.** [Archive]

Exercise 3.8 Adding a New Patient Record

1. Select the *New* menu at the top of the main *Practice View* screen.
2. Select the *New Patient* submenu.
3. Enter yourself as a patient. Complete as much information as possible. Please use the zip code: 77521. For security reasons, do not use your actual Social Security number for your profile. For the purpose of exercises later in the text, make yourself a female patient with an age somewhere between 21 and 30.
4. Save the information by clicking on the [Save] button.

SpringCharts Tip

When entering a patient's name in SpringCharts, the first name is entered first, and then the last name. If you enter the last name in the first name field, you will not be able to locate the patient's chart later, because the program searches for the patient by the *Last Name* field.

Exercise 3.9 Editing a Patient Record

1. Select the main *Edit* menu at the top of the main *Practice View* screen.
2. Choose the *Patients* submenu.
3. In the *Edit Patient* window, select *Zip Code* as the *Search* criterion and type "77521" in the *Search* field.
4. Click the [Search] button.
5. Select *Patti Adams.*
6. Add a made up *Work Phone* to her demographics.
7. Click the [Save] button, but do not exit the *Edit Patient* window.

SpringCharts Tip

When adding household members to the Spring-Charts database, the *Address* field must be the same for patients to be linked in the same household list.

Exercise 3.10 Exporting a Patient List

1. Within the *Edit Patient* window, which still shows a list of patients with the zip code of 77521, click the [Export] button in the bottom right corner.

Note: Depending on the size of your screen, you may have to use your scroll bars to locate the [Export] button.

2. Select *Export List.*
3. Choose the [Open in Word Processor] option from the *Export Patient List* window. SpringCharts will re-create the list of patients with a zip code of 77521 in your computer's default word processing program. In most cases, this will be Notepad. From here, the list can be printed out or saved on the computer. Notice that the date of birth is in the *yyyymmdd* format. Also, Notepad defaults to the last font size used on the computer. You may change the text size by selecting *Format* > *Font* in Notepad.
4. Print out the list of patients with the zip code of 77521, circle your name on the paper, and submit to your instructor.
5. Close the Edit Patient window by clicking the red 'X' in the upper right corner.

SpringCharts Tip

Reminder: Telephone numbers and Social Security numbers can be typed into the appropriate fields without punctuation. Once you tab off the field, punctuation is automatically inserted.

3.5 Insurance Data Setup

In this section, you will learn to add new insurance information to the Spring-Charts program and edit existing insurance information. Because SpringCharts is not a billing program, the insurance information database includes only the

chapter 3 summary

Learning Outcome	Key Concepts/Examples
3.1 Provide a brief history of SpringCharts EHR software and list three clinical and three administrative tools that it offers. **Pages 55–59**	Developed and implemented over a period of 12 years Designed to manage all nonfinancial activities of a medical practice Features combine robust clinical tools to enhance patient care and clerical tools designed to speed and streamline office communication and documentation 2007: SpringCharts was CCHIT-certified for ambulatory EHRs 2011: SpringCharts was ONC-ATCB certified, qualifying for stage one of MU program under the HITECH Act
3.2 Set up user preferences. **Pages 60–65**	User Preferences Location: *Practice View* screen > *File* menu > *Preferences* > *User Preferences* User Preferences set up in SpringCharts to customize program for each specific user: • *Your Provider* • *Your Practice* • *Appt Schedule* • *Tracker Group* • *OV Form View* • *Search Mode* • *PopUp Text Insert* • *Measurements* • *Time* • *Font* • *Rx Print Attending* • *Provider Role* • *Office Visit Orientation* • *Password* • *Signature*
3.3 Set up, edit, and print addresses in the physician, employee, pharmacy, and testing facility categories. **Pages 66–72**	New Address: • Location: *Practice View* screen > *New* menu > *New Address* • Data for pharmacies, testing facilities, referring physicians, vendors, etc. • Required fields: *Last Name* or *Company,* and *Category* • *Category* and *Specialty* list setup on SpringCharts server • Entities from the address book grouped by categories throughout the program • *Specialty* field used for physicians Editing Addresses • Location: *Practice View* screen > *Productivity Center* menu > *Address Book* • Locality for searching, editing, and printing address entries • Search by: name, company, specialty, or category
3.4 Set up new patients, edit patient information, and export patient lists. **Pages 72–77**	New Patient • Location: *Practice View* screen > *New* menu > *New Patient* • Required fields: *First Name, Last Name, Date of Birth* • Automatic punctuation for capitalization, Social Security and telephone numbers, and dates • Social Security number alert for duplicate patient entries • Category fields for in-house grouping of patients • Standard list for race and ethnicity established by OMB Editing Patients • Location: *Practice View* screen > *Edit* menu > *Patients* • Locality for searching, editing, and other functions regarding patient charts • Search by last name, zip code, Social Security number, home number, work number, patient number, birth date, and e-mail • Patient database can be exported to other programs
3.5 Set up new insurance companies and edit existing insurance company information. **Pages 78–79**	New Insurance • Location: *Practice View* screen > *Edit* menu > *Insurance* > *New Insurance Company* • Patient's primary insurance information is stored in patient's chart and added to physician's order form for outside testing facilities Editing Insurance • Location: *Practice View* screen > *Edit* menu > *Insurance* • *Details* window for communication and documentation

chapter 3 review

Name ______________________ Instructor ______________ Class ______________ Date ______________

Using Terminology

Match the terms on the left with the definitions on the right.

_____ 1. **LO 3.2** GUI

_____ 2. **LO 3.2** Imperial units

_____ 3. **LO 3.2** User preferences

_____ 4. **LO 3.2** Metric units

_____ 5. **LO 3.2** OV

_____ 6. **LO 3.2** Attending physician

_____ 7. **LO 3.5** Secondary insurance

_____ 8. **LO 3.1** End-to-end solution

_____ 9. **LO 3.5** Primary insurance

_____ 10. **LO 3.4** Demographics

A. Practitioners having final responsibility for patient healthcare, even when many of the medical decisions are made by subordinates like physician assistants, nurse practitioners, and medical interns.

B. This software industry term suggests that the vendor of an application program can provide all the hardware and software components to meet the client's requirement and that no other supplier need be involved.

C. Weights and measures that conform to standards legally established in Great Britain; still widely used in the United States.

D. Software program screen that can display icons, sub windows, text fields, and menus designed to standardize and simplify use of the computer program.

E. Choices the user makes in a software program to preset elements and features of the program that will be displayed when that specific user logs in to the program.

F. An insurance policy that pays for some of the patient's medical expenses that primary insurance does not pay.

G. Also known as the International System of Units, having to do with weights and measures based on the decimal system, which is mandatory in a large number of countries.

H. The acronym used in SpringCharts to designate the graphical user interface window in which the encounter note is created.

I. A program that covers a portion of a patient's incurred medical expense.

J. Statistical data of a person or population that is typically comprised of address, phone numbers, gender, age, marital status, and so on.

Checking Your Understanding

Choose the best answer and circle the corresponding letter.

11. LO 3.1 The abbreviation ONC-ATCB stands for:
a) Office of National Coordinator Authority for Testing Certified Programs
b) Office of National Coordinator Authorized Testing and Certification Body
c) Official National Coordinator for Authorizing Testing and Certification Bodies
d) Official National Center Authorized Technology for College Bodies

12. LO 3.1 In 2011, the first of three stages of the meaningful use (MU) program created by the ONC was rolled out. What will each stage require regarding EHR programs?
a) New criteria and functionality standards
b) More dollars and higher costs
c) More physicians in the workforce
d) Mandatory use

13. LO 3.2 Each user's role is defined in the *User Preferences* window. In what section of the patient's chart will the EHR program automatically and permanently stamp the staff's name and role?
a) Patient's chart screen
b) Office visit note
c) Face sheet
d) Patient demographics

14. LO 3.1 In the MU Core Measure: *Privacy and Security*, which of the following would *not* be required for an EP to qualify for this criteria?
a) Implement systems to protect privacy and security of patient data in the EHR program
b) Send staff members to the ONC certified training on HIPAA privacy and security regulations
c) Update EHR software and improve physical security
d) Conduct or review a security risk analysis

15. LO 3.4 The ONC has determined five essential patient demographics that should be recorded in a certified EHR program. Which of the following is *not* a required demographic?
a) Gender
b) Ethnicity
c) Social Security number
d) Date of birth

16. LO 3.5 The *Details* window in the insurance editing screen can be used for recording:
a) The patient's co-pays and deductibles
b) Financial information regarding insurance payment of the patient's claims
c) The patient's secondary and tertiary insurance companies
d) Other information about the insurance company such as contact personnel

17. LO 3.1 SpringCharts EHR program is designed to manage this side of a medical practice:
a) Financial
b) Nonfinancial
c) Accounts receivable
d) Accounts payable

18. LO 3.2 A practice that has several clinics in different locations and share the same database has the ability to:
a) View complete patient medical records stored at the central office only
b) View complete patient medical records at each location provided that the records are stored there
c) View complete patient medical records for any of the clinics from any location
d) A practice that has several clinics in different locations cannot share the same database

19. LO 3.2 When a clinic has several locations that share the same database, the *Tracker Group* option allows each clinic to display the list of patients for:
a) Its specific location separately
b) Only the combined patients from all locations
c) Patients attending competitors' offices in the same area
d) The waiting room only

20. LO 3.2 In the United States, the typical units of measure in which the vitals will be recorded are:
a) Metric
b) Imperative
c) Imperial
d) CCs

21. **LO 3.4** Capturing the preferred language of a patient is a requirement for a clinic to qualify for MU. However,
    a) The clinic should require the patient to speak in English.
    b) The clinic is not required to communicate with the patient in his or her preferred language.
    c) There should be designated clinics for patients who cannot speak English.
    d) The language needs to be tied to ethnicity.

22. **LO 3.3** Automatic capitalization and punctuation is a SpringCharts feature designed to:
    a) Ensure consistent documentation by physicians.
    b) Confuse the user.
    c) Be selected in the *Set User Preferences* window.
    d) Speed the data entry process.

23. **LO 3.4** A duplicate patient alert is triggered when the following patient information is duplicated:
    a) Social Security number
    b) Date of birth, zip code, and area code
    c) First name, last name, and date of birth
    d) Same household list

24. **LO 3.3** Why is the *Category* field required to be filled in when setting up an entry in the *New Address* window?
    a) So the program can display specific facilities throughout the program based on these categories
    b) So more information can be stored for companies
    c) To provide an alternative to the *Specialty* field
    d) So SpringCharts can run more detailed reports

25. **LO 3.5** A patient's primary insurance is stored in the patient's chart in SpringCharts so that:
    a) It can be used to bill insurance companies.
    b) It can be added to an order form for testing facilities.
    c) Patients can be reminded to file with their insurance companies.
    d) It only takes up a limited amount of space.

Applying Your Knowledge

Use your critical-thinking skills to answer the following questions.

26. **LO 3.3** The Address Book in the EHR program enables the user to record addresses, phone, fax, and cell phone numbers. It even enables the user to group the entries into categories and specialties. Why should the user not add patients to the Address Book?

27. **LO 3.4** Explain why some field names in the *New Patient* window are highlighted in red, some in yellow, and some in blue.

28. **LO 3.5** The SpringCharts program is only able to keep record of the patient's primary insurance plan. Why does this EHR program not record the patient's secondary and tertiary medical insurance policies?

4

The Clinic Administration

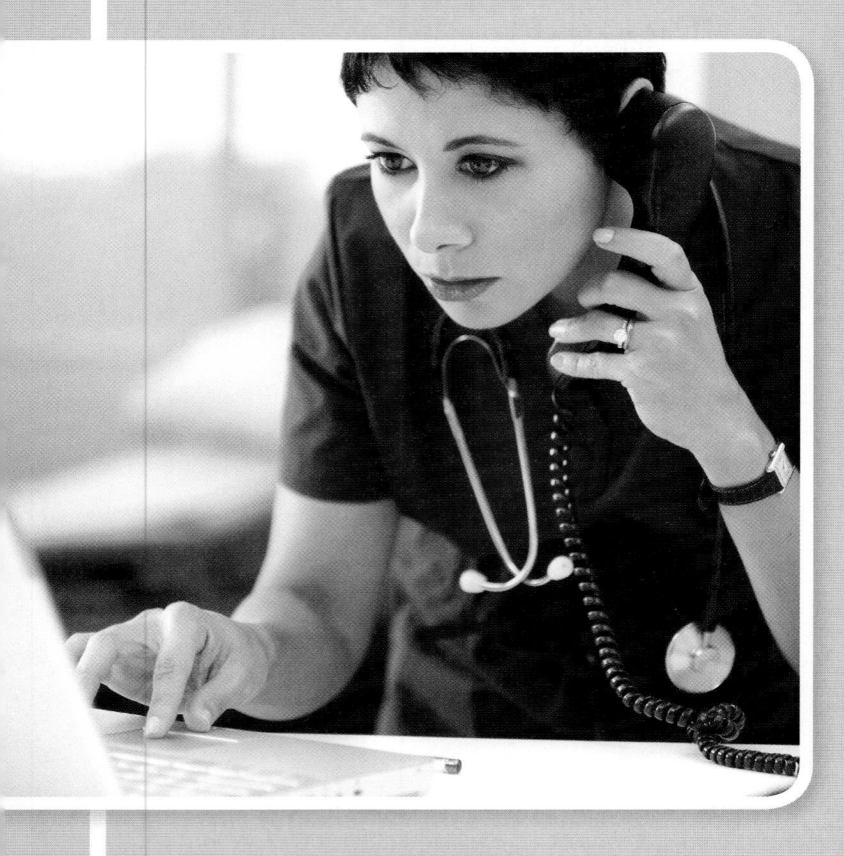

Learning Outcomes

After completing Chapter 4, you will be able to:

LO 4.1 Navigate the *Practice View* screen.

LO 4.2 Use the *Office Schedule* to add patients and notes to the schedule, add blocked time to the schedule, and chart "no shows."

LO 4.3 Use the *Patient Tracker* to perform tasks such as change a patient's location and status, assign color codes, move patients, and check out patients.

LO 4.4 Use the *To Do List* to set reminders and send to-do items to yourself and another user.

LO 4.5 Create internal messages, both nonpatient and those concerning patients.

LO 4.6 Demonstrate how to send and respond to an urgent message.

What You Need to Know

To understand Chapter 4, you will need to know:

- How to start the SpringCharts EHR program
- How to set individual user preferences
- How to set up addresses and edit address information
- How to set up new patients and edit patient information
- How to set up new insurance companies and edit company information

Key Terms

Appointment schedule
Message Archive
No show
Patient status
Patient Tracker
Pop-up text
Routing slip
Toolbar

Introduction

Although the main focus of electronic medical record systems is the storage and retrieval of patient healthcare data, EHR programs also offer features that enable clinical and clerical staff members to perform their day-to-day duties with greater efficiency and accuracy. These tools enhance patient safety and quality of care. Every medical practice employee, including the clinician, has administrative responsibilities as a member of the healthcare team. Whether it's a task as simple as documenting a telephone call from a patient or something more complex, such as transferring a patient's healthcare information from one provider to another, the ability to communicate clearly, complete assigned tasks, and execute administrative duties flawlessly is critical in a busy medical office. In your position as a healthcare professional, carrying out your assignments and duties effectively reflects directly on each staff member and the medical office as a whole.

EHR systems provide administrative functions, such as scheduling and tracking patients, creating personal to-do and reminder lists, and generating and receiving messages from co-workers, patients, and other healthcare providers. Some advanced EHR programs offer the ability to track a patient's location in a clinic and record what is happening with the patient at any given time. Some advanced features are specific to the user who is logged on, displaying only the user's self-entered information; other features are universal in nature and display updated information for all users.

EHRs have been designed to move medical offices toward a paperless environment. Many common administrative tasks and standard paperwork typically generated are now executed electronically via EHR programs.

4.1 The Practice View Screen

Most administrative tasks and communication are done from the *Practice View* window of the SpringCharts program (Figure 4.1). This is one of the three main screens from which clinical and administrative staff members can perform more than 90 percent of their duties. The *Practice View* window is the first screen displayed after a user logs on to SpringCharts. This main administrative screen provides an up-to-the minute overview of all office activity. Note the following at-a-glance features in Figure 4.1:

A. Office Calendar
B. Appointment Schedule
C. Patient Tracker
D. To Do List
E. Messages
F. Shortcut keys

The top left corner of the *Practice View* screen displays the current time and the user who is presently logged on to the SpringCharts program on that specific computer. The *Office Calendar* (A), *Appointment Schedule* (B), and *Patient Tracker* (C) windows are consistent for all users on the network; when an update is made to any of these features, it is seen by all users logged on to SpringCharts. On the other hand, the *To Do List* (D) and *Messages* (E) windows are user-defined and only show information relevant to the specific user who is logged on. When modifications are made in these two windows, only the user who makes the modifications can view the changes. All of these features are fully integrated with the program's patient charting feature, enabling the user to access the chart from multiple locations within the program.

Focal Point

Some features in the *Practice View* screen are network-defined; all users view and modify the same information. Other features are user-defined; only the user logged on views and modifies the information.

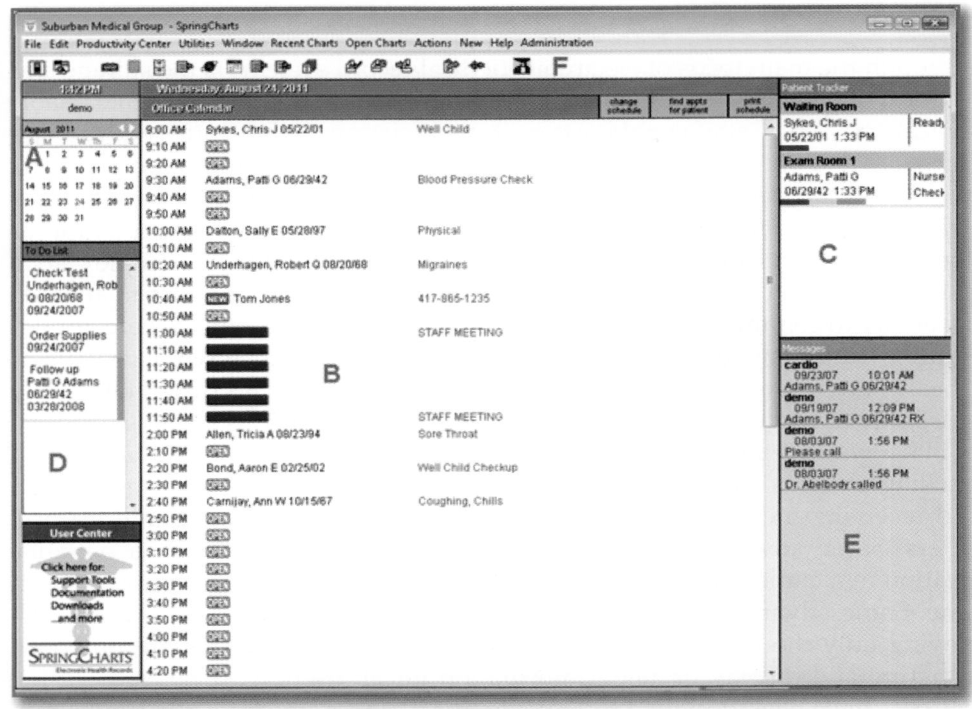

Figure 4.1 *Practice View* screen.

Toolbar

The Toolbar displays a lineup of icons that gives users shortcut access to the program's most commonly used functions.

The **Toolbar** (F) at the top *Practice View* screen (Figure 4.2) displays universal icons that are shortcuts to the program's most commonly used features, such as the urgent message function. When using the shortcuts with the program's Tap-N-Go navigation, tablet users can bypass using drop-down menus.

SpringCharts Tip

In most cases, when selecting an item in SpringCharts, a user simply needs to left-click the mouse once. The program's *Tap-N-Go* feature, used on a tablet, enables the user to tap the tablet screen once with a stylus pen to move to the next screen.

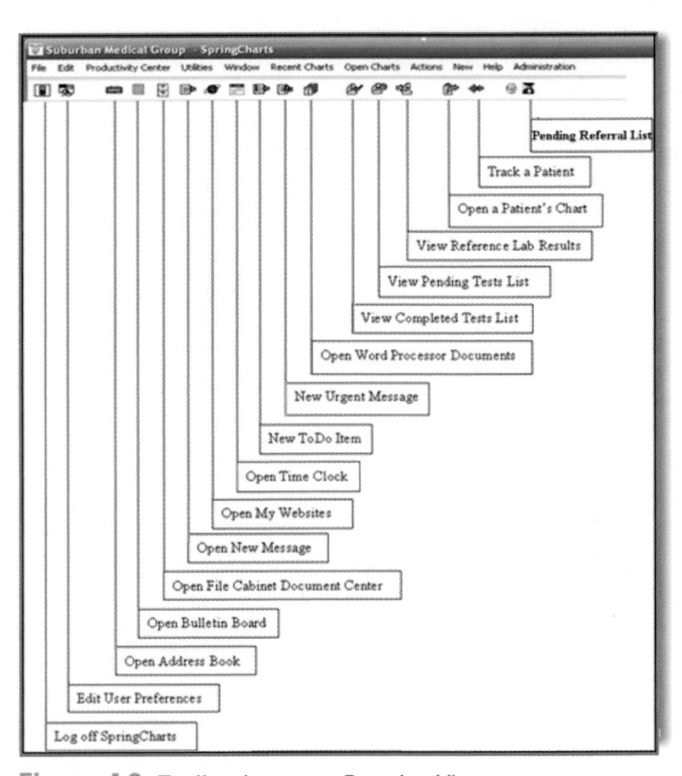

Figure 4.2 Toolbar icons on *Practice View* screen.

Concept Checkup 4.1

A. What is the common trait between the *To Do List* and the *Messages* center?

B. The following three icons on the *Practice View* Toolbar correspond to viewing what three tests?

Exercise 4.1 Becoming Familiar with the Toolbar

1. Log on to SpringCharts so the *Practice View* screen is open.
2. Click on the *New To Do Item* icon (shown in margin). A *New ToDo/Reminder* box appears.
3. Examine the *New ToDo/Reminder* window, and then close it.
4. Click on the *Open New Message* icon (shown in margin). A *Link Message to Patient* box appears.
5. Click the [No] button in the *Link Message to Patient?* window.
6. Examine the *New Message* window, and then close it.
7. Click on the *New Urgent Message* icon (shown in margin). A *Send Urgent Message* box appears.
8. Examine the *Send Urgent Message* window, and then close it.

New To Do Item icon

Open New Message icon

New Urgent Message icon

4.2 Appointment Schedule

Although patient appointment schedules have traditionally been part of PMS programs in medical clinics, they have now been incorporated in EHR programs so practitioners and office staff can view the schedules and see the patient load for any given day. Patient schedules change throughout the day for many reasons: Some patients may not show up for their scheduled appointments, patients are placed into the schedule at the last minute, physicians are called away for emergencies, and clinicians fall behind schedule. The EHR makes it possible for practitioners and staff to have the most recent, real-time information regarding the patient schedule. In EHR programs, a patient's name on the schedule is integrated with the patient's chart, messaging, referrals, and other features so clinicians can access linked material for the patient with one mouse click.

After logging on to SpringCharts, the *Practice View* screen appears, and the **appointment schedule** appears as the main window on the screen. From this main *Office Schedule* window, the user can view other office schedules for the same day by clicking on the [change schedule] button (shown in margin) on the menu bar in the upper right of the window. A *Choose Schedule* window displays, from which the user can select the desired schedule. The new schedule then becomes the main window schedule. The current schedule in the *Practice View* screen can be printed by selecting the [print schedule] button on the *Office Schedule* menu bar. Patient appointments and scheduled breaks can be easily scheduled by clicking on the appropriate time slot and completing the required information in the *Edit Appointment* window (Figure 4.3). Existing patients are then added to the appointment schedule by first selecting the [Choose Patient] button. Patients are chosen by typing the first few letters of the patient's last name in the *Choose Patient* window that appears, and then conducting a search.

Appointment schedule
The appointment schedule displays past, current, and future patient appointment schedules and time blocks for activities. Multiple appointment schedules can be created within the program to display patient appointments for different medical providers and other resources. Appointment schedules can show a variety of appointment-length slots.

change schedule	find appts for patient	print schedule

Office Schedule menu items

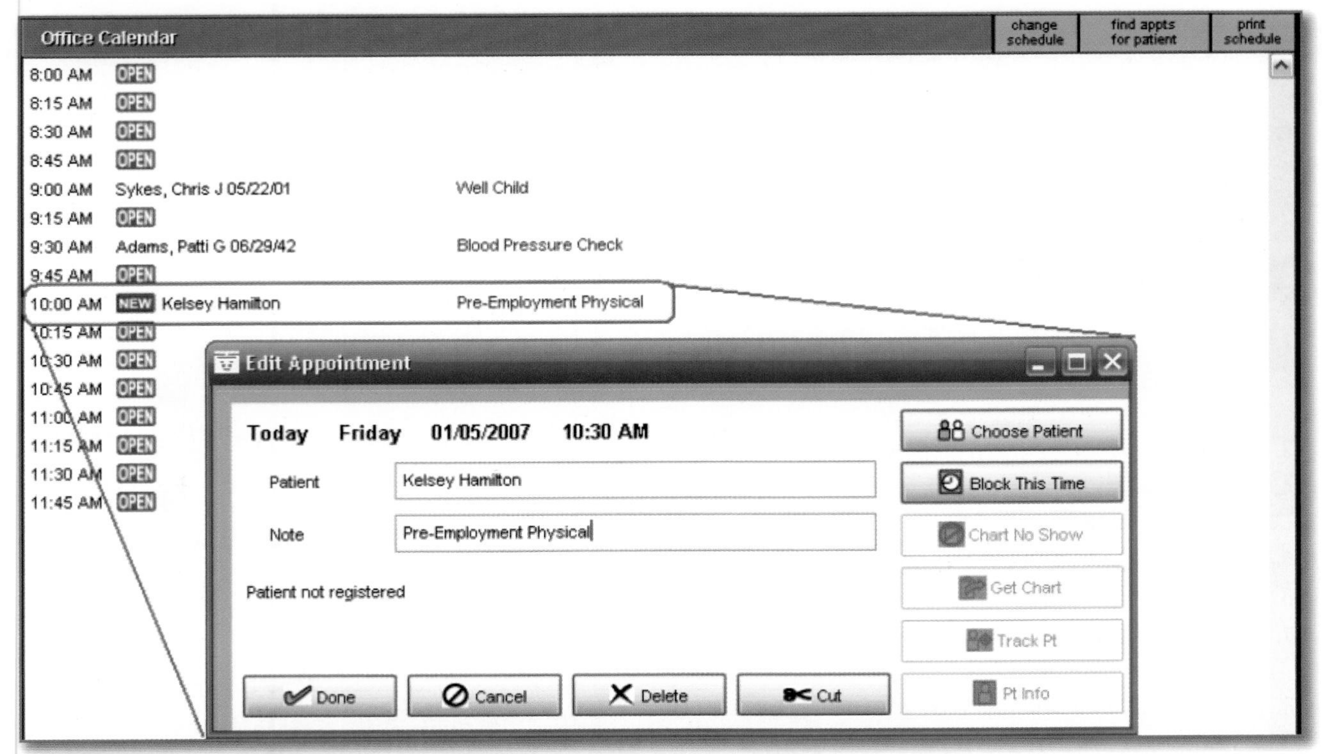

Figure 4.3 Adding a new patient to the appointment schedule.

NEW
New patient icon

Focal Point

For an *Existing/Registered* patient on the schedule, the user can access the patient's chart, change demographic information, move the patient to the *Tracker,* and chart a no show. These functions are not possible for *New/Unregistered* patients on the appointment schedule.

Focal Point

New and existing patients, scheduled breaks, meetings, and notes can be entered into the EHR office schedule.

To add a new patient to the appointment schedule without adding demographic information into the database, the user simply types the patient's name in the *Patient* field of the *Edit Appointment* window (see again Figure 4.3) without first selecting the [Choose Patient] button. After the user clicks the [Done] button, the *NEW* symbol (shown in margin) appears on the schedule beside the patient's name. This feature is suited for clinics that wait until a new patient arrives for the appointment before entering name and demographic information into database. Some clinics save time this way because, from time to time, new patients who are scheduled on the appointment schedule do not show for their appointments.

To block out time slots on the schedule for staff meetings and other activities, the user selects the [Block This Time] button in the *Edit Appointment* window. The user can enter the reason for the blocked time by filling in the *Note* field in the *Edit Appointment* window.

Past and future appointments for patients can be viewed and printed by selecting the [find appts for patient] button on the *Office Schedule* menu bar. The *Search for Pt Appt* window displays, and the user is given the choice to view appointments for either new or existing patients (Figure 4.4). A *New/Unregistered* patient is one whose name appears on the schedule but the demographics have not been entered into SpringCharts database, whereas an *Existing/Registered* patient is one whose information **has** been set up in SpringCharts database. When searching for a *New/Unregistered* patient on the appointment schedule, the user simply types the patient's name in the *Find New Patient* field. When searching for an *Existing/Registered* patient, the user types the first few letters of the patient's last name in the *Choose Patient* window. A printable appointment list appears, showing all past and future appointments for the selected patient (Figure 4.5).

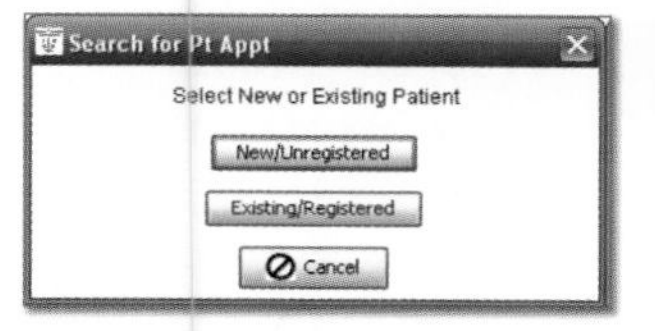

Figure 4.4 Searching for new or existing patient appointments.

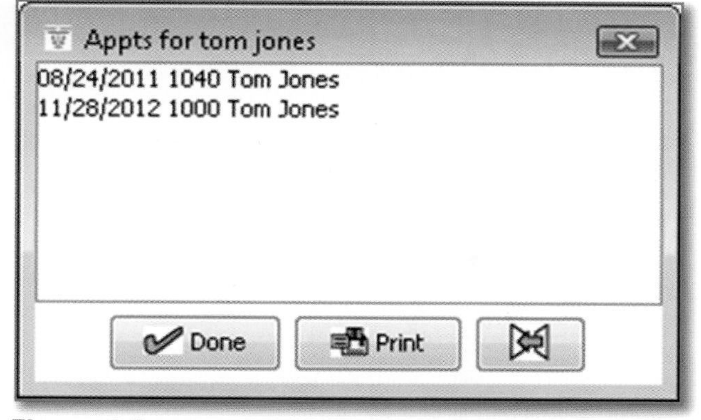

Figure 4.5 Scheduled appointments for a new patient.

No show
This term is used to indicate that a patient missed a scheduled appointment without calling in advance to inform the clinic or to reschedule.

The *Office Schedule* also includes the ability to document a **no show,** a patient who did not keep his or her appointment. When a patient misses a scheduled appointment, the receptionist clicks on the patient's name in the office schedule. The *Edit Appointment* window displays and the receptionist clicks on the [Chart No Show] button (shown in margin). This adds a note to the patient's chart documenting the no show. Patients who repeatedly cancel or do not keep scheduled appointments can then be tracked, enabling the clinic to enforce corrective policy.

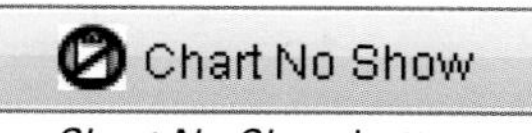

Chart No Show button

The *Edit Appointment* window also includes a [Cut] button, which enables the appointment to be "cut" from the existing schedule and "pasted" into another open time slot. After deleting the appointment with the [Cut] button, the same button changes to a [Paste] button when the user selects an open time slot in that day's schedule or another schedule. From the appointment schedule, the user can navigate to prior or future months by clicking on the left or right arrows on the month title bar of the *Office Calendar* found in the upper left corner of the *Practice View* screen (shown in margin). The current date in the monthly calendar is always displayed in red. Future patient appointment schedules can be displayed on top of the main *Office Schedule* window (Figure 4.6) by clicking on the appropriate date of the calendar. Multiple appointment schedules are stored within the program so users can view patient appointments for different medical providers and other clinic resources. Other providers'/resources' schedules can be selected and edited by using the drop-down menu in the *Schedule* field. Once opened and modified, future appointment windows can be closed by clicking on the red [X] in the upper right corner.

SpringCharts Tip

Patients who are new/unregistered on the schedule cannot be processed as a no show because an electronic chart has not been created for them in the database.

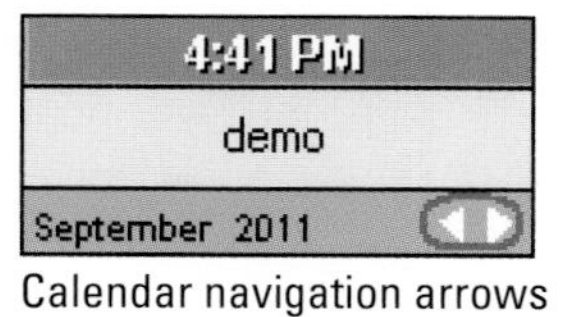

Calendar navigation arrows

Provider and resource schedules are set up on the SpringCharts server. In the *Appointment Setup* window on the server the administrator can choose the days of the week, the beginning and end time slot, and the appointment length for each provider. The time slot options range from 10 minutes to 60 minutes. The appointment intervals for the current SpringCharts schedule is 10 minutes.

SpringCharts Tip

The starting and ending time slots, as well as the appointment-length intervals, are established and modified in the administration panel of the single-user version of SpringCharts or on the SpringCharts server in a network environment.

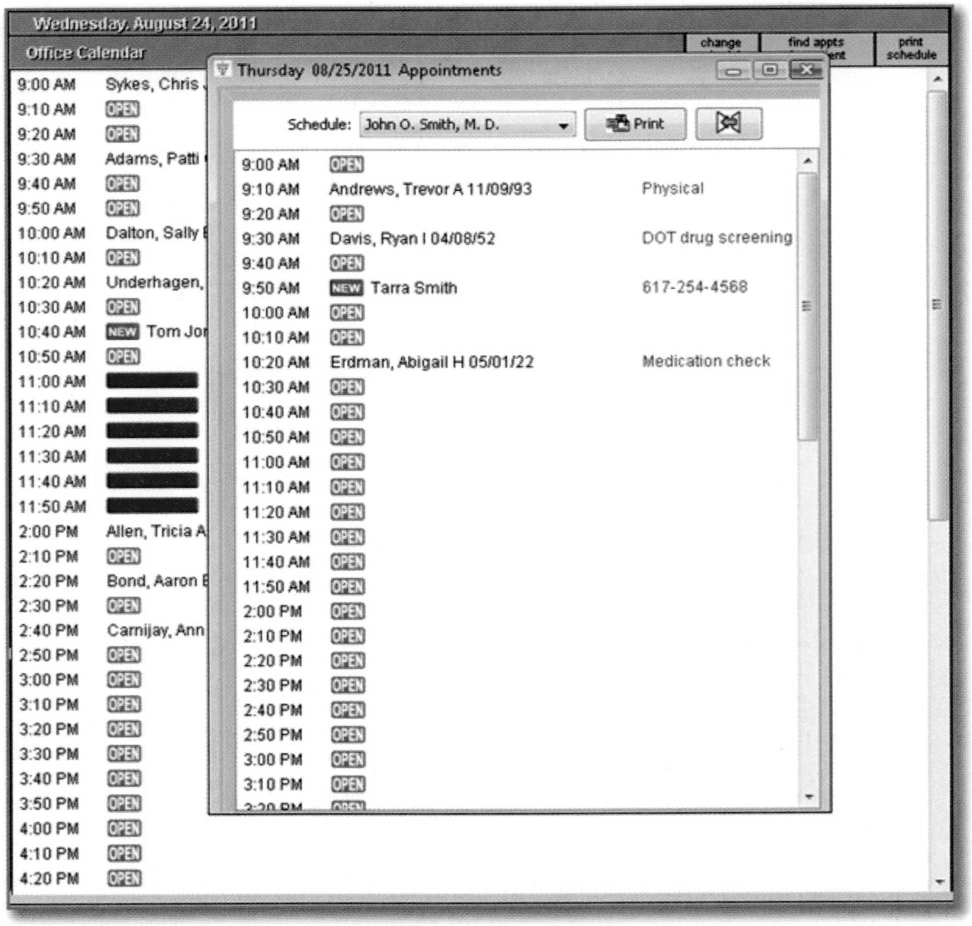

Figure 4.6 Opening additional appointment schedules.

Concept Checkup 4.2

A. For the *New* icon to appear beside a patient's name on the scheduler, how must the patient's name be added in the *Edit Appointment* window?

B. What is a *New/Unregistered* patient?

C. What button is selected in the *Edit Appointment* window to add a No Show note in the patient's chart?

Note: It is important to complete Exercises 4.2–4.9 in one day. Because SpringCharts EHR is an industry-standard program, patients placed on today's schedule will not appear on the schedule when you log in the next day.

Exercise 4.2 Adding an Existing Patient to the Schedule

1. Log on to SpringCharts. Close the *Tutorial* window.
2. Click on any *OPEN* icon on the appointment schedule.
3. When the *Edit Appointment* window displays, click on the [Choose Patient] button.
4. With the *Choose Patient* window open, type the first few letters of your last name, and then press the [Search] button.
5. Select your name from the list.
6. Enter a fictitious reason for your visit in the *Note* field of the *Edit Appointment* window.
7. Add your initials after the note.
8. Click the [Done] button.

Exercise 4.3 Blocking Out Time on the Schedule

1. Click on the *OPEN* time slot for the beginning of the last hour of the work day, where you will block out time on the schedule for a staff meeting. Depending on the day, you may have to use the scroll bar to slide down to the last hour on the Appointment Schedule.
2. Type *Staff Meeting* in the *Note* field of the *Edit Appointment* window.
3. Click on the [Block This Time] button.
4. Repeat this exercise for each 10-minute increment until the entire hour is blocked.

Exercise 4.4 Adding a New Patient to the Schedule

1. Click on any *OPEN* time slot on the appointment schedule.
2. When the *Edit Appointment* window displays, type *Jeremie Hill* in the *Patient* field.
3. Type in *Physical* for the visit reason in the *Note* field.
4. Add your initials after the note.
5. Click the [Done] button.

Note: You will notice that this patient's appointment will be scheduled with the *New* icon in the time slot because he is not currently in the database; this indicates that he is a new patient to the practice.

Exercise 4.5 Adding a Note to the Schedule

1. Add two established patients, *Sally Dalton* and *Robert Underhagen,* to the appointment schedule.

Note: Refer back to Exercise 4.2 if you need help adding existing patients to the schedule.

2. Add the reason note *UTI* (urinary tract infection) to Sally's appointment and the reason note *Lab* to Robert.
3. Add your initials after the notes that you add to the schedule.

Exercise 4.6 Adding Additional Patients to the Schedule

Add two new patients to the appointment schedule, along with the appropriate reason notes. You may make up the names of your patients and the reasons for their visits.

Note: Remember, these are *New/Unregistered* patients, so you will not be able to search for them in the database.

Exercise 4.7 Scheduling a Meeting in a Future Schedule

1. From the main *Practice View* screen, click on the last Friday of the month on the calendar in the upper left corner.
2. In the appointment window for that date, click on the 4:30 p.m. *OPEN* time slot.
3. When the *Edit Appointment* window appears, type *Staff Meeting* in the *Note* field.
4. Click on the [Block This Time] button.
5. Repeat this exercise for each 10-minute increment until an entire half hour is blocked for the staff meeting. (You do not need to repeat "Staff Meeting" for subsequent time slots.)
6. Block out time in the schedule for a half-hour staff meeting on the last Friday of each month for the next 3 months. Close the additional appointment windows by clicking the red [X] in the upper right corner of each window.

Exercise 4.8 Charting a No Show

1. Click on your name on the appointment schedule.
2. Click on the [Chart No Show] button in the *Edit Appointment* window.
3. Save the No Show documentation in the *Save As* window under the *Encounter* tab by clicking on the [Save] button.
4. The program will indicate the charting of the No Show.
5. Click on the [Get Chart] button in the *Edit Appointment* window.
6. Click on the "+" sign to the left of the *Encounter* tab in the upper right panel of the patient's chart to view the No Show entry.
7. Click on the No Show entry to view the details in the lower window.
8. The No Show note can be further modified by clicking on the [Edit] button in the lower right window of the patient's chart.
9. In the *Note* window, type a fictitious reason for the missed appointment after the phrase "Missed Appointment for:"
10. Click the [Done] button.
11. Resave the No Show note under the *Encounters* tab and select the [Save and Skip Billing] option key.
12. Close the patient's chart and close the *Edit Appointment* window

Exercise 4.9 Printing the Patient Schedule

1. Print the current patient schedule by clicking on the [Print schedule] button in the upper right corner of the office schedule.
2. Circle your name on the schedule.
3. Submit the printed schedule to your instructor.

4.3 Patient Tracker

Most ambulatory EHR programs record the location and status of patients as they transition from one area to another within the medical clinic. By recording this information electronically, the medical office also has a record of when the patient arrived and left the clinic. This is important not only as a historic record of when the patient was at the clinic, but also for legal verification. When a patient is on the clinic premises and under the supervision of clinical staff, the medical office carries limited liability for the patient's well being and safety. Being able to record dates and times when the patient was under direct healthcare supervision is critical for proving or refuting legal responsibility.

Another important purpose for being able to electronically display patient location and status in the clinic is to allow staff members to see at a glance on the computer screen where each patient is and what is happening to him or her at that time. Figure 4.7 shows the ***Patient Tracker*** window in the SpringCharts system. This function provides for greater efficiency in the office, reducing the need to locate staff members and to communicate verbally when and where the patient needs to be seen.

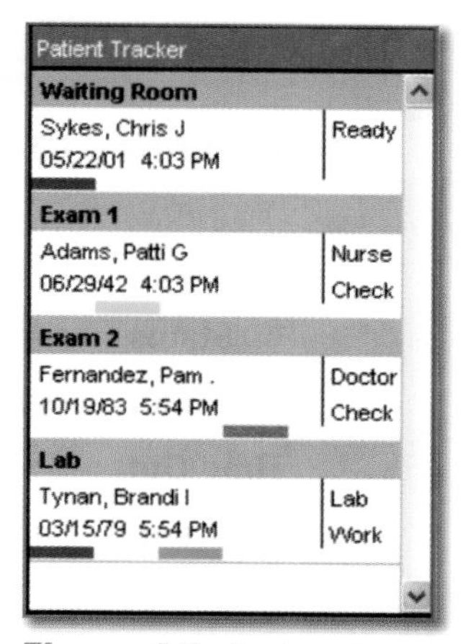

Figure 4.7 *Patient Tracker* window.

Patient Tracker
The *Patient Tracker* function enables all users across the network to see at a glance the current location and status of all patients in the clinic. It records the time each patient enters and leaves the clinic.

Focal Point

Only existing patients can be added to the *Patient Tracker* from the appointment schedule. New patients need to be set up in the database first before being added to the *Patient Tracker.*

The *Patient Tracker* window is located at the upper right side of the *Practice View* screen. Patients can be added to the *Patient Tracker* by clicking once on their name in the schedule. When the *Edit Appointment* window displays (Figure 4.8), the user selects the [Track Pt] button, and the patient is added to the *Patient Tracker* feature.

When the [Track Pt] button is selected, the *Edit Tracker* window appears; the first item in the *Location* list is highlighted by default. This is typically the *Waiting Room* (Figure 4.9). The front-office user clicks [Done] when this window opens to add the selected patient into the *Patient Tracker,* displaying the patient's location as the waiting room. The tracker feature also displays the patient's date of birth and the time he or she was added to the tracker (*Time In*) (Figure 4.9).

If an unscheduled patient comes into the office, the user clicks on the *Patient Tracker* title bar (shown in margin) and selects the patient by typing the last name in the search field of the *Choose Patient* window. This function is useful for clinics that allow walk-in patients. However, to add a walk-in patient to the tracker, whether from the schedule or by clicking on the *Patient Tracker* title bar, the patient first needs to be set up as an existing patient in the database; a *New/Unregistered* patient who has never been seen at the clinic will not be in the database.

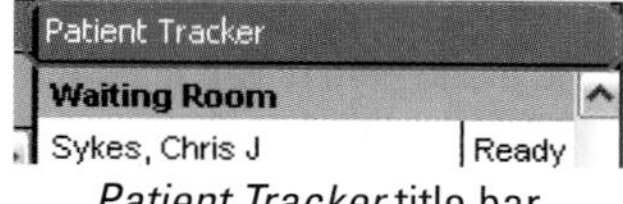

Patient Tracker title bar

SpringCharts Tip

It is important to add patients to the *Patient Tracker* as soon as they arrive in the clinic. The program time-stamps the tracker record when a patient is added. This information may be important at a later time when determining the exact time a patient was in the clinic. The program also time-stamps the tracker record when the patient is checked out of the clinic.

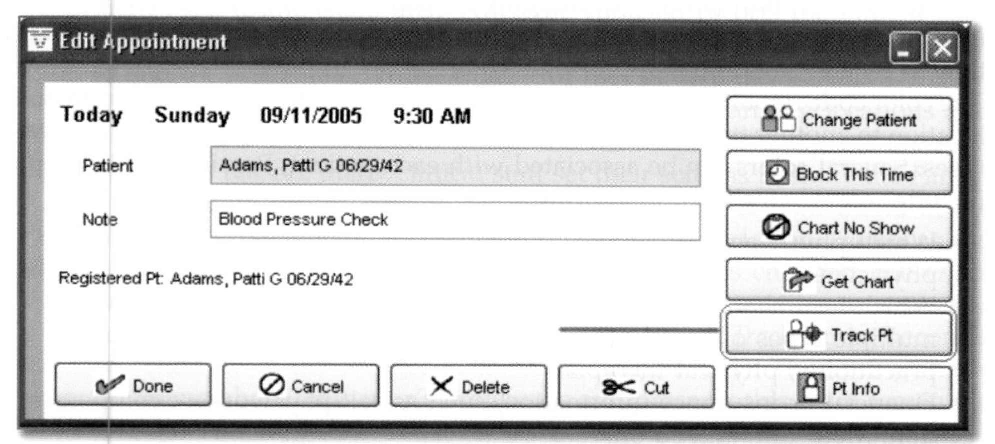

Figure 4.8 Tracking a patient from the *Edit Appointment* window.

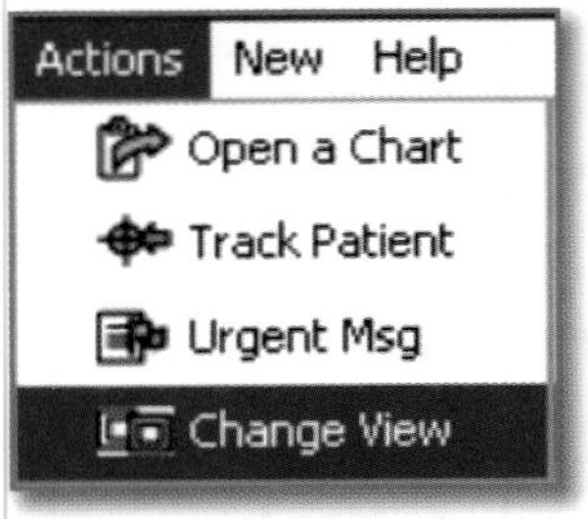

Figure 4.10 Changing the main view through the *Actions* menu.

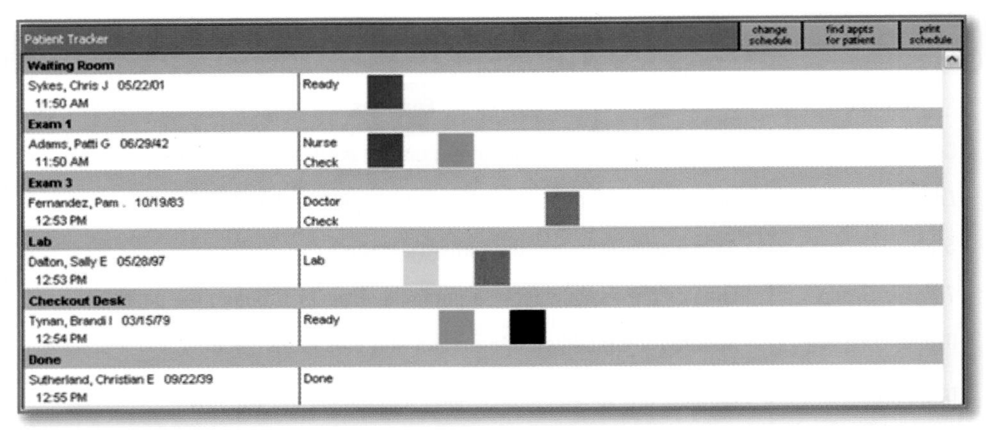

Figure 4.11 *Patient Tracker* window as the main screen.

SpringCharts Tip

Setting up distinct *Tracker Groups* may also be useful for single clinics that have more than one waiting area, for example, a pediatrician's office that has separate sick and well child waiting rooms. In this case, based upon the user logged on, the *Practice View* screen would show either the sick child tracker list or the well child tracker list.

Tracker Group

Clinics that have offices in more than one location usually operate from the same SpringCharts database, enabling all locations to access complete patient healthcare information via the Internet. For a clinic to track the location of each patient separately, *Tracker Groups need to be setup* on the SpringCharts server (e.g., Northside Clinic, Southside Clinic, and so on). Then a specific *Tracker Group* can be assigned to each patient, along with his or her *Location* and *Status*, in the *Edit Tracker* window (Figure 4.12). In the *Set User Preferences* window described in Chapter 3, the user chooses the appropriate default *Tracker Group*; once logged on to SpringCharts, the program only shows the patients from this specific *Tracker Group* in the *Patient Tracker* window for this user.

If *Show All* is selected in the *Tracker Group* field in the *Set User Preferences* window, the user sees a list of all patients presently in the *Patient Tracker* grid, including all clinics or all clinic areas.

Focal Point

The *Tracker Group* option can be set up for clinics that have separate locations but share the same EHR database, or for a single medical office with more than one waiting room.

Patient Info

Patient demographic information can be viewed, modified, and printed from the *Edit Tracker* window by clicking on the [Pt Info] button (Figure 4.12) which

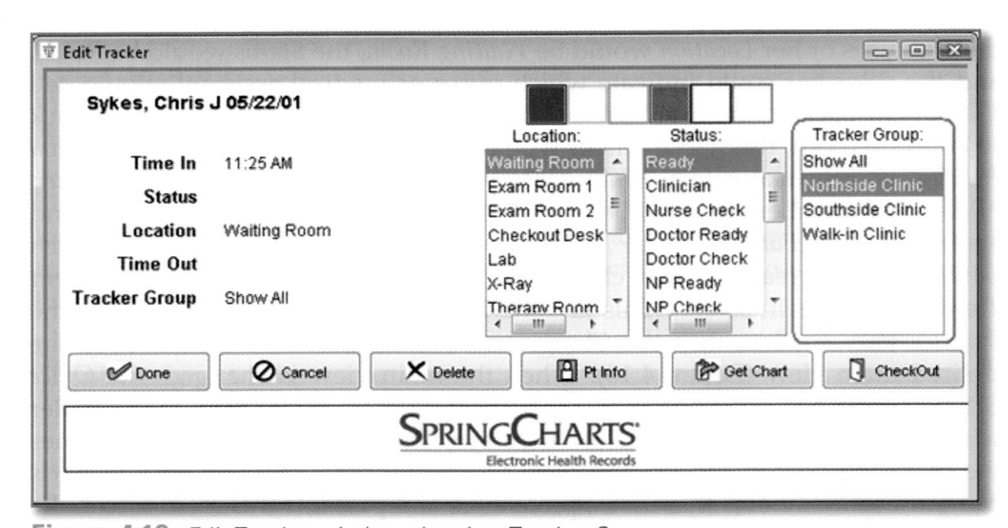

Figure 4.12 *Edit Tracker* window showing *Tracker Groups*.

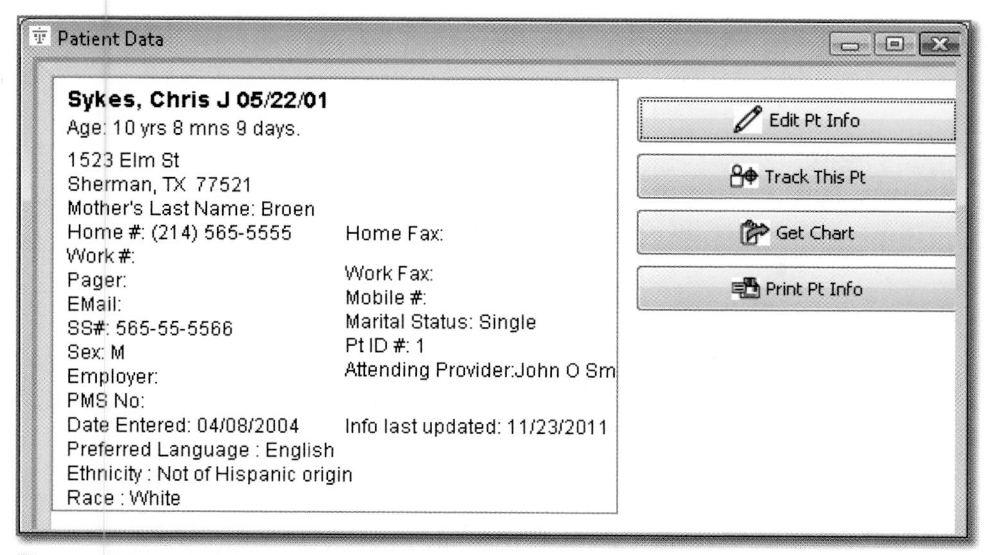

Figure 4.13 *Patient Data* window.

opens the *Patient Data* window. To edit the patient's information, the user clicks on the [Edit Pt Info] button in the *Patient Data* window (Figure 4.13) and make any necessary updates to the patient's demographics.

Check Out

When a patient is checked out of the facility, the receptionist selects the [Check Out] button in the *Edit Tracker* window (Figure 4.12). The patient's name moves out of the previous location heading in the *Patient Tracker* and moves to the *Done* category heading. The patient's status also changes to *Done* in the right column of the *Patient Tracker,* and the color codes for the patient are removed (Figure 4.14). The system then logs the checkout time for the patient, which can be viewed in the *Time Out* field of the *Edit Tracker* window for all "Done" patients.

In the *Patient Tracker* window, SpringCharts also displays a notification when a **routing slip** has been generated for the patient after a billed encounter. When a routing slip is created at the completion of a billable office visit, the tracker shows a pink checked *Routing Slip* stamp (Figure 4.14). The routing slips for billable encounters are located under the *Edit*

SpringCharts Tip

In a medical clinic that has an interface linking SpringCharts to a PMS program, patient information is often imported automatically into SpringCharts from the PMS. If this is the case, changes to the patient's demographics are entered in the PMS program, and the modifications are automatically updated in SpringCharts.

Routing slip

This charge ticket or superbill contains the healthcare codes, description, and charges relevant to a patient's visit.

Figure 4.14 *Patient Tracker* window showing a checked-out patient.

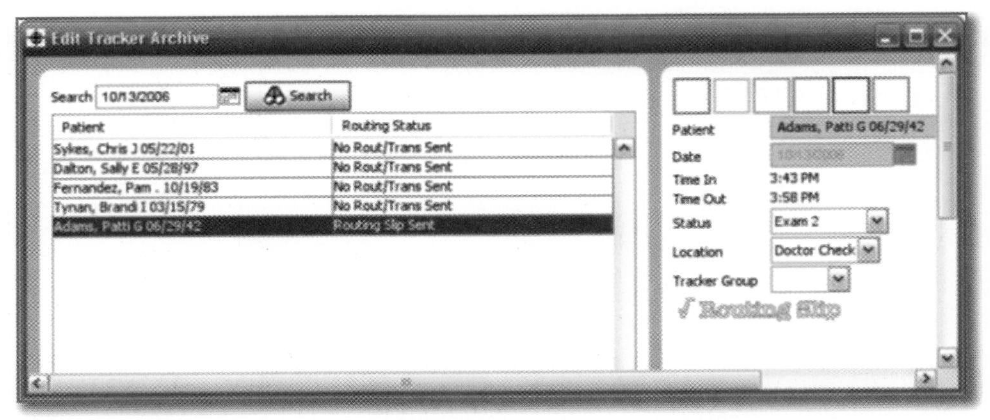

Figure 4.15 *Edit Tracker Archive* window.

menu at the top of the *Practice View* screen, under the *Routing Slips* submenu. From here, routing slips can be printed out and manually entered into the PMS program for billing or sent to a third-party billing company. When an EHR program is interfaced with a PMS program, billing transactions may be sent electronically to the PMS software; in this case a routing slip would not be created. (Routing slips will be discussed in more detail in Chapter 6.)

Tracker Archive

A record of patients who have been tracked through the *Patient Tracker* is maintained in the EHR system's *Tracker Archive.* To view these records, the user selects the *Tracker Archive* submenu from the *Edit* menu in the main *Practice View* screen. The *Edit Tracker Archive* window then appears (Figure 4.15). In the *Search* field, the user types the desired date or selects a date via the calendar icon, and all patients tracked for that date appear in the window, along with such details as times logged in and out of the tracker and whether a routing slip was created. The *Tracker Archive* feature is useful when determining what time a patient entered and left the medical clinic.

Concept Checkup 4.3

A. What two elements are staff able to see at a glance in the *Patient Tracker* concerning patients in the clinic?

B. What menu and submenu will a user select to set the *Patient Tracker* as the main screen?

C. Where is the *Tracker Archive* feature located?

Note: If you work the following set of exercises (4.10 through 4.21) on a different day to completing the previous set of exercises, you will need to complete Exercises 4.2 and 4.5 again before you begin.

Exercise 4.10 Changing the Status of a Patient in the Tracker

1. Log on to SpringCharts. Close the Tutorial window.
2. Click on the patient *Chris Sykes* in the *Patient Tracker* feature.
3. Change the *Status* in the *Edit Tracker* window to *Ready.*
4. Click the [Done] button.
5. Click on the patient *Patti Adams* in the *Patient Tracker* feature.
6. In the *Edit Tracker* window, change the *Status* of *Patti Adams* to *Nurse Ready.*
7. Click the [Done] button.

Exercise 4.11 Adding a Patient to the Tracker

1. Add *Sally Dalton* to the *Patient Tracker* by clicking once on her name in the *Office Schedule.*
2. Select the [Track Pt] button. Notice that the program automatically selects *Waiting Room* as the default location and stamps the time Sally Dalton was entered into the *Patient Tracker.*
3. Without selecting any information in this window, click [Done].

Exercise 4.12 Assigning Color Codes to Patients in the Tracker

Assume you are working in a clinic that has allocated color flags as follows:

- *Blue—A patient visit for Dr. Finchman*
- *Yellow—A patient visit for a nurse check only*
- *Green—A self-pay patient*
- *Red—A patient visit for lab work only*
- *Black—A patient visit for a specific office procedure*
- *Fuchsia—A Medicaid patient*

1. Click on Sally Dalton's name in the *Patient Tracker.*
2. In the *Edit Tracker* window, click on the appropriate color flags along the top of the window to indicate that Sally is coming in for a nurse check and has Medicaid as her primary insurance.
3. Assign her a *Ready* status.
4. Click the [Done] button.
5. Click on *Chris Sykes* in the *Patient Tracker.*
6. In the *Edit Tracker* window, change his location to *Exam Room 2.*
7. Give Chris a status of *Nurse Check.*
8. Click the [Done] button to save him back into the tracker.

Exercise 4.13 Communicating to Co-workers through the Tracker

As the clinician assigned to Patti Adams in Exam Room 1 you are recording the patient's chief complaints and taking her vital signs.

1. Open the tracker item and select *Nurse Check* as the status the click the [Done] button.
2. Now that you have finished with the initial intake, update the *Patient Tracker* by changing the status of *Patti Adams* to *Doctor Check* and click the [Done] button. Dr. Smith will notice the update on his *Patient Tracker* and know the location of the patient who now requires his attention.

Exercise 4.14 Moving a Patient into the Tracker

Robert Underhagen arrives at the clinic and is taken to the clinic's lab room for his appointment.

1. Select *Robert Underhagen* from the schedule.
2. Click the [Track Pt] button in the *Edit Appointment* window.
3. Place Robert in the *Lab Area* location with the status of *Clinician.*
4. Indicate by designating color codes that this is a *Nurse Check Only* and for *Lab Work Only.*
5. Click the [Done] button.

Exercise 4.15 Making the *Patient Tracker* the Main Screen

Assume you work in the clinic area of the medical office. You decide to make the *Patient Tracker* appear as the main screen on your computer.

1. Click on the *Actions* menu at the top of the *Practice View* screen.
2. Select the *Change View* option.
3. Select the *Tracker* option.

Exercise 4.16 Assigning a Walk-in Patient to the Tracker

A walk-in patient has arrived at the clinic. The patient is not on the schedule, but she is an established patient.

1. Click one time on the *Patient Tracker* title bar.
2. Type the last name *Zigman* in the *Choose Patient* window and conduct a search.
3. Select the patient *April Zigman.*
4. Click [Done] in the *Edit Tracker* window to add April to the tracker.

Exercise 4.17 Changing the Tracker Location and Status

Assume you are the doctor, and you are now finished with the patient examination in Exam Room 1.

1. Click on Patti Adams's name in the tracker.
2. In the *Edit Tracker* window, change the patient's location to *Checkout Desk.*
3. Change her status to *Ready.*
4. Click the [Done] button.

Exercise 4.18 Moving a Patient from One Location to Another in the Tracker

Exam Room 1 is now available for another patient.

1. Click on *Chris Sykes* in the tracker.
2. In the *Edit Tracker* window, change the status of the patient to *Doctor Check.*
3. Click the [Done] button.
4. Click on *Sally Dalton* in the tracker.
5. Move *Sally Dalton* into the *Exam Room 1* location.
6. Change Sally's status to a *Nurse Check.*
7. Click the [Done] button.

Exercise 4.19 Checking out a Patient in the Tracker

Patti Adams has been processed at the front desk by setting another appointment and paying her co-pay.

1. Click on Patti's name in the tracker.
2. Click on the [Check Out] button in the *Edit Tracker* window. Notice that the program changes the patient's location and status to *Done* and removes the color flags from the patient's listing. The window automatically closes.

Exercise 4.20 Adding More Patients to the Tracker

1. Add yourself to the *Patient Tracker* by first clicking on your name in the *Office Schedule* in the upper right corner of the screen.
2. Click on the [Track Pt] button.
3. Give yourself the location of *Waiting Room* and the status of *Ready.*

Exercise 4.21 Working with the *Tracker Archive*

1. Click on the *Edit* menu on the main *Practice View* screen.
2. Click on the *Tracker Archive* submenu. The *Edit Tracker Archive* window displays the patients who were processed through the *Patient Tracker* today.
3. Click on *Patti Adams* and notice the *Time In* and *Time Out* stamps on the right-side panel.
4. Click on the [Export] button (shown in margin).
5. Select the *Export List* option.
6. Select the *Open in Word Processor* button in the *Export Tracker List* window.
7. Select the *File* menu and then the *Print* option. Close the word processor window.
8. Print out the list of patients, circle your name, and submit the list to your instructor.
9. Close the *Edit Tracker Archive* window.

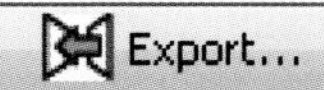

Export button

Focal Point

The *ToDo/Reminder* feature is a user-defined item that replaces the need for reminder notes.

4.4 To Do Lists and Reminders

Every member of a healthcare clinic staff is responsible for specific administrative duties in the medical office. The duties may be as simple as ordering sanitized hand wipes or as complex as discussing lab results over the telephone with a patient. Whatever the task, each staff member creates reminder notes and schedules future activities so that all actions, from the mundane to the more involved, are executed on time and with efficiency. Rather than adhering sticky notes to computer monitors throughout the office as reminders, SpringCharts provides each user with his/her own center for to-do lists and reminders so that all staff members can complete their duties with ease.

To Do List

To Do List title bar

The *To Do List* is located just below the calendar on the left side of the *Practice View* screen. This feature is user-defined, meaning that each user, when logging on to the system, only sees the items she or he entered previously. A user's to-do list is stored on the server, so the user sees the same exclusive to-do list from whichever computer in the network he or she uses to log on. A new to-do item can be created three ways: clicking once on the *To Do List* title bar (shown in margin), choosing *New ToDo* from the *New* menu on the main *Practice View* window, or selecting the *New To Do Item* speed icon on the Toolbar.

In the *New ToDo/Reminder* window (Figure 4.16), users can:

- Enter a *ToDo/Reminder* item and send it to the *To Do List.*
- Send the item to another co-worker.
- Link the item to a patient.
- Schedule the *ToDo/Reminder* item for themselves or a co-worker for a future date.

Focal Point

The *ToDo/Reminder* feature enables a user to send a reminder to him- or herself or a co-worker, link it to a patient, and schedule it for a future date.

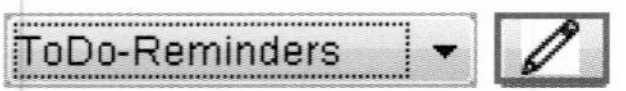

Pop-up text edit icon

In the *New ToDo/Reminder* window, the user enters the *ToDo/Reminder* message in the empty text field at the top of the window or selects **pop-up text** from the list in the right window. To add options to this pop-up text menu for current and future use, the user simply clicks on the *Edit* pencil icon to the right of the drop-down list (shown in margin). The link opens the *Edit PopUp Text* window, where the user can add, delete, or modify text in many different categories used in the system.

Pop-up text
Pop-up text is large groups of predefined text that SpringCharts users can rapidly select to complete office visit notes, letters, reports, messages, and to-do/reminder lists. The program includes 34 static categories and 20 categories of pop-up text that can be customized to suit the needs of each user. Each category has the capacity to hold 60 lines of customized type.

When a user sends a *ToDo/Reminder* item to him- or herself, it is stored in the personal *To Do List* (Figure 4.17), until the reminder item is completed.

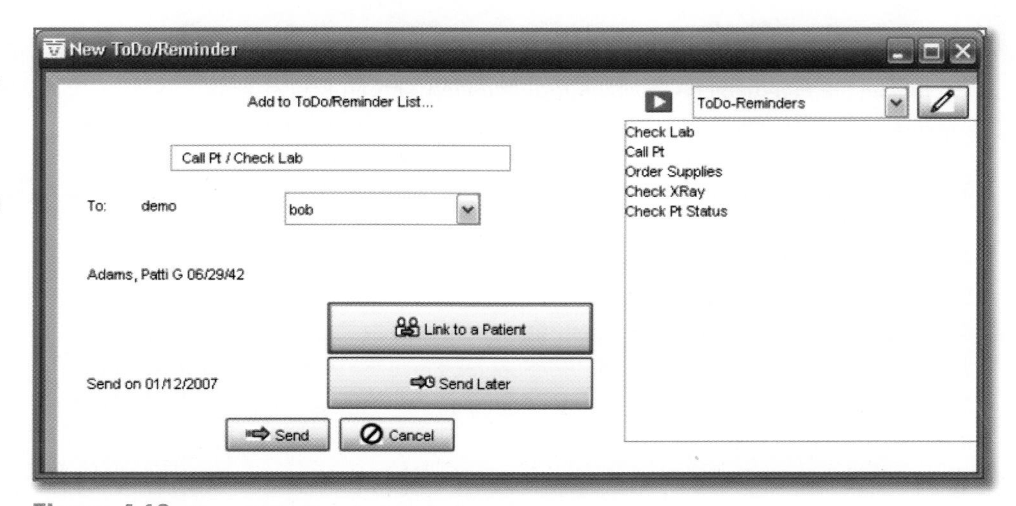

Figure 4.16 *New ToDo/Reminder* window.

When *ToDo/Reminder* items are saved, the program automatically assigns each item one of four possible color codes:

1. A *ToDo/Reminder* item with a green bar on the right is active and stays on the user's list until it is selected by clicking on the item. Doing so changes it from an active item to a completed one, indicated by a red checked box (Figure 4.17); clicking it again reactivates the to-do item with the original color bar.
2. A *ToDo* item with a blue bar on the right indicates that the item is linked to a patient. When this item is selected, the patient's chart opens automatically, and the item is checked as completed. Selecting the item again reactivates it with the original color bar.
3. A *ToDo* item with an orange bar indicates communication between a user and an administrator regarding requested changes to the time clock feature. (The time clock feature will be discussed in Chapter 10.)
4. A *ToDo* item with a red check is a completed item. The next time this user logs on, completed items with the check mark will not be included in the list. Clicking on a red check box before the user logs off activates the *ToDo* item again. All items without a red check box continue to roll over each day until completed.

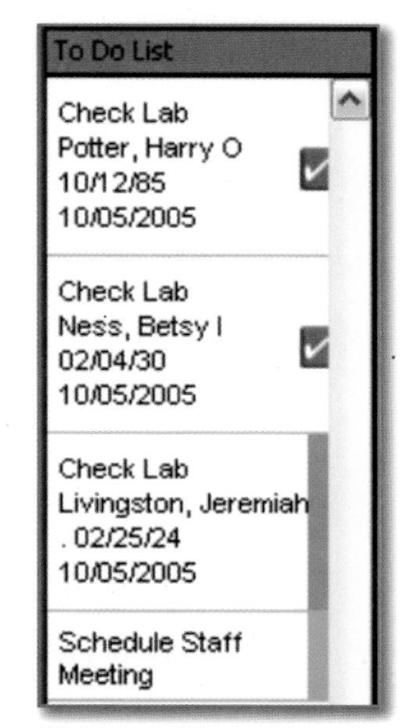

Figure 4.17 *To Do List* items.

ToDo/Reminders can be linked to a patient or a future date, and can be sent to another recipient, in which case the item appears on that colleague's *To Do List* on the selected date, indicating from whom the *ToDo/Reminder* came. An item linked to a specific patient is marked with a blue color bar and opens the patient's chart when the recipient clicks on the to-do item.

Essentially, *ToDo/Reminder* items are simple instructions and reminders of tasks that need to be performed. A user cannot respond back to a *ToDo/Reminder* item sent from a co-worker.

SpringCharts Tip

If co-workers need to communicate back to the sender regarding the task, they can do so via the SpringCharts EHR messaging system; the *ToDo/Reminder* system cannot be used for that purpose.

My ToDo List

Current and future scheduled *ToDo/Reminder* items can be accessed from the main *Practice View* screen by selecting *Edit* menu and then the *My ToDo List* submenu. In the *Edit ToDo* window (Figure 4.18), items can be reassigned to different users and/or reset to a different due date. Pop-up text can also be edited, and nonlinked items can be linked to a patient. Once modifications have been made, the user clicks the [Save] button, and the corresponding item in the user's *To Do List* is updated. New *ToDo/Reminder* items can also be created from the *Edit ToDo* window (Figure 4.18); the program automatically adds the newly created items to the user's *To Do List* on the main screen.

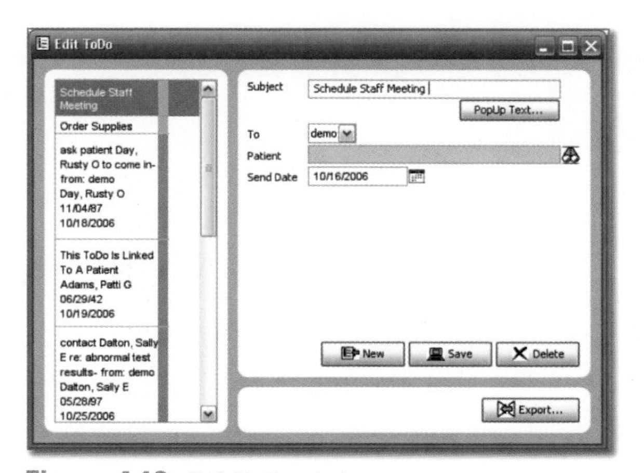

Figure 4.18 *Edit ToDo* window.

Concept Checkup 4.4

A. What occurs with a red-checked *ToDo/Reminder* item the next time the user logs back into SpringCharts?

B. What occurs when a user clicks on a *ToDo/Reminder* item marked with a blue bar?

C. A user can link a *ToDo/Reminder* item to a patient and assign a future date when it will show up in the *To Do List.* What else can a user do with a *ToDo/Reminder* item?

Exercise 4.22 Setting a Reminder

1. Click on the *To Do List* title bar.
2. At the top of the *New ToDo/Reminder* window, type *Schedule Staff Meeting* in the empty item field.
3. Click on the [Send] button. Notice that the new *ToDo* item has been added to your *To Do List,* with a green bar next to it.
4. Assume you have completed the task, and click the *Schedule Staff Meeting* to-do item. Notice the program adds a red check box to the item, indicating it has been completed. The next time you log on to SpringCharts, this item will have been removed from your *To Do List.*

Exercise 4.23 Setting a Patient Reminder

1. Click on the *To Do List* title bar.
2. In the *New ToDo/Reminder* window, select *Call Pt* and *Check Lab* from the pop-up text panel at right.
3. Click the [Link to a Patient] button.
4. In the *Choose Patient* window, type *"under"* and conduct a search.
5. Select *Robert Underhagen.*
6. Select the [Send] button. Notice that the new to-do item has been added to your *To Do List,* with a blue color bar beside it, indicating it is linked to a patient.
7. Assume you have completed the task. Click on the Robert Underhagen *ToDo* item. The patient's chart opens, enabling you to access his telephone number and other important information.
8. Close the patient's chart by clicking on the red [X] in the upper right corner of the chart. Notice the red checked box added to this item in your *To Do List.* The item will be removed when you log off SpringCharts and will *not* appear in your *To Do List* the next time you log on.

Exercise 4.24 Sending a *ToDo* Item to Another User

1. Open a *New ToDo/Reminder* window by clicking on the *To Do List* title bar.
2. From the pop-up text menu at right, select *Order Supplies.*
3. In the ToDo field, after the phrase *Order Supplies,* type bandages.
4. In the *To* drop-down list at left, select *Jan.*
5. Select the [Send Later] button and choose any date next month.
6. Click the [Send] button. This *ToDo* item will appear in Jan's *To Do List* on that specific date.

Exercise 4.25 Sending a Future *ToDo* Item to Yourself

1. Create a new, fictitious *ToDo/Reminder* for yourself by typing or selecting pop-up text in the right side of the *New ToDo/Reminder* window.
2. Link the item to the patient *Rusty Day* by clicking on the [*Link* to a Patient] button.
3. Send it to yourself on any day in the future by clicking on the [Send Later] button. Click the [Send] button.
4. Go to the main *Edit* menu and select the *My ToDo List* submenu item.
5. Find the item you scheduled for yourself.
6. Click on the red [X] in the upper right corner to exit this window.

4.5 Internal Messages

Another administrative function of EHR programs is the ability to send and receive internal office messages between co-workers. Sending messages electronically allows for greater versatility than writing and delivering a message in a paper format. First, an electronic message trail is created that can be archived and stored in the patient's chart. Second, many items can be attached and sent along with the message, such as a patient's chart, details about medications, and patient information. The *Messages* center is a user-defined area, meaning that the user only sees his or her messages. Regardless of what computer the user logs on to, only the specific messages related to that user are seen in this feature of the EHR program.

Focal Point

The *Messages* center in SpringCharts enables the user to send and receive messages from co-workers within the office or between offices if the clinic has more than one location.

Figure 4.19 *Messages* window.

The *Messages* window (Figure 4.19) is located in the lower right quadrant of the main *Practice View* screen. To view a specific message, the user clicks on it in the *Messages* list. Messages are organized with the most recently received message at the top. The display shows who sent the message, the date and time it was sent, and the subject line.

Nonpatient Messages

A user can create a new message in three different ways: Click on the *Messages* title bar, choose *New Message* from the *New* menu on the main *Practice View* screen, or select the *Open New Message* speed icon (fifth from left) on the Toolbar. A dialog box appears, asking if this message concerns a patient. If the message does not concern a patient, the user clicks on the [No] button and a *New Message* window appears (Figure 4.20).

The user enters a subject line in the *Re:* field and types a message into the blank text area or selects pop-up text from the window to the right. To add to the pop-up text list for current and future use, the user can click on the Edit pencil icon (shown in margin) in the top right corner of the window. The link opens the *Edit PopUp Text* feature, which enables the user to add, delete, or modify text in the many different categories used in the system.

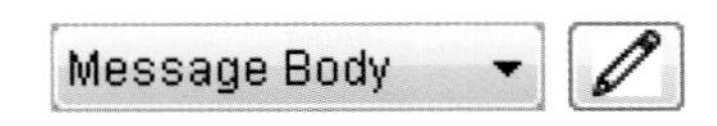

Edit PopUp Text icon

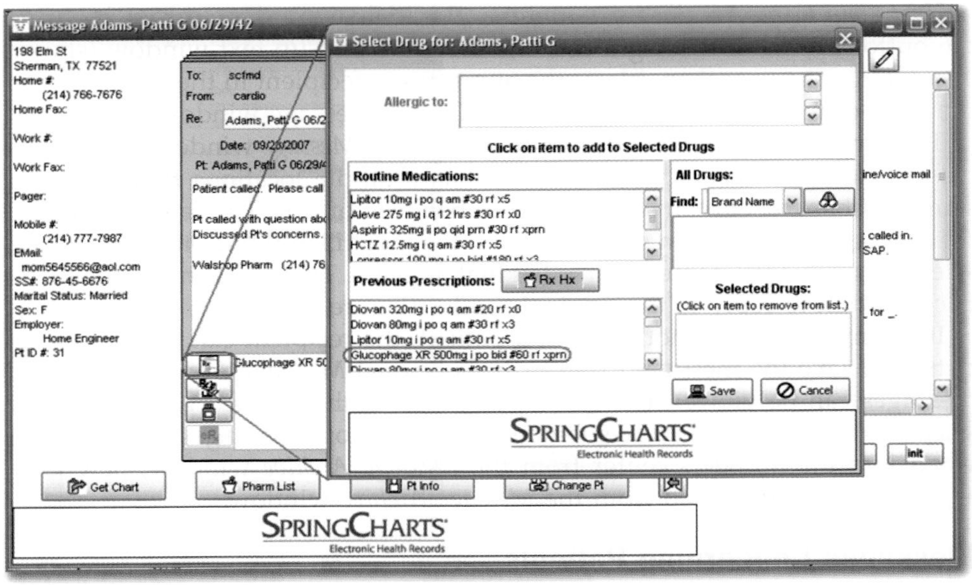

Figure 4.24 Access to the patient's medications.

might call the front office, wanting to discuss a medication with a nurse or request a medication refill. Rather than the staff member having to type the drug name and possibly misspelling it in a message to the clinician, the EHR program allows the user to select the medication from the patient's chart. The *Rx* icon button in the bottom section of the message window gives the user access to the patient's routine medications and previous prescriptions (Figure 4.24). In this window the user can also select additional medications from the program's database. Once the medication(s) is selected, the user clicks on the [Save] button, and it is added to the bottom section of the *New Message* window.

By clicking on the selected medication in the *New Message* window, the user can edit that specific medication (Figure 4.25), then click [Save]. Any changes

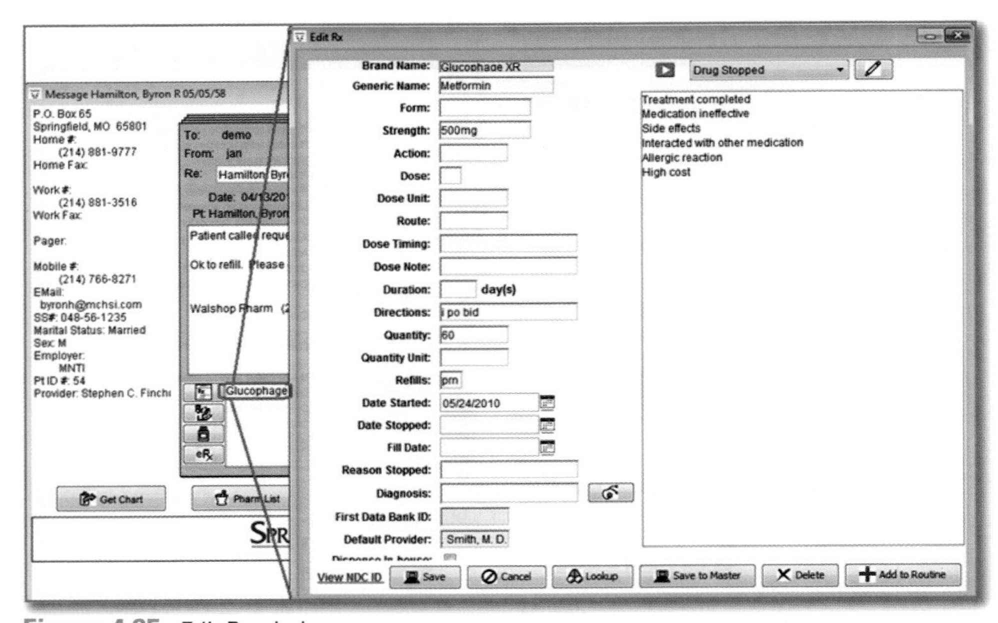

Figure 4.25 *Edit Rx* window.

only affect the medication information in the message; changes do not affect the original medication selected from the patient's chart. When the message is received, the recipient can print the prescription for the patient by using the prescription printer icon button (shown in margin) or electronically send the prescription to the pharmacy clearinghouse by using the electronic prescription icon button (shown in margin). Both are located in the bottom left corner of the message window.

(See Appendix A—*Sample Documents;* Sample 1. *Prescription Forms*).

When a message is finalized and no longer needed, the user clicks the [Chart It] button in the message window to automatically place the message into the patient's chart. An information window appears, notifying the user the message was charted in the patient's chart (Figure 4.26). The message is saved under the *Encounter* tab on the right side of the patient's chart by default or any other custom-designed tab selected by the user. To read or print the saved message at a later date, the user can access the message under the chart tab to which it was saved (Figure 4.27).

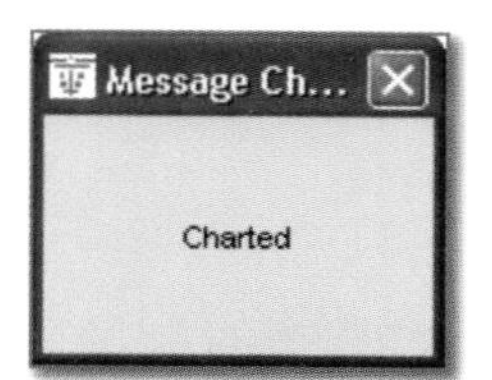

Figure 4.26 *Message Charted* notification.

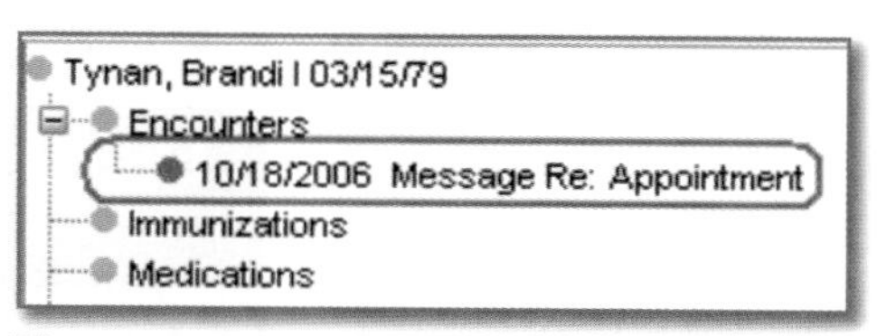

Figure 4.27 Message saved in patient's chart.

Concept Checkup 4.5

A. Identify the two types of messages that can be sent in SpringCharts.

B. What does the recipient have access to when a message is linked to a patient?

C. What button does the user click on to save a message to the patient's chart?

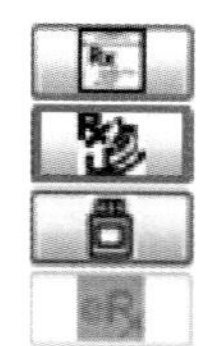

Prescription printer icon button in *New Message* window

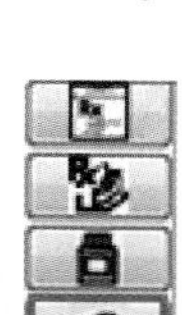

Electronic prescription icon button in *New Message* window

Exercise 4.26 Creating a Nonpatient Message

In this exercise, you are functioning as the office manager.

1. Click in the *Messages* title bar in the lower right quadrant of the main *Practice View* screen.
2. Click [No] to the *Link Message to Patient* dialog box question: *Does this message concern a Patient?*
3. In the subject line on the *New Message* window *(Re:)*, type *Staff Meeting.*
4. In the body of the message, write a note inviting staff to the meeting, giving the time and location.
5. Click the [MultiSend] button in the middle column of the *New Message* window.
6. Check all the staff including demo. Do not check the physicians.
7. Click on the [Send] button. Because you are logged in to the program as "Demo," note that the message appears in your own *Messages* center at the top of the list, including the subject, date, and time the message was sent.

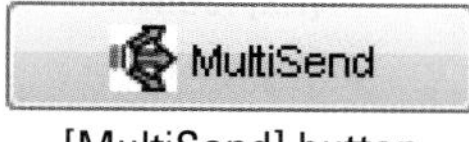

[MultiSend] button

Exercise 4.27 Archiving a Message

As the office manager, you would like to save the message created in Exercise 4.26 so you can send it out again next month.

1. Click on the *Staff Meeting* message in your *Messages* center.
2. Click on the [Save] button in the middle panel of the *Message* window. The program removes the message from the *Messages* center and indicates the message has been archived.

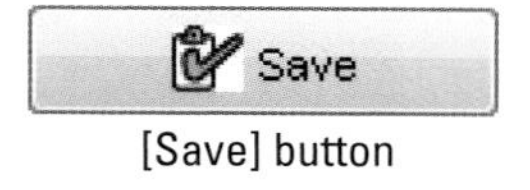

[Save] button

(continued)

Exercise 4.29 Sending an Urgent Message

New Urgent Message icon

1. Click on the *New Urgent Message* icon on the Toolbar of the *Practice View* screen.
2. From the *Send Urgent Message* window that appears, select *Demo* in the *To:* drop-down list.
3. Select *Urgent call from* in the pop-up text list. Add *Dr. Smith.* after the phrase *Urgent call from* in the message box.
4. Click the [Send] button. Typically the urgent message would be sent to the recipient's computer and appear on his or her screen. However, because you chose *Demo* as the recipient, the urgent message is delivered to your computer.

Exercise 4.30 Responding to an Urgent Message

Assume you are a practitioner who has received an urgent message on your computer screen.

1. In the pop-up text field of the *Urgent Message* window, select the following phrases: *OK. Thanks. Tell them I will call back later. Send me this info in a message.*
2. Click the [Send] button. Again, because you are in Demo mode, the reply to the urgent message is delivered to your computer.

Exercise 4.31 Creating a Regular Message from an Urgent Message

A practitioner has indicated that he or she cannot take a call now and wants you to forward an urgent message to him or her as a reminder to call Dr. Smith.

1. In the open *Urgent Message* window, click on the [Message] button.
2. Answer [No] to the question in the prompt window: *Does this message concern a Patient?*
3. In the subject line *(Re:)* in the *New Message* window that appears, type *Urgent Message.*
4. Select *Demo* in the drop-down *To:* field.
5. Click the [Send] button in the middle panel. The message will arrive at the top of your *Messages* center.
6. Retrieve the message from your *Messages* center by clicking on it.
7. Click in the body of the message under the phrase: *demo: Urgent call from Dr. Smith.*
8. Type your name in full.
9. Click on the [Print] button in the middle panel.
10. Click the [Print] button in the *Document Printing Options* window.
11. Print out the message, circle your name, and turn the page into your instructor.
12. Click on the red [X] in the upper right corner of the message window.

chapter 4 summary

Learning Outcomes	Key Concepts
4.1 Navigate the *Practice View* screen. **Pages 85–87**	The *Practice View* screen functions as an administrative center consisting of: • The *Appointment Schedule,* the *Patient Tracker, To Do List,* and the *Messages* center. • The *Appointment Schedule* and *Patient Tracker* are universal features. • The *To Do List* and *Messages* center are user-defined features. • The Toolbar displays speed icons to access most commonly used features.
4.2 Use the *Office Schedule* to add patients and notes to the schedule, add blocked time to the schedule, and chart "no shows." **Pages 87–92**	The appointment schedule gives clinicians real-time information regarding daily patient appointments schedule. The appointment calendar allows a user to: • Set up multiple office schedules. • Navigate to future and prior appointment schedules. • Add *Existing/Registered* and *New/Unregistered* patients to appointment schedule. • Block out events on the appointment schedule. • Locate past and future appointments for a patient.
4.3 Use the *Patient Tracker* to perform tasks such as change a patient's location and status, assign color codes, move patients, and check out patients. **Pages 93–101**	The *Patient Tracker* displays the location and status of each patient in the clinic. • Patients are added to the tracker from the appointment schedule or tracker header. • The tracker time-stamps each patient's entry of and departure from the clinic. • Location, status, *Tracker Group,* and color coding are elements of the tracker. • The *Patient Tracker* can be made into the main window in the *Practice View* screen. • The *Tracker Archive* feature keeps a history of patients who were placed in the tracker.
4.4 Use the *To Do List* to set reminders and send to-do items to yourself and another user. **Pages 102–105**	The *To Do List* is a user-defined feature that enables staff to easily execute administrative tasks such as: • Notate the *ToDo* item by typing or by using pop-up text. • Send a *ToDo* item to oneself or another co-worker immediately or for a future date. • Color bars indicate whether the *ToDo* item is linked to a patient or not. • Items linked to a patient will open the patient's chart once selected.
4.5 Create internal messages, both nonpatient and those concerning patients. **Pages 105–110**	The *Messages* center is a user-defined feature that enables clinicians to: • Create a message not related to a patient and send it to a co-worker(s). • Archive a nonpatient-related message. • Create a message related to a patient and send it to a co-worker(s). • Add a patient's medication to a message. • Chart a patient-related message in the patient's chart.
4.6 Demonstrate how to send and respond to an urgent message. **Pages 111–112**	• Urgent messages are created from the *Actions* menu or with a speed icon. • An urgent message is displayed on the recipient's computer screen. • Urgent messages can be saved in the regular *Messages* center.

chapter 4 review

Name ______________________ Instructor ______________ Class ______________ Date ______________

Using Terminology

Match the terms on the left with the definitions on the right.

_____ 1. **LO 4.2** No show

_____ 2. **LO 4.3** Patient status

_____ 3. **LO 4.3** Patient Tracker

_____ 4. **LO 4.1** Toolbar

_____ 5. **LO 4.4** Pop-up text

_____ 6. **LO 4.3** Routing slip

_____ 7. **LO 4.5** Message Archive

_____ 8. **LO 4.2** Appointment schedule

A. Offers a lineup of icons that gives the user shortcut access to the most commonly used functions of the program.

B. Where a sent or received message not regarding a patient is saved and can be reactivated.

C. A repository of text in SpringCharts enabling clinic staff rapid selection of predefined text.

D. Displays past, current, and future appointments for patients and time blocks for activities.

E. Indicates a patient missed a scheduled appointment without calling in advance to inform the clinic of his or her intentions or to reschedule.

F. Feature that enables all users across the network to see at a glance the current location and status of all patients in the clinic.

G. Allows the clinical staff to know in general terms what is currently happening with the patient or what needs to be done next.

H. Synonymous with a charge ticket or superbill and contains the healthcare codes, description, and charges relevant to the patient's visit.

Checking Your Understanding

Choose the best answer and circle the corresponding letter.

9. **LO 4.4** Which one of the following functions can be performed in the *New ToDo/Reminder* window?
   a) Send the item to another co-worker
   b) Change the location and status of the patient
   c) Send an urgent item to a co-worker
   d) Change the color code assigned to the patient

10. **LO 4.5** Two types of messages can be created from the *Messages* center. Select all that apply.
    a) Nonpatient message
    b) E-mail message to patient
    c) Patient-related message
    d) Urgent message

11. **LO 4.1** Which of the following features on the *Practice View* screen is user-defined?
    a) Office Schedule
    b) Patient Tracker
    c) ToDo/Reminder List
    d) Office Calendar

12. **LO 4.2** Which of the following features on the *Practice View* screen is network-defined? Select all that apply.
    a) Appointment Schedule
    b) ToDo/Reminder List
    c) *Messages* center
    d) Patient Tracker

13. **LO 4.6** To send an urgent message to a co-worker:
    a) Click on the *Actions* menu and select *Urgent Msg.*
    b) Yell with all your might in the co-worker's general direction.
    c) Create a message and click the [Send Now] button.
    d) Create a message from the *Messages* center then select the [Urgent] button.

14. **LO 4.3** A *Tracker Group* is best described as:
   a) Assigned staff who follow the patients around in the clinic to keep up with their whereabouts
   b) Categories given to patients in order to track various disease groups
   c) A classification assigned to a patient in clinics with multiple locations
   d) A collection of locations and statuses in a medical clinic

15. **LO 4.3** A color code flagging in the *Patient Tracker* can indicate certain things, such as:
   a) Which physician is scheduled to examine the patient
   b) Which insurance carrier a patient has
   c) Which clinician is working with the patient
   d) Any of these

16. **LO 4.2** By using the appointment schedule, the user can:
   a) Schedule personal appointments.
   b) Navigate to prior or future appointments.
   c) Get the patient's pending tests.
   d) Send a message about a scheduled staff meeting.

17. **LO 4.4** A *ToDo* item that has a blue color bar in the *To Do List* indicates:
   a) The item is associated with a patient.
   b) The item is *not* associated with a patient.
   c) The item has been completed.
   d) The item concerns a requested change to the time clock.

18. **LO 4.5** An internal message in the EHR program enables users to:
   a) Record their thoughts, feelings, and hunger cycle.
   b) Send messages within the program to other co-workers.
   c) Send e-mails to providers outside the network.
   d) Send urgent messages to physicians.

19. **LO 4.4** To check on future, scheduled *ToDo* items, the user must:
   a) Send a message to the supervisor who tracks all future ToDo items.
   b) Click on the future date on the calendar and view the scheduled item.
   c) A user can only schedule current *ToDo* items.
   d) Go to the *Edit* menu and select *My ToDo List*.

20. **LO 4.6** Urgent messages function like instant messaging because they:
   a) Are created in and sent to the *Messages* center where the recipient accesses them in a timely manner
   b) Have the ability to be sent to multiple recipients
   c) Pop up on the computer screen of the recipient
   d) Are able to be attached to a patient's chart

21. **LO 4.1** Identify this icon from the Toolbar:
   a) *New Patient Tracker Item*
   b) *New ToDo Item*
   c) *Open New Message*
   d) *New Urgent Message*

22. **LO 4.1** Identify this icon from the Toolbar:

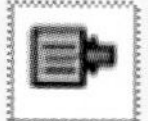

   a) *New Patient Tracker Item*
   b) *New ToDo item*
   c) *Open New Message*
   d) *New Urgent Message*

23. **LO 4.5** Identify this icon:

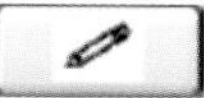

   a) *Edit Tracker Window*
   b) *Edit ToDo List Window*
   c) *Edit Message*
   d) *Edit PopUp Text*

24. **LO 4.5** Which button is found in the window of a message linked to a patient, but *not* in a nonpatient message window?
   a) [Chart It]
   b) [MultiSend]
   c) [Spell]
   d) [Send Back]

25. **LO 4.6** As a staff member, you receive a phone call the physician is expecting. You should:
   a) Create a new *ToDo* item and send it to the physician.
   b) Create a new message and send it to the physician.
   c) Notify the physician through the *Patient Tracker.*
   d) Create an urgent message and send it to the physician.

Applying Your Knowledge

Use your critical-thinking skills to answer the following questions.

26. **LO 4.4, LO 4.5** If you want to communicate to another co-worker that he or she needs to contact a patient regarding rescheduling an appointment and that you do not require a response, would you use the *ToDo/Reminder* system or the *Messages* system? Why would you use that feature instead of the other one?

27. **LO 4.2** You work as a front-office staff member in a family healthcare practice that allows "walk-in" patients. An individual enters the waiting room who is not scheduled on the appointment schedule, and you determine this person is a new patient. Do you enter the person as a "new patient" on the schedule, by typing his or her name directly in the *Patient* field of the *Edit Appointment* window, or do you first set this patient up in the database in the *New Patient* window, under the *New* menu of the *Practice View* screen? Please explain your answer.

28. **LO 4.3** You are working in the front office and an existing patient already in the EHR database enters the waiting room. You check the electronic appointment schedule and see that the patient is not on it. What is the quickest way you can place the patient in the *Patient Tracker* feature so the program records the exact time the patient entered the waiting room and became the clinic's responsibility?

5

The Patient Chart

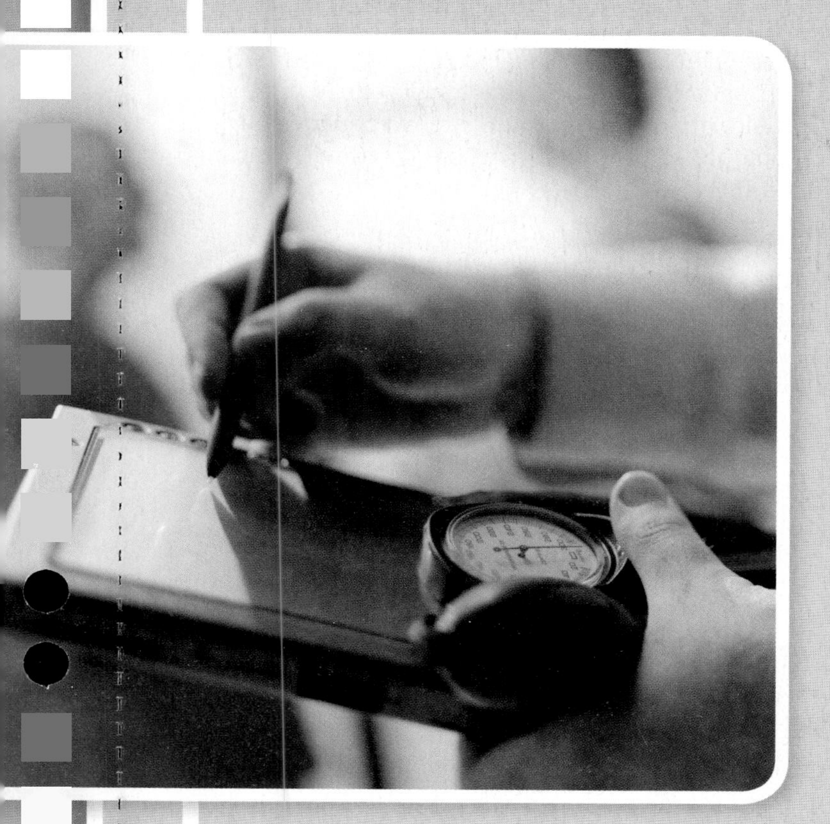

Learning Outcomes

After completing Chapter 5, you will be able to:

LO 5.1 Understand the layout of an electronic chart.

LO 5.2 Demonstrate how to build a patient's face sheet.

LO 5.3 Perform various procedures in a patient's chart.

LO 5.4 Create new documentation in a patient's chart.

What You Need to Know

To understand Chapter 5, you will need to know:

- How to start the SpringCharts EHR program
- How to set up new patients and edit patient information
- How to create an electronic patient chart
- How to enter and edit electronic pop-up text
- How to establish and edit electronic category preferences

Key Terms

Care tree

Category preferences

Chart Alert

Co-pay

Deductible

Encounters

Face sheet

Family medical history (FMHX)

Mandated reporters

Past medical history (PMHX)

Surveillance Reports

Introduction

The electronic chart is the repository for patient medical data created through computer automation in medical offices, clinics, and hospitals. Similar to the traditional paper chart, it holds static information, such as the patient's demographics, allergies, medical history, and medical problems, as well as dynamic, changing information, such as office visit notes, diagnostic tests, letters, and reports concerning the patient. *Static information* refers to information that is fixed and undergoes very little change, whereas *dynamic information* refers to information subject to change with each patient visit. This chapter describes the major parts of a patient's chart. You will learn how to create and store a patient's healthcare information and documentation, how to perform and document various procedures within the chart, and how to create new activities in the chart.

5.1 Overview of the Patient Chart

In EHR systems, electronic charts can be accessed from many different places in the program. In SpringCharts, the electronic chart can be accessed from the *Practice View* screen in several different ways by clicking on:

- The patient's name in the *Appointment Schedule* and selecting the [Get Chart] button
- The patient's name in the *Patient Tracker* and selecting the [Get Chart] button
- A *ToDo* item associated with a patient
- A message associated with a patient and selecting the [Get Chart] button
- The *Open a Patient's Chart* icon on the speed Toolbar (Figure 5.1)
- The *Actions* menu and then selecting *Open a Chart*
- The *Recent Charts* menu

Face sheet
This portion of the patient's chart contains relatively static patient information, such as allergies, problem list, past medical history (PMHX), and so on.

Care tree
This portion of the patient's electronic chart lists categories that store encounters (progress notes), tests, excuse notes, letters, reports, and other current records.

Encounters
This specific tab in the care tree of the patient's chart stores many of the documents created from encounters with the patient.

Figure 5.1 illustrates several options for accessing a patient's chart. The *Recent Charts* menu provides a drop-down window (Figure 5.2) that allows the user to access charts opened during the current log-on session.

Once the electronic chart is accessed by one of these methods, the *Patient Chart* window appears. A toolbar at the top of the patient's chart displays icons for the most commonly used chart features (Figure 5.3). These features can also be accessed from the main menu bar through drop-down menus. (*Note:* Some of the most common toolbar icons are featured in the SpringCharts Tips boxes in the margins throughout this text.)

The patient chart in the SpringChart EHR system is composed of the face sheet and care tree. The **face sheet** includes a series of panels on the left for displaying and editing comprehensive patient information that is relatively static, such as allergies, problem list, the patient's past healthcare issues, family medical issues, and so on (Figure 5.4). The dynamic **care tree** on the right side lists **encounters** (progress notes), tests, and other current records and documents.

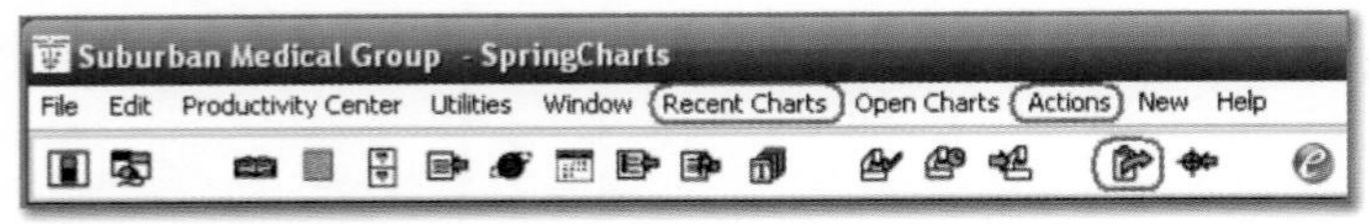

Figure 5.1 Examples of options for accessing a patient's chart from the *Practice View* screen.

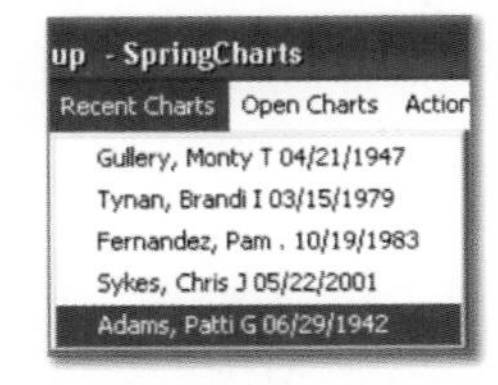

Figure 5.2 Accessing a patient's chart through the *Recent Charts* menu, opened during current log-on session.

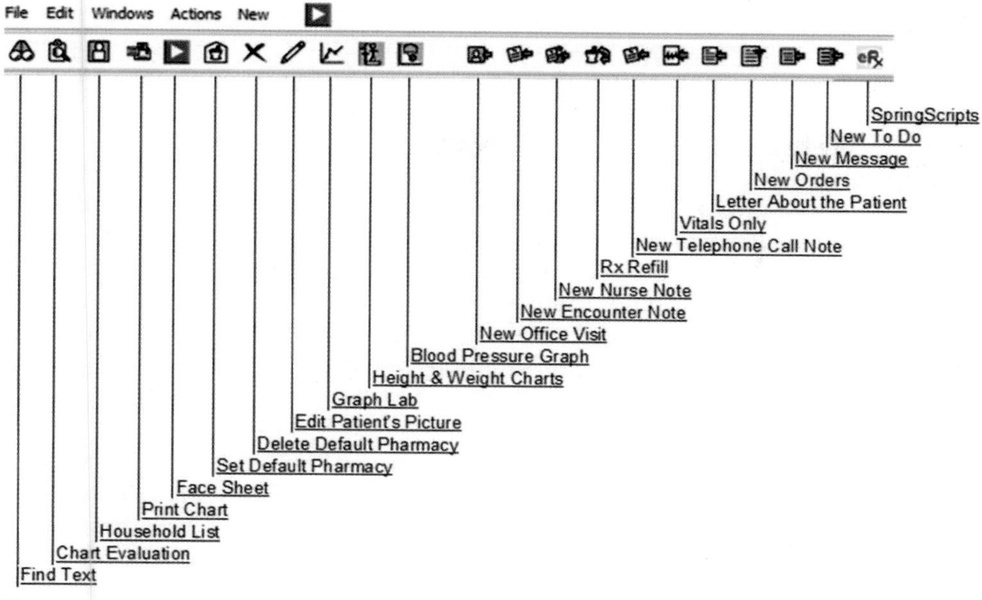

Figure 5.3 Patient chart toolbar with icon descriptions.

SpringCharts Tip

The *eRx* icon on the far right of the toolbar is only seen when the medical clinic has activated the e-prescribing feature of SpringCharts EHR.

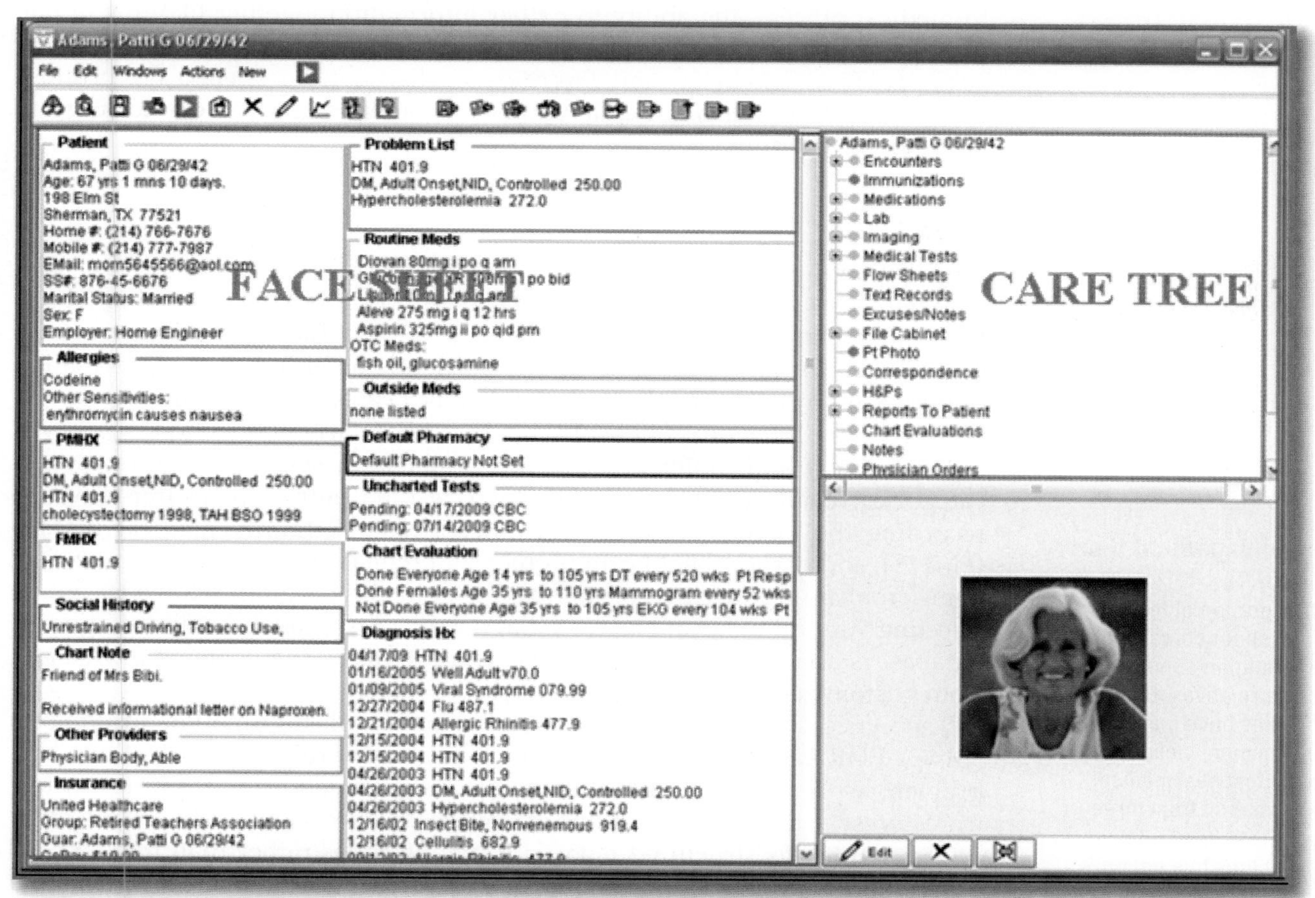

Figure 5.4 *Patient Chart* screen.

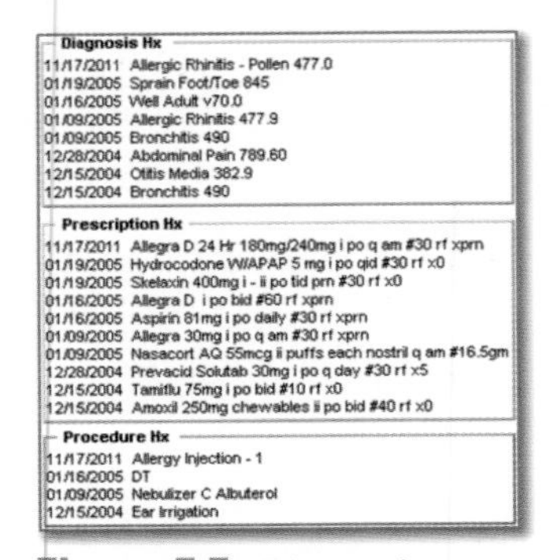

Figure 5.5 *Diagnosis Hx, Prescription Hx,* and *Procedure Hx* lists on the face sheet.

The program provides practitioners with a view of the entire chart at a glance—like having a paper chart open in front of you. All users can open—and edit—a patient's chart in the EHR program at the same time. However, data is protected because the same *specific area* of the chart cannot be edited simultaneously by different users. For example, one user can edit a patient's address while another enters lab results, but two users cannot edit the patient's address at the same time. In addition, the same user can open several different patient electronic charts simultaneously.

In interfaced environments with practice management system (PMS) software programs, patient demographics can be imported into SpringCharts EHR in real time. That is, when patient demographic information is added or modified in the PMS program, the information is sent electronically to the EHR program, creating a new patient chart there or modifying an existing patient's chart with the new information.

Three areas of the face sheet cannot be altered nor edited: the diagnosis history (*Diagnosis Hx*), prescription history *(Prescription Hx),* and procedure history *(Procedure Hx)* (Figure 5.5). The information contained in these areas is extracted from the patient's various encounters stored in the EHR program. As various diagnoses, prescriptions, and procedures are entered in the office visit note, they also appear on these lists in the face sheet, with the most recent item at the top. This function enables the practitioner to view the history of the patient's diagnoses, prescriptions, and procedures in one central place, rather than opening each encounter note and viewing the details of these areas. This is one of the significant benefits that EHR programs bring to medical offices—the ability to gather information together like this in one place is difficult, if not impossible, in a paper chart environment. The *Diagnosis Hx, Prescription Hx,* and *Procedure Hx* lists can be opened for printing by accessing the *Actions* menu within the patient's chart and selecting the appropriate heading.

Face Sheet

Open Face Sheet icon

Information can be added to or edited within the face sheet categories by clicking on the *Open Face Sheet* icon (shown in margin) on the chart menu bar (above the icon toolbar), in the *Patient Chart* screen. The *Edit Face Sheet* window allows clerical and clinical staff to quickly and efficiently enter healthcare information (Figure 5.6). Once the face sheet is open, the user can select any of the navigation buttons on the left side of the window to edit that particular section.

Pop-up text and preference lists are available in several of the face sheet categories to allow for quick and accurate data entry. For example, when recording the patient's personal healthcare history, **family medical history (FMHX)**, and chronic healthcare problems in the face sheet, the user can select items from user and clinic customized lists in the program. However, when selecting routine medications and diagnoses a drug database and diagnoses database is accessed for descriptions and codes rather than entered as free text from customized lists.

Family medical history (FMHX)
This portion of the patient's face sheet contains health information about a patient's close relatives. Because families have many factors in common, including genes and lifestyles, medical information from three generations of relatives can give clues to a patient's increased risk of developing a particular condition.

The Office of the National Coordinator for Health Information Technology (ONC) EHR regulations mandate that a patient's routine medications and problem list be transmitted to the SureScripts clearinghouse each time an electronic prescription is sent. For this reason, medications and problem lists must be transmitted as structured data with unique codes rather than free text. By transmitting these discrete values, the SureScripts interface is able to recognize the patient's routine medications and chronic medical problems. SureScripts

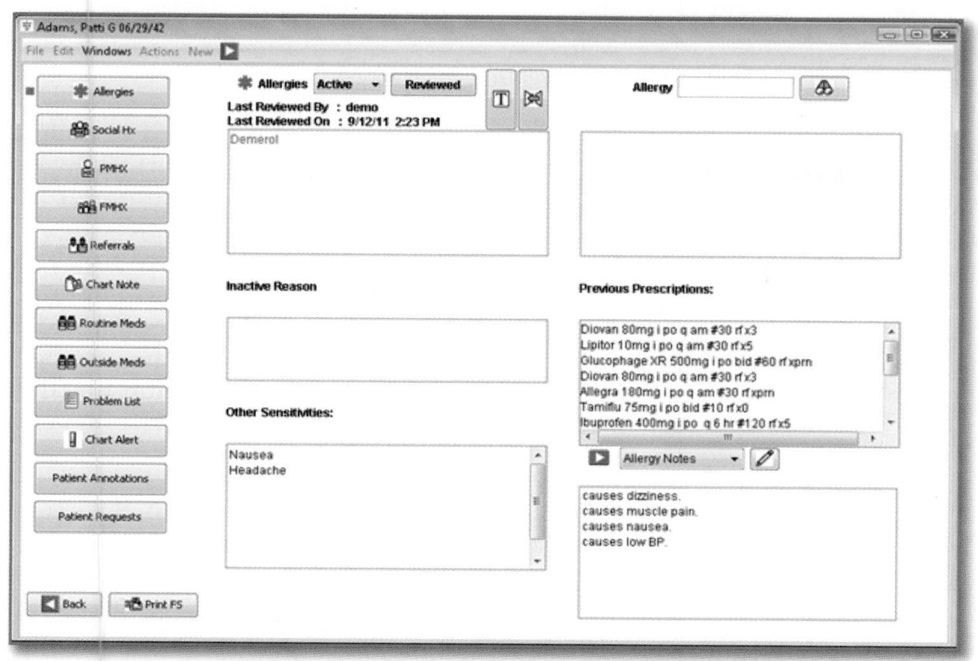

Figure 5.6 *Edit Face Sheet* window.

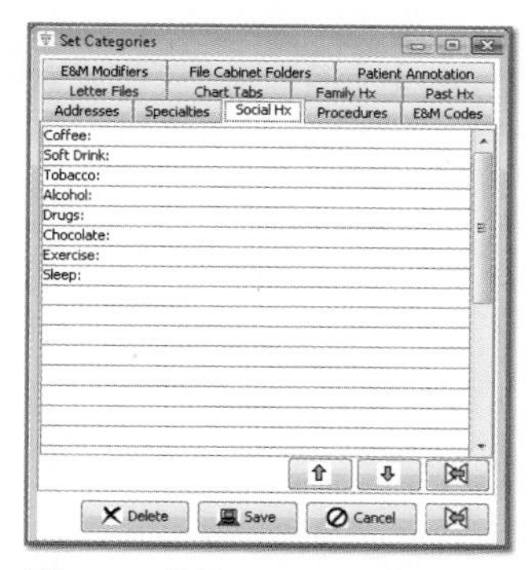

Figure 5.7 An example of a customized list in the category preferences table.

checks for drug interactions with medications the patient has been prescribed by other practitioners. Healthcare providers who use EHR programs to transmit electronic prescriptions help build collective databases that ensure patient safety and prevent substance abuse.

The social history, **past medical history (PMHX)**, and family medical history (FMHX) sections contain medical history lists that are set up in the **category preferences** table on the SpringCharts server (Figure 5.7) in a network environment or under the *Administration* menu on a single-user version. The category preferences table enables the clinic administrator to create customized lists of medical data. The lists are displayed in the EHR program, enabling users to rapidly select items with which to build the face sheet. These lists can be easily customized for each clinic based on the medical specialty, thereby displaying the most common items for that particular medical office. During initial setup on the SpringCharts server, the administrator may add up to 30 items in each category.

Past medical history (PMHX)
This portion of the patient's face sheet contains healthcare information gained by clinicians regarding the patient's major illnesses, previous surgeries/operations, and so on. This information is used to help in formulating a diagnosis and providing medical care.

Category preferences
This table on the SpringCharts server enables the clinic administrator to create customized lists of medical data. The lists enable users to rapidly select items to build the face sheet.

Care Tree

As mentioned above, the care tree is the section of the patient's chart that contains documents and records more dynamic in nature. Users add new notes to this area with each encounter with a patient. This is in contrast to the face sheet section, which contains healthcare information that seldom changes.

To edit an item on the care tree diagram, the user clicks on the "+" symbol to the left of the appropriate category to expand the list and then selects the specific "branch" item designated with a red bullet. The details of the particular item then display in the bottom right window. The "+" symbol turns into a "−" symbol when the category is expanded. To collapse the detailed list, the user simply clicks once on the "−" symbol; the category then closes, and the "+" symbol reappears. If a particular category does not display a "+" symbol, that means no documents are in that category for that patient. To edit an item in the care tree, the user clicks the [Edit] button at the bottom of the screen.

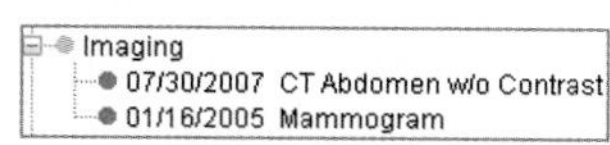

Branch items in the care tree

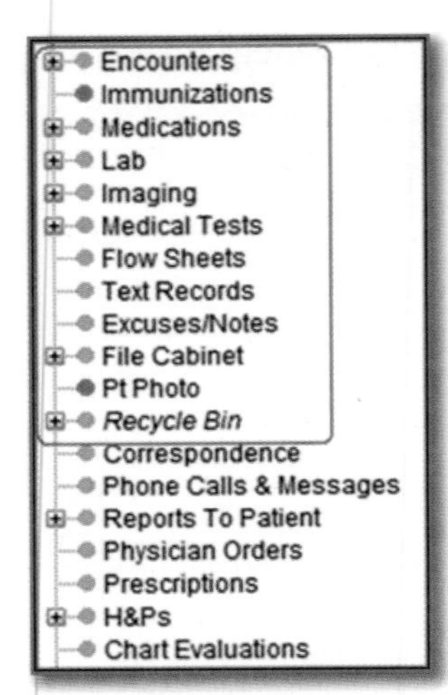

Figure 5.8 Permanent categories in the care tree.

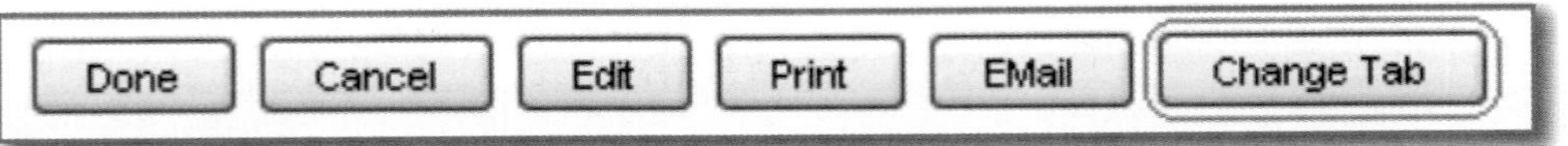

Figure 5.9 [Change Tab] button in the *Edit Document* window.

There are preset categories in the care tree that cannot be altered or edited. When certain documents and tests are saved in a patient's chart, they are automatically placed in the appropriate care tree categories. The preset list includes all categories from *Encounters* through *Recycle Bin* (Figure 5.8). An additional 30 customized categories can be added to the care tree list. This provides all users the opportunity to store created documents and imported files in the patient's chart under appropriate customized categories. Figure 5.8 also shows seven additional categories that have been added to the care tree. Customized categories for the care tree are added through the setup function of the SpringCharts server in *Category Preferences* in a network environment, or under the *Administration* menu item in the *Practice View* screen of a single-user computer version of SpringCharts.

Many of the newly created documents in the EHR program provide users an option to choose a care tree category before saving a document. Because many of the created forms are initiated from patient encounters, the *Encounters* category is displayed as the default place to store these documents. However, users can save documents under other additional category options. Even after a document has been saved in the care tree, the selected category can be changed by selecting the [Edit] button in the bottom window of the care tree screen. Once the window is reopened, the user chooses the [Change Tab] button (Figure 5.9) and selects another category. The program moves the document from the former category to the newly selected one in the care tree.

SpringCharts Tip

On a Mac computer the "+" sign appears as a side arrow beside the care tree categories. When the side arrow is clicked on to expand the category, it turns into a down arrow.

SpringCharts Tip

Once new items are added to the Spring-Charts server, each client version of SpringCharts on network workstations needs to be refreshed by shutting down and starting up the program in order for the changes to be seen.

Concept Checkup 5.1

A. An electronic chart created through computer automation in the medical clinic is the repository for what information?

B. Name three ways in which a user can access the patient's chart in the Spring-Charts program.

C. Can the same patient's chart be opened by multiple users at the same time?

D. Where would a user set up preference lists that are used in the social history, past medical history, and family medical history sections of the face sheet?

E. What information is stored in the care tree?

Exercise 5.1 Building Category Preferences

EHR programs can be customized for specific medical specialties. The major portion of customization occurs on the server.

1. Close any face sheet and patient's chart you may have open on your computer.
2. In the main menu of the *Practice View* screen, select *Administration*. From the drop-down menu, select *Category Preferences*.
3. In the *Set Categories* window that appears, locate the tab for *Social Hx*. Double-click to select each item in the list, and then backspace to remove the data. The *Social Hx* tab then should be blank, with no categories to select.
4. Add the following category preferences. [Because the list will appear as headings in the *face sheet* window, you need to place a colon (:) after each item.].
   - Alcohol Use:
   - Caffeine Use:
   - Education:
   - Occupation:
   - Living Arrangements:
5. Locate the *Family Hx* tab in the *Set Categories* window. Once again, double-click on each item to delete the existing list.

Exercise 5.1 (Concluded)

6. Create the following categories within the *Family Hx* tab, each on its own row. [Note: Some will have a colon; others will not]: *Father:, Mother:, Brother:, Sister:, Arthritis, Asthma, Cancer, Chemical Dependency, Diabetes, Heart Disease, High Blood Pressure, Kidney Disease, Tuberculosis, Died at Age:, Cause of Death:.*
7. Locate the *Past Hx* tab in the *Set Categories* window. Double-click on each item to delete the existing list.
8. Create the following categories within the *Past Hx* tab, each on its own row (there is no need to place a colon after each item): *Asthma, Bronchitis, Cancer, Diabetes, Gout, Heart Disease, Hernia, High Cholesterol, HIV Positive, Kidney Disease, Liver Disease, Migraine Headaches, Miscarriage, Mononucleosis, Pacemaker, Pneumonia, Prostate Problems, Stroke, Thyroid Problems, Tonsillitis, Ulcers, Vaginal Infections.*
9. Locate the *Chart Tabs* tab, and add the following categories: *Insurance Card, Reports to Patient* and *Letters.*
10. Locate the *File Cabinet Folders* tab, and add two categories: *Office Forms* and *Patient Forms.*
11. Press [Save] to save the amended categories.

5.2 Creating a Face Sheet

The information used to create electronic face sheets is typically taken from the paper intake forms patients fill out regarding their past medical history, routine medications, current medical problems, and so on. Traditionally, new patients have completed these forms in the waiting room, while waiting to be processed. However, with the introduction of ONC-certified EHR programs in 2011, many EHR vendors have added patient portals as a feature of their EHR programs. A patient portal allows patients limited access to sections of their electronic charts via a secure Internet log-in. Patients can then enter, update, and store their personal healthcare information directly on the medical facility's computer via their home computer.

Information to create a face sheet can also be obtained through a one-on-one patient interview. In this scenario, a medical office staff member sits with the patient and asks questions regarding allergies, past healthcare history, family medical history, routine medications, and so on, notating the patient's responses directly in the EHR program. The EHR program layout guides the staff member through all interview areas that need to be covered. To open the patient's face sheet, the user clicks on the *Show Chart/Face Sheet* icon to the right of the menu bar in the patient's chart.

HIPAA/HITECH Tip

A patient's authorization to release PHI is not needed when the purpose is for treatment, payment, or operations (TPO). However, because state laws vary, many practices will ask patients to sign releases.

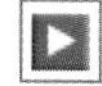

Show Chart/Face Sheet icon

Allergies

One of the 15 core ONC objectives for stage 1 of the EHR meaningful use (MU) measures involves recording allergies. During the 90-day time frame to report MU in 2011, eligible professionals (EPs) were required to record at least one allergy for 80 percent of patients seen during this time period (Table 5.1).

The allergy section of the patient's face sheet allows for adding and modifying/editing information about the patient's drug allergies and other sensitivities. The *Allergies* section opens by default when accessing the *Edit Face Sheet* window. Drug and non-drug allergens can be added by typing the first few letters of the allergen in the *Allergy* field in the top right corner of the window and then conducting a search. For established patients with a prescription history, drugs can also be pulled from the *Previous Prescriptions* field on the right side of the screen.

For the *Other Sensitivities* text field in the lower half of the *Allergies* window, pop-up text is available on the right side to choose the sensitivity or add descriptive text to a sensitivity specific to the patient's situation. Entries in the *Allergies* and *Other Sensitivities* fields can be removed from the patient's face sheet by highlighting and deleting them. If no allergies are entered into the patient's face sheet, the program will automatically enter *Patient Not Asked* into the *Allergies* section of the face sheet.

SpringCharts Tip

Many times, when an EHR program is implemented in a medical office, the paper intake forms are redesigned to cover the same categories and data flow that appears in the EHR face sheet. (See Appendix B. *Source Document 3—Patient Intake Sheet.*)

Table 5.1 Meaningful Use Core Measure

Active Medication Allergy List	
ONC Stage 1 Objective	**Meaningful Use Measure**
Maintain active medication allergy list. The list can be constructed through patient disclosure or through the regular course of treatment.	More than 80 percent of patients have at least one allergy entry recorded as structured data.

Notes:

- Medication allergies should be recorded as "structured" data so that the EHR program can compare prescribed medications with the patient's medication allergies and alert providers to possible conflicts.
- A physician is allowed to record that a patient has no known medication allergies.
- The MU measurement is based on number of unique patients seen by the physician, regardless of the number of times any individual patient is seen or the number of medication allergies per individual patient.

Details about the allergies can be added by clicking the specific allergy in the upper left field. In the *Edit* window allergies can be inactivated by first recording a reason for the inactive status in the *Inactive Reason* field and then selecting the [Inactive] button. An allergy may become inactive because the patient may no longer be intolerant to the allergen if he or she has moved to another part of the country and no longer has seasonal allergies, the patient may have had an operation to remedy the problem, the patient outgrew the allergy, and so on. Once saved, this allergy and its inactive reason can only be viewed if the user selects the *Inactive* or *All* option from the drop-down menu located at the top of the *Allergies* window (Figure 5.10).

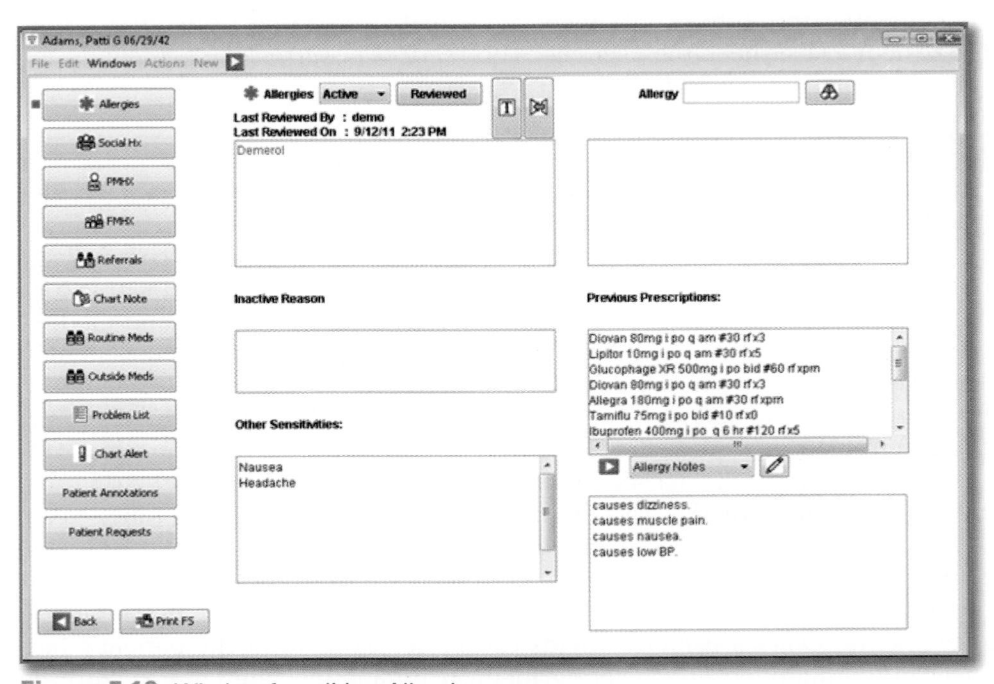

Figure 5.10 Window for editing *Allergies* category.

Table 5.2 Meaningful Use Core Measure

Smoking Status	
ONC Stage 1 Objective	**Meaningful Use Measure**
Record smoking status for patients 13 years of age and older.	More than 50 percent of patients 13 years of age and older have smoking status recorded as structured data.

Notes:

- Does not require a physician to offer tobacco cessation counseling.
- Specific to smoking. Other types of tobacco use and exposure to secondhand smoke do not need to be recorded.
- Smoking status does not need to be updated every time the physician sees the patient.
- A physician who does not see patients ages 13 and older is excluded from this measure.
- A physician does not need to obtain this information directly from the patient. Physicians who do not see the patient (e.g., radiologists) can receive this information from a referring physician.

When printing the patient's face sheet, the allergy name, details (if any), date and time entered, and the user who entered the allergy will be displayed. Once a patient's allergies are reviewed with the patient, the user selects the [Reviewed] button, which records the name of the staff member (based on the user logged on), the date, and time of the review in the *Edit* window.

Social History

Table 5.2 outlines the ONC objectives and meaningful use (MU) measures regarding social history. EPs were required to report the smoking status of 50 percent of their patients who were 13 years of age and older during the stage 1 period of 2011 and 2012. Because this information has to be reported electronically it cannot be entered into the EHR as free text. The user must select the patient's smoking status from a predetermined coded (or structured data) list in the EHR program.

To access the *Social History* section, the user clicks once on the [Social Hx] button of the *Edit Face Sheet* window. The window that opens allows for creating and editing the patient's social history. Social history is information a clinician gains by asking the patient specific questions related to topics such as drug use (including tobacco and alcohol), caffeine intake, living arrangements, occupation, number of children, recent foreign travel, exercise, pets, and so on. The information obtained under social history will vary from one medical specialty to another. It is useful in determining diagnoses and providing medical care.

Up to 30 common social history items can be chosen from a predetermined list in the *Preferences* field in the lower right of the *Edit Face Sheet* window. The preferences are set up under *Category Preferences* on the SpringCharts server or under the Administration menu on a single-user version. Additional defining text can be added to the preference categories selected in the *Preferences* field by selecting text from the pop-up text area above the *Preferences* field (Figure 5.11).

Smoking Status is a separate section within the *Social History* field, containing predetermined, discrete data that is used when creating **Surveillance Reports**. Because smoking status is selected from this area, smoking information does not need to be created in the *Preferences* window or the pop-up text

SpringCharts Tip

Before selecting pop-up text in the *Social History* window, place the cursor in the desired location where the pop-up text should appear. The program places the pop-up text where the cursor is located if this option has been chosen in the *Set User Preference* window.

Surveillance Reports
These reports provide information to the federal Centers for Disease Control and Prevention to enable effective monitoring of rates and distribution of disease, detection of outbreaks, monitoring of interventions, and prediction of emerging hazards.

In the *Completion Details* area—the bottom section of the *Referral Details* window—the user can record the appointment date and time for the referral, and then indicate the *Reason Of Referral* in the text box below. Once the appropriate fields are completed, the user clicks the [Save] button. The program then prompts the user to create a Continuity of Care Document (CCD) for the patient (see Chapter 1). If the "referred to" provider requires a CCD, the user can create a document that contains a core set of data reflecting the most relevant summary of a patient's medical healthcare. This XML file is stored on the computer, exported, and sent to the referral provider, where it is imported into that provider's EHR program for viewing and storage. If the practice to which the patient is being referred does not utilize an EHR program, then relevant portions of the electronic chart can be printed out and sent to the practice. This process will be discussed later in this chapter.

Show All Referrals

Show All Referrals option in *Edit Face Sheet* window.

To view all referrals for a particular patient in the *Edit Face Sheet* window, a user selects the *Show All Referrals* checkbox at the top of the screen; all referrals for this patient, both pending and completed, are displayed. Completed referrals are displayed in blue text. (By default, the window initially displays only pending, not completed, referrals). Once a patient completes a referral appointment and the medical office is notified, a user can open the patient's *Edit Face Sheet* window and select the pending referral in the *Referred To* field. The *Referral Details* window opens, and the user may input any comments and mark the referral complete by selecting the [Complete] button (Figure 5.14). All pending referrals for *all* patients can be tracked in the *Pending Referrals* window, by selecting the *Open pending referral list* icon on the *Practice View* Toolbar.

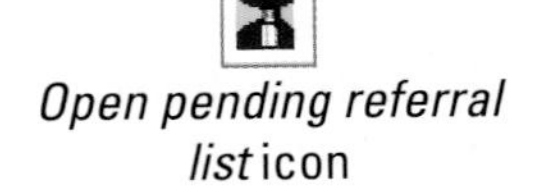

Open pending referral list icon

Chart Note

The *Chart Note* section of the face sheet includes important patient information that needs to be seen immediately when medical office staff open a patient's

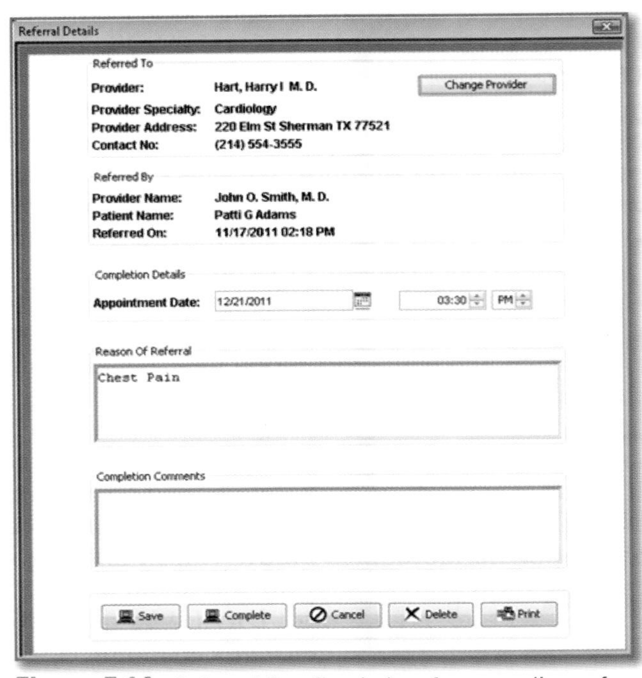

Figure 5.14 *Referral Details* window for a pending referral.

chart. A clinic might use this section to record specific medical history based on the clinic specialty. For example, an obstetrics and gynecology medical office might use the area to document menstrual history, menopausal history, births, types of deliveries, and miscarriages. Or a psychologist might use *Chart Note* to record previous psychiatric treatment, substance abuse treatment, history of harmful mood and behavior, and so on. This part of the face sheet enables a medical specialty clinic to capture healthcare history pertinent to their field that would not be part of the general past medical history section. Pop-up text is provided in this window to rapidly add predefined text.

Routine Medications

The ONC requires that EPs maintain an active list of prescription medication and over-the-counter medication for their patients (Table 5.3). To qualify for HITECH compensation in 2011, EPs had to report for a 90-day period that at least 80 percent of their patients who were seen had this data recorded. In 2012, EPs had to report for the full 12 months.

The *Routine Medications* section of the face sheet includes information about a patient's current routine medications and over-the-counter (OTC) medications. To access the *Routine Medications* section, the user clicks on the [Routine Meds] button in the *Edit Face Sheet* window. Displayed in red at the top of the screen in the *Allergic To* field are the *allergies* and *other sensitivities* that were chosen previously in the *Allergies* window. The patient's allergies and other sensitivities are displayed each time routine medications are accessed in SpringCharts. This enables the clinician to see at-a-glance any immediate concerns when discussing medications with the patient.

To add routine medications to a patient's chart, the user performs a search for the desired drug—by either brand name or generic name—in the upper right field of the screen, below the allergies notification panel. Medications can be edited by clicking once on their name in the *Routine Medications* field and amending any of the specifications in the *Edit Rx* window that appears (Figure 5.15). The changes affect only the patient whose chart is open, not the entire database.

In the *Edit Rx* window, the clinician can also add the date stopped and the reason the medication was stopped. When the clinician is reviewing the routine

SpringCharts Tip

The drug database in EHR programs is coded with discrete values so that e-prescribing clearinghouses like SureScripts can read the code and know precisely which medication, strength, dosage, and so on is being transmitted. In SpringCharts one can view the code for a particular drug in the *First Data Bank ID* field in the *Edit Rx* window.

Table 5.3 Meaningful Use Core Measure

Active Medication List	
ONC Stage 1 Objective	**Meaningful Use Measure**
Maintain active medication list that a patient is currently taking. The list will include both prescription medication and over-the-counter drugs.	More than 80 percent of patients have at least one entry recorded as structured data.

Notes:

- A physician is allowed to record that a patient has no current medications.
- The measure is based on individual patients seen by the physician, regardless of the number of times any individual patient is seen, or the number of medications any individual patient takes.
- This rule does not override a patient's right to privacy. A physician will not be held responsible for recording medications that the patient does not disclose.

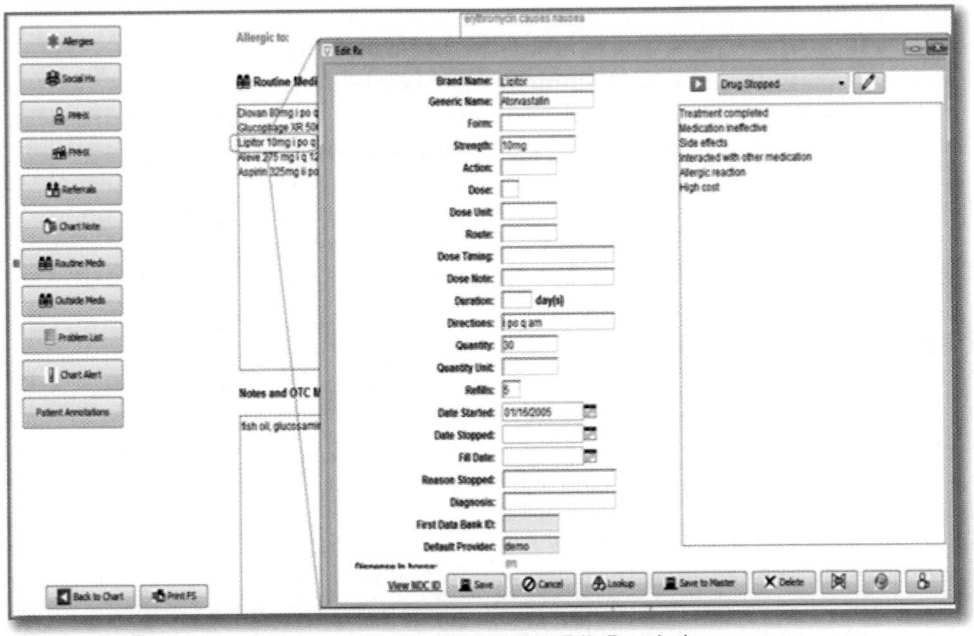

Figure 5.15 Editing medication information in the *Edit Rx* window.

medications with patients, patients can indicate if they are no longer taking a medication. Pop-up text is provided in the right side panel for easy selection of text for the reason stopped. The drug will remain in the routine medication list for history purposes, but will have a caption indicating the medication was stopped, the date stopped, reason, and the name of the practitioner who stopped it (Figure 5.16).

Physicians are licensed to dispense medication to their own patients, which is referred to as point-of-care medication dispensing. This was a common practice

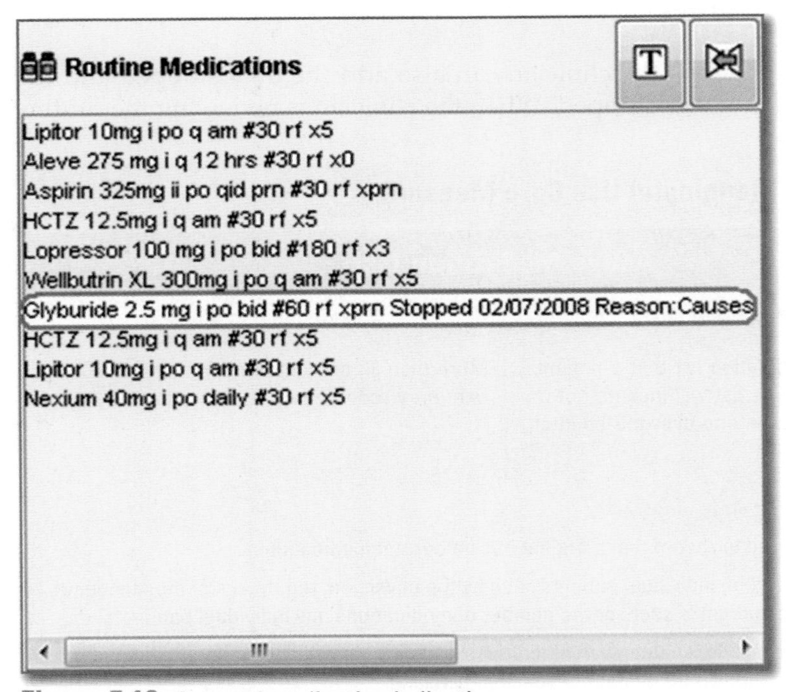

Figure 5.16 Stopped medication indication.

in the past, and is now regaining popularity due to higher prescription co-pays, the need for greater confidentiality, and the assurance that the patient actually receives their prescribed medication. Clinics that dispense medication to their own patients typically carry generic medication commonly used in their medical specialty. By dispensing directly to patients, the physician does not need to manually write or electronically transmit a prescription, and the patient does not need to wait for a pharmacy to fill the prescription.

When a physician prescribes multiple medications to a patient, some may need to be transmitted electronically and some may be dispensed directly by the physician. EHR programs allow for medications in the database to be flagged as dispensed by the clinic (Figure 5.17). Medications dispensed in-house are required to contain a lot number and expiration date. EHR programs create a warning message when the physician attempts to dispense a medication with an expired lot number. In the SpringCharts EHR system, when the in-house dispensing option is checked in the *Edit Rx* window, the program opens up fields to record the lot number and expiration date in the *Edit Rx* window (Figure 5.17). In-house medications are not transmitted through the e-prescribing channels.

In the *Routine Medications* section of the patient's *Edit Face Sheet* window the user can also record any over-the-counter (OTC) medications the patient is taking. Pop-up text allows for easy listing of OTC drugs and non-drugs the patient is obtaining from a pharmacy. Because the OTC section of the face sheet is created from pop-up text, the clinician can continue to build this database as necessary.

Outside Medications

The *Outside Medications* section of the face sheet, accessed via the [Outside Meds] button, automatically populates with drug data prescribed by other providers when the SpringCharts program sends e-prescriptions across the Internet to the clearinghouse. This window allows clinicians to see what medications are being prescribed by other physicians for this patient. Currently, physicians are not legally required to prescribe medication electronically; however, ONC-certified EHR programs must include this function, and physicians must demonstrate e-prescribing as part of the meaningful use criteria to qualify for ONC financial incentives through the Medicare or Medicaid programs. All e-prescribing across the nation goes through a centralized clearinghouse before prescriptions are sent to the indicated pharmacy. Therefore, each physician who participates in e-prescribing is able to view all medications that are electronically transmitted by other physicians for that specific patient. The provider cannot manually enter or alter information in the *Outside Medications* area of the face sheet.

Problem List

The *Problem List* area of the face sheet includes information about a patient's chronic medical problems. The ONC requires that EPs maintain an active list of patient problems. This list must be structured data, that is, coded rather than free text so that electronic reporting can be carried out. In 2011 and 2012, qualifying EPs had to certify that 80 percent or more of their patients had this data recorded in the EHR program (Table 5.4).

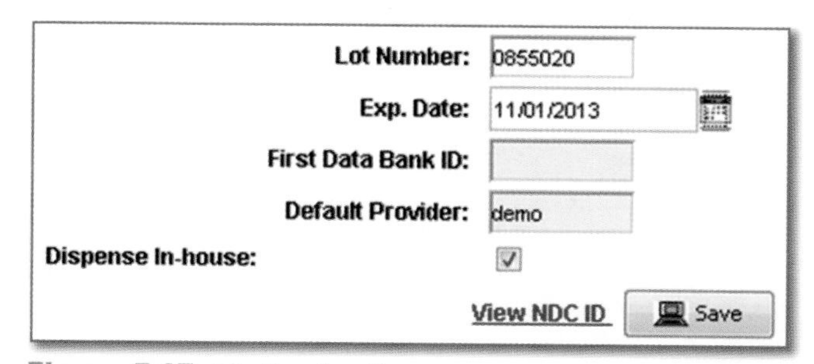

Figure 5.17 Medication flagged as in-house for direct dispensing.

Table 5.4 Meaningful Use Core Measure

Up-to-Date Problem List	
ONC Stage 1 Objective	**Meaningful Use Measure**
Maintain up-to-date problem list of current and active diagnoses.	More than 80 percent of patients have at least one entry recorded as structured data.

Notes:

- The term "up-to-date" means the most recent diagnosis known to the physician.
- The rule does not specify a standard that a physician must use in order to record a patient's diagnosis (i.e., the rule does not specify ICD-9-CM or SNOMED CT).
- A physician is allowed to record that a patient has no current diagnoses.
- The measurement is based on individual patients seen by the physician, regardless of the number of times any individual patient is seen.
- The list can include diagnoses from other physicians.

To access the *Problem List* section, the user clicks on the [Problem List] button of the *Edit Face Sheet* window. Entries are chosen by either diagnosis name or description from the *Dx* field at the top right of the window. The problem list is also transmitted with e-prescribing and is another reason why the problem list cannot be created with free text. EHR programs also pull data from patients' problem lists when creating Surveillance Reports. When a diagnosis is chosen in the *Office Visit* screen during a patient visit, the physician can add the diagnosis to the chronic *Problem List* at that time. For established patients who have been previously assigned a diagnosis in an office visit note, the diagnosis code and description can be selected for the *Problem List* from the *Previous Dx* field on the right side of the *Edit Face Sheet* window.

When reviewing the *Problem List* with a patient, the clinician will determine if the medical problem is active, resolved, or inactive. If a healthcare problem is *resolved,* the clinician selects the diagnosis from a patient's *Problem List,* which opens the *Diagnosis* window (Figure 5.18). The physician inputs a *Resolved Reason* and selects the [Resolved] button. An example of a resolved medical problem is a diagnosis that becomes obsolete after a patient undergoes surgery for the condition. If the healthcare problem is *inactive,* the user selects the entry from the *Problem List* and checks the [Inactive] checkbox in the *Diagnosis* window. An example of an inactive healthcare problem is a diagnosis controlled by medication, with the patient not experiencing any signs or symptoms of the condition.

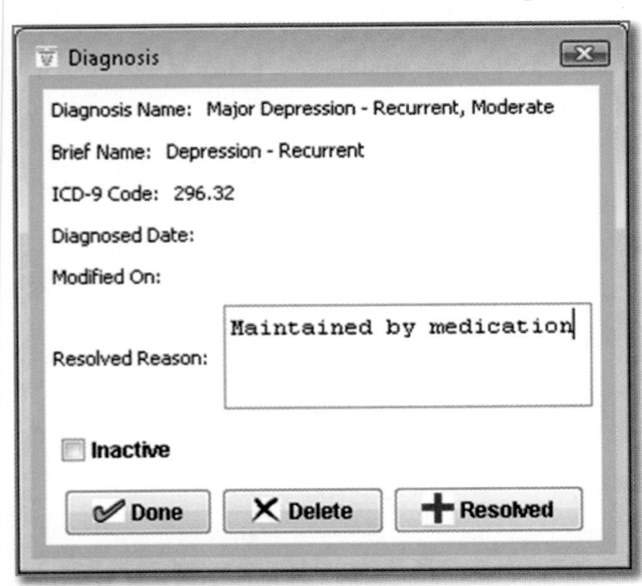

Figure 5.18 *Problem List* area's *Diagnosis* window with *Inactive* check box.

By default, the *Problem List* window displays all the patient's problem diagnoses regardless of the status: active, resolved, or inactive. If a user highlights a resolved diagnosis, the reason is displayed in the *Resolved Reason box* of the *Diagnosis* window (Figure 5.18). A user can view a patient's list of problems by those that are active, resolved, or inactive, or the entire list, by selecting a preference from the drop-down menu located at the top of the *Problem List* screen. A clinical staff member should check the *Problem List* with the patient at each encounter to ensure this important information is up-to-date.

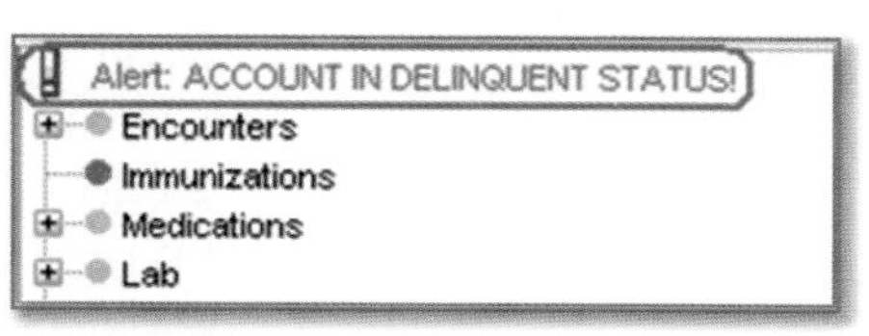

Figure 5.19 *Chart Alert* in a patient's care tree.

Predefined pop-up text is available to further explain or describe *Problem List* items. The pop-up text is not transmitted when e-prescribing and is not pulled into Surveillance Reports. SpringCharts automatically stamps the user ID and date at the bottom of the *Problem List* on exiting the *Edit Face Sheet* window. The program updates the user ID and date with each review of the *Problem List*.

Chart Alert

The ***Chart Alert*** area of the face sheet allows users to input important text that will appear in red above the *Encounters* category on the patient's care tree (Figure 5.19). The text can be typed in the *Chart Alert* window or selected from predefined text in the pop-up text field. Chart alerts enable clinicians to be attentive to important information regarding the patient, like special needs, English as second language, and so on. The chart alert may be medical or administrative in nature.

Chart Alert
Chart alerts in EHR programs highlight important text that appears in prominent areas of the patient chart or as warning pop-up messages when certain areas of the program are accessed.

Mandated reporters
These professionals have regular contact with children, disabled persons, older adults, and other identified vulnerable individuals. Such professionals are legally required to report any observed or suspected maltreatment or neglect to the appropriate authorities.

Patient Annotations

The *Patient Annotations* area of the face sheet includes any important additional explanations or statements a patient may provide during an encounter with a clinician or other staff member that are deemed important enough to be displayed on his or her face sheet. A patient may sometimes mention issues irrelevant to the current office visit, but still important to record. For example, the patient may be under stress from work or the family environment, which could have a bearing on his or her health.

Sometimes patients mention maltreatment by another individual. Physicians are considered **mandated reporters** who can be held liable by both the civil and criminal legal systems for intentionally failing to make a report whenever physical, sexual, or other types of maltreatment or neglect has been observed or is suspected. The *Patient Annotations* area of the face sheet provides a location to document a patient's comments regarding maltreatment, neglect, and other issues.

A user may input an annotation in the upper section of the screen by typing or selecting from the list of preferences. When a clinician returns to the patient's face sheet, the annotation is automatically saved. The next time the *Edit Face Sheet* window is opened, the annotation is displayed in the *Previous Annotation(s)* section and cannot be edited. All annotations will show on the face sheet of the patient's chart.

SpringCharts Tip
As is the case with other areas in the program, the *Patient Annotations* preferences can be customized under *Category Preferences* on the SpringCharts server.

Patient Requests

The *Patient Requests* section of the *Edit Face Sheet* window includes information about a patient's healthcare record request. Providers who meet ONC meaningful use criteria must demonstrate they are able to supply a patient with medical documentation from the EHR program. This action may be in response to a patient request for a copy of his or her lab results, a request for a copy of the office visit notes, and so on. The *Patient Requests* area of the face sheet documents these requests and enables the staff to track, process, and report that these requests have been fulfilled.

Saving and Printing

Not all areas of the patient's chart will be completed on the first visit. Other sections will be completed upon return visits. However, it is recommended that the details of the patient's face sheet be discussed with the patient upon each visit to the clinic. This practice ensures up-to-date healthcare information on the patient and is exemplary of quality patient care.

All new and modified face sheet information is saved in the patient's chart when the [Back] button is selected in the *Edit Face Sheet* window. In many cases, clerical staff build the electronic face sheet with information taken from the patient's paper intake forms. The newly completed face sheet can then be printed for new patients to review by pressing on the [Print FS] button in the *Edit Face Sheet* window. This gives patients the opportunity to review and revise their medical information. All information in the *Edit Face Sheet* window is printed except the *Chart Alert* and *Patient Requests*. Thus the patient does not see sensitive information recorded in these two areas of the face sheet. The patient's demographics and primary insurance details are also printed on the face sheet.

(See Appendix A—*Sample Documents*; Document 2. *Patient's Face Sheet*.)

Concept Checkup 5.2

A. Information gathered to complete the patient's past medical history, routine medications, current medical problems, and so on in the electronic face sheet can be collected from three different sources. What are these three sources?

B. What is the purpose of the *Outside Medications* section in the patient's face sheet?

C. Stage 1 of EHR MU requires that qualifying EPs maintain an active list of allergies, medications, and medical problems for what percentage of their patients?

D. Are patients restricted by HIPAA from providing complete medical history information on family members? Explain your answer.

SpringCharts Tip

Shortcut: 

Open a Patient's Chart

The third speed icon from the right on the Toolbar of the main *Practice View* screen enables the user to quickly open a patient's chart and bypass the *Actions* menu.

Hamilton, Byron R 05/05/58
File Edit Windows Actions New

Show Chart/Face Sheet icon

Exercise 5.2 Building a New Patient's Face Sheet

If your SpringCharts program was not shut down and reopened after completing Exercise 5.1, you may do so now. This will refresh the program to include the new items added in the *Category Preferences* window of the *Administration* menu in Exercise 5.1.

1. Open your own chart by selecting the *Open a Patient's Chart* icon (shown in margin) on the main menu. Type the first few letters of your last name in the search field of the *Choose Patient* window and click on the *Search* icon.
2. Select your name, and your chart will open. It will be empty except for your demographic information.
3. Within your chart, click on the *Show Chart/Face Sheet* icon, located at the far right of the menu bar, to open the *Edit Face Sheet* window.

Allergies

4. The window opens to the *Allergies* section.
5. In the *Allergy* field on the right side, type "peni" and press the *Search* icon.
6. Select *Penicillins* from the list. The program adds this drug to your allergy list on the left side.

Exercise 5.2 (Continued)

7. Repeat these steps to add the drug *Codeine* and the allergen *Peanut Containing Prod.*
8. In the *Other Sensitivities* field, in the lower part of the window, type the medication *Erythromycin.* Then select *causes nausea* from the *Allergy Notes* pop-up text (to the right).

Social History

9. Click on the [Social Hx] button to open the *Social History* window.
10. In the *Preferences* list in the lower right, select the *Alcohol Use:* category.
11. Select the appropriate item from the *Social Hx* pop-up text field in the upper window, for example, *Alcohol Use: NonDrinker.*
12. Repeat these steps to add information in the *Caffeine Use* and *Living Arrangements* preference categories, using the pop-up text of your choice.

Past Medical History

13. Click on the [PMHX] navigation button to open the *Past Medical History* window.
14. Select several items of your choice from the *Preferences* list to build your past medical history.
15. Add a medical condition that is not in the *Preferences* list by searching for a diagnosis in the *Dx* field in the upper right. Type *HTN* for hypertension, click the *Search* icon, and select the diagnosis.

Family Medical History

16. Click on the [FMHX] navigation button to open the *Family Medical History* window.
17. Select several medical conditions of your choice from the *Preferences* list to build your family medical history.
18. Select Father: Died At Age: and Cause of Death: from the *Preferences* list. Place your cursor at the end of the *Died at Age:* phrase in the *Other FMHX* field and then type a fictitious age. Hit the [Enter] key.
19. Place your cursor at the end of the *Cause of Death:* phrase and select a medical condition from the list.
20. In the *Parents Information* section in the lower left, check the box to indicate the father is deceased. Select the date from the calander icon: 6/9/1969.

Chart Note

21. Click on the [Chart Note] navigation button to open the *Chart Note* section.
22. Select *Prefers Hospital* in the pop-up text on the right side. Then select *St. Judes* from the right side.
23. Click in the *Chart Note* field on the left side of the window. Hit the [Enter] key to move your cursor to a new line.
24. Select *Religion* in the pop-up text on the right side. Place your cursor at the end of this word and type a specific religion (can be fictitious).

Routine Medications

25. Click on the [Routine Meds] navigation button to open the *Routine Medications* window.
26. In the upper right quadrant, search for and select each of the following medications: *Diovan, Glucophage,* and *Lipitor.* You can select the strength of your choice. All three medications should now appear on the left side of the window.
27. In the *Notes and OTC Meds* field, select several OTC (over-the-counter) items from the *Routine Meds* pop-up text in the lower-right quadrant.

(continued)

SpringCharts Tip

Remember that you only need to type the first few letters of the word to conduct a search. The more letters you type, the more likely you are to make a mistake, and the system will not be able to locate the term.

SpringCharts Tip

If you don't see the list of items you added under the *Social Hx* section of the *Category Preferences* window in Exercise 5.1, you may need to close SpringCharts and restart the program.

SpringCharts Tip

Place your cursor after the *Preferences* category item you selected and then click on the pop-up text item. The placement of the cursor determines where the pop-up text is inserted.

Exercise 5.2 (Concluded)

Problem List

28. Click on the [Problem List] navigation button to open the *Problem List* window.
29. In the *Dx* field in the upper right, type in htn (*for hypertension*) and conduct a search. Select *HTN 401.9 for hypertension.*
30. In the same field, type the code *250* and conduct a search. Select *Diabetes.*
31. In the *Dx* field, type *hypercholest* and conduct a search. Select *Hypercholesterolemia 272.0.*
32. Search for and select *Allergic Rhinitis—Pollen 477.0.*

Chart Alert

Chart Alert

Edit PopUp Text icon

33. Click on the [Chart Alert] navigation button (shown in margin) to open the *Chart Alert* window.
34. Click on the *Edit PopUp text* icon on the far right. Place your [Caps Lock] key on and type *SPANISH–ENGLISH IS SECOND LANGUAGE* on the next empty line in the *Edit Pop-up Text* window. Click the [Done] button.
35. Select *SPANISH–ENGLISH IS SECOND LANGUAGE* from the available pop-up text.

Printing the Face Sheet

36. Click the [Print FS] button in the lower left corner of the *Edit Face Sheet* window.
37. Click the [Print] button in the *Document Printing Options* window. Select the printer and print your documents.
38. Click on the [Back] button in the *Edit Face Sheet* window. All the data selected is now positioned in the various face sheet categories within your chart.
39. Close your patient's chart.
40. Collect your printed face sheet document and turn it in to your instructor.

5.3 Procedures in a Patient's Chart

EHR programs are designed to center all activities around the patient's chart. Although the patient is the focus of healthcare, the electronic chart is the focal point of the processes within EHR programs. Therefore the patient's electronic chart is opened first before any activity related to the patient is begun. With the chart opened, everything processed from that point on is saved in the patient's chart without the user needing to select the appropriate patient each time. This order of events safeguards against any activity being completed and then accidently saved into the wrong patient's chart. Remember, in an electronic chart environment, everything is done electronically—from documenting a phone call to recording lab results. EHRs are now advanced enough that even basic activities such as issuing an excuse note to a patient who missed work or school due to a medical appointment are now accomplished electronically.

SpringCharts Tip

SpringCharts EHR is not an insurance billing program; it is not necessary to add a patient's secondary or tertiary (third) insurance companies to the chart.

Adding the Primary Insurance

Chapter 3 described how to set up insurance companies in the SpringCharts EHR program database by accessing the *Edit* menu on the main screen and choosing *Insurance*. Now we need to link a specific insurance company to a patient's chart and add unique patient information. A patient's primary insurance company is added to his or her face sheet by right-clicking on the *Insurance* section at the bottom left of the chart and selecting *Edit*. The *Edit Patient Insurance* window displays (Figure 5.20), allowing the user to record such specific

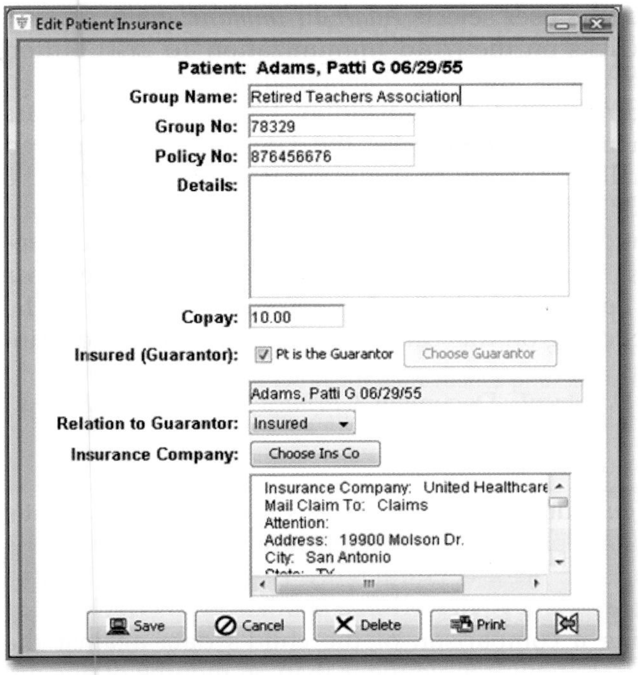

Edit Patient Insurance

Patient: Adams, Patti G 06/29/55
Group Name: Retired Teachers Association
Group No: 78329
Policy No: 876456676
Details:
Copay: 10.00
Insured (Guarantor): Pt is the Guarantor Choose Guarantor
Adams, Patti G 06/29/55
Relation to Guarantor: Insured
Insurance Company: Choose Ins Co
Insurance Company: United Healthcare
Mail Claim To: Claims
Attention:
Address: 19900 Molson Dr.
City: San Antonio

Save Cancel Delete Print

Figure 5.20 *Edit Patient Insurance* window.

patient information as group name and number, policy number, **co-pay** amount, and guarantor.

The *Details* field in the *Edit Patient Insurance* window enables the user to record additional information, such as the patient's **deductible** amount and how much of the deductible has been met for the current year. If the patient hasn't yet fully met the deductible, the medical office may be able to collect medical expenses directly from the patient. The *Details* field can also be used to document communication with insurance company representatives specific to the patient.

The [Choose Ins Co] button is selected to add the patient's primary insurance company from the EHR program database list. The patient's primary insurance information is then displayed on the face sheet and printed on the face sheet form and office visit routing slip. It also may be added to the physician's order form. Only one insurance company and the patient's personal insurance information can be added to a patient's chart in the SpringCharts program. The information can be viewed on the face sheet for reference purposes.

Entering Past Immunizations

Immunization is a simple, safe, and effective way to protect children and adults from a wide variety of potentially deadly diseases. For vaccines to be most beneficial, they need to be administered on time. EHR programs enable past immunization records to be entered into the patient's chart. By recording past and ongoing immunizations in the EHR program, the provider and staff have a complete record of each patient's vaccinations. After recording the patient's past immunizations, all future vaccines are automatically added to the immunization record when they are conducted and recorded in the office visit note.

Immunization information can be viewed, added, and edited in a patient's chart by accessing the *Actions* menu in the *Patient Chart* window and selecting submenu *Immunization*. To add a past immunization to a new patient's

Focal Point

The patient's co-pay and deductible amounts can be added via the *Insurance* section in the face sheet of the patient's chart.

Co-pay
This amount is paid by a policyholder for each medical office visit or other type of medical service obtained by a patient covered under a health insurance policy (for example, $25 per visit). The insurance company then pays the remainder of the healthcare expense, providing that the deductible has been paid.

Deductible
An annual amount of money the policyholder pays toward medical expenses before the insurance company pays its share, for example, $500 per year. Most medical insurance policies require a deductible.

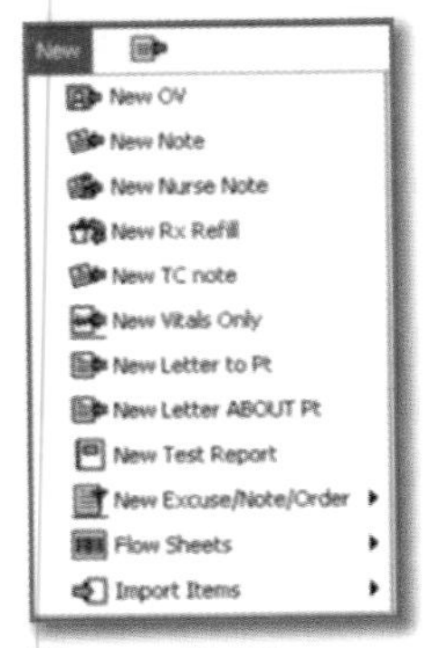

Figure 5.24 *New* menu in patient's chart.

5.4 New Activities in a Patient's Chart

The *New* menu in the *Patient Chart* view leads to several documents and reports that can be created and stored in a patient's chart (Figure 5.24). Once again, the patient's chart first needs to be opened to access and perform new activities for the patient. This enables documents and reports to be saved automatically in the correct chart, thus preventing possible misfiling.

New TC Note

Selecting the *New TC note* submenu from the *New* menu creates a new telephone call encounter form. From the *Telephone Call Edit* window that appears, a user can choose phrases from the *Notes Panel* pop-up text in the upper right quadrant of the window (Figure 5.25). Text from previous telephone call notes, in the lower right quadrant, can also be used by highlighting and copying into the *Notes* field in the lower left quadrant, using the *Copy Highlighted Text to Note* icon (shown in margin) in the left side of the *Copy Previous Notes* field. The date stamp and initial stamp icons are also available in this field, just below the *Copy Highlighted Text to Note* icon.

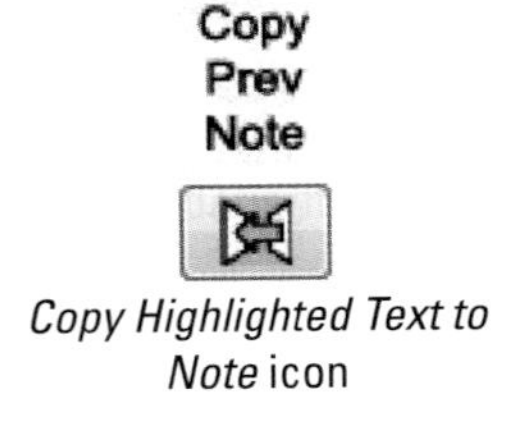

Copy Highlighted Text to Note icon

A tab with the *Rx* icon also appears in the upper right corner of the *Telephone Call Edit* window. Once accessed, the panel displays the patient's *Routine Medications* and *Previous Prescriptions* lists. If a medication needs to be refilled as a result of the telephone conversation, the provider can document and print the patient's prescription by selecting from these lists or adding the medication after searching the database. Thus, the provider can document the call and order the prescription without having to close one window and open another.

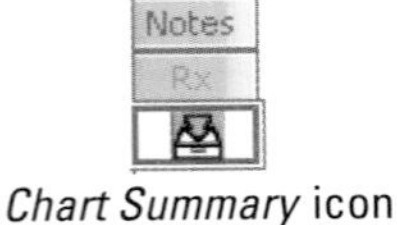

Chart Summary icon

The tab below the *Rx* tab, with the *Chart Summary* icon, opens the *Chart Summary* panel, which displays the patient's face sheet information. This feature enables the user to discuss items contained in the patient's face sheet without having to return to the patient's chart.

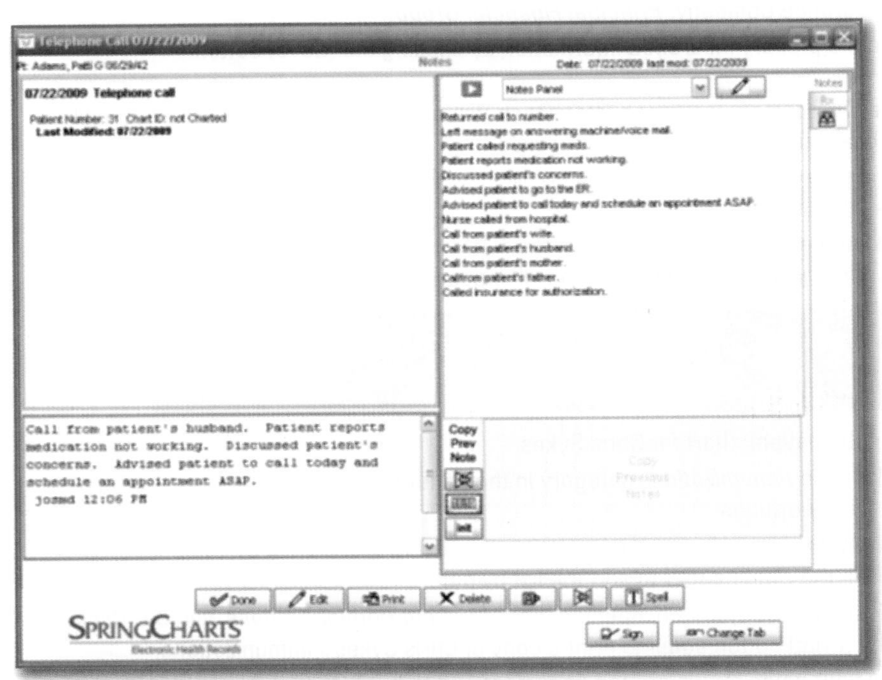

Figure 5.25 *Telephone Call Edit* window.

In the *Telephone Call Edit* window, the user can also convert a telephone call note into an office visit note. Once the *Convert This Note to an Office Visit* icon has been selected at the bottom of the window, text from the TC note appears on the *Objective* section of a new office visit note, and any prescribed medication appears in the *Plan* section of the SOAP note. (Chapter 6 covers SOAP—subjective, objective, assessment, and plan—in more detail.) This feature enables a patient to be seen by the physician on the same day the call was made. Details from the telephone conversation are then included in the office visit note, which the physician can complete on the patient's arrival at the clinic.

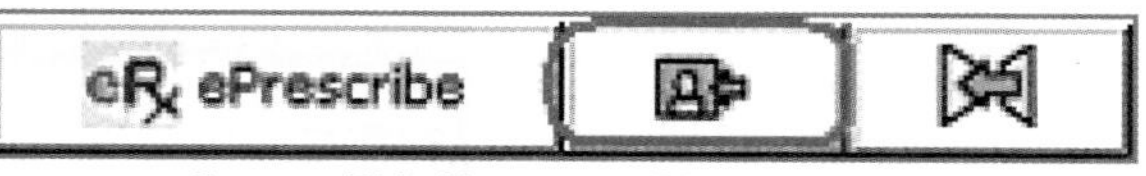

Convert This Note to an Office Visit icon

The [Sign] button in the bottom right of the *Telephone Call Edit* window gives the user the option to stamp his or her initials at the bottom of the note or to permanently initial and lock the note so modifications cannot be made.

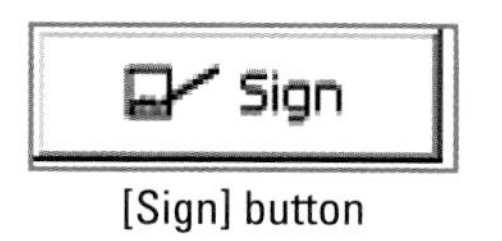

[Sign] button

When the TC note is completed and the user selects the [Done] button, the program offers the option to *Save and Edit Routing Slip* in order to bill for the telephone consultation (Figure 5.26). In several states, patient telephone consultations are a billable encounter. The TC note is saved under the *Encounters* tab in the patient's care tree unless the user selects a customized tab at the time the document is saved.

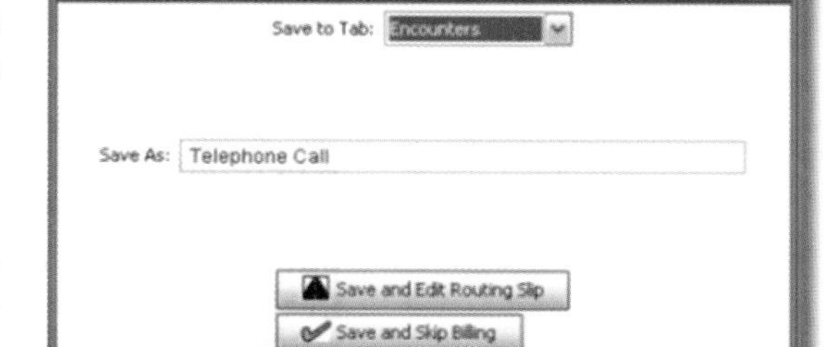

Figure 5.26 Saving a telephone call to a care tree.

New Vitals Only

Stage 1 of the meaningful use program requires EPs to record at least the height, weight, and blood pressure of patients two years of age or older in a certified EHR program (Table 5.5). More than 50 percent of a provider's patients had to have this data recorded to qualify for incentive payment in 2011 and 2012.

The *New Vitals Only* submenu in the *New* menu of the patient's chart creates a form only used when patients come to the medical clinic for the sole purpose of having their vital signs taken. (Vital signs are also taken during office visit encounters, which is described in Chapter 6.) The *New Vitals Only* window

Table 5.5 Meaningful Use Core Measure

Changes in Vital Signs	
ONC Stage 1 Objective	**Meaningful Use Measure**
Record vital signs and chart changes (height, weight, blood pressure, body mass index, growth charts for children).	More than 50 percent of patients 2 years of age or older have height, weight, and blood pressure recorded as structured data.

Notes:

- Certified EHR technology can calculate a patient's body mass index (BMI) and create a growth chart (for children and adolescents) based on the entered data.
- A physician who believes that recording a patient's height, weight, and blood pressure is not relevant to his or her scope of practice can attest to that fact.
- Physicians who do not see patients over the age of 2 are excluded from this requirement.
- The vital signs need not be updated at every patient visit.
- A patient's height can be self-reported.

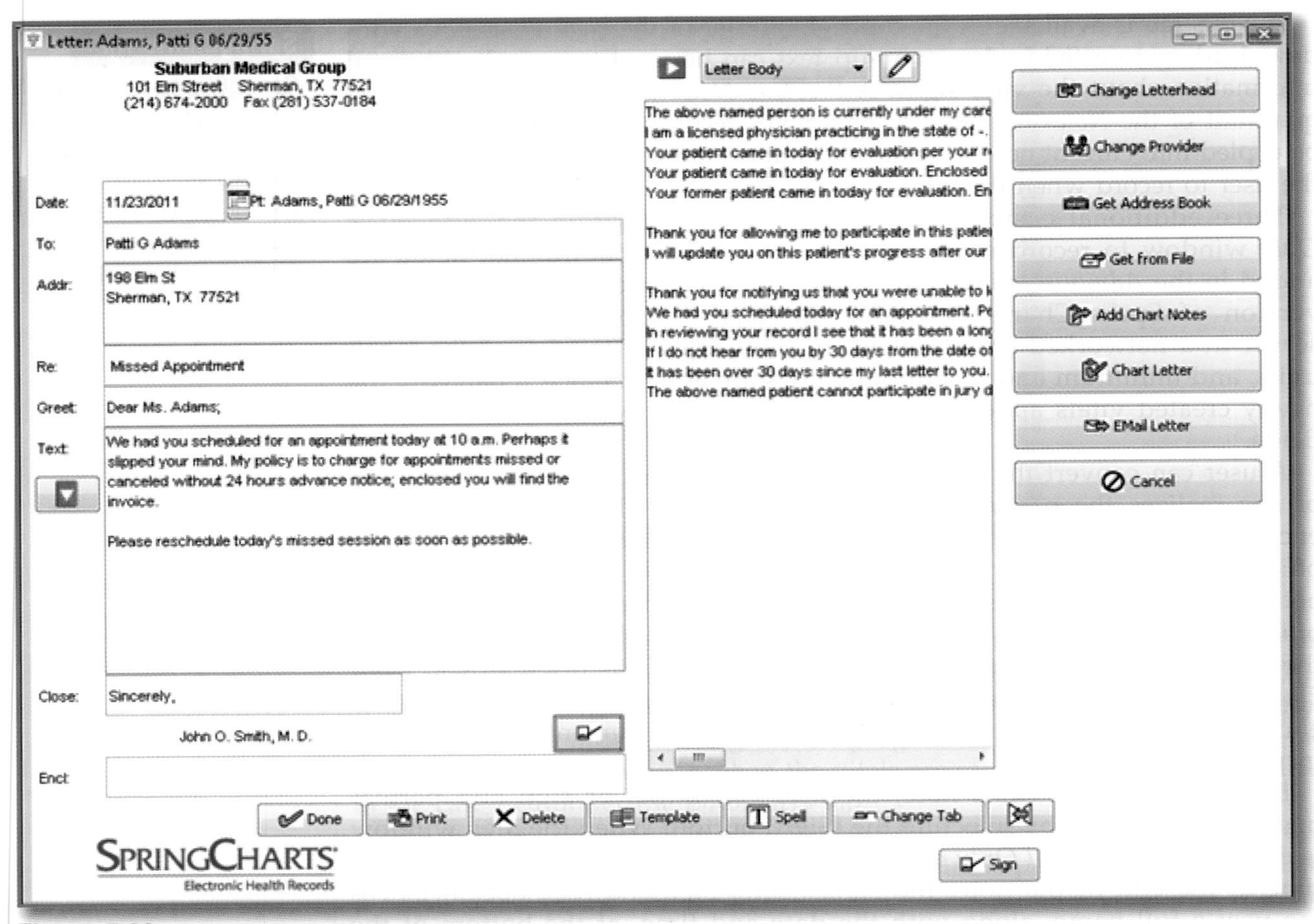

Figure 5.29 *Letter to the Patient* window.

New Letter about a Patient

The *New Letter about a Patient* feature creates a new letter concerning the patient (Figure 5.30). Letters concerning patients are frequently sent to third-party entities such as other healthcare providers, referring physicians, insurance companies, workers' compensation agencies, and so on. This feature is accessed under the *New Letter ABOUT Pt* submenu under the *New* menu in the patient's chart.

Letters *about* a patient do not automatically default to the patient's name and address, as is the case with letters *to* a patient. However, the patient's name and date of birth do automatically appear on the subject line (*Re:* field). The recipient name and address information can be retrieved from the [Get Address Book] button in the right-hand panel, and pop-up text is available in the middle *Letter Body* field. As with all pop-up windows, text can be modified and added by selecting the *Edit* (pen) icon. If multiple practices or physicians have been set up in the program, alternate letterheads and doctors' signatures can be chosen by selecting the appropriate navigation buttons to the right—the [Change Letterhead] and [Change Provider] buttons, respectively.

A template letter can be accessed via the [Get from File] button in the right-hand panel. These previously created letters can be added to the body of the letter. All items stored under the *Encounters, Lab, Imaging,* or *Medical Tests* categories of the patient's care tree are available to add to the body of the

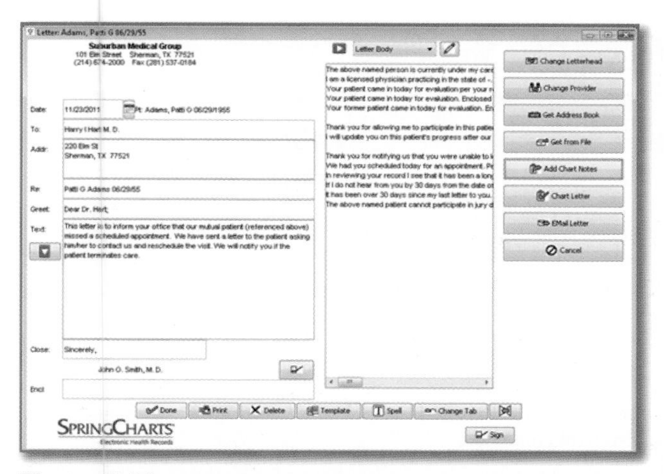

Figure 5.30 *New Letter about a Patient* window with data.

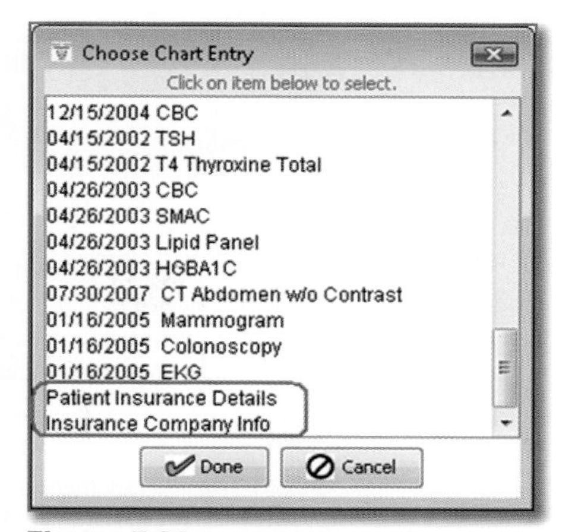

Figure 5.31 Insurance information added to a letter about a patient.

letter by selecting the [Add Chart Notes] button. This functionality is useful when sending office visit notes to a referring physician, such as test results and encounter notes. The user can also add the patient's personal insurance identification information and insurance company demographic details to the letter in the *Choose Chart Entry* window (Figure 5.31), again via the [Add Chart Notes] button. This functionality is useful when sending letters to insurance companies of behalf of the patient.

Add Chart Notes

[Add Chart Notes] button

The [Chart Letter] button saves a copy of the letter to the care tree, although this automatically happens when selecting the [Done] button at the bottom of the window. To activate the spell checker for the letter content, the user clicks on the [Spell] button. The letter can be printed out or e-mailed to a recipient by using the [Print] and [EMail letter] buttons, respectively. The *Copy or Export This Data* icon (shown in margin) enables the user to export the letter to another word processing program, where it can be reformatted, if necessary.

Copy or Export This Data icon

Selecting the *Signature* icon (shown in margin), located at the bottom of the letter just below the *Close* field, enables the user to choose which signature to place in the letter. The options are the user's name or the default doctor's name chosen in the *User Preferences* window during setup, located as an option under the *File* menu on the main screen. If a user wants to permanently lock a letter so no changes can be made to it after it is sent, the [Sign] button at the bottom of the *New Letter about a Patient* window needs to be clicked and the [Permanently Sign and Lock] button option activated. Once a letter has been signed, locked, and saved, it can be viewed but not edited, even by the author.

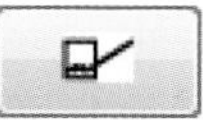

Change Signature of Letter icon

(See Appendix A—*Sample Documents*; Document 5. *Letter about a Patient*.)

New Test Report to the Patient

The ONC requires that EPs provide patients with a copy of healthcare information from a certified EHR program within 3 business days of the patient's request (Table 5.6). The *New Test Report to Pt* submenu under the *New* menu in the patient chart leads to a blank test reporting form that enables physicians to fulfill this meaningful use requirement. Any completed tests for this patient can be added to the report from the *Select Test* list in the upper right corner of the *New Report* window (Figure 5.32). The program comes preloaded with simplified explanations for many of the tests. These explanations are automatically incorporated into the left-hand report field below the test results when the test is selected.

SpringCharts Tip

For new tests the clinic has created and added to SpringCharts, descriptions can be created by accessing the *Edit* menu in the main *Practice View* and selecting submenu *Test Explanations.*

Table 5.6 Meaningful Use Core Measure

E-Copies of Health Information	
ONC Stage 1 Objective	**Meaningful Use Measure**
On request, provide patients with an electronic copy of their health information (including diagnostic test results, problem list, medication lists, and medication allergies).	More than 50 percent of requesting patients receive an electronic copy within 3 business days.

Notes:

- If a physician has no requests from patients for their health information during the reporting period, that physician is excluded from this objective.
- Physicians are allowed to withhold information that would potentially be harmful to the patient.
- Physicians are allowed to charge a fee for copying information, per HIPAA regulations.
- Patients are allowed to choose the format in which they receive their information.
- Disclosure of the information to a parent, family member, or caretaker is allowed under this objective.

Identified *Problems* and *Recommendations* can be added to the left-hand field from the pop-up list in the lower right of the window (the list defaults to the *Report-Probs* pop-up text category). The user places the cursor under the *Problems* heading in the body of the report and then selects the appropriate pop-up text. Next the user selects the *Report-Recs* heading by clicking on the down arrow to the right of the pop-up text category heading (Figure 5.33). Then, placing the cursor under the *Recommendations* heading in the report body, the clinician can select appropriate recommendations from the new set of pop-up text.

Multiple tests can be added to one report for the patient, and the completed report can be printed out and mailed to the recipient. When printing the

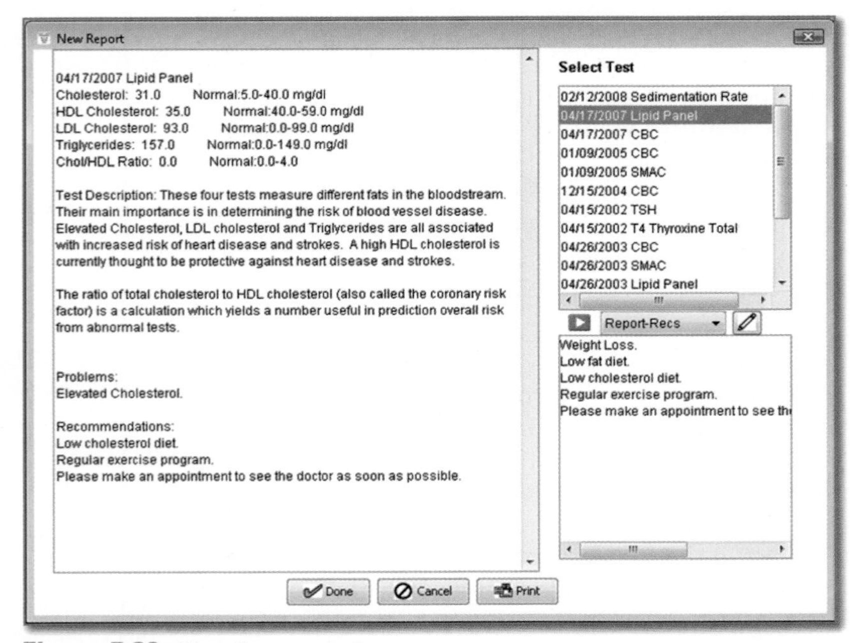

Figure 5.32 *New Report* window.

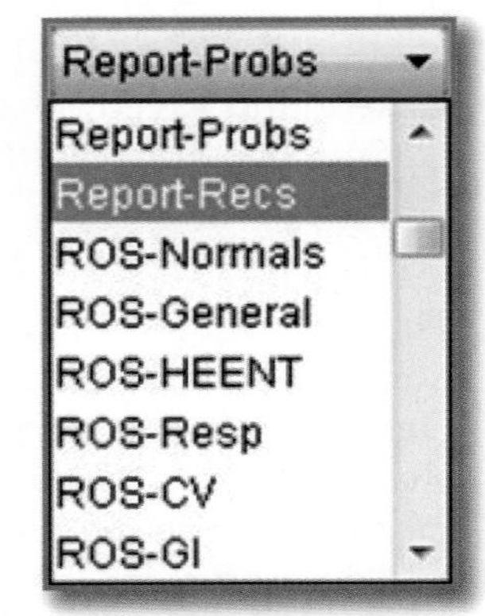

Figure 5.33 Selecting the *Report-Recs* pop-up text.

report, the EHR program automatically places the clinic's letterhead at the top. The current date, patient's name and address, salutation, and an introductory sentence are also automatically added. The incorporation of the clinic's letterhead and the clinician's digital signature in the report are optional check boxes at the time of printing (Figure 5.34).

(See Appendix A—*Sample Documents*; Document 6. *Test Report to a Patient*.)

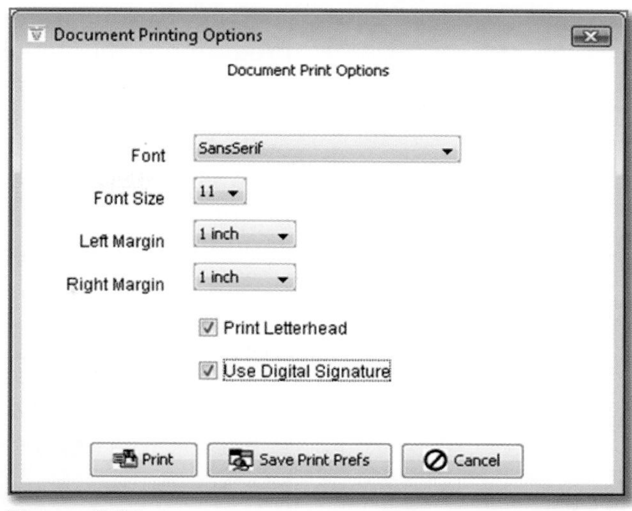

Figure 5.34 *Document Printing Options* window.

New Excuse/Note/Order

The *New Excuse/Note/Order* submenu under the *New* menu of the patient's chart allows the user to create printable forms for work or school excuses, notes, and orders. Once again, all new documents created for a patient are initiated from within the patient's chart. This method allows the patient's demographic information to be automatically included in the document and enables the item to be saved into the appropriate chart automatically.

After choosing the *New Excuse/Note* window option under the *New Excuse/Note/Order* submenu, the user types the name of the recipient (e.g., patient's school or employer) in the window's upper *To* field and then either manually types the note or uses pop-up text. The [Sign] button enables the user to either add initials to the note or permanently sign and lock the excuse note. Once locked, no user can open or modify the note. Excuse notes can be printed or faxed to the recipient. Once the [Done] button has been selected, excuse notes are automatically saved under the *Excuses/Notes* category of the care tree. There is no need for the user to select the category when saving an excuse note.

[Sign] button

(See Appendix A—*Sample Documents*; Document 7. *Patient's Excuse Note*.)

To create a new order form, the user selects the *New Orders* option under the *New Excuse/Note/Order* submenu under the *New* menu of the patient's chart (Figure 5.35). Order forms are used to record a physician orders for lab, imaging, and other medical tests typically conducted at a different facility. Within the order window, the user can select a diagnosis(es) from the patient's *Previous Dx* window, thus associating a relevant diagnosis and code with the ordered test(s). The program automatically prints the ordering provider's name on the order form. Pop-up text is also available for the user to select defining text for the order form, such as instructions for the patient or testing facility. Pop-up text can be modified by selecting the *Edit PopUp Text* (pencil) icon (shown in margin).

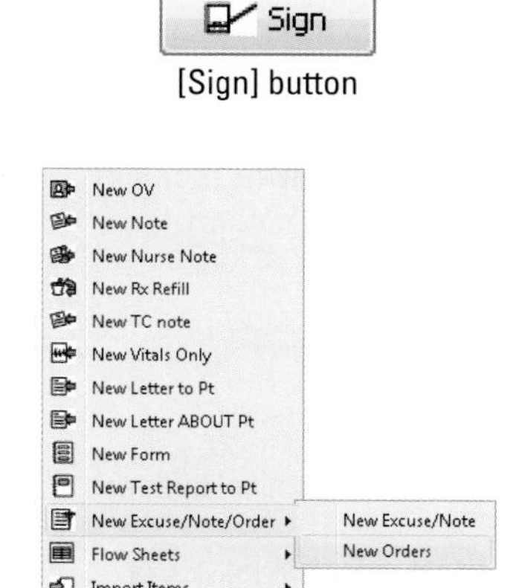

Figure 5.35 *New Orders* option under *New* menu > *New Excuse/Note/Order* submenu.

Edit PopUp Text icon

The patient's primary insurance information can be added to the order form by selecting the [Add Pt Ins] button (shown in margin) in the order window. The EHR program automatically adds the patient's personal insurance ID information, as well as demographic details of the insurance claims department from the patient's face sheet. Many testing facilities require that the patient's insurance information be sent along with the order form so the facility can bill the insurance company for the service. As with the test reports, when printing the order form, the user has the option to include the clinic's letterhead and digital signature (Figure 5.34). Once printed, the user can chart the order in the patient's care tree. Although the order form defaults to the *Encounters* tab when being saved, the user can choose another custom tab from the list.

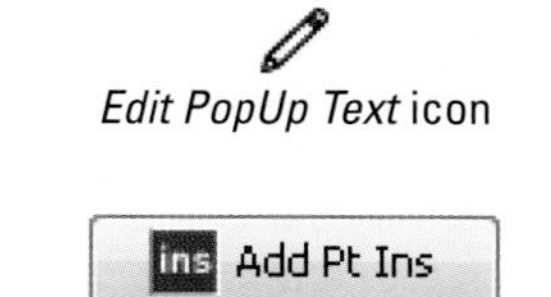

Add patient's insurance button

Users can create order forms in two places in the SpringCharts EHR program: in the patient's chart and in an office visit note. Orders created in the office visit note become part of the note and are printed on the routing slip for billing purposes. Orders created within the patient's chart, as outlined above, are not placed on the routing slip; therefore, no billable form is created for the orders. Clinicians who create order forms for tests performed outside the clinic and therefore not billed by the clinic can generate the order form from the patient's chart.

Concept Checkup 5.4

A. What does the *New TC note* function create?

B. When is the *New Vitals Only* submenu feature in SpringCharts used?

C. What navigation button is used in the *New Letter ABOUT a Patient* window to include test results and encounter notes in the letter?

D. When would the *Convert This Note to an Office Visit* icon be used in a TC note?

SpringCharts Tip

Shortcut:

Vitals Only

The fifth speed icon from the right (not counting the *eRx* icon) in the *Patient Chart* toolbar, *Vitals Only,* enables the user to access a New *Vitals Only* window without having to use the *New* menu in the patient's chart.

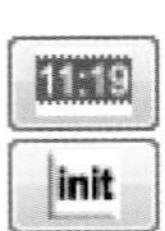

Time and initial buttons

Exercise 5.5 Recording and Viewing Vitals

1. Open Patti Adams's chart. Click on the *Vitals Only* speed icon (shown in margin) in the *Patient Chart* toolbar.
2. In the *New Vitals Only* window, record the following data: *Temperature 98.6, Respiration 17, Pulse 69, Blood Pressure 129/70, Height 64 inches,* and *Weight 163 pounds.*
3. Click on the *Notes* tab in the upper right and select any verbiage from the pop-up text. Add the time and your initials by clicking on the time and initial icon buttons (shown in margin), located in the lower middle section of the window.
4. Click the [Done] button and [Save and Skip Billing].
5. Open the *Actions* menu within the patient's chart. Select *Graph Vital Signs* and view the various graphed vitals.
6. Click on the [Body Mass Index] button and the [Blood Pressure] button and print a copy of the BMI and BP graphs. Write your name on the sheet and submit it to your instructor. Close all open windows.
7. Close the *Graph* window and the patient's chart.

SpringCharts Tip

Shortcut:

Letter about the Patient

The fourth speed icon from the right (not counting the *eRx* icon) on the *Patient Chart* toolbar enables the user to access the *New Letter about a Patient* window without needing to use the toolbar's *New* menu.

Edit PopUp Text icon

Exercise 5.6 Creating a Letter about a Patient

1. Open Patti Adams's chart. Under the *New* menu of the patient's chart, select *New Letter ABOUT Pt.*
2. Select the referring physician, *Dr. Harry Hart,* from the [Get Address Book] button on the window's right side.
3. Choose the pop-up text that begins with: *Thank you for allowing me to participate . . .*
4. Click on the *Edit PopUp Text* icon (shown in margin). Add the following sentence on an empty line: *Below please find a copy of the patient's recent lab results.* Click on the [Done] button.
5. Place the cursor in the letter body on a new line and select the newly added pop-up text sentence.

Exercise 5.6 (Concluded)

6. Click on the pop-up text sentence—*I will update you on this patient's progress after our next appointment*—to add this phrase to the letter as well.
7. Click on the [Add Chart Notes] button and select the *Lipid Panel* results from the *Choose Chart Entry* window. The lab test results will be added to the body of the letter.
8. Select the *Change Signature of Letter* icon (shown in margin) and select a signature.
9. Print the letter on the clinic's letterhead and submit to your instructor.
10. Click on the [Done] button and select *Letters* as the category where the letter will be stored in the patient's care tree.
11. On the patient's chart, click on the "+" expand symbol beside the *Letters* category in the care tree to see the saved copy of the letter.

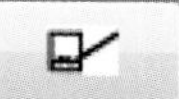

Change Signature of Letter icon

Exercise 5.7 Creating a Test Report for a Patient

1. In Patti Adams's chart, select the submenu *New Test Report to Pt* located under the *New* menu.
2. Highlight the *Lipid Panel* in the *Select Test* list. Note that the program automatically adds the test description to the bottom of the test results.
3. Place your cursor in the body of the report under the section heading *Problems*. Select *Elevated Cholesterol* from the pop-up text in the lower right panel.
4. Click on the down arrow in the pop-up text category field to reveal the list of pop-up text categories. Select *Report-Recs*.
5. Place your cursor under the heading *Recommendations* in the body of the report. Then select the following pop-up text line items from the right panel: *Low cholesterol diet. Regular exercise program. Please make an appointment to see the doctor as soon as possible.*
6. Print the test report and hand it in to your instructor.
7. Click on the [Done] button and store a copy of the report under the *Reports to Patient* category in the care tree. Note that a "+" expand symbol has been placed beside the *Reports to Patient* header in the care tree. Click the "+" symbol to see the saved report.
8. Close the patient's chart.

SpringCharts Tip

Shortcut:

New Message

The second speed icon from the right on the *Patient Chart* toolbar enables the user to create a new message about the patient that automatically references the patient and contains the patient's demographics. This pink speed icon bypasses the need to close the patient's chart, create a new message, and reference the patient.

SpringCharts Tip

Shortcut:

New ToDo

The last icon on the right of the *Patient Chart* toolbar enables the user to create a new to-do item that automatically references the patient. The icon with a blue bar to the right side bypasses the need to close the patient's chart, access the to-do header, and link a new to-do item to the patient.

chapter 5 summary

Learning Outcomes	Key Concepts/Examples
5.1 Understand the layout of an electronic chart. **Pages 118–123**	A patient's chart can be accessed from many places within an EHR program. An electronic chart can be opened by multiple users at the same time. The SpringCharts patient chart is composed of a face sheet and care tree. The face sheet houses more static information about the patient. The care tree contains more dynamic information about the patient.
5.2 Demonstrate how to build a patient's face sheet. **Pages 123–136**	Face sheet information is taken from intake sheets, the patient portal, or a patient interview: • Allergies • Social history • Past medical history • Family medical history • Referrals • Chart note • Routine medications • Outside medications • Problem list • Chart alert • Patient annotations • Patient requests
5.3 Perform various procedures in a patient's chart. **Pages 136–139**	Processes and documents are always started with the patient's chart open. The primary insurance is added to the patient's chart in SpringCharts EHR. The patient's past immunizations are added to the chart to create a complete list of vaccinations. EHR programs automatically graph a patient's vital signs, including height, weight, blood pressure, and body mass index. EHR programs automatically graph vitals of minors on growth charts.
5.4 Create new documentation in a patient's chart. **Pages 140–149**	A patient's chart must be open to create new documentation for the patient. The *New TC note* submenu displays a window to document telephone conversation, view face sheet information, and order new prescriptions. The *New Vitals Only* window documents vitals, provides face sheet information, and records vital notes. The *New Letter to the Patient* window automatically adds the patient's name and address, creates a letter from pop-up text, and adds items from the patient's chart. In the *New Letter about a Patient* window, you must select the addressee from the EHR *Address Book.* The *New Test Report* submenu enables you to select the patient's test results and create a report to the patient, detailing test results and a test description.

chapter 5 review

Name ______________________ Instructor ____________ Class ____________ Date ____________

Using Terminology

Match the terms on the left with the definitions on the right.

_____ 1. **LO 5.1** Care tree
_____ 2. **LO 5.1** Category preferences
_____ 3. **LO 5.2** Chart Alert
_____ 4. **LO 5.1** Electronic chart
_____ 5. **LO 5.1** Encounters
_____ 6. **LO 5.3** Deductible
_____ 7. **LO 5.1** Face sheet
_____ 8. **LO 5.3** Co-pay
_____ 9. **LO 5.2** Surveillance Reports

A. Information generated in an EHR that is provided to the Centers for Disease Control and Prevention, enabling effective monitoring of rates and distribution of disease.

B. The portion a medical insurance policyholder pays for each medical office visit or a specific type of medical service covered under the health insurance policy.

C. The portion of a patient's chart that displays the patient's demographics, medical history, and healthcare information.

D. The portion of the patient's chart that lists progress notes, tests, and other records; located on the right side in an EHR.

E. An annual amount of money a policyholder pays toward medical expenses to cover the patient's expenses, before the insurance company pays its contracted share.

F. A window on the SpringCharts server that enables the clinic administrator to create predetermined customized lists of medical data.

G. Allows for the inclusion of important text that appears in red at the top of the chart's care tree.

H. A category in the care tree that stores many of the documents created from contact with the patient.

I. The digital equivalent to a patient's paper chart, containing initial healthcare information and ongoing medical encounter documentation.

Checking Your Understanding

Choose the best answer and circle the corresponding letter.

10. LO 5.1 SpringCharts EHR provides practitioners a unique electronic view of the patient's chart similar to a:

a) Practice management system
b) Paper chart layout
c) Patient's intake sheet
d) Physician's order form

11. LO 5.1 All of the preset categories in the care tree:

a) Cannot be altered or edited
b) Can be altered and edited
c) Can be customized to the clinic's needs
d) Match the categories in the face sheet

12. LO 5.4 A new TC note stands for:

a) Technical committee note
b) Tissue culture note
c) Telephone call note
d) Total cholesterol note

13. LO 5.1 Three areas of the face sheet cannot be altered or edited. Select the one that *can* be altered.

a) Prescription history
b) Diagnosis history
c) Problem list
d) Procedure history

14. LO 5.3 Before creating new documentation or activities for a patient, the patient's chart must be:

a) Opened
b) Closed
c) In the *Recent Charts* list
d) Not in use by another clinician

15. LO 5.2 The information needed to complete the patient's face sheet is typically taken from which of the following? Select all that apply.

a) The patient's intake sheet
b) A family member
c) The Patient Portal
d) A one-on-one interview with the patient

Introduction

The most common encounter with patients in an ambulatory setting is the office visit (OV). An office visit is an outpatient encounter with a healthcare provider to receive health advice or treatment for a symptom or condition. A patient typically presents with a healthcare concern (complaint) or question. A clinician measures and records the patient's vital signs and may, under a physician's authority, perform diagnostic tests. A physician performs a diagnostic inquiry, which generally includes obtaining a history of the present illness or chief complaint, description of the signs and symptoms, previous state of health, social conditions, and family healthcare issues. The physician then inquires about the patient's body systems, often following a set of ordered questions about each major body system. Next, the physician performs a physical examination, after which he or she may order additional medical tests. The recording of this process and the subsequent results constitute an office visit note or progress note.

The findings from the history of the present illness, vital signs, review of body systems, and physical examination typically lead the physician to assign a diagnosis or multiple diagnoses. The clinical staff then enlists the patient's agreement to a management plan, which may include medication, medical procedures, and other therapies. The physician and clinical staff educate the patient about the causes, progression, outcomes, and possible treatments for the diagnosis(es), as well as give advice for maintaining health. A follow-up appointment is set, if necessary.

In this chapter we will learn the various components of an office visit note and learn how to create a detailed note. The skill of accurately recording a patient's chief complaint, history of the illness, vital signs, and test results is critical to a medical assistant's success. The EHR program allows the MA to collaborate with other providers and the physican to create a comprehensive analysis of the patient's current health situation and a plan for appropriate care.

SpringCharts Tip

If your SpringCharts *Office Visit* screen doesn't look like Figure 6.1, you need to adjust your *User Preferences* setting. Refer to Figure 3.6 in Chapter 3 to select the "large screen" view of the office visit note.

6.1 Components of the Office Visit

A new medical office visit encounter in SpringCharts EHR is created by selecting the *New* menu on the *Patient Chart* menu bar and then clicking on *New OV*. The *OV* screen appears (Figure 6.1).

The *OV* window has three main sections, left to right: the face sheet overview, office visit note section, and the pop-up text window with the navigation panel.

The left side panel displays an overview of the patient's face sheet. This panel allows users to view the patient's face sheet information without having to exit the office visit display. Later we'll learn how any face sheet categories can be added to the office visit note to document that a clinician discussed these issues with the patient.

The middle panel is the area where the notes from the office visit will be documented and stored. Information is entered in the **SOAP** format, which includes the subjective, objective, assessment, and plan components, outlined in Table 6.1. All of the text items selected from the office visit pop-up text categories or manually added to the text fields automatically save into one of these areas of the SOAP note. Below the OV note section is a box in which text can be created and modified.

The right side of the *OV* window contains the pop-up text window and a navigation panel with tabs to access information for the office visit note (Figure 6.1). When the user selects text from any of the 12 office note categories, the program automatically inserts the text into the appropriate segment of the SOAP note.

SpringCharts Tip

Shortcut:

New Office Visit Note

The first speed icon in the last set of icons in the patient's chart enables the user to open a new office visit note without accessing the *New* menu on the *Patient Chart* toolbar.

SOAP

An acronym for *subjective, objective, assessment,* and *plan.* The SOAP note is a convenient format for healthcare providers to document a patient's healthcare evaluation in a typical office visit.

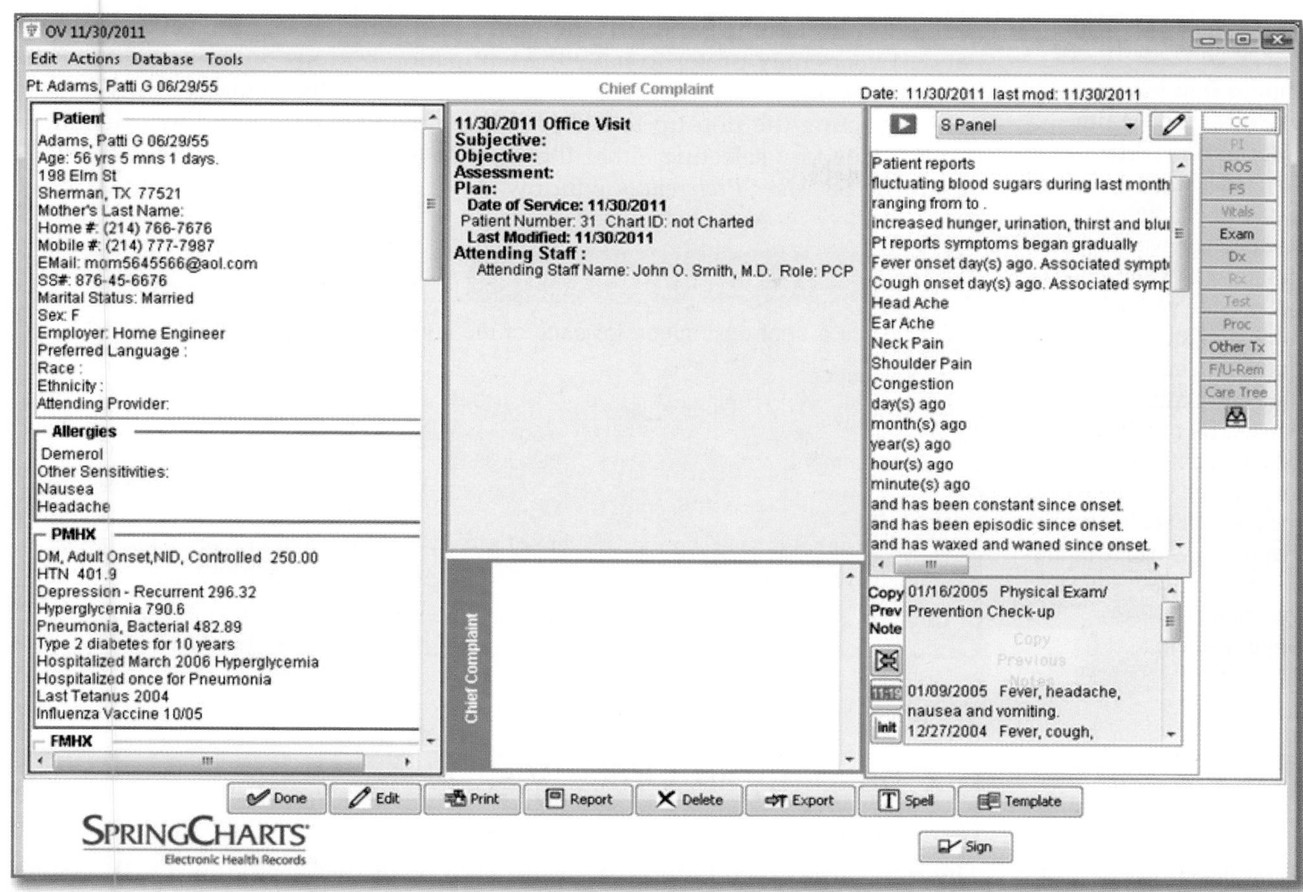

Figure 6.1 *New Office Visit* window with face sheet panel.

Table 6.1 SOAP Format for Documenting Medical Office Visit Notes

Component	Description
Subjective	The patient's current medical condition from the patient's point of view. It generally includes the signs and symptoms, history of the present illness, and a review of the patient's body systems (i.e., what the patient thinks and feels).
Objective	The patient's condition from the practitioner's perspective. It generally includes the vital signs and findings from the physical exam (i.e., what the physician sees, feels, hears, etc.).
Assessment	The physician's diagnosis(es) based on the objective findings. Possible diagnoses are usually listed in order of the most likely to the least likely.
Plan	What the physician will do to test and treat the patient's symptoms. It may include medications, diagnostic tests, counseling and advice, and scheduling of a follow-up visit.

SpringCharts Tip

Remember that all activities regarding a patient can only be documented once the patient's chart is opened. Therefore the patient's chart must be open in order to create an office visit note.

Focal Point

The SOAP note is only one of several methods of documentation used by healthcare providers to notate patient encounter observations.

HIPAA/HITECH Tip

Public Disclosure of Protected Health Information (PHI)
Don't talk about a patient's condition or treatments, even in general terms, to any individual outside your clinic. It is very difficult to keep a patient's identity anonymous no matter how hard you try. Be careful not to communicate healthcare information on social media like Facebook and Twitter; however, sharing any PHI may put you in violation of HIPAA's privacy ruling.

The left and right panels in the *Office Visit* window can be reversed. Left-handed users may prefer to have the navigation buttons on the left side of the screen, especially when using a tablet, so their hand doesn't cover the OV note when selecting the pop-up text. Recall that the *Office Visit* window orientation is determined by selecting either the right or left options under the *Preference 2* tab in the *Set User Preferences* window.

Concept Checkup 6.1

A. Provide a brief description for each of the components of the SOAP format.

Subjective:

Objective:

Assessment:

Plan:

B. What panel is seen on the left side of the *OV* screen when first entering the window?

C. What screen must be opened first before the *OV* screen can be opened?

Review of systems (ROS)
A review of systems is a structured technique used by providers to gather healthcare history covering the organ systems from a patient. It is therefore a component of the 'subjective' portion of the SOAP note. There are 14 body systems recognized by the CMS.

6.2 Building an Office Visit Note

Overview

The navigation panel along the right side of the screen (Figure 6.2) enables the user to proceed through the office visit note in a logical order; however, the tabs can be chosen in any order. Included in the panel are chief complaint [CC], history of present illness [PI], **review of systems [ROS]**, face sheet [FS], [Vitals], [Exam], diagnosis [Dx], prescriptions [Rx], tests [Test], procedures [Proc], other treatment [Other Tx], and follow-up and reminders [F/U-Rem]. The [Care Tree] tab allows the user to view the care tree portion of the patient's chart while still in the *OV* screen (for example, to view a document or spreadsheet in the patient's *File Cabinet* while discussing issues with the patient during the office visit). Finally, the *Show Chart Summary* tab (shown in margin), at the very bottom, allows the user to enter all text into the SOAP note and view the entire note.

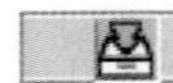
Show Chart Summary tab

When a tab is selected, a list of relevant pop-up text appears in the third panel of the screen (Figure 6.1). Data can be entered into the office visit note by:

1. Tapping on the pop-up text with a stylus tool (as with a tablet)
2. Clicking on pop-up text items with a mouse
3. Typing directly into the text box at the bottom of the middle panel
4. Dictating through a third-party voice recognition program, causing the dictated text to enter the text box

Although there are many ways in which text can be added into the office visit note, the use of pop-up text is the most rapid way of building documentation for an office visit note.

Focal Point

The use of pop-up text and templates provides for a rapid way to populate an OV note.

Chief Complaint, Present Illness, Review of Systems, and Exam

The chief complaint [CC], present illness [PI], review of systems [ROS], and examination [Exam] tabs displays text notes from previous encounters with the patient in the bottom right panel. A user can highlight any previous note text and copy it to the present note by clicking on the *Copy Highlighted Text to Note* icon (shown in margin). Notes from previous encounters are dated and organized in chronological order with the most recent first. These notes enable clinicians to refresh their memory regarding past visits and copy any similar notes quickly into the current office visit box, if necessary, without opening up previous SOAP notes. The previous note panel only displays the previous documentation specific to the area (tab) selected on the navigation panel.

To the left of the previous note panel are time and initial buttons (shown in margin) that enable the user to time- and initial-stamp that portion of the office visit note. This feature allows multiple medical providers to be involved in the same patient encounter. For example, a medical assistant may record the patient's symptoms when first admitting the patient to the exam room. The user's identification and the time can be recorded in the *chief complaint* portion of the OV note. Similarly, a nurse may administer an injection after the physician has completed the examination and then initial- and time-stamp that procedure. In this way, one OV note can document the actions of several users in addition to those of the primary physician.

Although the program defaults to the appropriate pop-up text category when a specific navigation tab is selected, additional pop-up text can be accessed from other categories in the pop-up text header field at the top of the right panel (Figure 6.3). Here, the user can choose from multiple categories of text. Any selected text from these fields is added to existing text in the open text box. For example, a practitioner may create a new category of text specific to a certain procedure he or she performs or to a unique review of systems, or the practitioner may create a category specifically for chief complaints. Regardless of what category the pop-up text is chosen from, it will always go into the appropriate *SOAP* format section based on the navigation panel open at the time of text selection. The program offers an additional 20 user-defined categories that can be added to the pop-up text feature.

The [Dx], [Rx], [Test], and [Proc] navigation tabs operate differently than the ones already mentioned by offering a search feature of the database rather than using pop-up text. Because information from these categories is transmitted electronically from the EHR to clearinghouses, insurance companies, and testing facilities, it has to be in a structured or coded format rather than in free text. The diagnosis, prescription, and procedures panels also offer the user a choice of items from previous chart entries.

Copy Prev Note

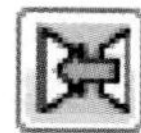

Copy Highlighted Text to Note icon

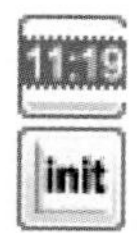

Time and initial buttons

Focal Point

Multiple users can work on the same OV note. A medical assistant may be first to document medical information and then hand off the OV note to be completed by another provider.

HIPAA/HITECH Tip

Persons or entities that perform activities that involve the use or disclosure of PHI on behalf of a covered entity are considered *business associates* under HIPAA regulations and must follow the practice's guidelines to ensure that patients' PHI remains secure and private.

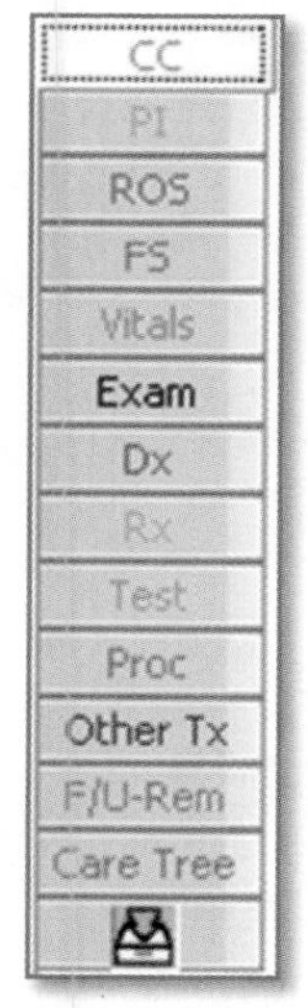

Figure 6.2 Navigation panel in the *Office Visit* screen.

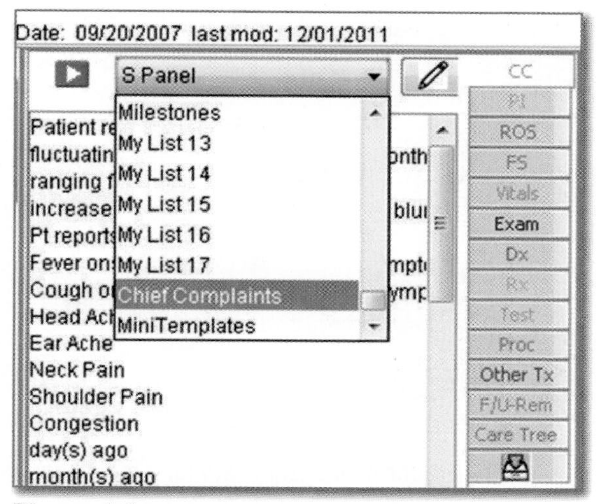

Figure 6.3 Pop-up text category list.

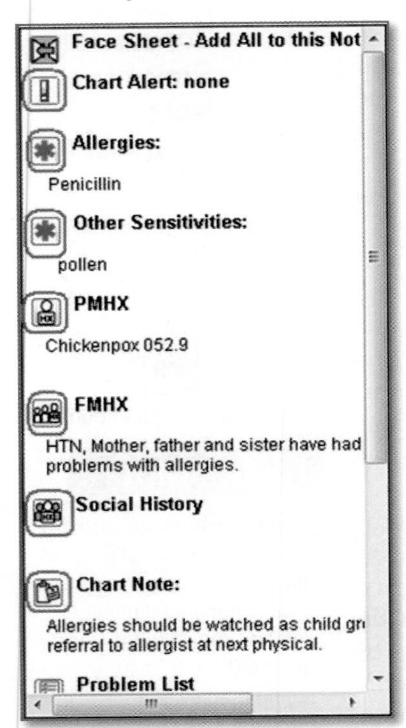

Figure 6.4 Category listing for face sheet information.

Face Sheet

The [FS] navigation tab allows the user to add a portion of or the entire face sheet to the office visit note by simply clicking on one or more of the category icons (Figure 6.4). The selected face sheet information is placed in the *Subjective* area of the OV note. If the provider wants to add the entire face sheet to the office visit note, he or she clicks on the icon at the top of the screen beside *Face Sheet—Add All to this Note* header (shown in margin).

Vitals

Vital signs are usually taken before the physician examines the patient. By recording the vitals in the office visit note, the medical assistant provides the physician with valuable information about the patient's overall condition. Along with nine basic vital signs that appear by default in SpringCharts (temperature, respiration, pulse, blood pressure, height, weight, head circumference, **body mass index (BMI)**, and body fat), three additional custom vital signs can be added to the program, such as peak flow rate, oxygen saturation of the blood, and so on. These are added at the SpringCharts server in a network environment and will appear in the *Vitals* section of the *Office Visit* window and in the *New Vitals Only* screen of the patient's chart, as discussed in Chapter 5. The patient's body mass index (BMI) is automatically calculated for the user based upon the patient's height and weight. SpringCharts displays four vital sign charts (height, weight, blood pressure, and BMI) by accessing the graph icons at the top right in the *Vitals* panel (shown in margin). The graph backgrounds differ by patient age and gender, for the purpose of showing appropriate national percentiles for children. Figure 6.5 displays graphs for a boy between the age of 2 and 18 years (except HC, which displays for patients 0 to 3 years).

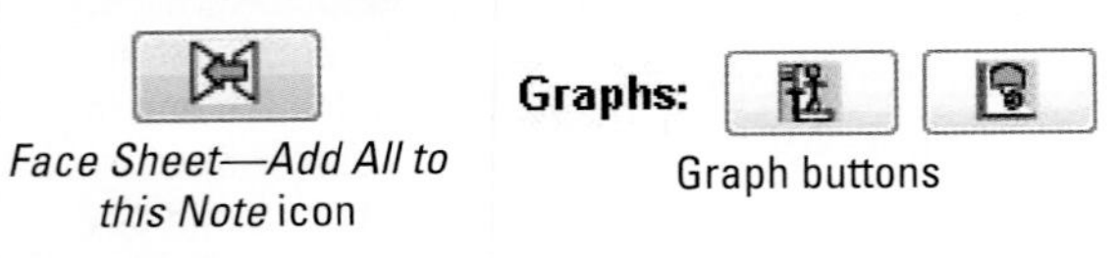

Face Sheet—Add All to this Note icon

Graph buttons

SpringCharts Tip

The patient's face sheet can also be accessed while in the office visit note by right-clicking (or CTRL-Click on a Mac) on the particular section of the face sheet panel in the *OV* screen and selecting *Edit*.

Body mass index (BMI)
BMI is a measure of body fat based on height and weight that applies to adult men and women. BMI is the measurement of choice for studying obesity. It is calculated by a mathematical formula that divides a person's weight in kilograms by their height in meters squared (BMI = kg/m^2).

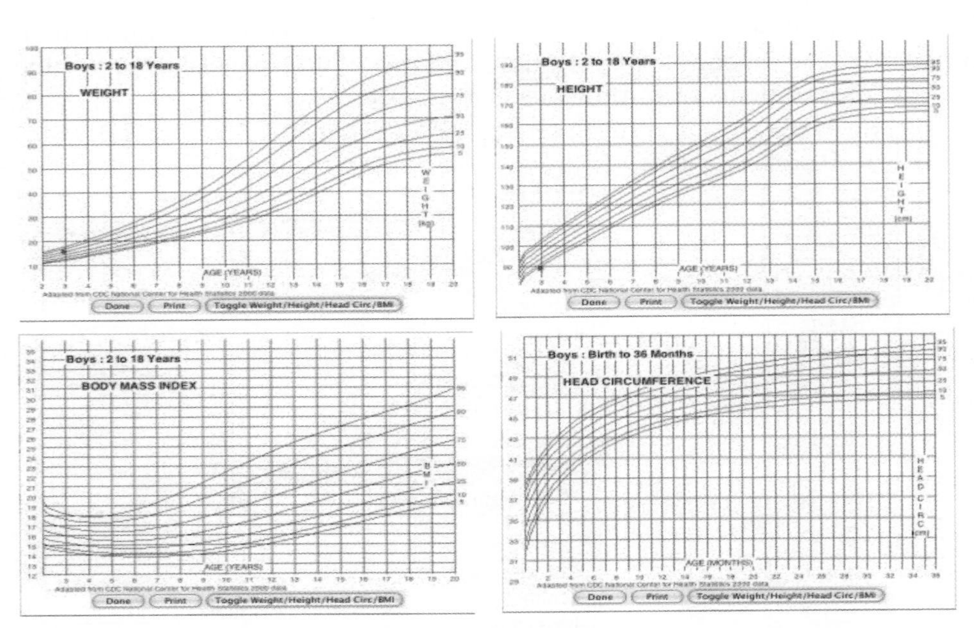

Figure 6.5 Graphs of vital sign data for a male between ages 2 and 18 (HC = 0 to 3 years).

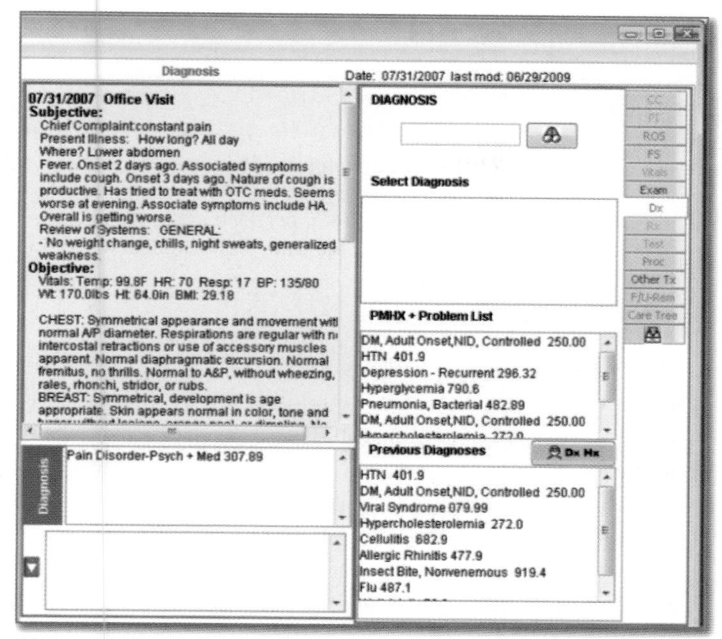

Figure 6.6 *Diagnosis* panel showing diagnoses from previous visits.

> **SpringCharts Tip**
>
> In the *Office Visit* screen, the provider can view the information already collected by the medical assistant. This can be done even before the provider opens up the office visit note by clicking on the OV note in the *Encounters* tab of the care tree and viewing the summary at the bottom of the screen.

Diagnosis

Selecting the [Dx] navigation tab produces a dialog widow that allows the user to choose diagnoses from the *PMHX + Problem List* and *Previous Diagnoses* fields (Figure 6.6). The *PMHX + Problem List* field displays diagnoses from the *PMHX* and *Problem List* areas of the patient's face sheet, whereas the *Previous Diagnoses* window displays all of the diagnoses from previous encounters with the particular patient. These features enable the rapid selection of diagnoses, drugs, and procedures within the *Office Visit* screen; many times patients are seen in the clinic for the same diagnoses, receive the same medications, and undergo the same procedures as previous visits.

Prescriptions

Under the HITECH ruling, ONC-certified EHR programs must be able to transmit prescriptions electronically. During the meaningful use (MU) stage 1 reporting period, physicians demonstrated that at least 40 percent of all prescribed medications were transmitted electronically from the clinic in any consecutive 90-day period. Table 6.2 outlines the ONC objectives and MU measures regarding e-prescribing. Because some pharmacies do not have the software necessary to receive prescriptions electronically, the MU requirements only specify the transmission of electronic prescriptions from the healthcare provider, not the receipt of them electronically.

The [Rx] navigation tab allows the user to view information fields from the patient's chart related to *Allergies* and *Other Sensitivities* in the upper section of the window. This information is useful for review when the physician is prescribing medication. New prescriptions can be chosen from the *Routine Medications* and *Previous Prescriptions* windows. This section provides practitioners with valuable information from which to make informed medical decisions.

Medication prescribed during the office visit can be added to the patient's routine medication list by clicking on the chosen medication in the lower

Table 6.2 Meaningful Use Core Measure

E-Prescribing	
ONC Stage 1 Objective	**Meaningful Use Measure**
Generate and transmit prescriptions electronically.	More than 40 percent of prescribed medication needs to be transmitted electronically using certified EHR technology.

Notes:

- Schedule II medications (i.e., drugs and other substances that have a high potential for abuse) are now permitted to be transmitted electronically as of 2010.
- Transmission of schedule II medications is not counted in the calculation as permissible prescriptions for the MU requirement.
- A prescription only needs to be transmitted electronically to qualify for this MU measure. The pharmacy can receive it in any format (e.g., fax).
- A physician may use "stand-alone" e-prescribing systems, however; for an EHR program to be certified by the ONC, it must have the capability to e-prescribe.

Focal Point

Creating a report from the OV note provides the patient with a record of the provider's notations of the exam, along with the diagnoses and treatment plan.

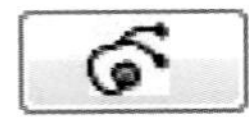

Diagnosis Search icon

middle area of the face sheet in the *Office Visit* screen and selecting the [Add to Routine] button in the *Edit Rx* window that appears (Figure 6.7). The strength, dosage, and other details can be edited for this specific prescription without changing the system's original medication information in the database. In the *Edit Rx* window, the provider can also associate the medication with diagnoses by clicking on the *Diagnosis Search* icon to the right of the *Diagnosis* field. A single diagnosis or multiple diagnoses can be selected from

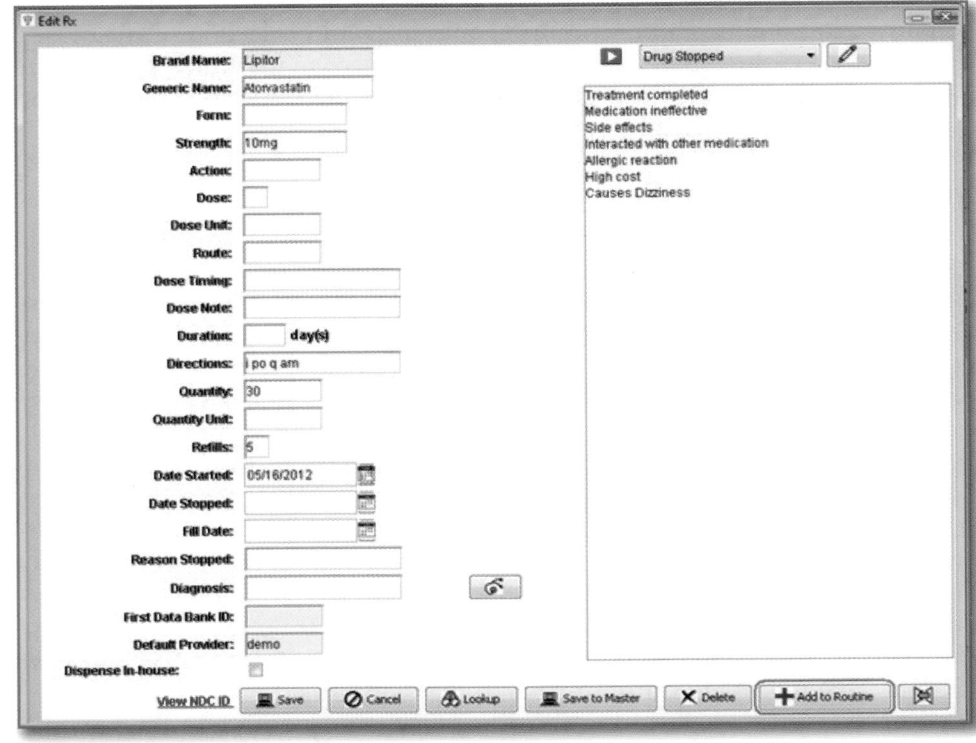

Figure 6.7 *Edit Rx* window.

Figure 6.8 *Prescription Printing Options* window.

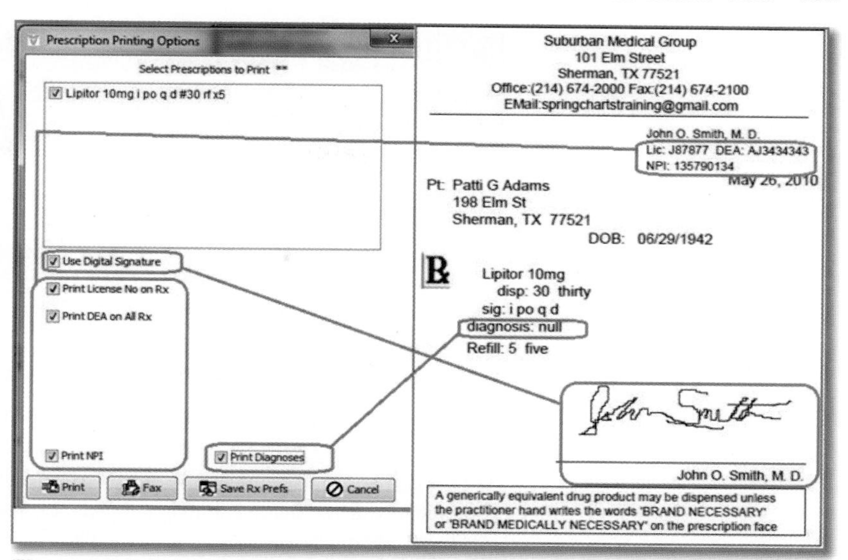

Figure 6.9 *Prescription Printing Options* window and hard copy of prescription.

any of the patient's past medical history, problem, or previous diagnoses lists, or a new diagnosis(es) can be selected from the program's activated database.

The printer icon in the lower middle panel (shown in margin) allows for the printing or faxing of prescriptions from the *Office Visit* screen. Once the data filter preferences have been selected in the *Prescription Printing Options* window, the [Print] or [Fax] button can be selected to produce the prescription form (Figure 6.8).

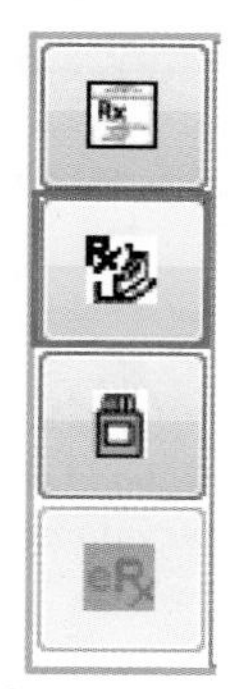

Printer icon in prescription text window

If the prescription is created by a user not set up in SpringCharts as a provider, the prescription will need to be printed and manually signed. Only users set up as providers in the EHR program have the *Use Digital Signature* check box option available in the *Prescription Printing Options* window. If the provider has added his/her signature into SpringCharts in the *Set User Preferences* window, the digital signature prints on the prescription(s). If the provider has not added his/her signature into SpringCharts and the *Use Digital Signature* box is checked, the prescription form prints *Electronic Signature Verified* above the provider's name on the script form. The form can then be sent electronically directly to the pharmacy's fax machine from SpringCharts. The *Electronic Signature Verified* phrase informs the pharmacy the prescription was sent by the provider, even though it doesn't display the digital signature.

If the provider has also selected an attending physician in the *Set User Preferences* window, this physician's name and ID information will also appear on the prescription form (see Figure 3.7 in Chapter 3). Also available in the *Prescription Printing Options* window is the choice to have the provider's license, Drug Enforcement Administration (DEA) number, National Provider Identification (NPI) number, and the diagnosis(es) printed on the prescription(s) (Figure 6.9). These various choices can be set as defaults for future prescriptions by selecting the [Save Rx Prefs] button before the scripts are printed.

(See Appendix A—*Sample Documents*; Document 1. *Prescription Forms*.)

Drug allergies can cause patient injuries and fatalities. Because EHRs store information about patients' allergies, sensitivities, and routine medications, they can effectively prevent reactions by performing drug-to-drug checking and drug-to-allergy checking in the patient's chart and display warnings for any allergy-related adverse interactions for the provider. Although ONC-certified

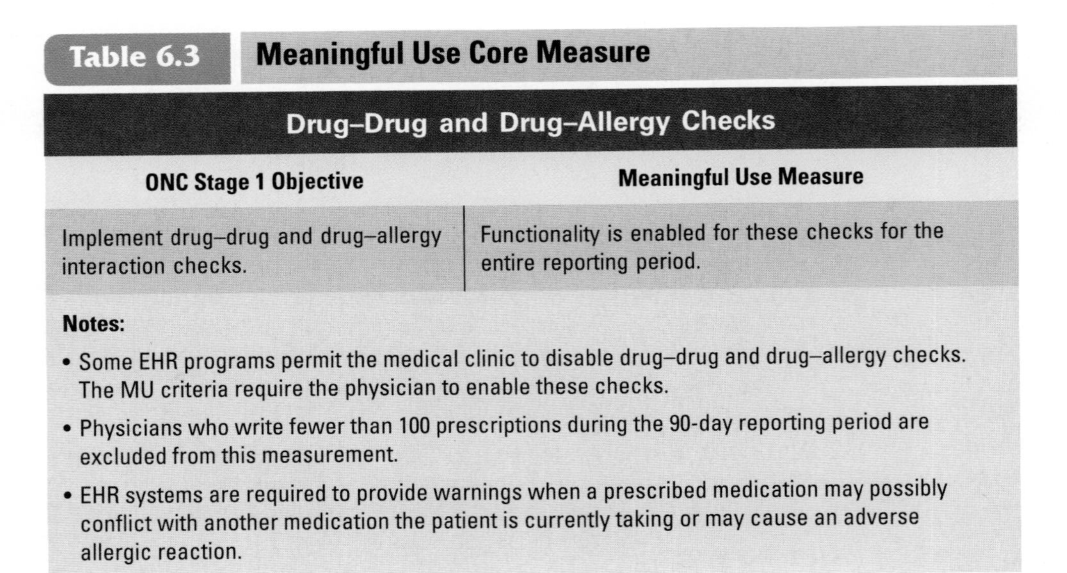

Table 6.3 Meaningful Use Core Measure

Drug–Drug and Drug–Allergy Checks	
ONC Stage 1 Objective	**Meaningful Use Measure**
Implement drug–drug and drug–allergy interaction checks.	Functionality is enabled for these checks for the entire reporting period.

Notes:

- Some EHR programs permit the medical clinic to disable drug–drug and drug–allergy checks. The MU criteria require the physician to enable these checks.
- Physicians who write fewer than 100 prescriptions during the 90-day reporting period are excluded from this measurement.
- EHR systems are required to provide warnings when a prescribed medication may possibly conflict with another medication the patient is currently taking or may cause an adverse allergic reaction.

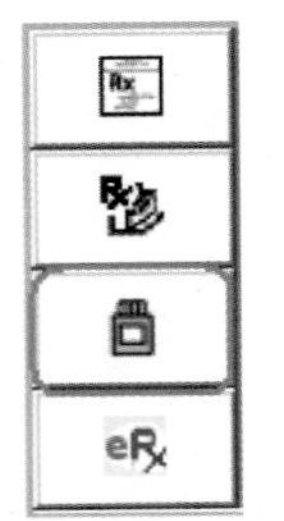

Drug Interactions and Allergy Checking icon

EHR programs are required to perform drug–drug and drug–allergy checks, stage one of the MU program only required eligible professionals (EPs) to have this function turned on. Table 6.3 outlines the ONC objectives and MU measures regarding drug–drug and drug–allergy checks.

The Drug Interactions and Allergy Checking icon is the third button in the prescription text window. When the user selects this button, the program checks any new drug that appears in the window against the patient's allergies and current medications for any adverse reactions. This option is available throughout the EHR program in any window in which a medication can be prescribed. The resulting window, seen in Figure 6.10, shows the details of the prescriptions checked against the patient's current medications and allergies. Any potential allergic reactions or drug interactions are listed in this window, along with the severity level of the interaction. This information enables the physician to

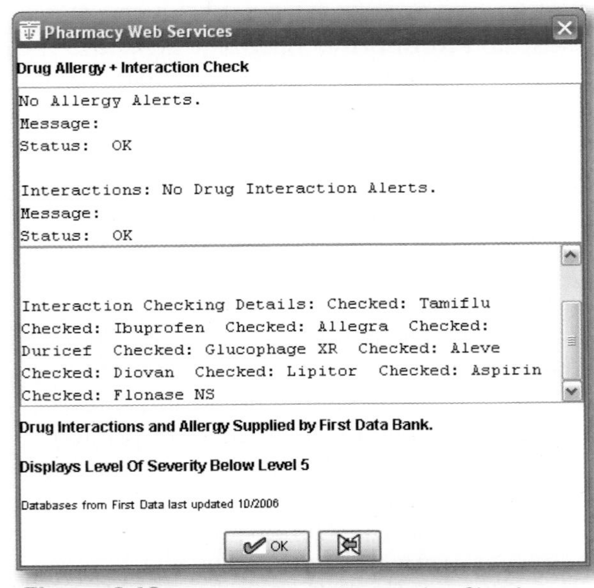

Figure 6.10 *Drug Allergy + Interaction Check* information.

determine if the prescribed medication should be given to the patient. However, the program allows the physician to prescribe the medication even if there is an alert.

The *Send Prescriptions Electronically* icon at the bottom of the prescription window allows for the prescription to be sent electronically to SureScripts, the Web-based e-prescribing clearinghouse, and then on to the pharmacy. The *Drug Interactions and Allergy Check*ing icon described above does not need to be used when transmitting e-prescriptions because the clearinghouse conducts its own drug–allergy interaction check. When the prescribed medication is electronically transmitted, SpringCharts also sends the patient's routine medications, allergies, and current medication lists to SureScripts. The clearinghouse analyzes this information as well as prescribed medications from other providers transmitting electronic prescriptions. The SureScripts clearinghouse provides information regarding drug formularies, correct dosage, drug–drug interaction, and drug–allergy interaction.

Send Prescriptions Electronically icon

Tests

The vision of an integrated electronic healthcare system is that all healthcare providers will be able to transmit, receive, store, and analyze all medical services related to a patient's healthcare. To this end, the ONC requires that all certified EHR programs have the functionality to generate computerized provider order entry (CPOE). The CPOE feature in EHR programs enable physicians to document orders for labs, imaging studies, medical tests, and medication in the patient's electronic chart and maintain a record of that order. Stage one of the MU requirement in 2011 and 2012 only required EPs to demonstrate the ordering and storage of one medication for the patient. Table 6.4 outlines the ONC objectives and MU measures regarding CPOE.

Tests are ordered within the *Office Visit* screen by clicking on the [Test] navigation tab. In the upper portion of the *Test* window the user types the first few letters of the test name and conducts a search. From the search results list the user can select the appropriate test. Multiple tests can be

SpringCharts Tip

SpringCharts EHR has an add-on feature that provides prebuilt office visits notes, orders, and letters, as well as pop-up text for specific specialists. Installing these templates saves time and facilitates more complete patient documentation with a minimum of effort. Some of the specialty templates includes family practice, gastroenterology, internal medicine, pediatric, psychiatry, and pulmonary medicine.

Table 6.4 Meaningful Use Core Measure

Computerized Provider Order Entry	
ONC Stage 1 Objective	**Meaningful Use Measure**
Provide computerized provider order entry (CPOE) for medication orders, lab services, imaging studies, and other services and store in EHR.	More than 30 percent of patients must have at least one medication in their medication list and at least one medication ordered through CPOE.

Notes:

- Physicians who write fewer than 100 prescriptions during the 90-day reporting period are excluded from this MU objective.
- Although the CPOE function should handle all physician orders, this MU objective in Stage 1 is limited to only medication orders.
- It is only required that the physician enter the order using CPOE and store a copy in the patient's chart. The electronic transmission of the order is not required for Stage 1 of MU.
- The measure is based on individual patients, regardless of how many times an individual patient is seen or how many orders are generated for an individual patient.

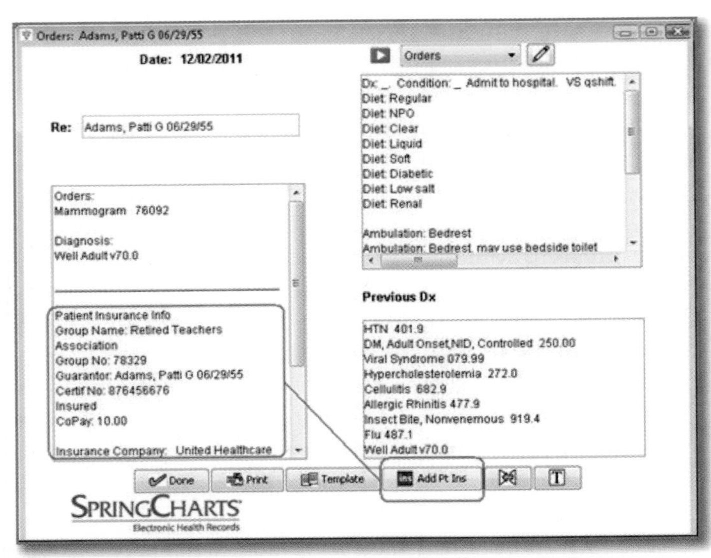

Figure 6.11 Order form showing patient's primary insurance.

SpringCharts Tip

For a nonphysician user to order tests in the *Office Visit* screen, the user must have first selected a physician in his/her *Set User Preferences* window *(File > Preferences > User Preferences)*. Once set up, the program will also allow the nonphysician user to order tests.

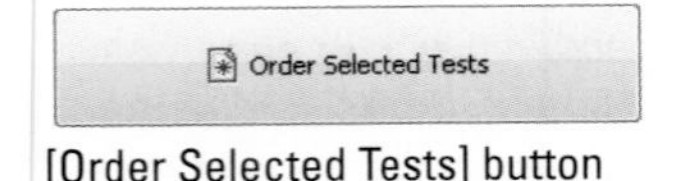

[Order Selected Tests] button

Write and Print Orders icon

selected at the same time. Once all the applicable tests have been chosen, the user clicks the [Order Selected Tests] button to send the tests to the *Tests* text box in the lower middle panel of the *OV* screen. The tests can then be printed or faxed as a physician order by selecting the *Write and Print Orders* icon in the lower left corner of the *Tests* text box. The resulting *Orders* window automatically adds the selected test(s) and diagnoses from the office visit note. Tests that will be conducted in the clinic can be deleted from the CPOE form, leaving only the tests to be conducted at an outside testing facility.

In the *Orders* window, the user can add pop-up text from the *Orders* category at the top right of the screen. The patient's primary insurance information can be added to the order form by selecting the [Add Pt Ins] button (Figure 6.11). The CPOE form for tests conducted at a third-party facility can then be printed and given to the patient.

(See Appendix A—*Sample Documents*; Document 8. *Test Order Form*.)

The order form can also be used as a referral form. Because the program automatically places the diagnosis codes from the OV note on the form and provides the user with pop-up text and templates, a referral form can be created quickly, printed for the patient, and stored in the patient's chart. The form is printed with the clinic's letterhead and contains the patient's name, address, and date of birth.

When the order form is printed, the user is given the option to save a copy of the order in the patient's chart. This feature enables the form to be reprinted if necessary.

SpringCharts Tip

Although the SpringCharts program contains the entire set of procedure codes, not all are activated in the drop-down lists. When the program is initially set up, only those procedure codes the clinic commonly uses are activated for the clinicians to see. Limiting the number of codes to those the clinic uses most often enables speedier selection.

Procedures

Procedures can be added to an OV note by first selecting the [Proc] navigation tab in the *Office Visit* screen and then the correct procedure category (for example, *Immunization, Surgery, Dermatology)* (Figure 6.12). Once selected, each category displays only the specific procedures activated for that category. (See Chapter 9 for further discussion on activating new procedure codes.) The user may also select procedures from the *Previous Procedure* text box in the lower right corner. These procedures are ones conducted during previous encounters with the patient. Once a procedure has been selected, additional notes can be manually added to the procedure, such as injection sites, medication strengths, procedural notes, and so on, by clicking on the procedure in the text box in the *OV* screen's lower middle panel.

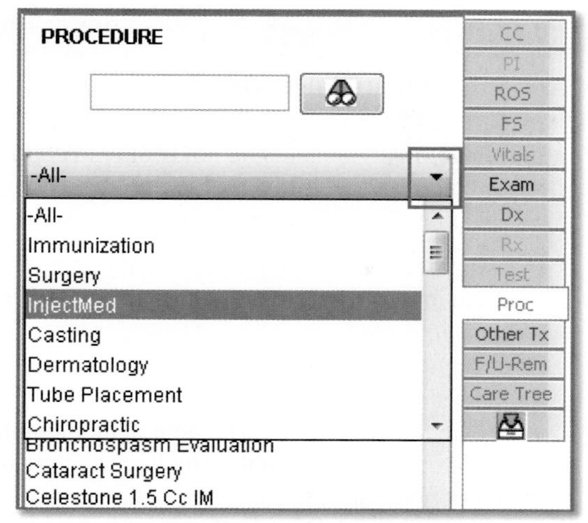

Figure 6.12 Prodcedure categories in the procedure section.

Other Treatment

The [Other Tx] navigation tab allows the provider to select text from the default pop-up *Other Treatment* category for counseling and **coordination of care** items. Once again, text used in previous encounters with the patient relevant to the *Other Tx* section is available in the lower right window for previewing and copying into the current visit. If the same counseling is conducted, the physician simply highlights previous text (not including the date) and then selects the *Copy Highlighted Text to Note* icon (shown in margin) to add this note to the existing office visit.

Follow-up

The [F/U-Rem] navigation tab allows a user to select a follow-up period and create reminder/referral notes. Text can be chosen from the pop-up text or selected from the previous note window, which contains text for this section from prior encounters. In the lower middle text box of the *OV* screen, the user can find a *Create a Reminder* icon (shown in margin) that enables the provider to send a *ToDo/Reminder* item to another person in the clinic or to him- or herself. Clicking on the icon activates the *New ToDo/Reminder* window (Figure 6.13). The *ToDo/Reminder* feature in the OV screen enables providers to communicate with other staff members regarding scheduling follow-up appointments, making a call, setting reminders for a patient's lab or procedure, and so on. Because this window was activated from within a specific patient's office visit note, the dialog box automatically links to the patient's chart. Pop-up text is available for rapid text selection. The [Send Later] button can be used to send the reminder to another staff meeting on

Figure 6.13 *New ToDo/Reminder* window in *Office Visit* screen.

Focal Point

Procedure categories are first set up on the SpringCharts server. When procedures are activated in the program, they are activated under these categories.

Coordination of care

Coordination of care comprises making available all resources to ensure healthcare providers have access to all required information on a patient's conditions and treatments and that the patient receives appropriate healthcare services.

Copy
Prev
Note

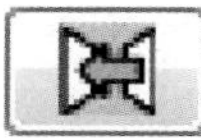

Copy Highlighted Text to Note icon

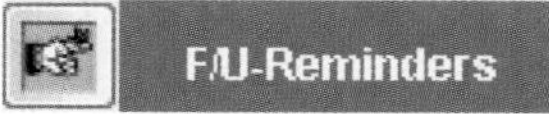

Create a Reminder icon

HIPAA/HITECH Tip

Faxing Healthcare Information
Disclosure of PHI via fax machine is permitted by HIPAA/HITECH between group healthcare providers and facilities as necessary to support patient diagnosis, prognosis, treatment, and care. It is allowed to third-party payers as required for certification of a hospitalization. The following procedures must be observed:

1. The fax cover sheet must be used with an approved confidentiality statement.
2. Limit the information being faxed to the minimum information necessary to serve the purpose intended.
3. Establish that the receiving fax machine is secure or attended at the time of transmission.
4. Verify the fax number before sending documents. Use a preprogrammed fax number to send faxes when feasible. The law requires preprogrammed numbers be reconfirmed periodically for accuracy.
5. Log all fax transmissions in the record, including the fax number, recipient, date and time, and specific material sent.
6. Pick up and distribute received faxes as soon as possible after receipt.

Focal Point

Before completing an OV note, the provider can send a follow-up note regarding the patient to him- or herself or to another co-worker.

a future date. When the recipient clicks on the item in his or her *To Do List* the patient's chart opens, providing all necessary information to execute the scheduled activity.

Signing and Dating an OV Note

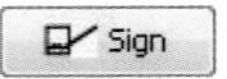

[Sign] button in OV note

Finalizing the follow-up section of the OV note completes the notation on the *Office Visit* screen. The provider then either initials the note or signs and locks the note. Selecting the [Sign] button at the bottom of the *OV* screen provides the practitioner, via the *Sign* dialog window, with the opportunity to [Initial Only] or [Permanent Sign and Lock] the office visit (Figure 6.14). The [Initial Only] button allows the office visit note to be recalled for further edits by anyone with chart editing privileges. Portions of the office visit note can be completed and saved into the patient's chart without the entire note being finalized. This enables various healthcare providers to take responsibility for segments of the healthcare process. For example, a nurse or medical assistant may document the chief complaints and record the vital signs in an office visit note and save the partial note into the patient's chart. A physician may then open the same note, accessed from another computer, complete the exam, assign diagnoses, prescribe medication, and so on, and then create a **routing slip** for billing purposes. The office visit note is placed in the patient's chart by selecting the [Done] button at the bottom left of the *OV* screen.

Routing slip
The routing slip is a form that contains the medical office's most common procedure and diagnosis codes and descriptions. It also contains the patient's name, demographics, and billing information and may or may not include pricing. In a paper environment the physician usually indicates on the routing slip which procedures and diagnoses were used in the office visit. With an EHR program only the codes and description that were selected in the office visit will print on the routing slip. Some other names for a routing slip are superbill, encounter form, charge ticket, and fee ticket.

Editing an unlocked office visit note at a future date updates the *Last Modified* date. The *Date Created*, *Date of Service*, and *Last Modified* date are recorded automatically at the bottom of the office visit note (Figure 6.15). The *Date of Service* automatically defaults to the date the office visit note is first created. If a doctor wants to chart an office visit note on a day following the actual encounter, the *Date of Service* must be changed. For example, a physician may visit a long-term care facility on a certain day, but enter encounter notes in the EHR program the following day. Because the date of service defaults to the date the encounter note is created, the date of service in this example will need to be corrected. To do so, the physician would select *Tools* > Date Of Service from the OV note main menu. The desired date of service would be chosen in the dialog box, causing the office visit to be saved in the care tree

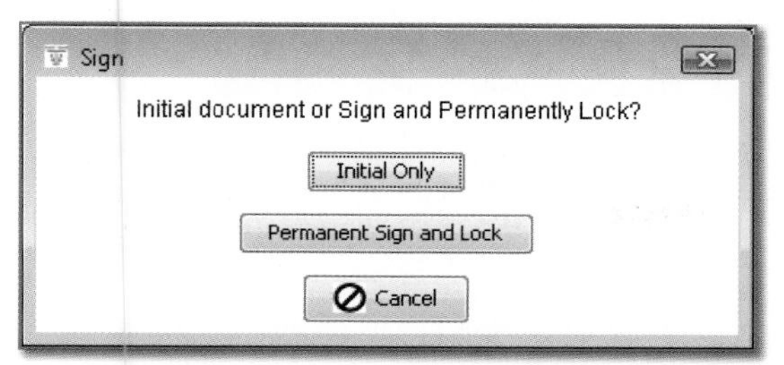

Figure 6.14 *Sign* window from the office visit note.

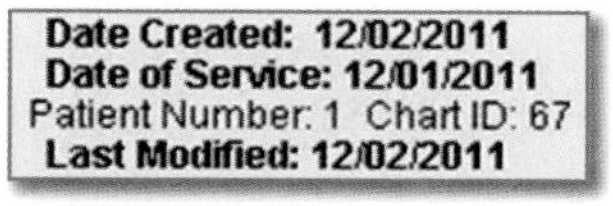

Date Created: 12/02/2011
Date of Service: 12/01/2011
Patient Number: 1 Chart ID: 67
Last Modified: 12/02/2011

Figure 6.15 Dates automatically recorded in the office visit note.

Encounters category with the accurate date of service. This date would be transferred to the PMS software for billing or printed on the routing slip, regardless of the date on which the office visit note was created.

Concept Checkup 6.2

A. When certain navigation tabs are selected in the *Office Visit* screen, (for example, CC, PI, ROS, and Exam), what will appear on the bottom right side of the screen?

B. What does the *Copy Highlighted Text to Note* icon in the *OV* window enable a clinician to do?

C. Along with 9 basic vitals, how many additional custom vitals can be added to the SpringCharts EHR program?

D. Rather than free text (pop-up text), what do the diagnosis [Dx], prescription [Rx], tests [Test], and procedures [Proc] navigation buttons allow the user to access?

Exercise 6.1 Building an OV Note (Part 1—MA)

Note: For this exercise, you will use your own chart but also assume you are the medical assistant.

1. Open your own patient chart and select the *New Office Visit* icon (shown in margin) from the chart menu. In the *Office Visit* screen notice the face sheet information on the left side of the window, which was pulled from the chart. Also note that the [CC] (chief complaint) navigation tab is already highlighted on the right.
2. Click on the down arrow of the pop-up text header (shown in margin) and scroll down until you find the pop-up text heading, *Chief Complaints* (see marginal illustration and Figure 6.3 for further help).
3. In the *Chief Complaints* pop-up text list, click on *Allergies, Itchy eyes,* and *Runny nose.* The words will be added to the lower middle *Chief Complaint* text box in the *OV* screen.
4. Click in the *Chief Complaint* text box and hit [Enter] to start a new line. Click on the time and initial buttons in the lower right section to add the time and your initials to the note.
5. Select the [Vitals] navigation tab on the right. Notice all previously created text is now added to the *SOAP* format. Add fictitious vital sign information for the patient, including a normal temperature using the SpringCharts Tip in the margin.

(continued)

New Office Visit icon

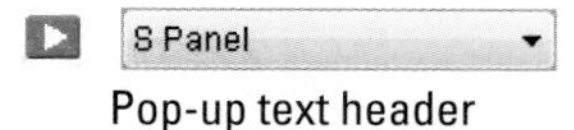

Pop-up text header

SpringCharts Tip

Normal Vital Ranges
Temp: 98.6
Resp: 12–20
Pulse: 66–100
BP: Systolic: 100–140
Diastolic: 60–90

SpringCharts Tip

HC stands for head circumference and is used by pediatricians to record head measurements for developing infants. *BMI* (body mass index) is grayed out because the program will calculate this item from the height and weight measurements

Exercise 6.1 (Concluded)

6. Click on the [Done] button and then, in the *Save As* window, the [Save and Skip Billing] button. (You will come back later, finish the note, and create a routing slip for this office visit.) The OV note has been added to the list of *Encounters* in the care tree of your chart.
7. Close the chart.

Exercise 6.2 Building an OV Note (Part 2—Provider)

Note: Now that a medical assistant has completed the initial assessment, the office visit is handed over to the physician or another healthcare provider. Rather than start a new office visit note, the provider edits the existing note.

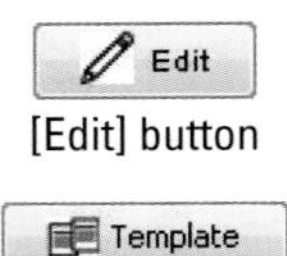

[Edit] button

[Template] button in *OV* screen

1. Open your chart.
2. Click on the "+" sign beside the *Encounters* heading in the care tree and select the office visit entry you started in Exercise 6.1.
3. Click on the [Edit] button (shown in margin) at the bottom of the window.
4. Click on the [Template] button in the bottom right corner of the *Office Visit* screen and, from the displayed list, select *Allergic Rhinitis.* Notice that the entire note has been built very quickly in the SOAP panel.
5. Click on the [PI] (history of present illness) navigation tab. The text from the template appears in the lower middle work text box of the OV note.
6. Move the scroll bar to the top of this panel and complete the following sentence: *Pt c/o red, itchy eyes, congested, itchy and runny nose (clear fluid), post nasal drip, sneezing, itchy ears, scratchy throat and occasional cough for the past _ weeks.* Place your cursor in front of the word *weeks*, highlight the underscore mark, and enter *3*.

Note: The physician would continue this way through the entire note, making changes and additions where necessary to reflect this specific patient's condition.

7. To add a diagnosis, click on the [Dx] navigation tab.
8. Look in the *Previous Diagnoses* box at the bottom of the right panel to determine if the patient has been in the clinic for this diagnosis in the past. Select *Allergic Rhinitis - Pollen 477.0* from the *PMHX + Problem List* window.
9. To prescribe a medication, click on the [Rx] navigation tab.
10. In the *Prescription* field, search for *Allegra 180 mg.* Click on the medication to add it to the text box in the bottom middle of the screen.
11. Search for and select *Flonase 50 mcg* to add it to the text box as well.

Note: Always refer to potential allergies at the top of the *Prescription* panel before prescribing medication and shots.

12. The physician asks you to come back into the exam room to administer a subcutaneous allergy shot. To order the injection, select the [Proc] navigation tab.

Exercise 6.2 (Concluded)

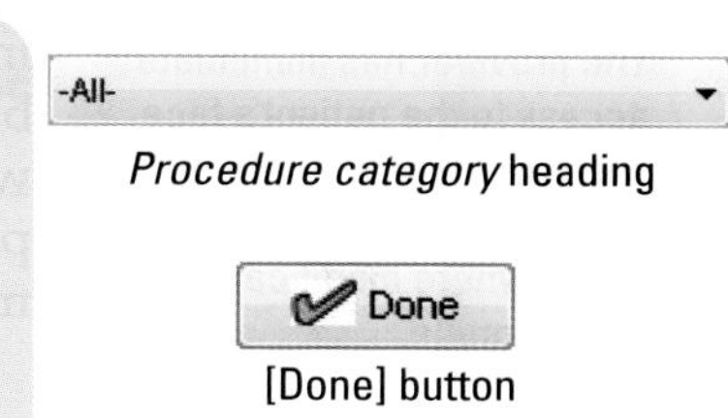

Procedure category heading

[Done] button

13. Click on the *Procedure Category* drop-down menu and select the category *InjectMed*. Choose *Allergy Injection—1* from the list.
14. Click on the [Done] button at the bottom of the *OV* screen, and choose the [Save and Skip Billing] button in the *Save As* window. (Later, the medical assistant will re-open this office visit note to document the administration of the allergy injection. The OV note has been added to the list of encounters in the care tree of your chart.)
15. Close the chart.

Exercise 6.3 Building an OV Note (Part 3—MA)

Note: The physician communicates with the medical assistant regarding administering the allergy shot. This may be done via the *Patient Tracker* by changing the *Tracker Status*. As the medical assistant, you administer and document the injection.

1. Open your chart. Click on the "+" sign beside the *Encounters* heading in the care tree and select the office visit entry you amended in Exercise 6.2.
2. Click on the [Edit] button at the bottom of the *OV* window.
3. Click on the [Proc] navigation tab and select *Allergy Injection—1* in the lower middle text box of the OV note.
4. In the *Edit Procedure* panel, document the administration of the injection. Choose the pop-up text *Lot#* and type in the lot number: 65894. Select the *Expiration date* pop-up text and add the date: 9/15/2015.
5. Hit [Enter] to move your cursor to the next line and choose the pop-up text *Site: Left arm*. Scroll down in the pop-up text window and select Route and add the appropriate route for the injection.
6. Place your cursor on the next line and click on the [D & T] and [Initials] buttons to add the date, time, and your initials to the notation.
7. Click on the [Save] button.
8. Click on the [Done] button in the *OV* screen, followed by [Save and Skip Billing] in the *Save As* window. The physician will now complete the routing slip and bill for the encounter. The OV note has been added to the list of encounters in the care tree of your chart.
9. Close the chart.

6.3 Activities within the Office Visit Screen

Editing the Patient's Face Sheet

Because the face sheet items from the patient's chart are displayed on the left side of the office visit note, users can review and edit the patient's face sheet information while in the OV note. Often, clinicians discuss past healthcare issues, routine medications, and family medical history issues with patients while documenting within the OV note. The ability to modify and update face sheet information while in the *OV* screen is an efficient way of updating patient information.

The *Edit* menu in the *Office Visit* screen provides quick access to the face sheet categories (Figure 6.16). By selecting any of these face sheet items, the

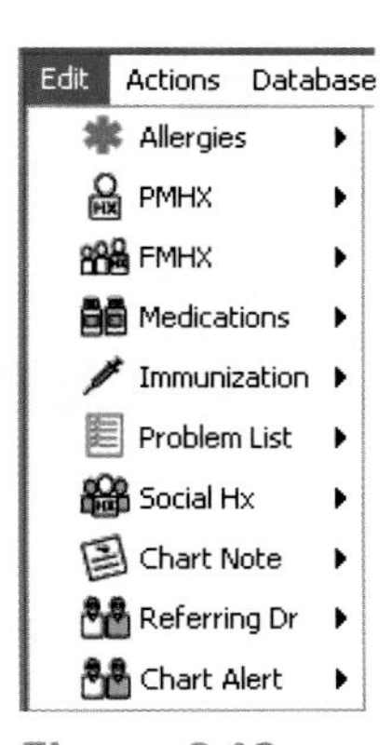

Figure 6.16 *Edit* menu in *Office Visit* screen.

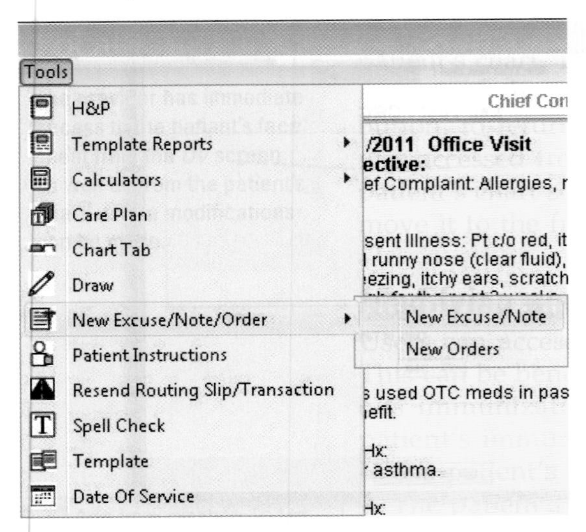

Figure 6.21 Creating an excuse note from the *OV* screen.

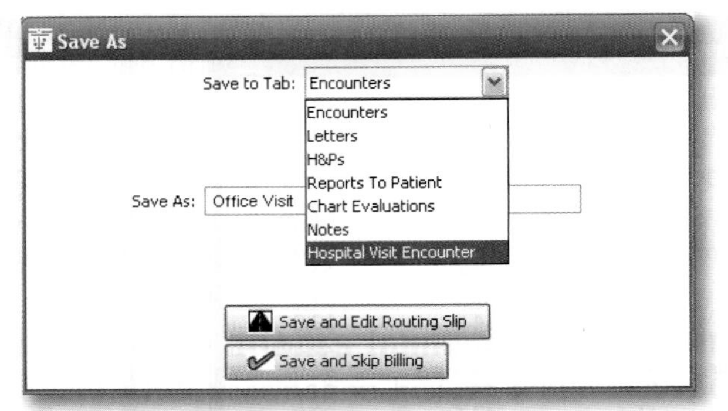

Figure 6.22 Saving office visit notes to specific care tree categories.

printed or faxed to the recipient. After the [Done] button has been selected the excuse notes are automatically saved under the *Excuses/Notes* category of the care tree in the patient's chart.

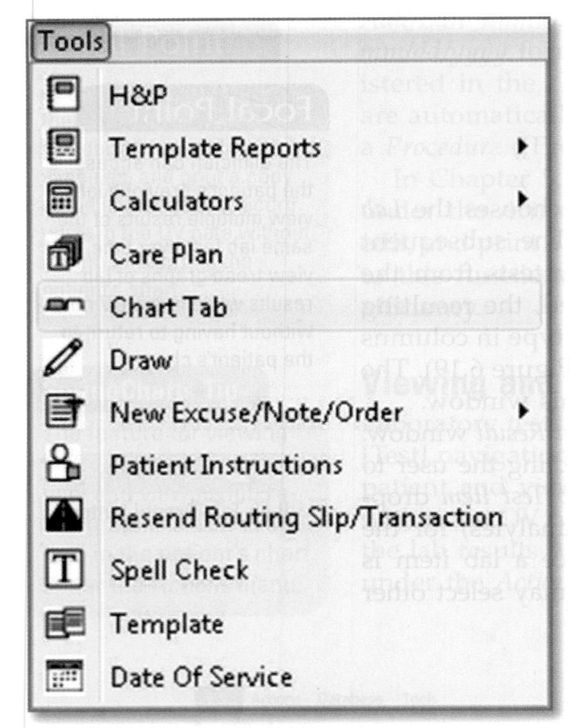

Figure 6.23 *Chart Tab* submenu to change care tree category in *Office Visit* window.

Changing the Chart Tab

Office visit notes are typically saved under the *Encounters* category in a patient's care tree. However, the SpringCharts EHR program also allows users to create customized tabs in the care tree that can be used to store documentation. If a customized tab has been created to store specific types of office visit notes, the user chooses that category in the drop-down menu of the *Save As* window after selecting [Done] in the main *OV* screen (Figure 6.22). The program also allows for OV notes initially saved under the *Encounters* category to be moved to a different category of the care tree.

To save an existing office visit note under a different care tree category, the user opens the OV note by highlighting the entry in the care tree and selecting the [Edit] button. Once the *OV* screen is open, the user selects the *Tools* menu and the *Chart Tab* submenu (Figure 6.23). The *Save As* window will appear, and the user can select an alternate tab in the care tree under which to store the OV note. The note will be removed from the former *Encounters* category.

Focal Point

Editing the face sheet, adding past immunizations, viewing past lab results, and creating an excuse note can all be conducted in the *OV* screen as well as in the patient's chart.

Concept Checkup 6.3

A. How does a user re-save an OV note so that it is stored under a customized category in the care tree rather than the *Encounters* category?

B. What are the two places where the patient's face sheet can be edited?

C. Why is it important to see a history of a patient's lab results from several different dates?

HIPAA/HITECH Tip

Fax Cover Sheet

A confidentiality statement must appear on a fax cover sheet when transmitting PHI. A sample confidentiality statement is as follows:

> *"The documents accompanying this facsimile transmission may contain confidential information belonging to the sender or recipient that is protected by federal law. This information is solely for the use of the addressee named above. You may be exposed to legal liability if you disclose this information to another person.*
>
> *If you are not the intended recipient, you are hereby notified that any disclosure, copying, distribution, or other use of the contents of this faxed information is strictly prohibited. If you have received this facsimile in error, please notify the sender immediately by telephone and confidentially dispose of the material."*

Focal Point

OV notes can be stored by default under the *Encounters* category in the patient's care tree or saved to a customized category in the care tree.

Exercise 6.4 Creating an Excuse Note

1. Open your chart and select the most recent office visit note. Click on the [Edit] button to open the OV note.
2. Select the *Tools* menu inside the *OV* screen. Select the *New Excuse/Note/Order* submenu and then *New Excuse/Note.*
3. In the *To* field, type the name of your college.
4. In the *Note* field, select pop-up text from the Excuse Text category to excuse your absence from college for the time period you were at the doctor's office, for example, 10:00 am to 12:00 pm.
5. On the next line add your initials to the note by using the [Sign] button.
6. Print the excuse note and submit it to your instructor.
7. Click the [Done] button in the *Note* screen.
8. Click the [Done] button in the *OV* screen. Click the [Save and Skip Billing] button.
9. In the care tree, click on the "+" sign to the left of the *Excuses/Notes* category to see the saved note. The note is also displayed in the lower right window. Close your patient's chart.

Exercise 6.5 Adding an Immunization

Note: As you review face sheet information during an office visit, your patient informs you he or she received a DT (Diphtheria and Tetanus Toxoids) shot about this time last year.

1. Open your chart and select the most recent office visit note under the *Encounters* category in the care tree.
2. Click on the [Edit] button to open the office visit note.
3. Under the *Edit* menu, select *Immunization* and then the *Add/Edit Immunization Archives* option.
4. Select [Add Immunization To List] to display the *Add Immunization* window in which you will add the past vaccination to the patient's chart.
5. Select *DT* from the *Select Immunization* drop-down menu.

(continued)

E&M Code Factors

Additional History Reviewed: Reviewed PMHx. Reviewed FMHx. Reviewed SocialHx. Reviewed Routine Meds.
Body Areas Examined: Head Face. Chest. Extremities.
Organ Systems Examined: Ears Nose Mouth Throat. Musculoskeletal. Hematologic Lymphatic Immunologic.
E&M Code Recommended based on:
History Level = Detailed
Exam Level = Detailed
Decision Complexity: Low Complexity
Est Pt Code = = 99214

OK

E&M Code Factors

E&M Code Recommended based on: Established Patient Counseling/Coordination of Care for 40 minutes.

OK

Figure 6.27 The different *E&M Code Factors* windows based upon level of care or time.

the *Yes* radio button activated. The *E&M Code Recommended* field then shows the new recommended E&M code based upon the time factor of the patient encounter. The provider must choose one or the other method of calculating the E&M code. The two different criteria for recommending an E&M code (that is, office visit note and time frame) are seen in Figure 6.27.

After confirming or selecting the E&M code, the user clicks the [Send] button to send the routing slip to the PMS interface (if available) or place the routing slip on file within SpringCharts. Stored routing slips can be accessed under the *Edit* menu on the main *Practice View* screen, from where they can be printed or faxed to a third-party billing company, as seen in the *View Routing Slips* window (Figure 6.28).

SpringCharts Tip

The codes for the alternate E&M codes are set up in the *Set Category Preferences* window on the SpringCharts server in the *E&M Codes* subwindow.

HIPAA/HITECH TIP

The HIPAA electronic claims form generated by a physician is called the HIPAA 837P (professional services). An electronic claim form generated by a dentist is the HIPAA 837D (dental services). A HIPAA electronic claim form generated by a hospital is called the HIPAA 837I (institutional services).

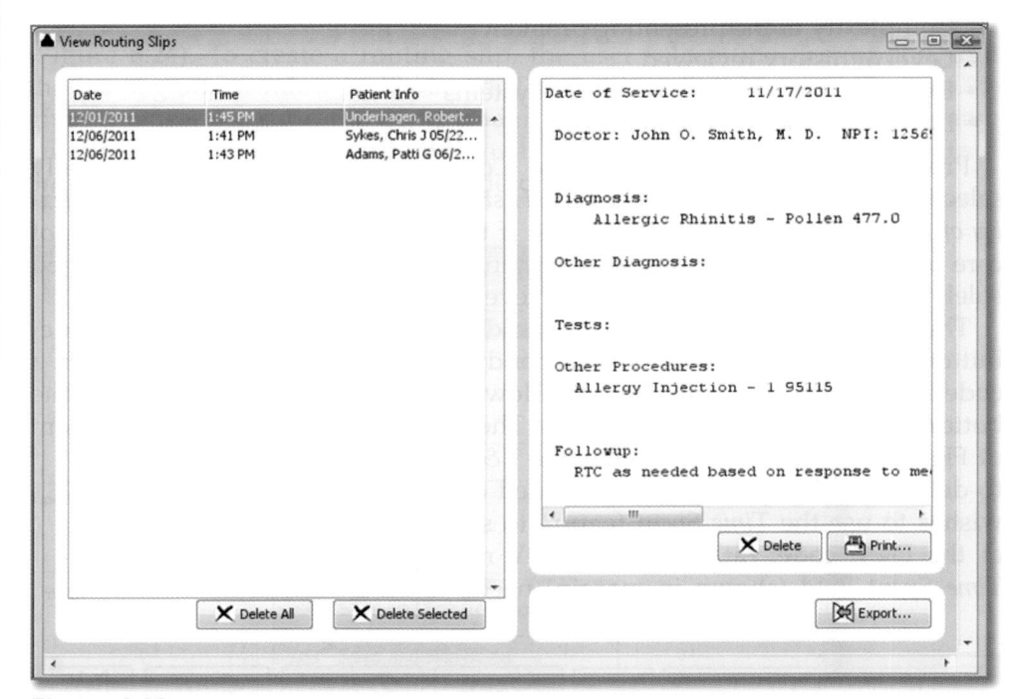

Figure 6.28 *View Routing Slips* window.

(See Appendix A—*Sample Documents*; Document 9. *Routing Slip*.)

Routing slips can be resent from the *OV* screen. This feature is useful if the original routing slip needs to be deleted due to errors or insufficient codes were documented in the OV note. If new information needs to be added to the OV note, the user simply reopens the *OV* screen and adds the required information in the appropriate section. When the user clicks on the [Done] button in the OV note screen, the option to save the note and edit the new routing slip appears. If no more information needs to be added to the OV note, the user can open the note and select *Resend Routing Slip/Transaction* from the *Tools* menu within the *OV* screen (Figure 6.29). The *Routing Slip* window appears, bypassing the *Save As* window. After the E&M code has been revised, the new routing slip can be processed by selecting the [Send] button.

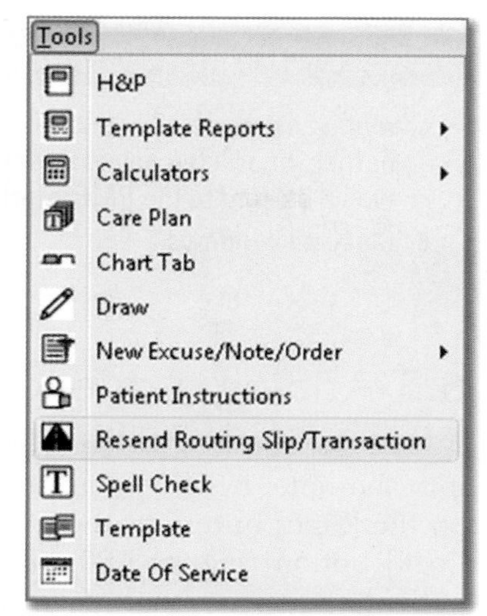

Figure 6.29 *Resend Routing Slip/Transaction* submenu option.

HIPAA/HITECH TIP

A clinician cannot code or bill for services not supported by the office visit note documentation, even if instructed to do so by a physician.

Concept Checkup 6.4

A. Why does an insurance company require codes rather than free text when a medical clinic documents procedures and diagnoses?

B. What five criteria are used by the *E&M Coder* to determine the appropriate E&M code for a routing slip?

C. What are the two means by which a E&M code can be chosen?

Exercise 6.6 Creating a Routing Slip

1. Open your patient chart and select the most recent office visit note from the care tree. Open the office visit by using the [Edit] button.
2. Click on the *Tools* menu and select *Resend Routing Slip/Transaction*. In the *Routing Slip* window, you should see the diagnoses and follow-up information recorded from the OV note. The *E&M Coder* in the middle section recommends the E&M code of *99215*.
3. Click on [Details] at the bottom of the *Routing Slip* window and read the factors considered by the E&M coder to choose the appropriate code about the body systems and areas reviewed during the office visit.
4. Click [OK] and then [Use Code] to use the recommended E&M code.
5. Print the routing slip and submit it to your instructor.
6. Click on the [Send] button and close the chart. Close your patient's chart.
7. In the main *Practice View* screen, select the *Edit* menu and choose the *Routing Slips option*. In the *View Routing Slip* window you should see the routing slip you just created at the bottom of the list. This is where billing personnel retrieve the

(continued)

Exercise 6.6 (Concluded)

routing slips each day in order to bill the insurance companies or other responsible parties. In a linked environment to a PMS program, this routing slip information would be sent to the PMS interface.

8. Close all windows.

6.5 Adding Addenda to an Office Visit Note

Focal Point

Addenda are only added to OV notes that have been signed and permanently locked.

Addendum
An addendum is a notation added to an office visit note, after it has been permanently signed and locked, to supplement the information in the original note.

A provider can lock office visit notes so no additional material can be entered into the note, even by the provider. Office visit notes are locked by clicking on the [Sign] button in the *OV* screen and selecting the [Permanent Sign and Lock] option (Figure 6.30). The locked office visit note then appears in the patient's care tree with a locked symbol beside the entry (Figure 6.31). OV notes that have *not* been signed and locked can be reopened and edited, such as adding information to the SOAP note.

Although office visit notes that have been permanently signed and locked cannot have new material added, they can be amended. In an existing signed and locked office visit note located in the care tree, the user selects the [Edit] button in the lower right panel of the patient's chart. A *Not Editable* dialog box appears, giving the user the option of adding an **addendum** to the office visit note (Figure 6.32). The addendum note will be placed at the bottom of the existing office visit note (Figure 6.33). The program automatically date-, time-, and initial-stamps the addendum when it is saved. Multiple addenda can be added to the same locked office visit note.

Concept Checkup 6.5

A. Office visit notes that have been *permanently signed and locked* cannot be edited. However, what can be added to a locked OV note?

B. What is automatically added to an addendum when one is saved?

C. How would a user distinguish between locked and unlocked office visit notes in the patient's care tree?

Exercise 6.7 Creating an Addendum

1. Open Robert Underhagen's chart by using the *Open a Patient's Chart* speed icon on the main *Practice View* screen.
2. In the *Encounters* category of the patient's care tree, highlight the office visit note that has a lock icon associated with it and click on the [Edit] button.
3. Answer [Yes] to the question, *Do you want to add an addendum?*
4. In the *Office Visit Addendum* window, type the following: *Patient developed allergic reaction of hives to the allergy injection. Allergy noted in patient's chart.*
5. Click the [Done] button in the *Office Visit Addendum* window and again in the OV note.
6. Scroll to the bottom of the OV note in the patient's chart and view the addendum. Close the patient's chart.

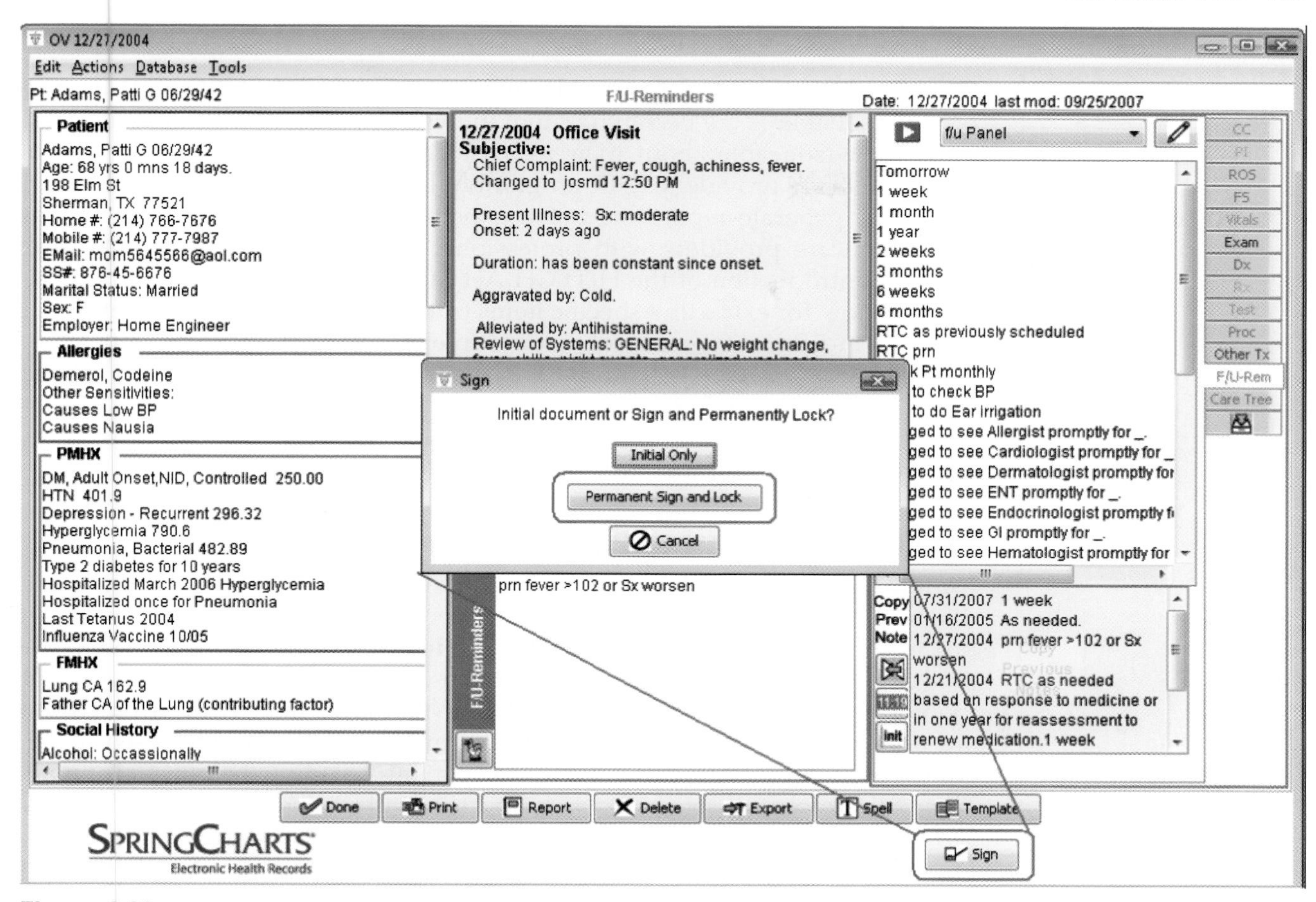

Figure 6.30 Permanently signing and locking office visit notes.

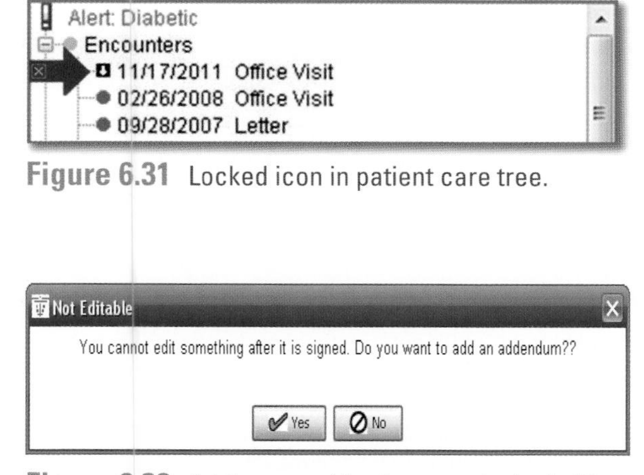

Figure 6.31 Locked icon in patient care tree.

Figure 6.32 Adding an addendum to a locked office visit note.

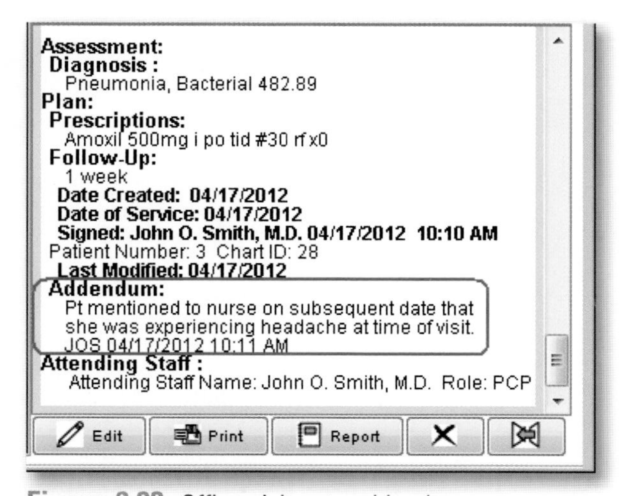

Figure 6.33 Office visit note addendum.

6.6 Office Visit Reports

Office visit notes contain valuable information useful to both patients and providers. Patients are becoming more involved in their healthcare issues and more knowledgeable about their rights to request personal medical reports from healthcare providers. EHR programs allow medical offices to quickly and accurately generate reports from the patient's chart that provide the patient and healthcare providers with professional documentation of medical care. With the introduction of the HITECH Act in 2009, EHR programs were modified to allow for extracting specific items from OV notes that the patient might request. An EP had 90 consecutive days in either 2011 or 2012 to demonstrate proficiency on an ONC-certified EHR program to qualify for stage 1 of the MU requirements and receive remuneration through the Medicare or Medicaid program. Table 6.5 outlines the ONC objectives and MU measures regarding provision of clinical summaries.

Examination Report to Patient

Examination reports detail the examination notes of an office visit and include diagnoses, tests, procedures, and prescriptions. Any test results that have been processed, the results entered into the pending tests, and then saved into the patient's chart are printed on the report, along with the names of the tests and the normal ranges of results. Ordered tests that have not yet been processed are also listed in this report, with the term *pending* beside the test's name. Examination reports are designed for the patient, detailing the office visit note. They are created by selecting the [Report] button at the bottom of the *Office Visit* screen (Figure 6.34). The pop-up text categories to the right, like *Report-Probs* (identified problems) and *Report-Recs* (suggested recommendations), can be used to add text for further clarification (Figure 6.35).

Table 6.5 Meaningful Use Core Measure

Clinical Summaries	
ONC Stage 1 Objective	**Meaningful Use Measure**
Upon request, the clinic must provide patients with clinical summaries for each office visit.	Clinical summaries must be provided to patients for more than 50 percent of all office visits within 3 business days.

Notes:

- Clinic must be able to provide healthcare summaries of OV notes containing reason for visit; vitals; procedures; updated problem list; updated current medication list; immunizations or medications administered during visit; patient instructions; time and location of next appointment/testing if scheduled, or a recommended appointment time if not scheduled; and list of other appointments and testing patient needs to schedule, with contact information.
- Physicians are allowed to withhold information that would potentially be harmful to the patient.
- Patients are allowed to choose the format in which they receive their information: paper copy, CD, USB device, or secure e-mail, or through a patient portal.
- Physicians who have no office visits during the EHR reporting period of 90 days are excluded from this rule.

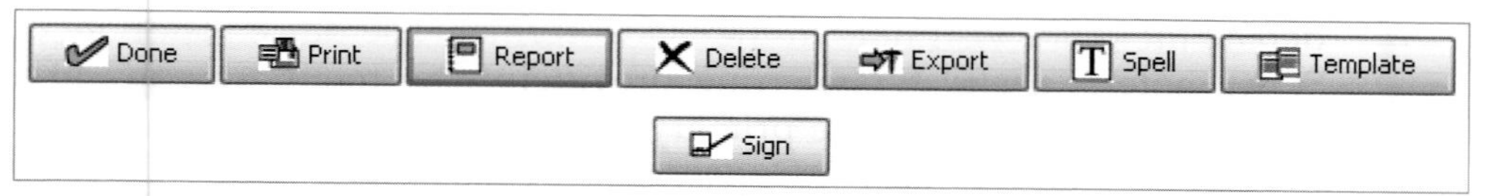

Figure 6.34 [Report] button in speed button bar in *Office Visit* screen.

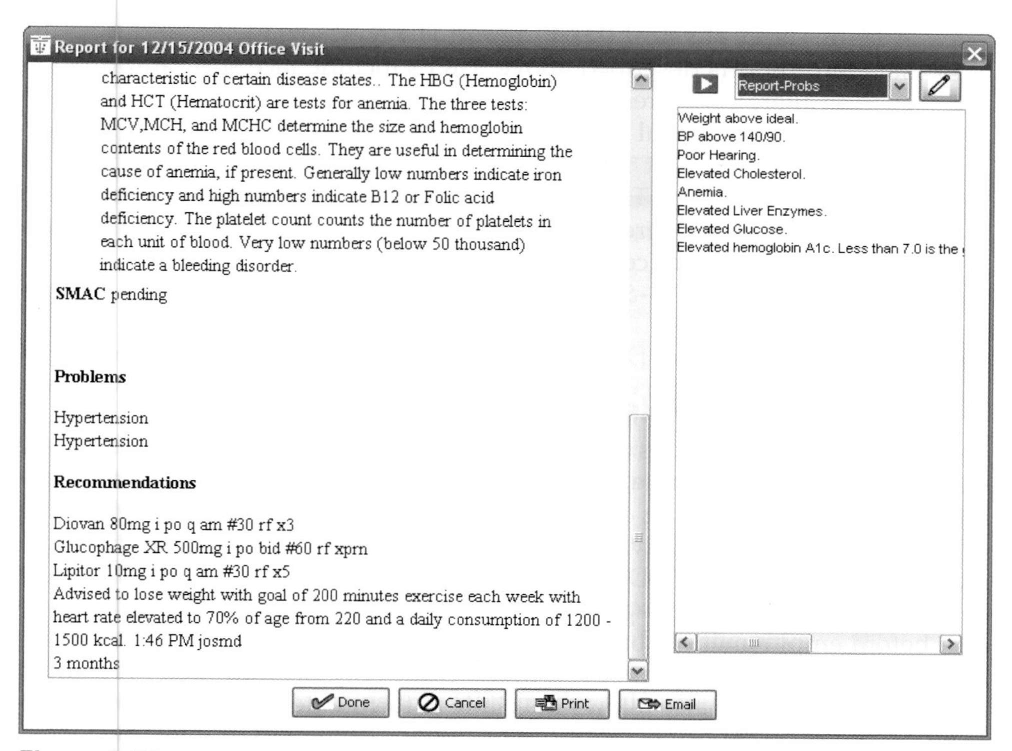

Figure 6.35 Creating an exam report from an office visit note.

An alternative way to create an examination report for a patient is to click the [Report] button in the lower right corner of the patient's chart once the office visit note has been selected in the care tree (Figure 6.36). This enables the user to create a report without having to open the *OV* screen.

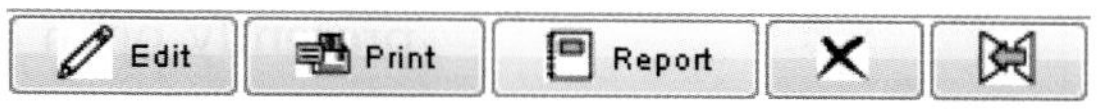

Edit Print Report

Figure 6.36 [Report] button in patient's chart.

(See Appendix A—*Sample Documents*; Document 10. *Examination Report to Patient*.)

Office Visit (SOAP) Note

The entire office visit note can also be printed or faxed by selecting the [Print] button at the bottom of the *Office Visit* screen (Figure 6.37) or the [Print] button at the bottom of the patient's chart when the OV note is highlighted in the care tree. The office visit note does not include tests' results or allow for the use of pop-up text to tailor the note to the recipient. Rather, it simply

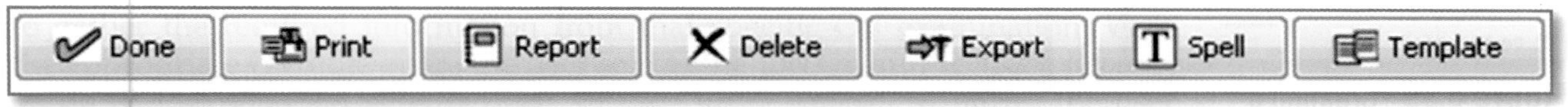

Figure 6.37 [Print] button in *OV* screen.

19. **LO 6.6** The purpose of the office visit template report is to:
    a) Create an office visit note that can be used for other patients.
    b) Have a standard report to send to hospitals when the patient is admitted.
    c) Provide patients with a copy of their recent examination report, required by the ONC.
    d) Create customized reports of specific elements from the office visit note.
20. **LO 6.3** The *Lab* submenu under the *Actions* menu in the *OV* screen enables the provider to:
    a) Order new labs for the patient.
    b) View previous labs for the patient.
    c) Connect to SureScripts across the Internet to send the patient's labs.
    d) Access the patient's pending labs.
21. **LO 6.4** The electronic routing slip is displayed for the provider:
    a) Only when the user selects the *Save and Edit Routing Slip* option
    b) Every time the OV note is saved
    c) By accessing the *Tools* menu in the *OV* screen
    d) In the PMS program
22. **LO 6.3** The patient's name is always automatically defaulted into the excuse note because:
    a) Patients' names are often difficult to spell.
    b) It saves the provider time in not having to type the name.
    c) It is created within the patient's chart screen or the patient's OV note screen.
    d) The checkout desk needs to know which patient the excuse note is for.
23. **LO 6.6** The OV note report that provides information on just the physical examination and test results for the patient is called:
    a) History & Physical
    b) OV note report
    c) OV note template report
    d) Examination Report to patient
24. **LO 6.5** When a provider signs and permanently locks an OV note:
    a) Only that provider can enter data into the OV note.
    b) No one can enter data into the OV note, not even the provider.
    c) Only that provider can unlock the OV note.
    d) A new OV note will have to be started to include addenda.
25. **LO 6.6** The H&P report:
    a) Stands for History & Problems
    b) Enables the user to create customized reports from the OV note
    c) Combines information on the patient's healthcare history and current examination
    d) Is received from the hospital when the patient comes for follow-up work

Applying Your Knowledge

Use your critical-thinking skills to answer the following questions.

26. **LO 6.2** Group the following eight activities that occur in a typical OV by the provider responsible for each activity, either clinician or physician:

    Completing routing slip; Ordering a test; Recording chief complaints and vital signs; Documenting ROS and exam; Documenting the administration of an injection; Reviewing face sheet information; Assigning diagnosis and medication; Entering in-house test results.
27. **LO 6.2** Why is it beneficial to the provider that the *Chief Complaint, Present Illness, Review of Systems, Examination, Procedure, Other Treatment,* and *Follow-up/Reminder* areas of the *OV* screen display additional notes from previous encounters with the patient?
28. **LO 6.3** If a user accidentally saved an OV note under the wrong category in the care tree of the patient's chart, how would the user get the document under the correct category?

7

Clinical Tools

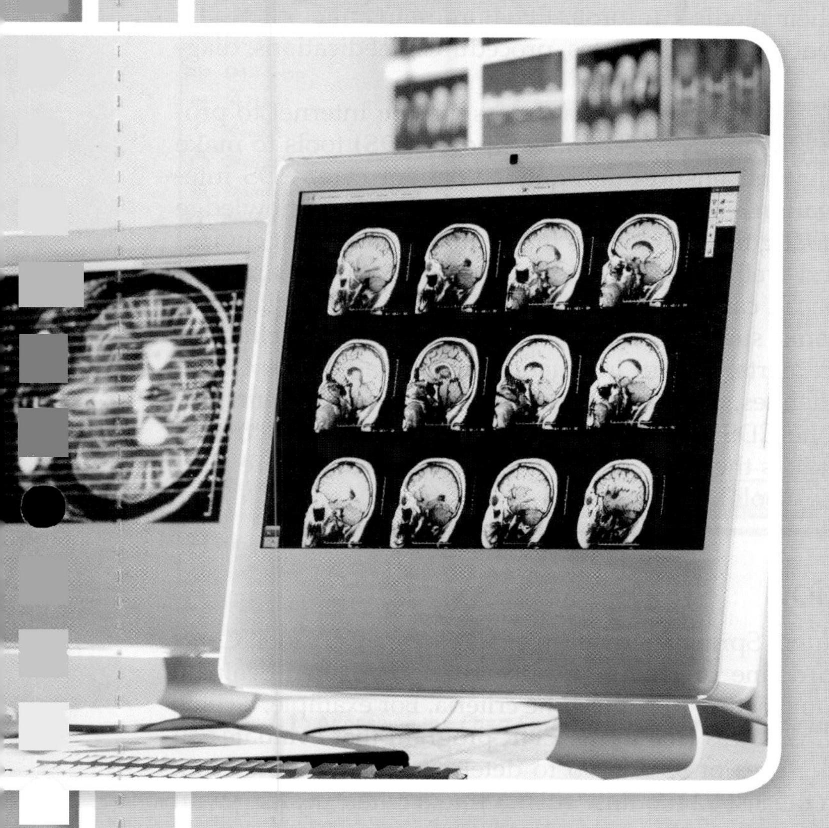

Learning Outcomes

After completing Chapter 7, you will be able to:

LO 7.1 Create and conduct a chart evaluation.

LO 7.2 Demonstrate how to order a test in the *Office Visit* screen.

LO 7.3 Describe the function of the *E&M Coder.*

LO 7.4 Demonstrate how to add items to a superbill.

LO 7.5 Create and administer a patient instruction sheet.

LO 7.6 Describe how to add a care plan to an office visit.

LO 7.7 Explain the purpose of the *Draw* program.

LO 7.8 Demonstrate how to import a document to a patient's chart.

What You Need to Know

To understand Chapter 7, you will need to know how to:

- Open an electronic patient chart.
- Open a new office visit note within a patient chart.
- Navigate within the *Office Visit* screen.
- Add new pop-up text.
- Create a routing slip.

Key Terms

Care plans and practice guidelines

Chart evaluation

Clinical decision support (CDS)

Draw program

National Guideline Clearinghouse (NGC)

Patient Instructions Manager

Rich text format (RTF)

Superbill

Wellness screenings

Well patient visit

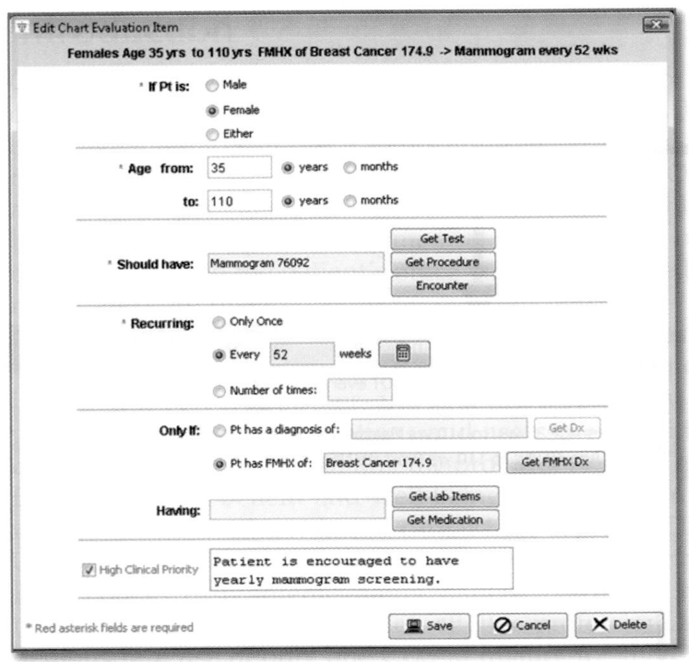

Figure 7.2 *Edit Chart Evaluation Item* window.

program flags the clinician when either of these diagnoses is selected in the OV note.

6. *Having Lab or Medication:* Select a lab item or medication from the EHR database. If the *High Clinical Priority* box is checked, the program flags the clinician and displays a warning message when this lab or drug is selected in the OV note.
7. *High Clinical Priority:* The priority box is checked to create an automatic warning in OV notes, triggered by the assigned diagnosis, lab, or medication selected in one of the preceding fields. The desired warning message is created in the blank text box to the right.

Linking the wellness screenings to a diagnosis, lab, or medication from the patient's chart is optional. Only the line items marked with a red asterisk in the *Edit Chart Evaluation Item* window are mandatory when setting up chart evaluation criteria. These guidelines can be accessed on the SpringCharts server and modified at a later time, if necessary.

Individual patient charts can be screened by accessing the *File* menu and selecting the *Evaluate Chart* submenu within the patient's chart. This opens the *Evaluate Chart* window, which lists each evaluation screening not up-to-date in the patient's chart. (Figure 7.3). The clinician recommends the identified health screening(s) to the patient; however, the patient may decline to have the test, injection, or procedure done on that day. Under each recommendation is a *Pt Response* field in which the user documents the patient's response. If a verbal recommendation is made to the patient, the clinician clicks the *Mark this 'Completed'* radio button. When the [Done] button at the bottom of the window is selected, the patient's response and a summary of the evaluation item(s) are recorded and dated in the patient's care tree under the *Encounters* category. It is recommended that clinic personnel run chart evaluations with each patient encounter.

SpringCharts Tip

Shortcut:

Chart Evaluation

The second icon in the toolbar at the top of the patient's chart is a rapid way to perform a chart evaluation for the patient.

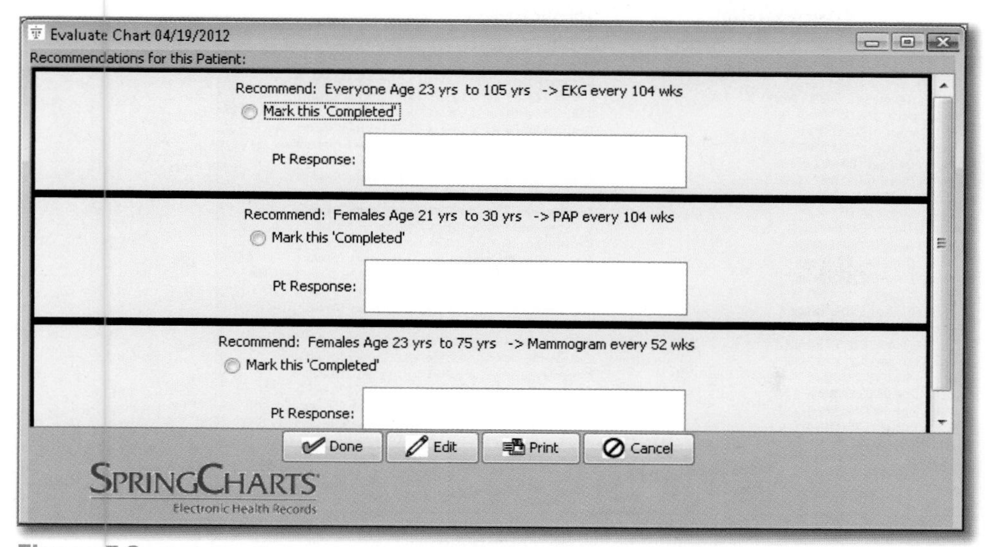

Figure 7.3 *Evaluate Chart* window in patient's chart.

If the patient is up-to-date with evaluations and wellness screenings, the user receives the message, *Pt up to date with recommendations,* when the *Evaluate Chart* feature is activated. If the user receives the message, *No criterion set,* it indicates that no chart evaluations have been set up on the SpringCharts server.

SpringCharts can also scan the entire patient database, applying the chart evaluation criteria to all patient charts. To do so, the administrator clicks on the *Utilities* menu at the top of the main *Practice View* screen and selects *Evaluate All Charts*. This opens the *Chart Evaluation Results* window, where the user can select the [Evaluate All Charts] button to choose individual evaluation items (Figure 7.4) or direct the program to evaluate the entire patient database for all chart evaluation items. The program then lists all

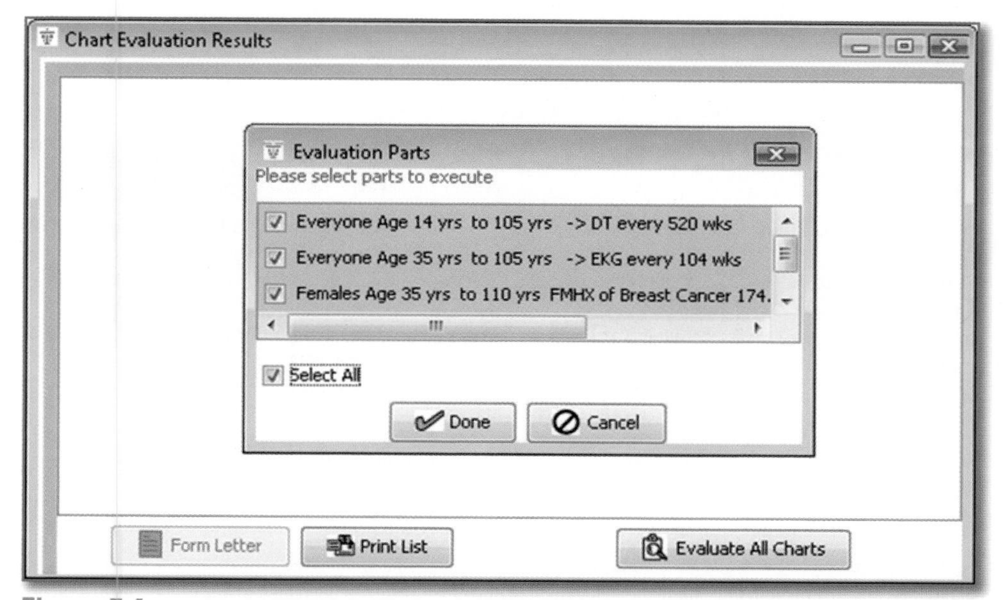

Figure 7.4 Selecting specific evaluation items in the *Evaluate All Charts* feature.

Focal Point

Chart evaluations should be performed each time a patient has an office visit, to ensure he or she is up-to-date with wellness screenings.

Focal Point

Chart evaluation criteria change from clinic to clinic based on a clinic's specialty.

SpringCharts Tip

Because all charts are evaluated, the *Evaluate All Charts* process can be time consuming and is typically run after hours.

Focal Point

SpringCharts can conduct a chart evaluation on specific patients or run an evaluation on the entire patient database.

SpringCharts Tip

The *communication preference* for each patient is initially chosen in the *Edit Patient* window. The *Communication Pref.* radio button choice is used by the EHR program to determine whether to communicate with the patient via regular mail or e-mail.

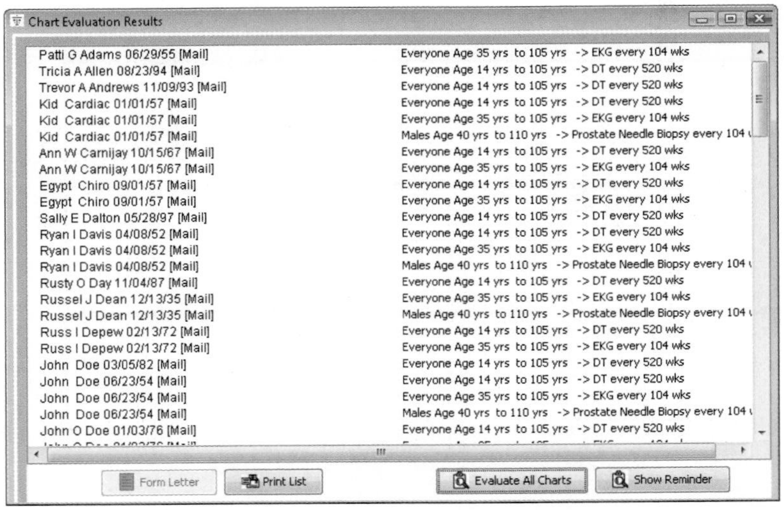

Figure 7.5 *Chart Evaluation Results* list from database.

patients who are not up to date with wellness screenings along with the specific wellness criteria (Figure 7.5). The *Chart Evaluation Results* window also displays the communication preference for each patient beside his or her name.

Wellness screenings are critical elements in preventative healthcare, particularly for the older and younger patients in the community. EHRs now provide the ability to track the age of patients, scan the patient database for wellness screenings that aren't up to date, and send reminder notices to patients to schedule appointments for various healthcare issues. The ONC requires all certified EHR programs to have the ability to send appropriate healthcare reminders to patients 65 years and older and patients who are 5 years of age and younger. This meaningful use (MU) objective is one of the 10 menu criteria from which an EP must choose five features in order to demonstrate MU and thus qualify for remuneration under the HITECH Act (Table 7.2). The ability

Table 7.2 Meaningful Use Menu Measure

Reminders Sent to Patients	
ONC Stage 1 Objective	**Meaningful Use Measure**
Send reminders to patients (via patient preference) for preventive and follow-up care, such as an office visit checkup, wellness screening, or renewal of a prescription.	More than 20 percent of patients 65 years of age or older or 5 years of age or younger are sent appropriate reminders.

Notes:

- The reminder can be delivered electronically or by hard copy, depending on the patient's preference.
- If a physician has no patients over the age of 65 or under the age of 5, this objective does not apply to that physician.
- The 20 percent measure is based on the total number of patients 65 years or older or 5 years old or younger.

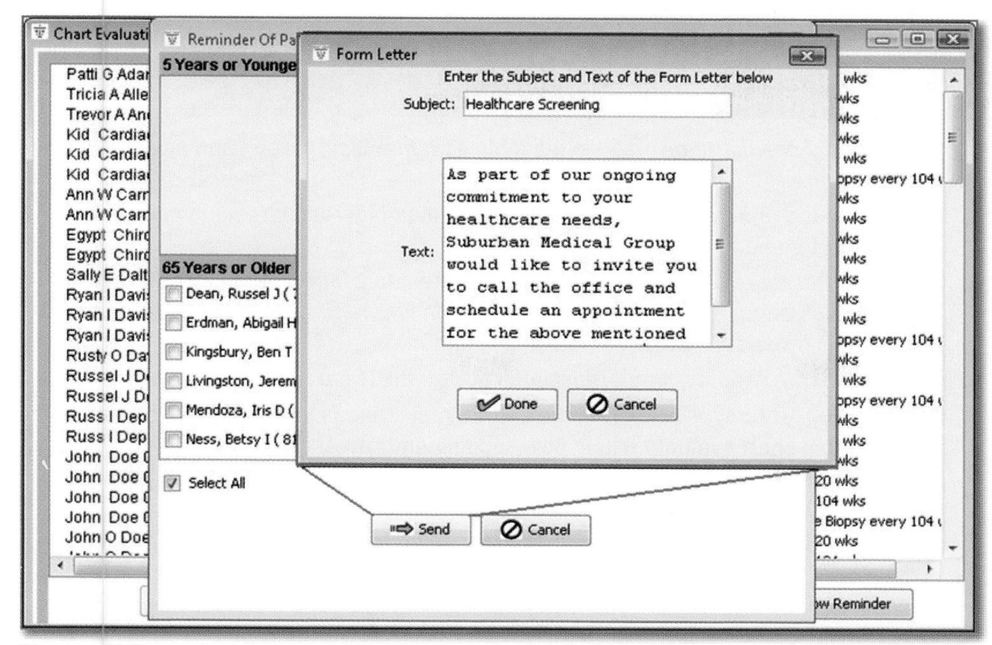

Figure 7.6 Creating a *Form Letter* in the *Chart Evaluation* feature.

to communicate with patients regarding necessary healthcare screenings in an automated fashion is a major reason the federal government got involved in promoting EHR program adoption. These healthcare reminders are powerful tools for helping patients to take responsibility for their own wellness.

In the *Chart Evaluation Results* window, the user can send reminder messages to patients 65 years and older and patients 5 years of age and younger regarding outstanding health screening items by clicking on the [Show Reminder] button. The resulting *Reminder Of Patients* window lists all patients in these age ranges. The user can select all identified patients, or individual patients, to receive reminders from the clinic. Once patients have been selected, the user clicks the [Send] button to create a form letter (Figure 7.6). When the form letter is completed, the user selects [Done] to print the letters.

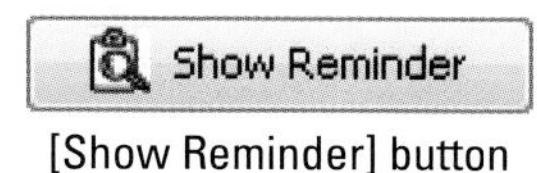

[Show Reminder] button

Concept Checkup 7.1

A. What does the chart evaluation feature in SpringCharts allow users to do?

B. What does the message *No criterion set* indicate?

C. What message window is displayed in the patient's chart when a patient is current with all the chart evaluation items?

D. The chart evaluation feature can be run for a specific patient's chart. How else can the chart evaluation feature be used?

Exercise 7.1 Creating and Conducting a Chart Evaluation

1. Open the *Administration* menu in the main *Practice View* screen and select *Chart Evaluation.*
2. Highlight the chart evaluation item regarding mammogram screening and click the [Edit] button.
3. Narrow the screening criteria by linking this item to a family medical history diagnosis. Click on the *Pt has FMHX of* radio button (in the *Only If* field) and select a diagnosis by selecting the [Get FMHX Dx] button.
4. In the *Search* window, type *breast* and click on the [Search] button.
5. Select *Breast Cancer 174.9* from the search results and click the [Save] button. Notice this chart evaluation item now recommends an annual mammogram for female patients between 35 and 110 years if their chart shows a family medical history of breast cancer.
6. Now add a new wellness screening item for a Pap test. Click on the [New] button in the *Chart Evaluation Items* window and add the following details. This test will be for all female patients, between the age of 21 and 30 years who should have a Pap test—PAP 88150—every two years (104 weeks). (Note: A Pap smear is considered a test, not a procedure). We will not link a Pap smear to any specific diagnosis.
7. Save the new item and close the *Chart Evaluation Items* window.
8. Because chart evaluations are typically conducted in a network environment, close SpringCharts and reopen it to see the changes made on the server.
9. Once the program is rebooted, open your own patient chart.
10. Locate the *Perform Chart Evaluation* icon on the toolbar and conduct a chart evaluation.
11. Check all the *Mark this 'Completed'* radio button(s) and add the following patient responses. In the DT recommendation: *The patient declines the DT shot and will schedule on the next visit.* In the Pap recommendation: *The patient has agreed to have the Pap smear test done today.*

Note: If your patient's demographics (age, sex, and so on) do not match the Pap test evaluation that you set up, then you will not get a chart evaluation warning for the Pap test.

12. Click the [Done] button.
13. Click on the "+" sign to the left of the *Encounters* category in the patient's care tree to see the addition of the chart evaluation screening(s), with details seen below.
14. Close your patient chart.

7.2 Test Orders

Tests performed in medical offices can be conducted by trained clinical staff (e.g., by medical assistants), by nurses, or physicians, depending on the specific test. For example, a clinic may allow MAs to perform a throat swab for patients whose chief complaint is a sore throat. A throat swab can be conducted during the initial patient intake period when the MA records chief complaints and vitals. Performing such a test before the physician sees the patient enables the throat culture results to be available when the physician is ready to determine the diagnosis and prescribe medication, creating greater efficiency in the medical office. It is critical that all tests be documented in the patients' charts.

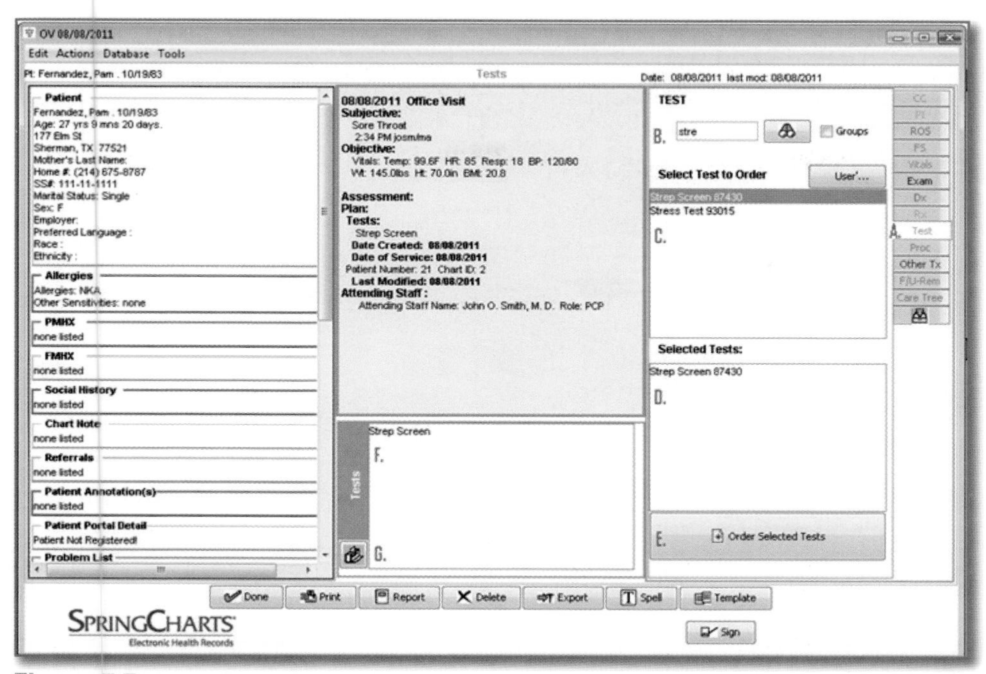

Figure 7.7 Ordering a test in an OV note.

In the SpringCharts EHR program, the clinician initially records the patient's symptoms and complaints under the chief complaint [CC] tab of the office visit note. The clinician then records vitals by switching to the [Vitals] tab. If the specific chief complaint is one that typically requires an in-house test to determine the diagnosis and the clinician has been authorized to do so, the [Test] tab (A)—seen in Figure 7.7—can be selected and a search conducted for the test name from the database in the upper right field (B.). The clinician types the name of the test (or a portion of the name) and conducts a search. If the search result lists several tests in the *Select Test to Order* field (C.), the appropriate test is selected, and the test name and code moves to the lower *Selected Tests* field (D.). Several tests can be ordered in this fashion. Once the appropriate test or tests are located in the lower window, the clinician selects the [Order Selected Tests] button (E.). The tests are then sent to the lower middle panel of the *Office Visit* screen (F.), where they become part of the official OV note. All ordered tests are also sent to the *Pending Tests* area of the EHR program, where they wait for the results to be posted.

Tests also can be ordered by a physician the same way during the examination process. Tests that need to be performed at an outside testing facility are created as CPOE orders and electronically sent to the testing facility; a paper copy is typically printed for the patient. A physician's order is created by clicking on the printer icon in the lower middle *Tests* panel (G). The diagnosis(es) from the office visit note is automatically added to the order, and the user can add additional pop-up text and the patient's primary insurance information before the order is printed. Remember that SpringCharts does not contain the patient's secondary insurance, so all insurance information will be the patient's primary insurance.

Once a clinician records the in-house test results in the *Pending Tests* area of the program, the results can be viewed in the office visit note. In the test portion of the *Office Visit* screen, the user clicks on the test name in the lower middle *Tests* panel, and a test results window appears (Figure 7.8). (Creating tests and processing test results are further explained in Chapter 9.)

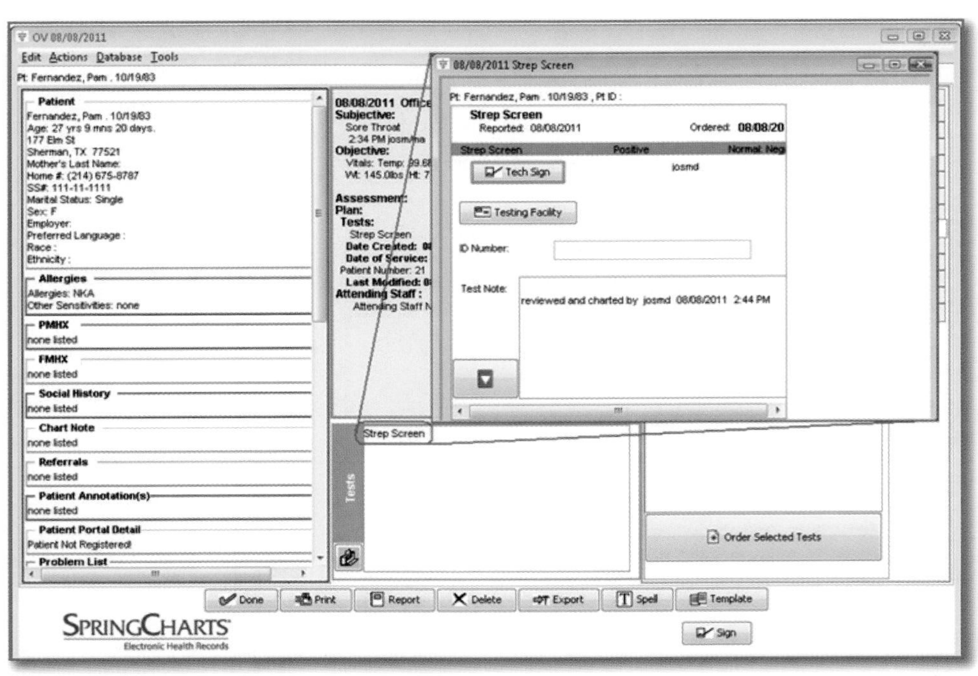

Figure 7.8 Viewing test results in the OV note.

Concept Checkup 7.2

A. All ordered tests in the OV note are also sent to a particular area of the EHR program, where they wait for the results to be posted. What is this area called?

B. What is created within the EHR when a test must be conducted at an outside testing facility?

Exercise 7.2 Ordering a Test in an Office Visit

Well patient visit
The focus of a well patient visit is regular preventive care. Such healthcare measures include routine immunizations to prevent disease for children and adolescents and screening procedures for early detection and treatment of illness for adults. There is typically no treatment for a specific medical condition during a well person healthcare visit and the CPT and ICD codes reflect a wellness visit.

1. Open a new *office visit* note in your chart. We will create a **well patient visit.**
2. Under the chief complaint [CC] navigation tab, select the *Well Visit* pop-up text.
3. Open the *Vitals* tab and record normal vital signs.
4. Select the diagnosis code for a *Well Woman* by searching for a new diagnosis under the [Dx] navigation tab.
5. Open the [Test] tab and type *pap* in the search field.
6. Select *PAP 88150,* and notice the test appears in the lower panel.
7. Click the [Order Selected Tests] button; the test is added to the lower middle field of the OV note.
8. To print the order for the test, click on the printer icon below the *Tests* field in the lower middle panel. Notice the diagnosis has been added to the *Orders* window from the OV note.
9. Add the patient's insurance information to the order form by clicking the [Add Pt Ins] button.
10. Click on the [Print] button, select the *Use Digital Signature* check box, print the order, and submit it to your instructor.

Exercise 7.2 (Concluded)

11. Click the [Done] button inside the *Orders* window and chart the order under the *Encounters* category in the patient's care tree.
12. Open the [F/U-Rem] tab to record a 3-year follow-up for the patient. (If you do not have 3 years in your pop-up text, add it by clicking on the *Edit PopUp Text* icon, find an empty line, type in *3 years,* then move it to its appropriate position by using the up and down arrows to the left.
13. Return to the *OV* screen and select the 3 year pop-up text.
14. Send a *New ToDo/Reminder* to Jan at the front desk to schedule an appointment in 3 years by using the *Create a reminder* icon.
15. Close the office visit note and create a routing slip.
16. Choose the recommended E&M code in the *Routing Slip* window.
17. Use the [Print] button and print the routing slip and submit it to your instructor.
18. Click the [Send] button to send the routing slip. Close the patient's chart.

Create a reminder icon

7.3 Evaluation & Management Coder

The SpringCharts *E&M Coder* helps the physician determine the correct Evaluation & Management code for office visit encounters. To set up this feature, the administrator selects *E&M Coder* from the *Administration* menu of the main *Practice View* screen on a sinlge user version of SpringCharts or on the SpringCharts server in a network environment. In the *E&M Coder Setup* window (Figure 7.9), the provider adds keywords for review of systems and examination of body areas and organ systems. For example, under the respiratory system header the provider would include words like *lung, breath, cough, chest,* and so on. The *E&M Coder* uses these keywords to search office visit notes to determine if a body system or area has been reviewed or examined. It is important that any words or abbreviations added to the *E&M Coder* are also set up as text in the pop-up text fields used in the office visit note. When the

SpringCharts Tip

In a networked environment, the *Administration* menu is accessible on the SpringCharts server. Once selected, the *E&M Coder Setup* window displays.

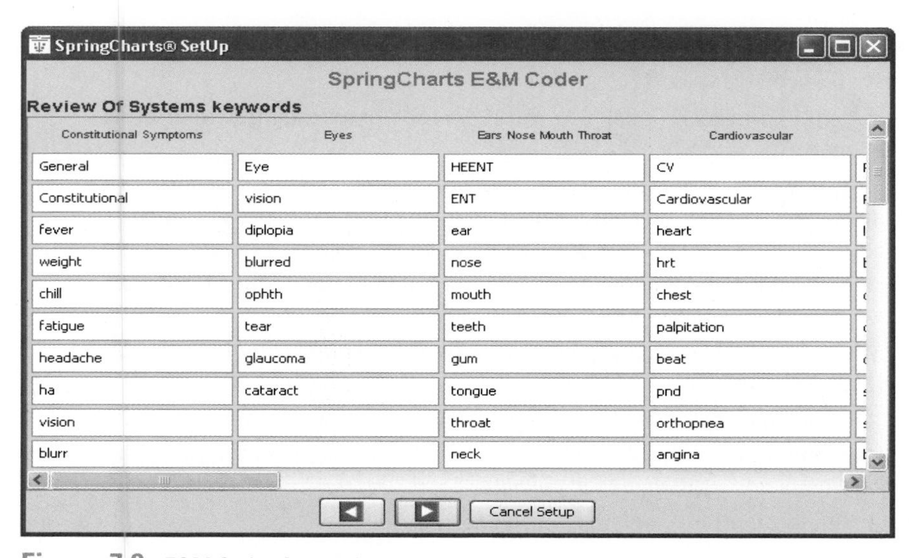

Figure 7.9 *E&M Coder Setup* window.

E&M Coder matches these words, it gives the practitioner "credit" for examining that specific body area or system to help determine the level of evaluation & management. The coder comes with a comprehensive list of terms and abbreviations, so it is only necessary to add terms for specialties that focus on specific body areas.

The *E&M Coder* determines an appropriate E&M code based on the following:

1. Thoroughness of terms and phrases used in the ROS and Exam portions of the OV note that match key terms in the *E&M Coder*
2. Number of diagnoses used
3. Number of procedures conducted
4. History of encounters in the patient's care tree

Based on an analysis of these findings, the program evaluates the type of patient encounter as new, established, or consultation; suggests the complexity of the present illness/problem; and calculates the complexity of medical decision making. From this information, the routing slip recommends the appropriate E&M code.

Focal Point

Key terms and phrases are set up in the *E&M Coder* on the SpringCharts server. The program analyzes the review of systems and exam verbiage in the OV note for these terms and then gives the provider "credit" for reviewing the body areas.

Focal Point

The number of encounters, number of diagnoses, extent of the history in the [CC] and [PI] tabs of the OV note, number of tests ordered, and number of body areas examined, as documented in the OV note, all have bearing on the suggested E&M code.

Concept Checkup 7.3

A. What items are setup in the *E&M Coder* in order for the correct E&M code to be recommended in the *Routing Slip* window?

B. What areas of the SOAP note is examined by the *E&M Coder* to locate key words which will aid in determining the correct E&M code recommendation?

Exercise 7.3 Adding Items to the E&M Coder

1. Click on the *Administration* menu on the main *Practice View* screen and select *E&M Coder.*
2. In the *SpringCharts Setup* window, click on the forward arrow button two times to confirm that you want to use the *E&M Coder.*
3. Read *SpringCharts E&M Coder—How It Works* and press the forward arrow button once again.
4. In the *Review of Systems keywords* window, drag the horizontal scroll bar to the right to view all 14 body systems, from *Constitutional Symptoms* to *Allergic Immunologic.* Note the keywords and phrases for each system.
5. Click the forward arrow button to view the *Examination Body Areas keywords* window and note the keywords in this section.
6. Click the forward arrow once again to view the *Examination Organ Systems keywords window.*
7. Drag the horizontal scroll bar to the right until you can view the *Skin* column.
8. Under the four items in the skin column, add the terms (one per row): *rosacea, hives, spider veins, stretch marks, cellulite.*
9. Click the forward arrow one last time and select [Finish].

7.4 Superbill Form

SpringCharts provides a customized **superbill** that can be set up to contain all additional and ancillary codes not typically selected within the *Office Visit* screen. For example, it can display procedures and codes such as venipuncture, administration of injections, surgical trays, splints, and other billable items that may not have been addressed during the encounter. The *Routing Slip* window is used to view the superbill; to identify any items that may need to be added to the routing slip. The superbill is set up on the SpringCharts server under the *Administration Panel*, or the *Administration* menu on the single computer version (Figure 7.10). The administrator simply adds the category heading and lists the code and item (e.g., *29515, Splint Short Leg).* The superbill items are then displayed in a gray panel in the *Routing Slip* window. From here, items can be clicked on and added to the routing slip.

Superbill
This form includes the medical office's most common procedure and diagnosis codes with descriptions. It is used to record procedures and diagnoses and for billing purposes. In SpringCharts, the superbill displays billable codes and other items often overlooked or not available in the OV exam.

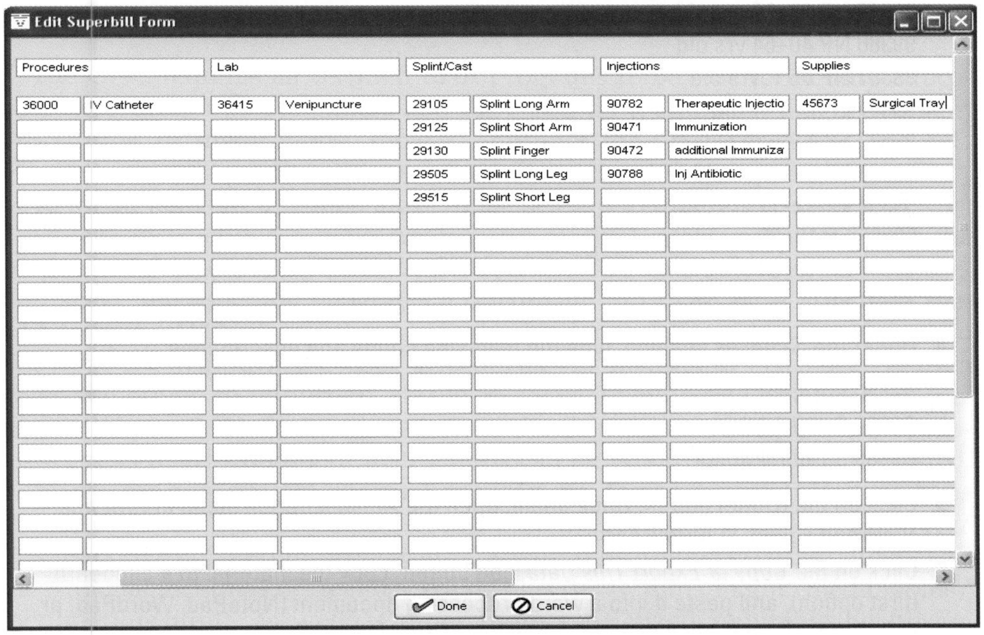

Edit Superbill Form

Procedures		Lab		Splint/Cast		Injections		Supplies	
36000	IV Catheter	36415	Venipuncture	29105	Splint Long Arm	90782	Therapeutic Injectio	45673	Surgical Tray
				29125	Splint Short Arm	90471	Immunization		
				29130	Splint Finger	90472	additional Immuniza		
				29505	Splint Long Leg	90788	Inj Antibiotic		
				29515	Splint Short Leg				

Done Cancel

Figure 7.10 *Edit Superbill Form* window.

Concept Checkup 7.4

A. What is the purpose of the superbill?

B. What two items appear in the superbill under each category heading?

Exercise 7.4 Adding Items to the Superbill

1. Open the *Administration* menu in *Practice View* and select *Superbill Form.* Notice a list of E&M codes and descriptions in the left column of the *Edit Superbill Form* window. Assume your physician performs preventive wellness exams for Medicaid patients. Currently the superbill is displaying additional E&M codes for inpatient

(continued)

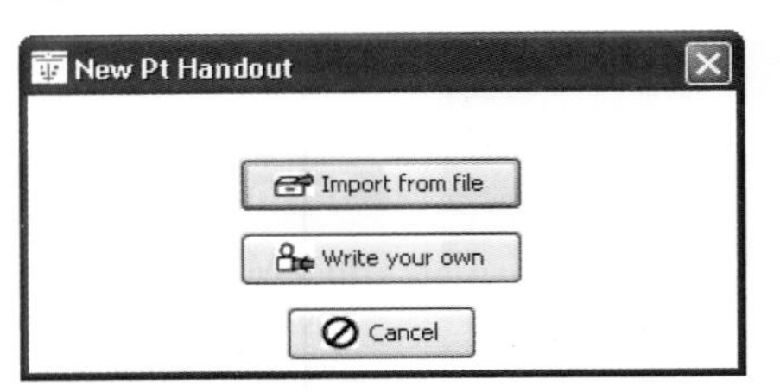

Figure 7.11 Creation option for a patient instruction resource.

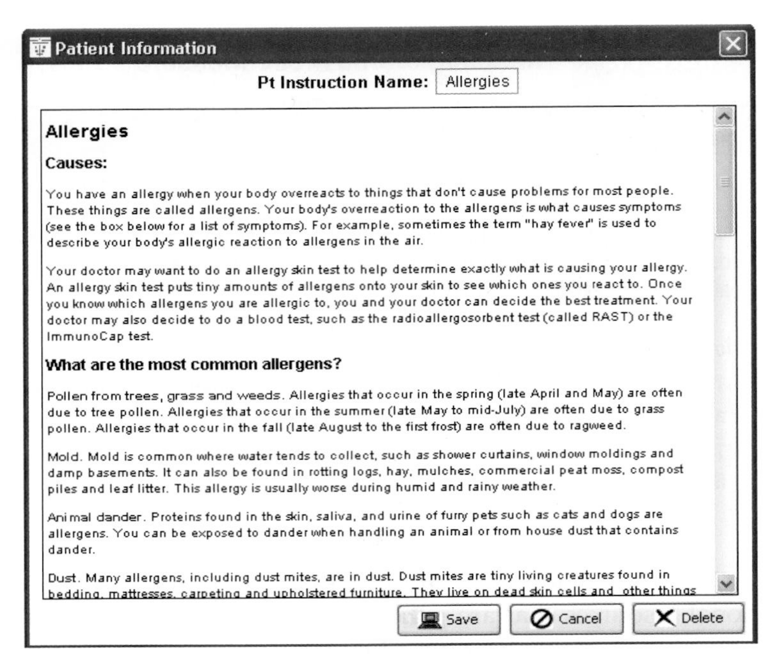

Figure 7.12 Newly imported patient instruction sheet.

To map a patient instruction document to a healthcare item, the user selects the [Map PI] button in the *Edit Patient Instruction* window (Figure 7.13). The resulting *Map Patient Instruction* window allows the user to choose problems (diagnoses), labs (lab tests), procedures, and medications from the EHR database. The first few letters of the item is typed into the *Find* field, and a search of the database is conducted. Multiple variables of that healthcare item can be selected (Figure 7.14). Once the [Done] button is selected, the resulting items are mapped to the patient instruction document.

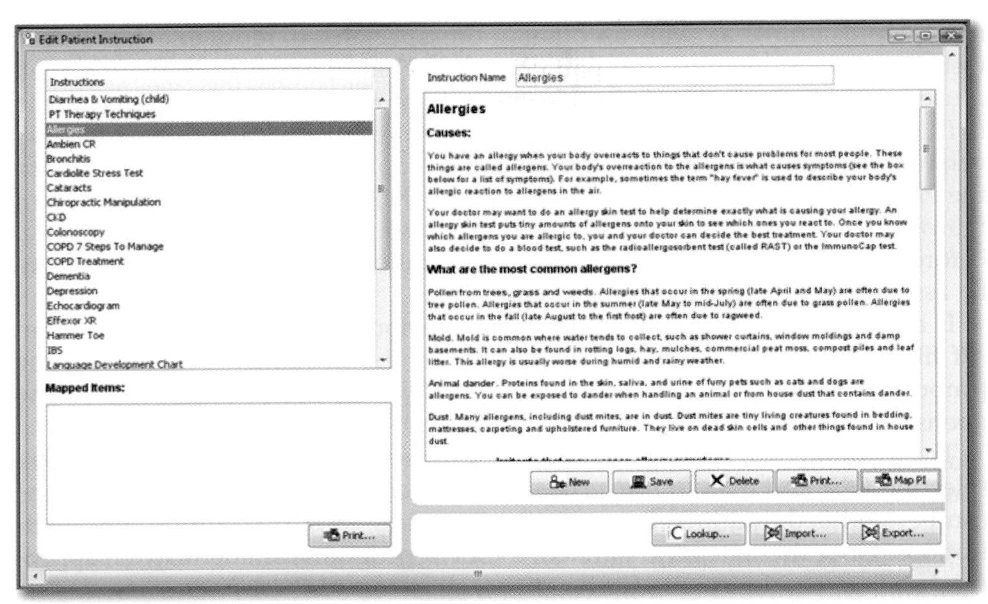

Figure 7.13 *Edit Patient Instruction* window.

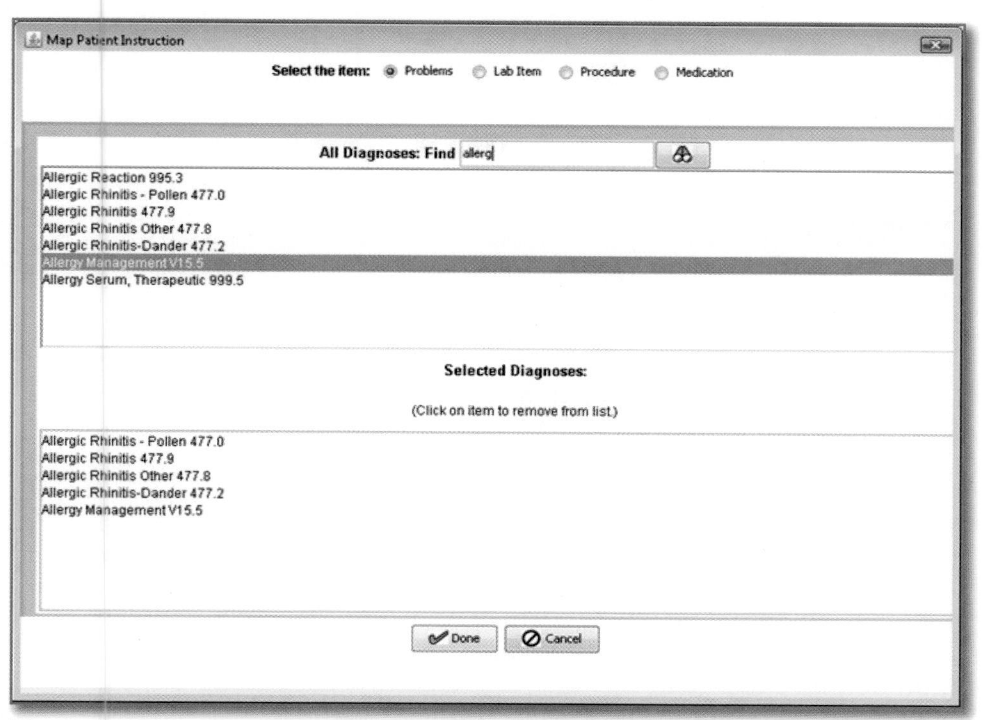

Figure 7.14 Selecting diagnoses for mapping to a PI document.

To administer a patient instruction, the user opens a new or existing office visit note from a patient's chart. Patient resources mapped to a new diagnosis, lab test, procedure, or medication will be triggered for the user when one of these items is documented in the OV note. The *Information Available* window then instructs the user that one or more resource documents are available that address that specific issue (Figure 7.15). To print or e-mail a

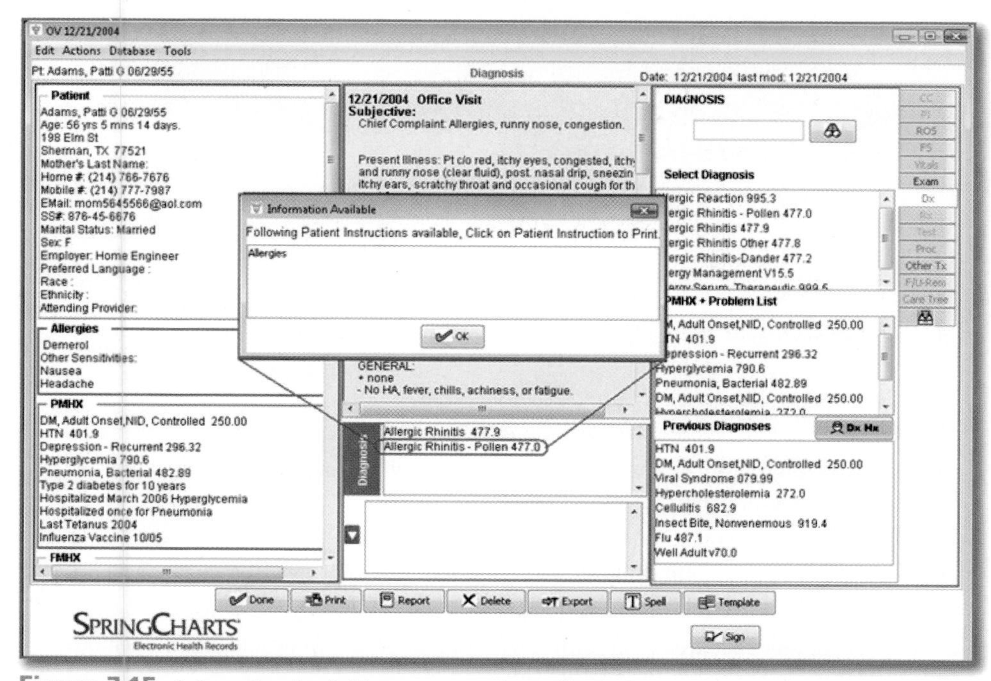

Figure 7.15 *Information Available* note mapped to a diagnosis.

Tools
- H&P
- Calculators
- Care Plan
- Chart Tab
- Draw
- New Excuse/Note/Order
- Patient Instructions
- Resend Routing Slip/Transaction
- Spell Check
- Template
- Date Of Service

Figure 7.16 Administrating a patient instruction sheet.

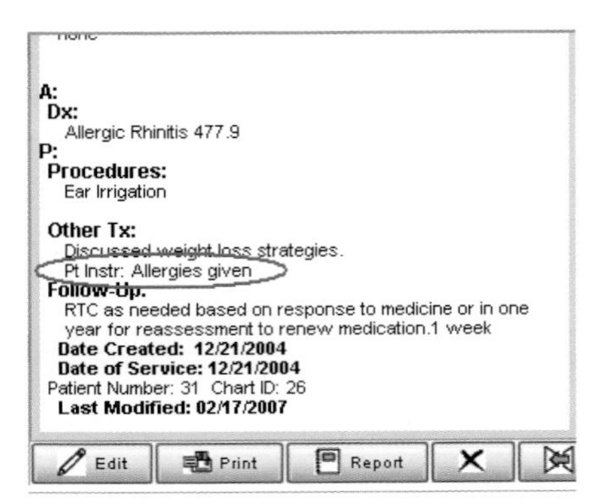

Figure 7.17 Record of patient instructions given to patient.

Focal Point

Patient instruction sheets are administered in the *OV* screen. When printed for a patient, the program adds a notation in the OV note that the information was provided to the patient.

resource document for a patient, the user selects the *Tools* menu in the *OV* screen, followed by the *Patient Instructions* submenu (Figure 7.16). Lists of all instructions that have been created in SpringCharts are displayed, and the user can print or e-mail the selected patient instruction sheet. Once printed, the OV note documents in the *Other Treatment* (Other Tx) portion of the *Plan* section of the SOAP note that the resource was given to the patient (Figure 7.17).

Concept Checkup 7.5

A. To import an existing patient instruction document into SpringCharts, it needs to be saved in what format?

B. In what screen are patient instruction sheets accessed for the patient?

C. To which items are patient instructions mapped, causing the EHR program to trigger an *Information Available* note for the clinician?

Exercise 7.5 Creating a New Patient Information Sheet

1. Click on the *New* menu in the main *Practice View* screen and select the *New Pt Instruction.*
2. Click [OK] in the information window and select the [Write your own] button.
3. Open your web browser and type in the URL address: *www.familydoctor.org.*
4. In the *Search* field in the top right of the web page, type *Pap Smears* and conduct a search.
5. Select the article *Cervical Cancer/Overview.*
6. Click on the *Print: Whole Article* option.
7. To highlight the article, press the [Ctrl] key and hold it down while pressing the [A] key. Release both keys.
8. Right-click on any highlighted area and choose *Copy.*
9. Close the web page and return to the SpringCharts program.
10. Click in the patient instruction window.
11. Using your key pad, press the [Ctrl] + [V] keys, to paste the article into the window.

Exercise 7.5 (Concluded)

12. At the end of the article add the following phrase: *For more information, contact our office at (214) 674-2000.*
13. At the top of the article, delete the statement, *Familydoctor.org—Return to Web version.*
14. Change the *Patient Instruction Name* field to *Pap Smears* and click the [Save] button.
15. To view all of the patient instructions in the program, select the *Edit* menu and choose *Pt Instructions.* Notice the new Pap Smears instruction sheet listed here. In this window, instruction sheets can be modified, exported, and deleted, and new ones can be created. Close the window.

Exercise 7.6 Administering a Patient Instruction

1. Open your chart.
2. Locate the office visit note in the *Encounters* category of the care tree that included the well adult visit created in Exercise 7.2. Highlight the OV note and click [Edit] in the lower window.
3. In the *OV* screen, select *Tools* and then *Patient Instructions.*
4. Click on the Pap Smears instruction sheet in the *Choose Patient Instruction* window.
5. At the top of the *Patient Instruction* window, type your name on the first line. Print the instruction sheet and submit it to your instructor.
6. Close the OV note and click [Save and Skip Billing].
7. Notice the phrase: *Pt Instr: Pap Smears given* recorded at the bottom of the OV note. This now becomes a permanent record in the patient's chart.
8. Close the patient's chart.

7.6 Care Plans and Practice Guidelines

Practitioners can also attach a text document outlining **care plans and practice guidelines** to a patient's office visit note. This document then becomes a permanent record attached to the OV note. To access a care plan, the user selects the *Tools* menu in the *Office Visit* screen and chooses *Care Plan* (Figure 7.18). The *Care Plan/Guideline* window opens, enabling the user to import a care plan document stored on the computer. Care plans and practice guidelines may be designed by the clinic or found at Internet sites such as the *National Guideline Clearinghouse* (NGC), accessed by clicking on the [NGC] button.

Care plans and practice guidelines
Specific documents that guide all individuals involved in a patient's care, outlining the appropriate treatment that will ensure the optimal outcome. A caregiver unfamiliar with a patient should be able to find all of the information needed to care for the patient in these documents.

The NGC website holds numerous medical treatment plans containing objective, detailed clinical information for physicians, nurses, and other healthcare professionals. The user simply searches for and highlights the specific document then pastes it into the patient's *Care Plan/Guideline* window using the [Ctrl]+[V] keys. Figure 7.19 shows a saved care plan. The selected care plan document becomes a permanent record associated with this office visit. It can be viewed at the bottom of the office visit note when selected in the patient's care tree (Figure 7.20).

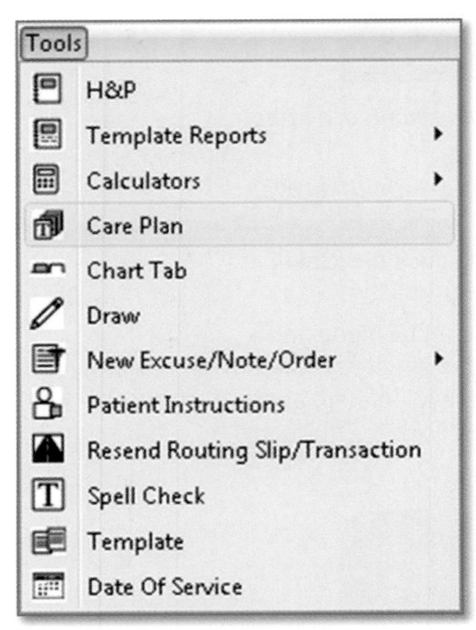

Figure 7.18 Accessing care plans in *OV* screen.

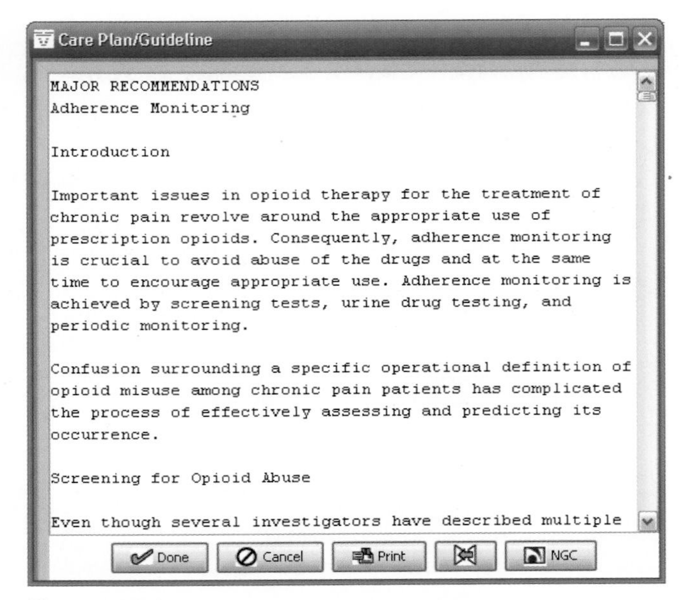

Figure 7.19 Sample care plan selected either from computer or NGC website.

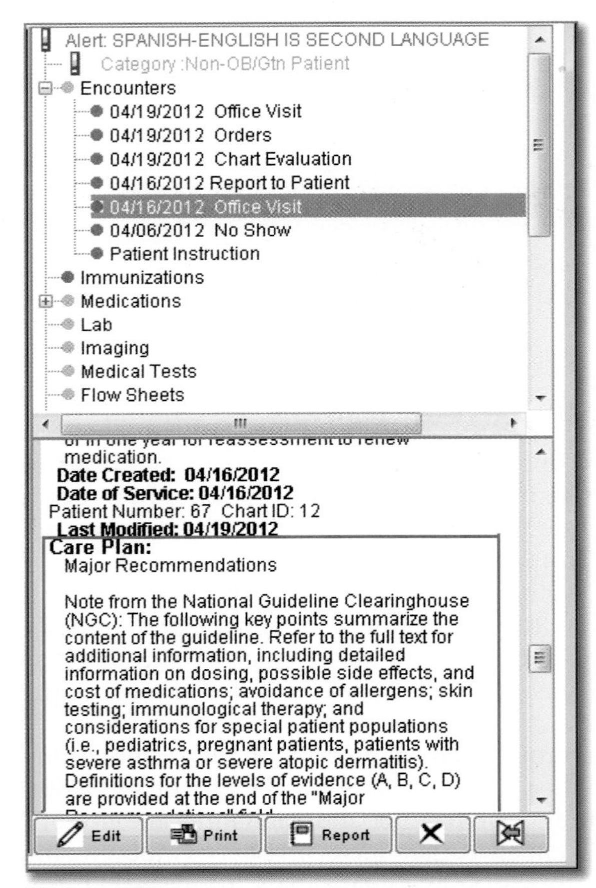

Figure 7.20 Care plan attached to office visit note.

Concept Checkup 7.6

A. What type of information can be retrieved from the National Guidelines Clearinghouse?

B. What information does a care plan include?

Exercise 7.7 Adding a Patient's Care Plan

1. Open your patient chart.
2. Select the OV note in the care tree that addresses allergy symptoms, and click on [Edit].
3. In the *OV* screen, select *Tools* > *Care Plan* from the main menu.
4. In the *Care Plan/Guideline* window, click on the [NGC] button.
5. On the NGC website, enter *seasonal allergies* in the *Search* field and search for the care plan. Locate and open the *Allergic Rhinitis* plan. In the *Jump To* section, locate and click *Recommendations.* Highlight and copy sections titled: *Major Recommendations*, *Diagnosis*, and *Therapy.* Close the web browser. Paste the material into the *Care Plan/ Guideline* window by using the [Ctrl]+[V] keys.
6. Click the [Done] button, close the *OV* screen, and click [Save and Skip Billing]. Notice the care plan has been added to the bottom of the OV note.
7. Print the OV note and submit it to your instructor.
8. Close the patient chart.

7.7 Drawing Program

The old adage, "A picture is worth a thousand words," can be applied to health record documentation. Photographs and drawings may be a useful supplement to OV notes, to document patients' wounds, skin disorders, pain sources, and so on. Photographs and sketches provide additional information in the physician's notes.

The *Office Visit* screen provides access to a basic **draw program** that enables the provider to draw on templates of body diagrams and add this visual information to the OV note. Within the *OV* screen, the provider accesses the *Tools* menu and selects the *Draw* option. From the *Templates* menu in the *Simple Draw* window, the user selects the desired body section and then uses the draw tools on the left to mark the illustration (Figure 7.21). Only one draw item can be added to each office visit note. The *Edit* menu inside the draw program enables the cutting, copying, pasting, and clearing of the *Simple Draw* screen.

Existing illustrations can be imported into the drawing program (Figure 7.22), by selecting *Background Image* on the menu bar of the *Simple Draw* window and then selecting a .jpg image already existing on the computer or a computer in the network. In addition, digital photographs can be taken of the patient's body area and imported to the draw program to document a patient's condition or treatment. Text can be added to the image to clarify content; the text font, accessed via the [T] button, is set at a default of 10-point plain. To increase the size or bold the font, the user can set the font size and style before

Draw program
The Draw program accessed in the *OV* screen enables providers to document injuries, pain locations, skin abnormalities, and so on, on templates of body areas or imported images. The completed drawing remains a permanent part of the OV note.

SpringCharts Tip
In many windows accessed within the patient's chart, like the *Simple Draw* window, the EHR program places the patient's initials in the header of the window. For example, a window accessed from within Patti G. Adams's chart displays (PGA) in the header.

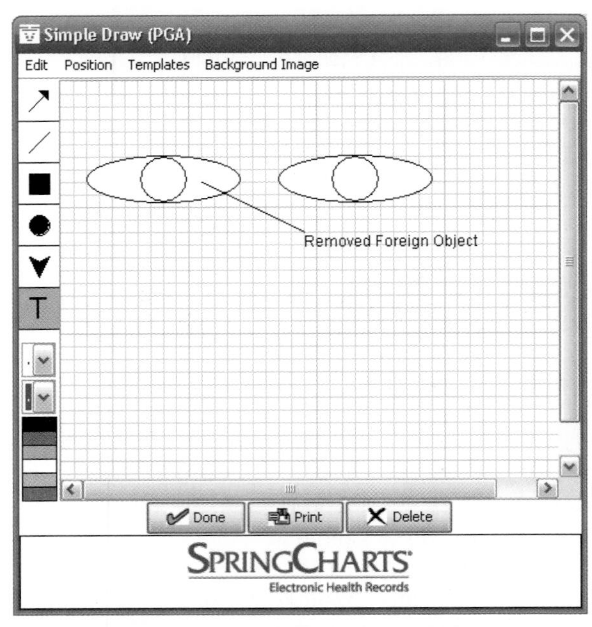

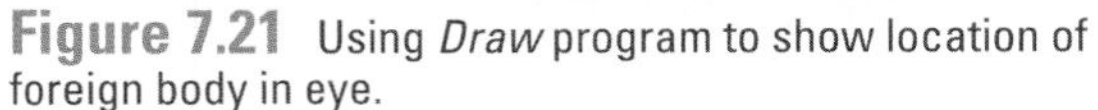
Figure 7.21 Using *Draw* program to show location of foreign body in eye.

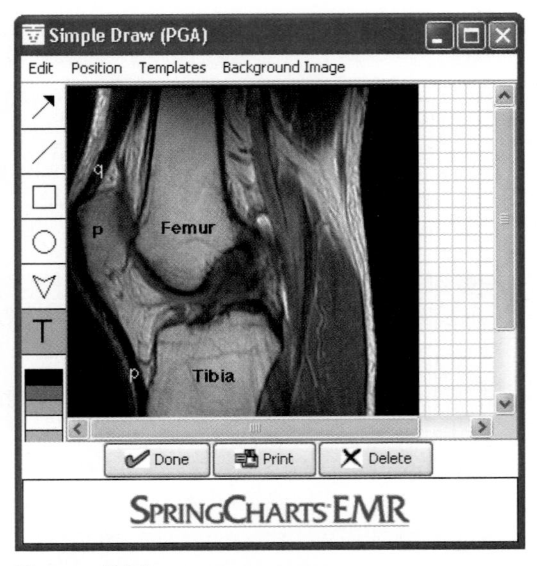

Figure 7.22 Imported images in the *Draw* program.

selecting the [T] button. The font size and style buttons are located below the [T] button.

The draw item is stored with the office visit note, and the *Follow-Up* segment on the note is stamped with the word *Graphic.* To view a graphic that has been added to an OV note, the user selects the specific office visit in the care tree and clicks on the word: *****Graphic***** in the lower right panel of the chart; the draw item window then displays, along with the accompanying OV note.

Concept Checkup 7.7

A. In what menu is the *Draw* feature located in the *Office Visit* screen?

B. Where is the draw item stored in the SpringCharts EHR program?

7.8 Importing Documents

Some documents cannot be created in an EHR program. For example, a patient's healthcare records may be sent from another physician who does not use an EHR program. In this case, the documents are sent through the mail and need to be scanned into the patient's chart within the EHR program. In another example, the clinic may want to scan a copy of the patient's driver's license and insurance card into the EHR program for future reference.

The *Import File Cabinet Document* option in the SpringCharts program allows users to attach documents to patient charts. This means the program creates a link to the document; the actual electronic file is stored in a separate folder in the SpringCharts server directory. The *File Cabinet Document* window is located under the *New* menu of the patient chart, under the *Import Items* submenu (Figure 7.23). This feature allows the user to add any type of document to a chart, including files ending with: .doc, .xls, .html, .xml, .pdf, .jpg, .tiff, and DICOM. Because the electronic documents are stored in a database folder separate from the patients' charts, the user can import multiple documents and graphics without compromising the performance or speed of the EHR program. When the document is accessed within the patient's chart, it is opened in the original program, for example Excel, Word, Acrobat Reader, and so on.

Within the *File Cabinet Document* window, the user needs to record several pieces of information, beginning with the name of the document. The patient's name is automatically added into the *Patient* field because the window was accessed from the patient's chart. To store a document in the *File Cabinet* section of the care tree, the user selects the *File Cabinet* option in the *Chart Tab* field. Next, a folder within the *File Cabinet* needs to be selected in which the document can be stored.

Some medical offices choose to store imported documents under a different tab than the *File Cabinet* tab, in the care tree. For example, if the document is accessed often, it may be placed under its own category so it can be located more quickly. If this is the case, the clinician would select one of the customized tabs in the care tree, listed in the drop-down menu of the *Chart Tab* field. Finally, a description of the document is added in the *Description* field. The user should always select the [Sign] button to time- and initial-stamp the operation.

SpringCharts Tip

A new folder category can be created by accessing the SpringCharts server and adding a new item in the *File Cabinet Folders* list in the *Category Preferences* window.

The user then selects the [Attach] button and chooses the *Existing* option (shown in margin). A standard file dialog appears for users to select a document stored on the network. The file name appears in blue type in the import window (Figure 7.23). Once the document is attached, the user selects the [Done] button to store the document in the patient's file cabinet or other customized tab within the patient's care tree. The program creates a copy of the original document, places it in a folder on the SpringCharts server, and creates a link to it in the patient's chart. The original document is still available on the network to be copied to other patients' charts.

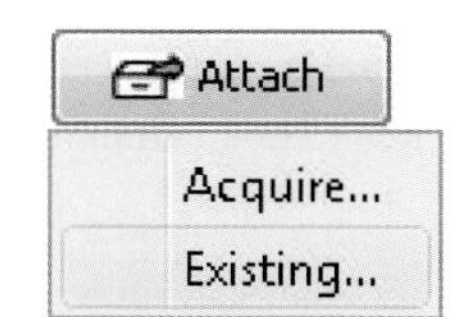

Attaching an existing document option

The second option for importing a document into a patient's file cabinet is through an interface with another piece of equipment. In this case, the user

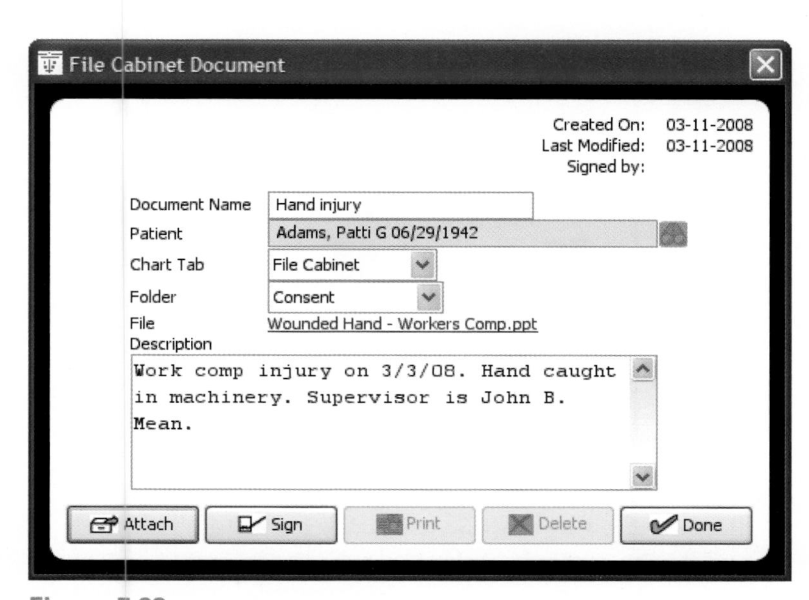

Figure 7.23 *File Cabinet Document* window.

SpringCharts Tip

TWAIN technology has been incorporated into equipment manufactured since the year 2000 and operates in Windows and Macintosh OS environments.

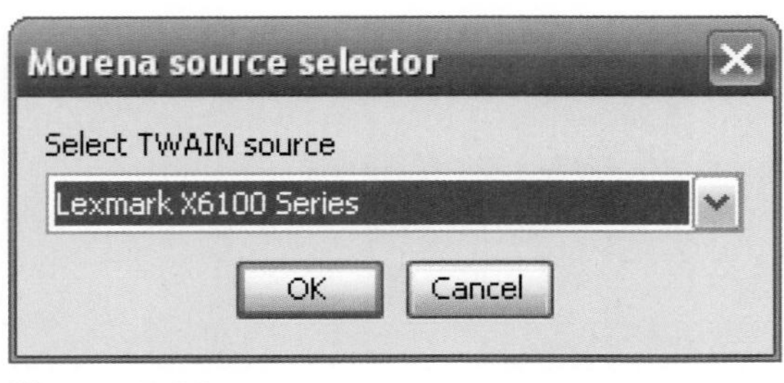

Figure 7.24 TWAIN source selection window.

selects the [Attach] button and chooses the *Acquire* option (shown in margin). This enables communication between image-capturing devices such as scanners, cameras, webcams, and computer programs.

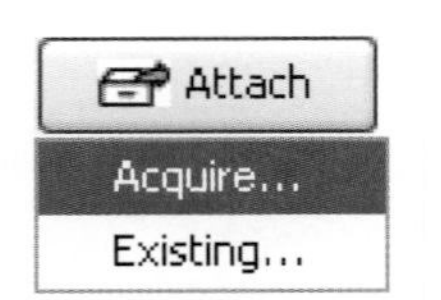

Acquire option to import a file.

After selecting the *Acquire* option, the user selects the appropriate source in the *Morena source selector* window (Figure 7.24). The drop-down menu in this window lists the equipment connected to the user's computer and available on the network (e.g., scanner, webcam, or other device). When the device is selected, the appropriate graphic user interface (GUI) dialog box opens (Figure 7.25). From this window, the user can activate a scanner or extract an image from a device like a webcam or a digital camera. The GUI screen looks different for each of the devices. This one-touch scanning feature enables the user to operate the scanner directly from SpringCharts.

A scanned document or image can be resized before attaching it to the patient's care tree. The user selects the [Done] button to store the document in the patient's chart.

To view a document attached to a patient's chart, the user highlights the appropriate document in the category of the care tree. A summary of the document will be seen in the lower right-hand window. As much detail as necessary can be added into the summary, enabling the provider to view information without opening the document. To open the document the user clicks the [Doc] button (shown in margin) at the bottom of the screen (Figure 7.26). The document opens in the native program in which it was originally created. Once opened within the patient's chart, any document can be edited and resaved. The file is dated by SpringCharts and can be signed by the doctor. Figure 7.27 and Figure 7.28 illustrate two different file types that can be

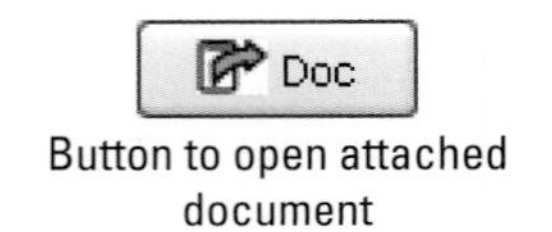

Button to open attached document

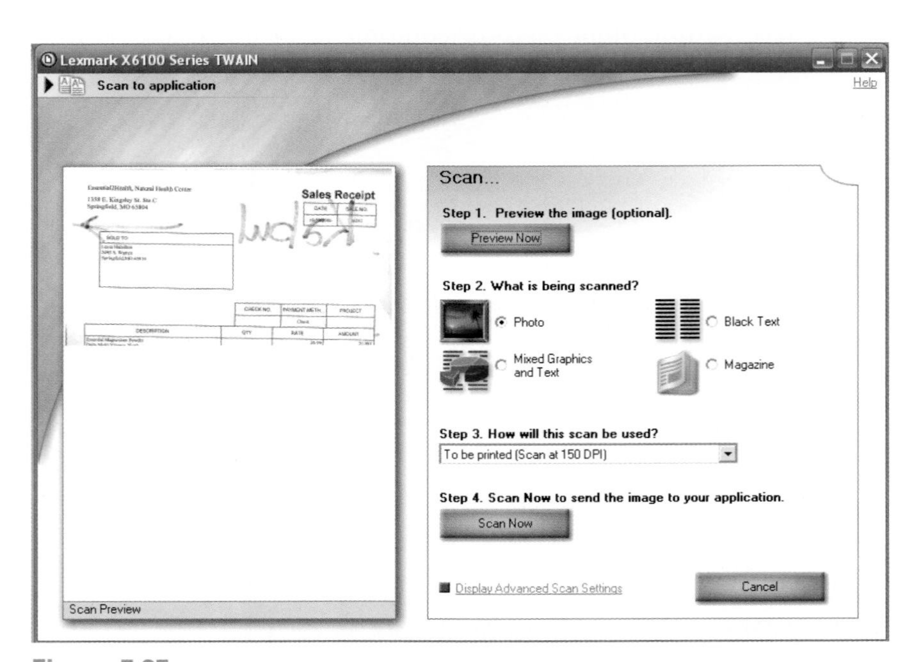

Figure 7.25 Specific operating window of TWAIN device.

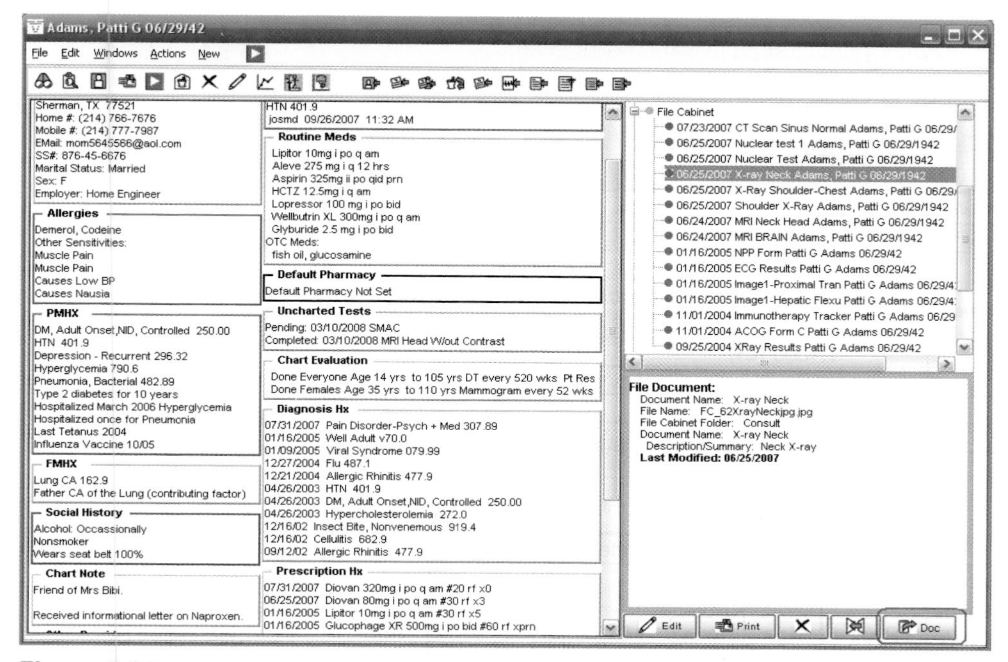

Figure 7.26 File document in care tree of patient's chart.

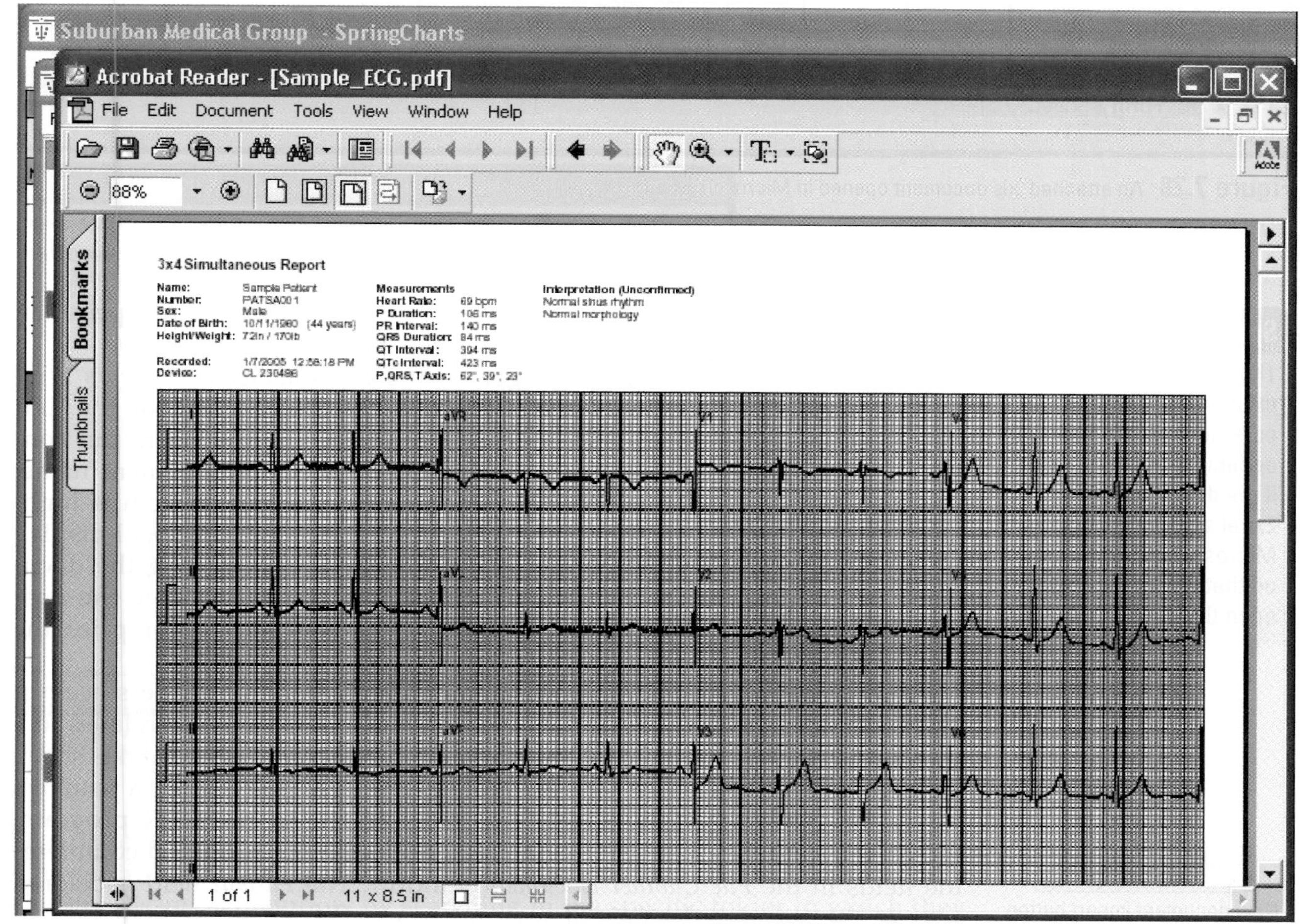

Figure 7.27 A scanned document as a .pdf file opened in Acrobat Reader.

Concept Checkup 7.8

A. Where are *File Cabinet Documents* stored?

B. What types of documents and files can be imported through the *File Cabinet Documents* window?

C. To view a document or file that has been imported into SpringCharts, what must be installed on the computer or workstation on which the file is opened?

Exercise 7.8 Importing A Document

1. Open your chart and select *Import Items* from the *New* menu.
2. Select the *Import File Cabinet Document* option.
3. In the *Document Name* field of the *File Cabinet Document* window, type *Insurance card.*
4. In the *Chart Tab* field, select the option *Insurance Card.*
5. In the *Folder* field, select *Consent.*
6. In the *Description* box, type *Galaxy Health Network—Primary Ins.*
7. Click the [Sign] button and add your initials only.
8. Click on the [Attach] button and choose the *Existing* option.
9. Within the *Open* dialog box, find your *EHR Material* folder. Your instructor will inform you where the *EHR Material* folder is located. Open the folder and select the *Ins Card.jpg* file. Make sure the file name shows in the File name field.
10. Click the [Open] button to attach the file. If you were successful, the file name should appear in blue type in the *File Cabinet Document* window.
11. Click the [Done] button. The newly imported file should display under the *Insurance Card* tab in the care tree.
12. Click on the [Doc] button in the lower right of your patient's chart to view the document. You may have to expand the window to see the entire image.
13. Print the document, write your name on it, and submit it to your instructor.
14. Click the [Done] button in the *Graphic* window. Close the patient's chart.

chapter 7 summary

Learning Outcomes	Key Concepts
7.1 Create and conduct a chart evaluation. **Pages 190–196**	Define preventive health criteria and then evaluate patients' charts by these criteria. Criteria set by *Gender, Age, Healthcare actions, Recurring event, Diagnosis(es), Lab or Medication,* and *High Clinical Priority.* Information windows will appear if the patient has outstanding screenings, is up-to-date with screenings, or if no chart evaluation criteria have been set. Chart evaluations can be performed on individual patients or on the entire patient database. Reminder notices can be sent regarding patients 65 years and older and 5 years and younger concerning necessary wellness screenings.

Learning Outcomes	Key Concepts
7.2 Demonstrate how to order a test in the *Office Visit* screen. **Pages 196–199**	Tests ordered in the OV note are sent to the *Pending Tests* area where they wait for results to be entered. Tests that need to be conducted at an outside testing facility require that a physician's order form be created. Test results are entered in the *Pending Tests* area and are available to be viewed in the OV note.
7.3 Describe the function of the *E&M Coder.* **Pages 199–200**	The *E&M Coder* uses keywords to search an office visit note and determine if a body system or area has been reviewed or examined. Based on terms and phrases used in the OV note, the number of diagnoses, the number of procedures, and the history of encounters in the patient's care tree, the *E&M Coder* recommends a code. It is not mandatory that the provider use the recommended E&M code.
7.4 Demonstrate how to add items to a superbill. **Pages 201–202**	The superbill contains additional billable terms and codes that may not have been selected in the OV note. Items from the superbill can be added to the routing slip.
7.5 Create and administer a patient instruction sheet. **Pages 202–207**	Providing patient's with educational material is an ONC MU menu measure. Patient instruction sheets can be created in the EHR program or imported. Patient instruction sheets are accessed and printed in the OV note. Patient instructions can be mapped to specific diagnoses, labs, procedures, or medications. An information window is displayed when one of these items is used in the OV note. When a patient instruction sheet is printed, the OV note will record that the information sheet was given to the patient.
7.6 Describe how to add a care plan to an office visit. **Pages 207–209**	Care plans are created and administered within the OV note. The care plan becomes part of the OV note record.
7.7 Explain the purpose of the *Draw* program. **Pages 209–210**	The *Draw* program provides a supplement of illustrations for the OV note. Draw templates can be used within the program to illustrate findings; illustrations and photos can also be imported into the *Draw* program. The illustration is stored in the OV note under the *Follow-Up* section.
7.8 Demonstrate how to import a document to a patient's chart. **Pages 210–216**	The *Import File Cabinet Document* allows the user to import any type of document to a chart. The originating program for the document must be on the computer to view and edit the document. Documents can be imported into a patient's chart or stored outside a patient's chart. A document can be imported from the computer or from any image-capturing device. A link to the document is created in the patient's chart because the document is stored on the server, not actually in the chart.

chapter 7 review

Name ______________________ Instructor ______________ Class ______________ Date ______________

Using Terminology

Match the terms on the left with the definitions on the right.

_____ **1. LO 7.4** Superbill

_____ **2. LO 7.1** Wellness screenings

A. A health insurance plan that pays for some of the patient's medical expenses that primary health insurance does not pay, for example, the deductible and co-payments.

B. A feature in which patient instructions can be modified and new ones created.

_____ 3. **LO 7.6** Care plans and practice guidelines
_____ 4. **LO 7.1** Chart evaluation
_____ 5. **LO 7.2** Secondary insurance
_____ 6. **LO 7.5** Patient Instructions Manager
_____ 7. **LO 7.1** NGC
_____ 8. **LO 7.1** CDS
_____ 9. **LO 7.2** Well patient visit
_____ 10. **LO 7.1** FMHX
_____ 11. **LO 7.7** Draw program
_____ 12. **LO 7.5** RTF

C. A comprehensive database of evidence-based practice guidelines.
D. An EHR integrated system designed to assist physicians and other health professionals with decision-making tasks concerning the healthcare of patients.
E. Specific documents that provide a "road map" to guide all involved with a patient's care.
F. Diagnoses from this section of the patient's face sheet contain health information about a patient's close relatives and can be linked to wellness screening criteria.
G. Periodic medical checkups to test for or inoculate against significant diseases.
H. A feature in the *Tools* menu of the *Office Visit* screen that enables the provider to illustrate procedures on built-in templates.
I. A SpringCharts feature used to establish criteria for medical checkups and appraise patients' charts for needed health screenings and tests.
J. Format in which new patient instructions must be created in order to to save into SpringCharts.
K. A routine patient encounter that may include an annual Pap smear and be recorded in an office visit note.
L. A panel in SpringCharts that contains codes that can be added to the routing slip for billing purposes.

Checking Your Understanding

Choose the best answer and circle the corresponding letter.

13. **LO 7.5** Patient instructions and educational documents can be created in SpringCharts or imported into the program. Which screen in the program can these documents be accessed for printing or e-mailing?
    a) *Office Visit* screen
    b) *Patient Chart* screen
    c) *Practice View* screen
    d) *Edit* menu

14. **LO 7.4** What type of codes are displayed on the customized superbill that are not usually selected within the *Office Visit* screen?
    a) Diagnosis
    b) Procedure
    c) Additional and ancillary
    d) Evaluation & Management

15. **LO 7.3** What type of code in the E&M Coder helps the physician determine the correct code for office visit encounters?
    a) Diagnosis
    b) Procedure
    c) Additional & Ancillary
    d) Evaluation & Management

16. **LO 7.1** What three items can be chosen in the chart evaluation wellness screenings that will create a *High Clinical Priority* message in the *OV* screen?
    a) Encounter, lab, medication
    b) Gender, age, procedure
    c) Test, procedure, encounter
    d) Diagnosis, lab, medication

17. **LO 7.2** What area of the EHR program are ordered tests sent to where they wait for results to be posted?
    a) *Completed Tests*
    b) *Pending Tests*
    c) *Stored Tests*
    d) *Physician Order Forms*

18. **LO 7.6** In what screen are care plans created and selected?
    a) *Office Visit*
    b) *Patient Chart*
    c) *Patient Instructions*
    d) *New Care Plan*

19. **LO 7.1** In the chart evaluation setup, the administrator will define what mandatory criteria for wellness screenings? Select all that apply.
    a) Gender (male, female, or either)
    b) Age range
    c) Actions (test, procedure, or encounter)
    d) Recurring

20. **LO 7.6** Once a practitioner attaches a plan of care in the *Office Visit* screen, it becomes:
    a) A temporary document that is deleted after 90 days
    b) A permanent part of the office visit note
    c) Unusable—a care plan cannot be attached to an office visit note
    d) Linked to the diagnosis, lab, and medication

21. **LO 7.1** The National Guidelines Clearinghouse website contains:
    a) National conference dates on a centralized calendar for physicians
    b) Detailed clinical information for nurses only
    c) Numerous medical treatment plans
    d) Electronic prescriptions from physicians across the nation

22. **LO 7.7** The *Draw* program feature of SpringCharts gives providers the ability to:
    a) Document a patient's wounds, injuries, skin disorders, and pain sources.
    b) Enable young patients to draw for psychological testing.
    c) Doodle while they wait for the MA to finish with the patient.
    d) Store documents in the patient's filing cabinet.

23. **LO 7.3** Key terms and phrases are set up in the *E&M Coder* on the SpringCharts server. The program analyzes the review of systems and the exam verbiage in the OV note for these terms and then gives the provider credit for reviewing the body areas. The number of body areas examined affects:
    a) The level of E&M code recommended by the program
    b) The price of the OV visit
    c) The number of diagnoses assigned
    d) The number of items selected from the superbill

24. **LO 7.5** The ONC requires that all certified EHR programs have the function of identifying patient-specific educational resources based on:
    a) Whether the patient requests an instruction sheet or not
    b) Their availability on the NGC website
    c) Whether the patient is over 65 years of age or under 5 years of age
    d) Identifiable diagnoses, labs, procedures, or medications of the patient

25. **LO 7.8** SpringCharts enables the user to import what type of document into the patient's file cabinet?
    a) Only .pdfs
    b) Only Microsoft files: .doc, .xls, and .ppt
    c) Any type of file
    d) Documents transmitted via a certified EHR program

Applying Your Knowledge

Use your critical-thinking skills to answer the following questions.

26. **LO 7.2** Describe a situation in a medical office in which an MA would order a test for a patient before the patient is seen by the physician.

27. **LO 7.8** The *File Cabinet Document* feature allows the user to import many different types of documents into a patient's chart. How would you store a general form, such as the original medical release form, unrelated to any specific patient?

28. **LO 7.4** The physician has chosen two diagnoses, a procedure, and an injection as part of the OV note. These billable items have been automatically added to the routing slip. The physician has also chosen an E&M code for the routing slip. The provider realizes that a venipuncture can also be added to the routing slip. What is the best way for the provider to add this charge to the routing slip?

8

Creating Templates

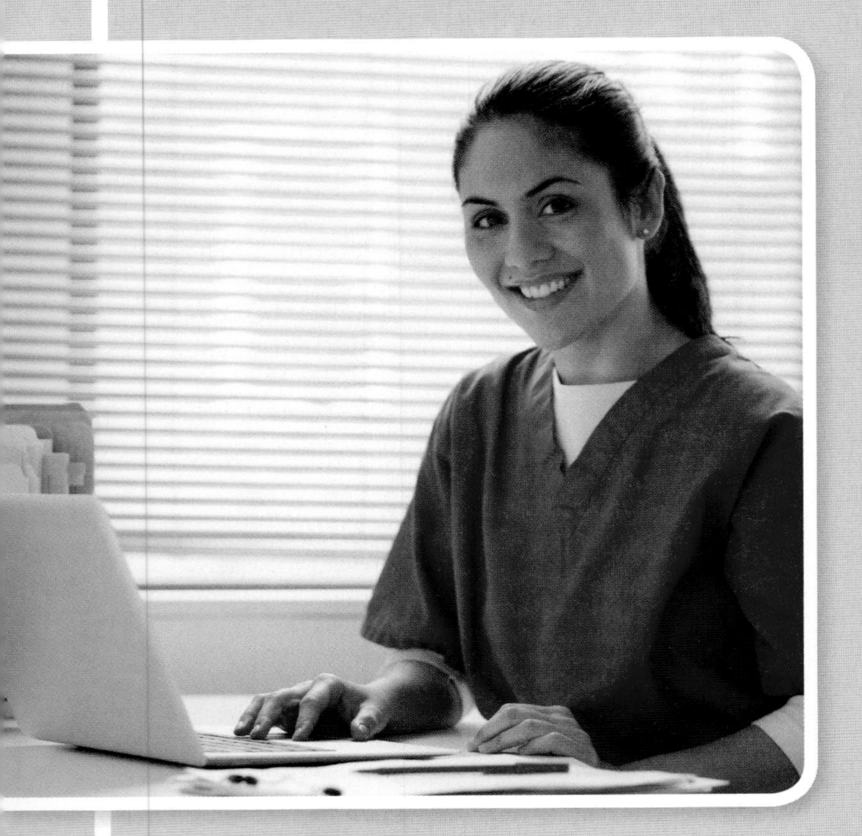

Learning Outcomes

After completing Chapter 8, you will be able to:

LO 8.1 Create and activate an office visit template.

LO 8.2 Create and use a physician order template.

LO 8.3 Create and use a letter template.

LO 8.4 Explain the function of the template manager.

LO 8.5 Create and use a procedure template.

What You Need to Know

To understand Chapter 8, you will need to know how to:

- Open an electronic patient chart and navigate within it.
- Open a new or established office visit note.
- Navigate within the *Office Visit* screen.
- Add new pop-up text.

Key Terms

Letter templates

Office visit templates

Order templates

Procedure templates

Template manager

Introduction

Templates have been used in clerical work for many years to help reduce the time it takes to produce multiple documents that follow a similar format. Rather than recreating the same information many times, templates, or pre-designed documents with a set format, structure, or "chunks" of text, can be used. In medical offices, templates can be used to efficiently create letters, reports, orders, and office visit notes. They are incorporated in EHR programs to reduce time, improve efficiency, and help to ensure accuracy in documentation in medical offices. Accurate, consistent templates also assist in legally protecting the physician and the practice by using uniform documentation when applicable. They can be used in the front office for clerical work and in the clinical area to document notes regarding common patient encounters.

The templates in SpringCharts can be created and customized to minimize the amount of data that needs to be added when working in the program. SpringCharts templates are simple to create, edit, and use. The **template manager** includes three template types: office visit notes, orders, and letters.

In addition, smaller templates can be created containing common verbiage that can be added to an OV note each time certain procedures are documented. This ensures that complete and consistent information about procedures, including their potential risks and complications, is provided to all patients.

Template manager
The template manager in the SpringCharts EHR program allows for the creation, editing, and storage of three template types: office visit notes, orders, and letters.

8.1 Creating Office Visit Templates

Office visit templates are used for the most common types of encounters. They should be designed to fit at least 90 percent of patients with any given ailment and diagnosis. The specific details relevant to each patient are added in the OV encounter itself, and then "fed" into the template. The OV template layout corresponds to the navigation categories in the *Office Visit* screen, making it simple to build the template. Its layout allows users to manually type text or add pop-up text data in the template fields.

To create a new office visit template, the user selects the submenu *New Template* from the *New* menu of the main *Practice View* screen, and then *New Office Visit Template* (Figure 8.1).

In the *Template Name* field of the *Office Visit Template* window, the user inserts the title for the template; the title is often the patient's chief complaint being addressed in the office visit. The provider then completes the template as if creating an office visit note. Any form of data input can be used, including selections from pop-up text, typing, handwriting recognition on a tablet, or third-party speech recognition software. The pop-up text is accessed by clicking on each side navigation tab and selecting appropriate text.

The OV template is organized with the same segments as the navigation tabs in the *Office Visit* screen in which the OV note is created (Figure 8.2). It is important to place the desired text into

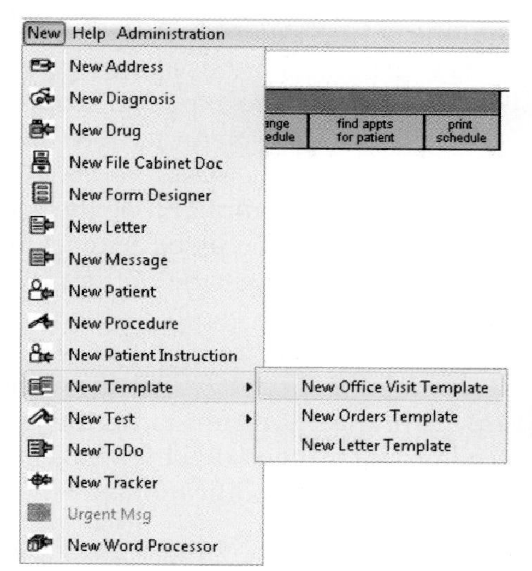

Figure 8.1 Accessing the *Office Visit Template window* from the *Practice View* screen.

Office visit templates
These templates allow users to create the majority of an office visit note that includes text common to all patients with the same ailment. When the OV template is selected in the *OV* screen, the provider only needs to add limited detail for a specific patient.

SpringCharts Tip
Data input in the *Office Visit* screen is added to the office visit template wherever the cursor is positioned, if the *Insert at Cursor* option has been chosen in *PopUp Text Insert* in the *Set User Preferences* setup.

SpringCharts Tip
TemplateWare, an add-on feature for SpringCharts, offers templates and pop-up text tailored for specific medical specialties.

SpringCharts Tip

Spring Medical Systems Inc. has developed templates as an add-on feature to SpringCharts for different medical specialties including pediatrics, family practice, internal medicine, gastroenterology, psychiatry, and pulmonary medicine. These templates come with prebuilt office visit, orders, and letter templates, as well as pop-up text tailored to each specialty. These add-ons enable providers and staff members to more rapidly and efficiently complete patient documentation.

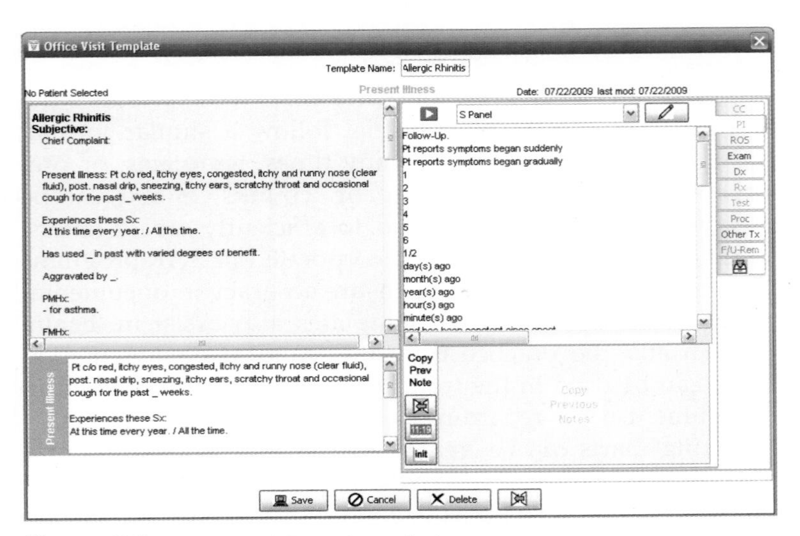

Figure 8.2 *Office Visit Template* window.

the proper template section so it will correspond to the correct navigation tab in the OV screen. There is no place for recording vitals or face sheet information in an OV template, because this information is added during, and specific to, the patient's actual visit. If the clinic has previously created office visit notes in a digital format prior to obtaining an EHR program, these notes can be copied and pasted segment by segment into a SpringCharts OV template. Once the [Save] button is clicked, the newly created template is added to the list of OV templates in the *Templates* window, accessed via the [Template] button at the bottom of the *OV* screen.

A template can also be created by saving an existing office visit note as a template. Within the *Office Visit* screen, the user selects the *Database* menu and then chooses *Copy OV to Template* (Figure 8.3). The entire OV note the provider has created for a real patient is then placed in an OV template format, with each portion of the note going into the appropriate segment. (Once again, vitals and face sheet information are not copied into the template.) The user then inserts a title for the new template in the *Template Name* field. The number of OV templates that can be created is not limited.

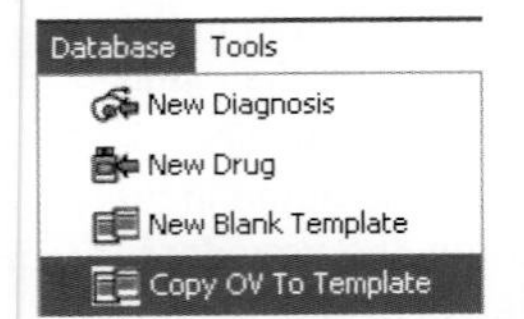

Figure 8.3 *Database* menu in the *Office Visit* screen.

Focal Point

OV templates can be created from scratch, or an existing OV note can be copied into a template.

OV templates are used to rapidly populate a new *OV* window. To use an office visit template, a provider opens a patient's chart and selects *New* > *New OV Note* from the menu to open the *Office Visit* screen. When the practitioner has determined the nature and cause of the patient's chief complaint(s), the list of OV templates can be accessed by clicking on the [Template] button at the bottom of the window (Figure 8.4). The user then selects the desired template from the list (Figure 8.5). The program populates all the various segments of the *SOAP* format in the *OV* screen. The provider then adds the vitals and makes any necessary modifications to the note for the specific patient.

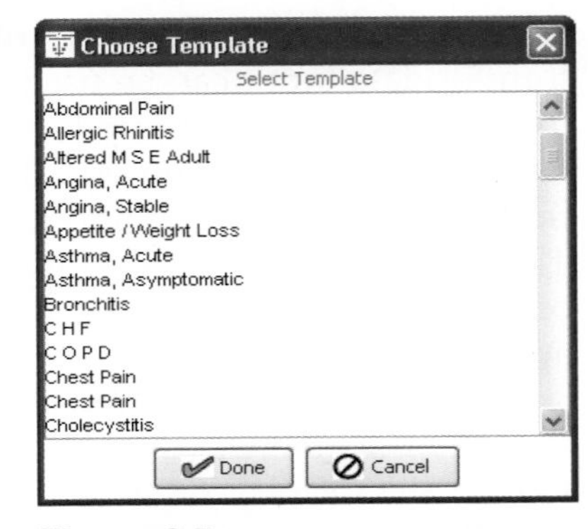

Figure 8.5 List of OV templates that can be accessed via the *OV* window.

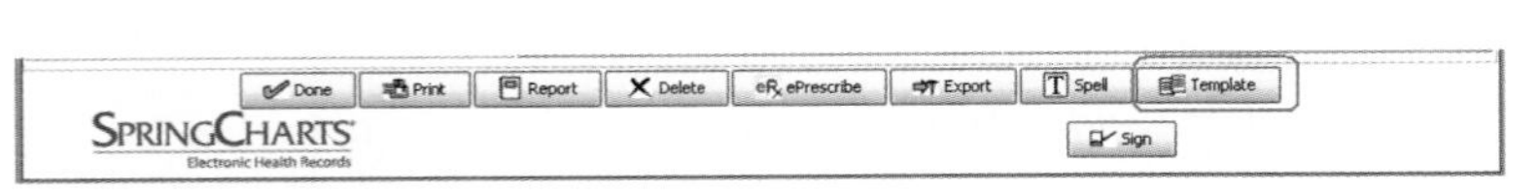

Figure 8.4 Template button at the bottom of the *Office Visit* screen.

Concept Checkup 8.1

A. What screen in SpringCharts is similar to the way the OV template is organized?

B. What two segments of an OV note are not included when building an OV template?

C. The purpose of adding templates to EHR programs is to (select all that apply):

1. Reduce time
2. Improve efficiency
3. Reduce surgical complications
4. Ensure accuracy

Exercise 8.1 Creating and Editing an Office Visit Template

1. Open your chart, using the *Open a Patient's Chart* icon.

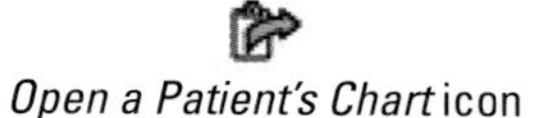

Open a Patient's Chart icon

2. Open the existing office visit note created for the complaints of allergies, runny nose, and itchy eyes (in Chapter 6), by selecting the [Edit] button.
3. Select the *Database* menu and choose *Copy OV To Template.*
4. Name the new template *Adult Allergies,* and [Save] it.
5. Close the *Office Visit* screen, select [Save and Skip Billing], and close the chart.
6. Click on the main *Edit* menu of the main *Practice View* screen and select *Templates.*
7. Select the [Office Visit Templates] button.
8. Choose the *Adult Allergies* template in the *Templates* window.
9. Remove all of the chief complaints (allergies, runny nose, etc.) and the user's initials and time in the *Chief Complaint* section.
10. Click on the [F/U-Rem] navigation tab. Remove the verbiage in the *F/U-Reminders* field that asks the patient to return to the clinic as needed.
11. Save the edited template and close the *TEMPLATES* window.

Exercise 8.2 Activating an Office Visit Template

1. Open Patti Adams's chart.
2. Open a new *OV* screen from the *New* menu.

   (Patti mentions that she has a runny nose and congestion. She believes she has allergies again.)
3. Look in the lower right field and find a notation that Patti was in your office on 12/21/2004 with the same complaints. Highlight the words *Allergies, runny nose, congestion.* (Do not highlight the date.)
4. Click on the *Copy Highlighted Text to Note* button to add the previous chief complaints into the new OV note.

Copy Highlighted Text to Note button

5. Open the [*Vitals]* tab and enter fictitious vital signs for Patti, including a normal temperature. Match her latest height and weight.
6. Click on the [Template] button at the bottom of the window and choose *Allergic Rhinitis.* The template content is added to the OV note to augment the chief complaints and vitals you've already added.

   (Patti mentions that her cough started about 7 days ago and she tells you she does not have a headache.)

(continued)

Exercise 8.2 (Concluded)

7. Click on the [PI] tab, and notice the content in the *Present Illness* field. Change the statement in the first paragraph—*and occasional cough for the past _ weeks*—to *7 days.*

Note: Remember to use the [Delete] key on your keyboard, not the [Delete] button in the OV screen.

8. Click on the [Dx] navigation tab. In the upper right *Diagnosis* field, type *allergic* and conduct a search.
9. Select *Allergic Rhinitis 477.9.*
10. In the *Information Available* window, select the *Allergies* patient instruction sheet.
11. Type your name at the top of the instruction sheet. Print a copy of the instruction sheet for the patient and hand in to your instructor.
12. Close the *Information Available* window.
13. The doctor prescribes *Flonase.* Open the [Rx] tab.
14. Scroll down to the bottom of the *Previous Prescription* field in the lower right corner of the *OV* window, and select *Flonase.*
15. Select the print prescription icon button - (Second down on left). Choose the boxes to print the physician's license and NPI numbers on the prescription form.
16. Print the prescription, write your name on it, and submit it to your instructor.
17. Save the office visit and edit the routing slip.
18. Use the recommended E&M code and [Send] the routing slip.
19. Notice the completed OV note saved under the *Encounters* category in the care tree of Patti Adams's chart. Close the chart.

8.2 Creating Physician Order Templates

Order templates
These templates store orders commonly used in a medical office. For example, physician order templates can be created for the most common laboratory, imaging, and medical tests and procedures.

Order templates are used to rapidly create orders for outside tests and other referrals. To create an order template, the user selects *New* > *New Template* > *New Orders Template* from the *Practice View* screen menu. The *Orders Template* window displays (Figure 8.6). The order information is entered as needed. If the order form is created in the *OV* screen, the diagnosis(es) and the ordered tests are automatically added to the order form from the OV note. Therefore, when creating an order template, this information is not included because it is patient-specific. Order templates can be designed with instructions, prompts, and specific questions to guide the practitioner to provide the necessary information for outside testing facilities. Once completed, the order template is given a title in the *Template Name* field (Figure 8.7). The newly saved order template is added to the list of available templates.

Focal Point

Order templates are typically used to create orders sent to outside testing facilities. When selected within the *OV* screen, they automatically include the diagnoses and tests from the OV note.

Order templates also can be selected from within a patient chart or the office visit screen. In a patient's chart, the user selects *New* > *New Excuse/Note/Order* > *New Orders* from the menu. The order forms would only be selected from within the patient's chart if the patient were not being seen by a physician as part of a normal office visit encounter. A patient could be seen in a medical office by a clinician for a follow-up visit to complete a test, for which an order form needs to be created, without having to start an actual office visit note.

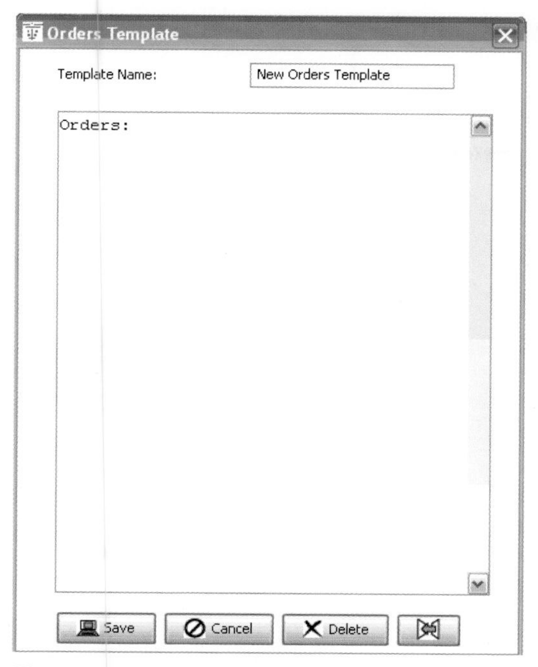

Figure 8.6 *Orders Template* window.

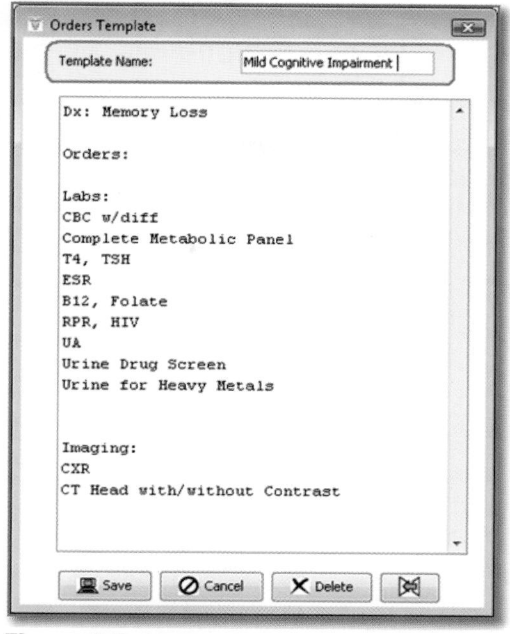

Figure 8.7 Naming a new order template.

Clicking the [Template] button (Figure 8.8) shows the available order templates in the *Choose Template* window (Figure 8.9). The user highlights the desired template, and the program populates the order window. From this window, the user also may add additional line items from the upper right pop-up text field and diagnoses from the patient's *Previous DX* field (lower right). The new order can then be printed or charted by clicking the [Done] button.

Order templates can also be used within the *Office Visit* screen. When this is done, the EHR program automatically displays the diagnosis(es) and ordered tests from the open office visit note. To create this type of order, the user opens the [Test] tab, enters the test name in the *Test* field, searches for and chooses the

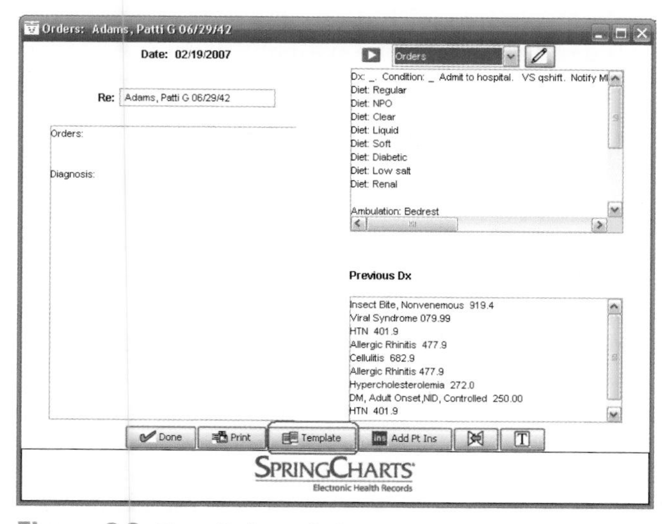

Figure 8.8 New *Orders* window.

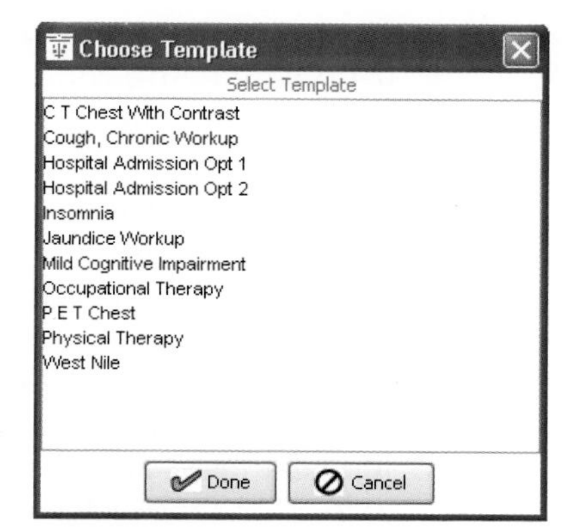

Figure 8.9 *Choose Template* window.

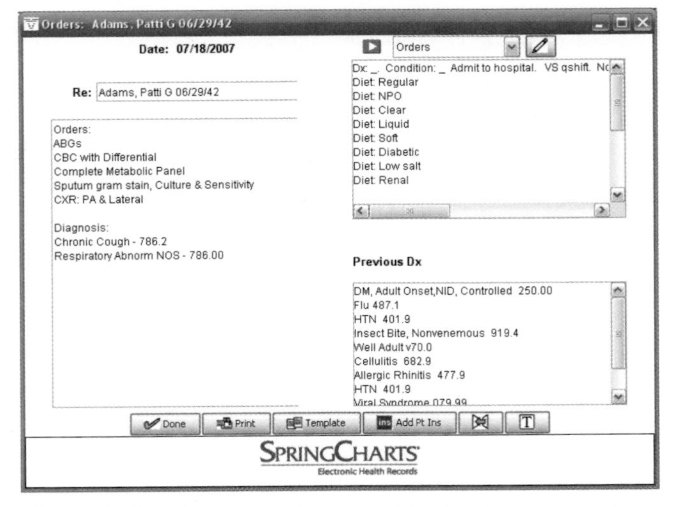

Figure 8.10 *Orders* window populated with orders and diagnosis.

Print order form button

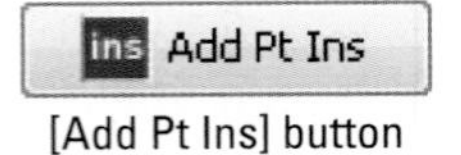

[Add Pt Ins] button

Focal Point

Orders are created from either the patient's chart or from within the *OV* screen. Orders created within the patient's chart will not automatically contain diagnoses or medical tests.

test(s), then clicks on the [Order Selected Tests] button. Once the test(s) have been ordered, the user clicks on the printer icon located below the *Tests* panel in the lower middle quadrant of the screen (shown in margin). The order window opens, showing the diagnosis(es) and test(s) already populating the OV note (Figure 8.10). The user can then add text to the order form by selecting pop-up text or typing directly into the form.

The [Add Pt Ins] button (shown in margin) is available in the *Orders* window regardless of whether the form was created in the patient's chart or in the OV note screen. Once the button is clicked, the program adds the patient's primary insurance (from the patient's face sheet) to the order form. Many third-party testing facilities require that the patient's healthcare insurance information be included on the physician's order form because the testing facility bills the insurance company for tests conducted outside the provider's medical office.

The computerized provider order entry (CPOE) can be printed or faxed by clicking on the [Print] button in the *Orders* window. Once the order is printed or faxed, the user selects the [Done] button and is presented with the option to save a copy of the order form in the patient's chart (i.e., "chart the order"). If test(s) are being conducted at an outside testing facility, it is appropriate to save a copy of the order form in the patient's chart. If the test(s) are being conducted onsite in the physician's office then it is unnecessary to print the order form; the notation of the test in the OV note is sufficient documentation.

The vision of an integrated electronic healthcare system is that all healthcare providers will be able to transmit, receive, store, and analyze all medical services related to a patient's healthcare. To this end, the ONC requires that all certified EHR programs have the functionality to generate computerized provider order entry (CPOE). The CPOE feature in EHR programs enable physicians and other providers to document orders for labs, imaging studies, medical tests, and medication in the patient's electronic chart and maintain a record of that order. Stage 1 of the MU requirement in 2011 and 2012 only required EPs to demonstrate the ordering and storage of one medication for the patient. Table 8.1 outlines the ONC objectives and MU measures regarding computerized provider order entry.

Table 8.1 Meaningful Use Core Measure

Computerized Provider Order Entry	
ONC Stage 1 Objective	**Meaningful Use Measure**
Provide computerized provider order entry (CPOE) for medication orders, lab services, imaging studies, and other services, and store in EHR.	More than 30 percent of patients with at least one medication in their medication list and who have at least one medication ordered through CPOE.

Notes:

- Physicians who write fewer than 100 prescriptions during the 90-day reporting period are excluded from this MU objective.
- Although the CPOE function should handle all physician orders, this MU objective in Stage 1 is limited to only medication orders.
- It is only required that the physician enter the order using CPOE and store a copy in the patient's chart. The electronic transmission of the order is not required for Stage 1 of MU.
- The measure is based on individual patients, regardless of how many times an individual patient is seen or how many orders are generated for an individual patient.

Concept Checkup 8.2

A. In which two screens can the physician order forms be created?

B. What is CPOE an abbreviation for?

C. When the order templates are used in the OV screen, which two items are automatically added from the OV note?

Exercise 8.3 Using an Order Template

1. Open Patti Adams's chart, and expand the *Encounters* category in the care tree by clicking on the '+' symbol.
2. Highlight the recent OV entry that contains the allergy template, and click the [Edit] button at the bottom of the window to open the OV screen.
3. Click the [Test] navigation tab on the right side.
4. In the *Test* field, type *all* and conduct a search.
5. Click on *Allergen Profile* to move the test to the lower window.
6. Click on [Order Selected Tests] button to move the test to the lower middle window.
7. Click on the print icon in the lower middle window to create a CPOE. Notice the EHR program has automatically added the ordered test and diagnosis from the patient's OV note.
8. Click on the [Add Pt Ins] button in the *Orders* window to add the patient's primary insurance to the order form.
9. Type your name at the top of the order form. Click on the [Print] button and hand in to your instructor.
10. Click the [Done] button and answer [Yes] to the question, *Do you want to chart this order?*
11. Save the order under the *Encounters* category of the patient's care tree.
12. Close the patient's OV note by clicking on the [Done] button of the *OV* window.
13. Choose the [Save and Skip Billing] button and close the chart.

Order Selected Tests

[Order Selected Tests] button

8.3 Creating Letter Templates

Letter templates
These templates allow users to create form letters that can be used as a *Letter to the Patient* or *Letter About a Patient*. Only the body of the letter template and the subject line need to be added; SpringCharts automatically completes the appropriate recipient's name, address, and greeting.

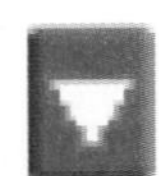

Access PopUp Text icon

Letter templates are created in the same way as office visit and order templates. The user selects the *New* > *New Template* > *New Letter Template* from the *Practice View* screen menu, and a blank letter template appears. The user enters the name of the letter template in the *Template Name* field, the subject of the letter in the *Re:* field, and then the narrative or body portion of the letter in the *Text* field (Figure 8.11). The SpringCharts program will populate the remaining fields when using this feature in a patient's chart. The program automatically includes the word *Sincerely,* as the *Close* unless different text has been entered in the template.

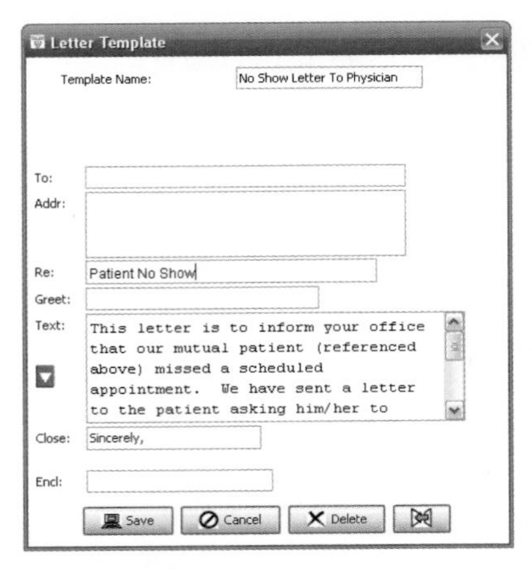

Figure 8.11 *Letter Template* window.

Pop-up text is available for use in letter templates by clicking on the *Access PopUp Text* icon (shown in margin) to the left of the *Text* window. Once completed, the new letter template is added to the list of templates. Letter templates to patients and letter templates to other providers about patients are both created in this window.

Letter templates can be accessed from within a patient chart by selecting the *New* menu and then *New Letter to Pt* or *New Letter ABOUT Pt.* A letter screen appears (Figure 8.12). When a user needs to generate a letter for which a template letter has already been created, he or she selects the [Template] button within the *Letter* window and chooses the desired template from the list (Figure 8.13). The letter can be revised by using line items from the pop-up text panel to the right or manually entering new content in the *Text* field on the

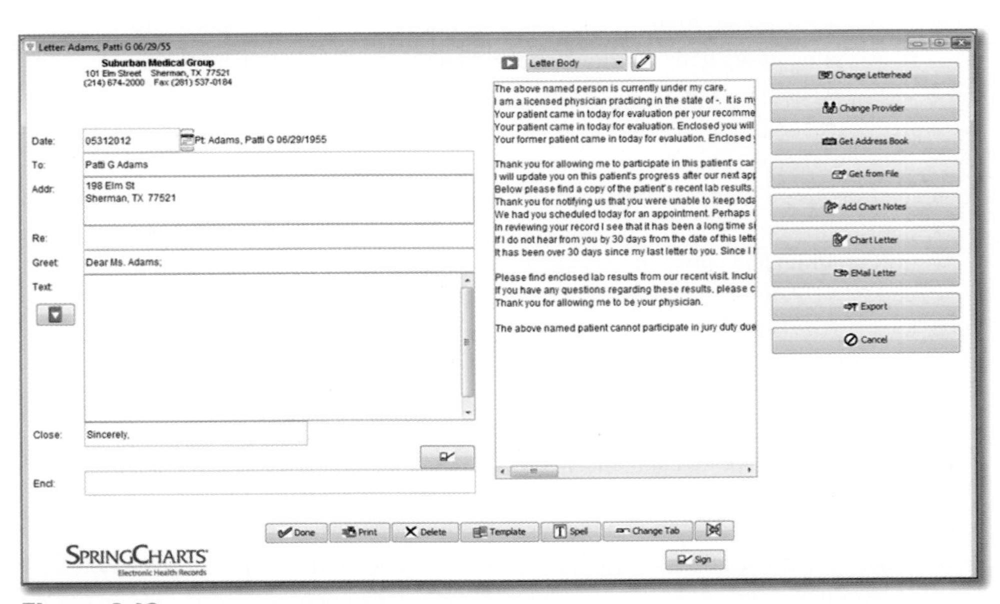

Figure 8.12 *New Letter* window.

left. When generating a letter to a patient from within the patient's chart, the program automatically adds the name, address, and greeting portions of the letter. When generating a letter to another provider *about* the patient, the user adds the address by selecting the [Get Address Book] button (shown in margin) to the right. This feature allows access to all referring physicians, pharmacies, testing facilities, and so on that have been set up in the SpringCharts *Address Book.*

Letters can be printed or e-mailed to their recipients. If additional formatting or color needs to be added to the letter, the document can be exported to the word processor by selecting the *Copy or Export This Data* icon (shown in margin) in the bottom of the *Letter* window. Copies of all created letters are automatically saved into the patient's chart. Customized categories in the patient's care tree can be used to store these letters.

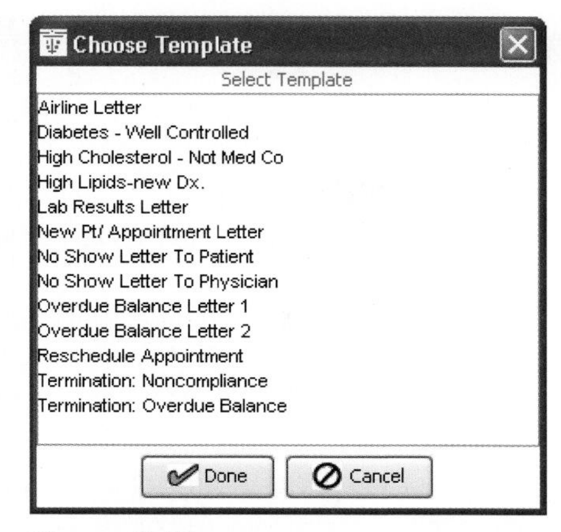

Figure 8.13 List of letter templates in the *Choose Template* window.

Focal Point

Letter templates can be used to create letters either to or about a patient. They are selected within the patient's chart, modified, printed, or e-mailed, and a copy is saved into the patient's care tree.

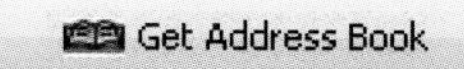

[Get Address Book] button

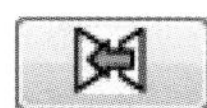

Copy or Export This Data icon

Concept Checkup 8.3

A. What three portions of the template must be completed when creating a letter template?

B. Letter templates are available to be used when creating what two types of letters in the patient's chart?

Exercise 8.4 Creating and Using a Letter Template

1. Create a new letter template by accessing the *New* menu in the *Practice View* screen and choosing *New Template > New Letter Template.*
2. In the *Letter Template* window, type the subject (*Re:*): *Welcome.*
3. In the body of the letter (*Text*), create a brief letter that welcomes new patients to the clinic and includes the following names and telephone numbers: *Office Manager: Donna Baird (417) 880-1327* and *Nurse Supervisor: Lissa Raines (417) 866-0062.* The program will automatically add a *Close* to the letter.
4. Name the letter template *New Patient Letter* and click the [Save] button.
5. Open your patient chart.
6. Click on the *New* menu and select *New Letter to Pt.* Notice that the letter is already addressed to the patient and is complete with greetings and closure.
7. Click on the [Template] button at the bottom of the screen and select *New Patient Letter.* Notice that the letter you just created has been added into the body of the letter. Format the template text so that the layout is acceptable.

(continued)

Exercise 8.4 (Concluded)

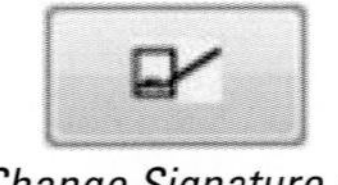

Change Signature of Letter icon

8. To add a signature to the bottom of the letter, click the *Change Signature of Letter* icon (shown in margin) at the bottom of the letter and select a signature line. You will be given the option of your default doctor (this was set up initially under *User Preferences*) or your name. Because you are logged in as *John Smith* in the demo program, you see the name twice.
9. If you used your proper e-mail address when setting up this patient, e-mail the letter to the patient by clicking the [EMail Letter] button to the right of the letter.
10. Print the letter by selecting the [Print] button at the bottom and checking the *Print Letterhead* and *Use Digital Signature* boxes. Submit the letter to your instructor.
11. Click the [Done] button and save the letter under the *Letters* tab in the care tree. Save the letter as: *New Patient Letter.* Notice the letter displayed in the lower right window of the patient chart and stored under the *Letters* category.
12. Close the patient's chart.

8.4 Template Manager

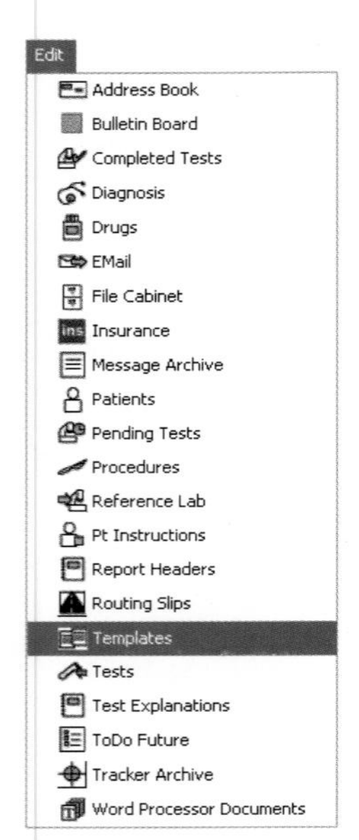

Figure 8.14 Accessing templates in the *Edit* menu of the main *Practice View* screen.

All the templates for office visit notes, physician orders, and letters can be accessed in the template manager from the *Practice View* screen by selecting the *Edit* menu and choosing the *Templates* option (Figure 8.14). The resulting *Templates* screen offers a list of templates for each of the three categories. The user selects the appropriate category button to view each list. To edit any of the templates, the user highlights the desired template and begins to make modifications. Templates also can be created from this window by selecting the [New Template] button. A window displays, allowing the user to choose which type of template to create (Figure 8.15). Once selected, the corresponding template window opens, and the user can create the new template.

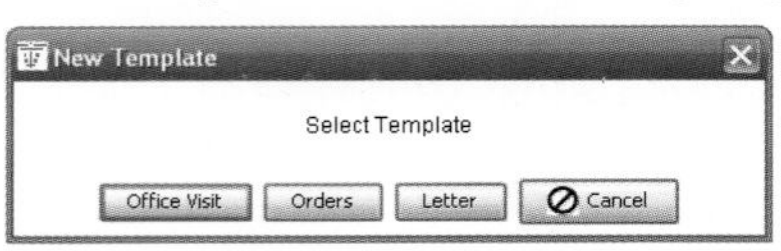

Figure 8.15 *New Template* window, from which three types of templates can be selected.

Concept Checkup 8.4

A. What are the three types of templates that are stored in the template manager?

B. What two things can be done with templates in the template manager?

Exercise 8.5 Modifying an OV Template

1. In the main *Practice View* screen, click on the *Edit* menu and select the *Templates* submenu.
2. In the *Templates* window select the [Office Visit Templates] button.
3. In the displayed list of OV templates, locate and select *Conjunctivitis.*
4. In the *Office Visit Template* window, select the [PI] navigation tab.
5. In the *Present Illness* text box located in the lower left corner, move the scroll bar to the top of the window.

Exercise 8.5 (Concluded)

6. At the top of the text window type the following: *Pt noted crusted eyelashes, eye redness and itching _ days ago.*
7. Click on the [Save] button and close the *Templates* window.

8.5 Creating Procedure Templates

Physicians and other clinicians are legally and ethically required to explain the risk factors of certain procedures to patients. Patients need to understand the possible complications, potential risks, and potential changes to their quality of life after the procedure in order to give informed consent. **Procedure templates** are very useful when documenting procedural text in the OV note because they ensure the same explanation and discussion are provided for each patient undergoing the same procedure. For this reason EHR programs allow providers to create text associated with specific procedures. Each time the procedure is documented in an OV note, the text associated with the procedure becomes a permanent part of the OV note as well. The provider uses this text to verbally describe the procedure's potential complications and risks to the patient (or guardian, if patient is a minor) and then the patient signs a consent form. The consent form typically includes the procedure description (including complications/risks) as well.

Procedure templates These templates are used to ensure that complete and consistent information about procedures, including their potential risks and complications, is provided to all patients.

Focal Point

Many procedures require the same explanation and discussion with the patient. Template verbiage is helpful to ensure that consistent and complete information about procedures is included in OV notes.

Procedure templates are created by accessing the *Edit* menu in the *Practice View* screen and selecting the *Procedures* submenu. In the *Edit Procedure* window, new procedure information can be created and existing procedure information edited (Figure 8.16). In the lower right quadrant of the *Edit Procedure* window is a *Detail* field in which text can be added to describe a specific

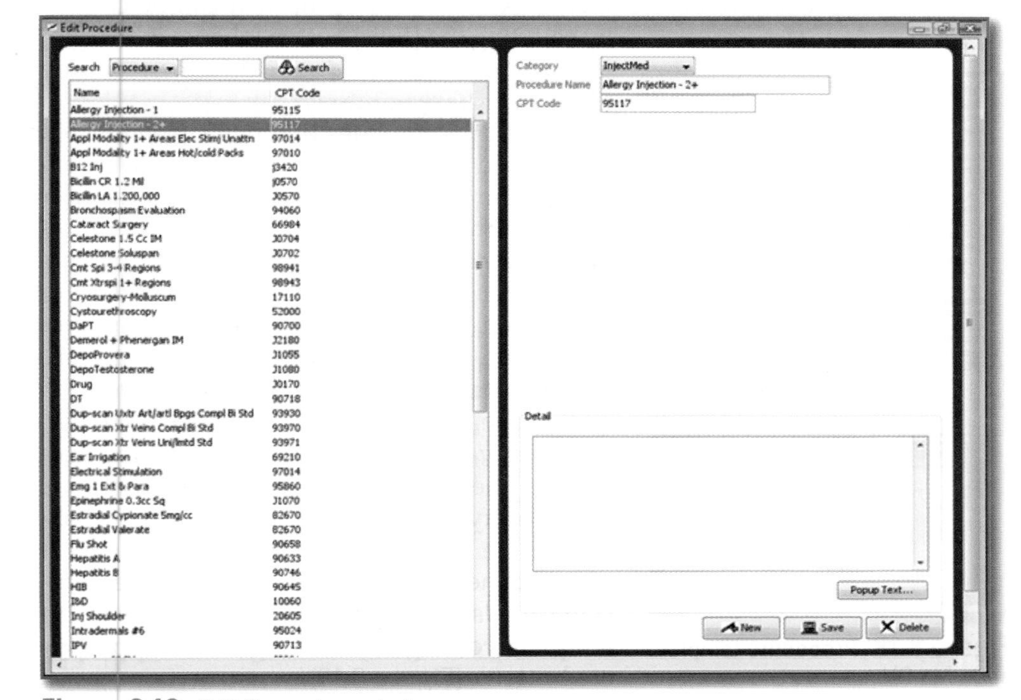

Figure 8.16 *Edit Procedure* window.

21. **LO 8.5** The *Edit Popup Text* window allows the user to:
   a) Create and modify customized text
   b) Delete error codes
   c) Add and send personal messages to other users
   d) Create templates that pop up in the OV note

22. **LO 8.5** Procedure templates are created by:
   a) Selecting the [Proc] tab of the *OV* screen, selecting the procedure, then modifying the text
   b) Accessing the *Edit* menu, selecting the *Procedures* submenu, then choosing the procedure
   c) Opening the *Tools* menu in the *OV* screen, selecting *Database*, then *Procedure Templates*
   d) Selecting *Previous Procedures* in the [Proc] tab of the *OV* screen

23. **LO 8.2** To print an order in the *OV* screen, the clinician needs to be working under what tab?
   a) Proc
   b) Other Tx
   c) Orders
   d) Tests

24. **LO 8.5** The procedure and any accompanying template text are automatically added into what area of the SOAP note when saved?
   a) *Subjective*
   b) *Objective*
   c) *Assessment*
   d) *Plan*

25. **LO 8.3** Office visit, order, and letter templates can be modified and new ones created in the template manager located in the:
   a) *Practice View* screen > *Edit* > *Templates*
   b) *Patient Chart* > *New* > *Templates*
   c) *Office Visit* screen > *Tools* > *Templates*
   d) *Practice View* screen > *New* > *Templates*

Applying Your Knowledge

Use your critical-thinking skills to answer the following questions.

26. **LO 8.2** A physician order form can be created and order templates used in the patient's chart as well as in the OV note. Why is the EHR program designed to create physician orders in either place?

27. **LO 8.1, LO 8.2, LO 8.3, LO 8.5** Provide a brief explanation of when and how you would use the following:
   Office visit template
   Order template
   Letter template
   Procedure template

28. **LO 8.1** A user can open the *Edit Popup Text* window and create new pop-up text and modify existing pop-up text. Does this activity affect the pop-up text of other users? Explain your answer.

9

Tests, Procedures, and Codes

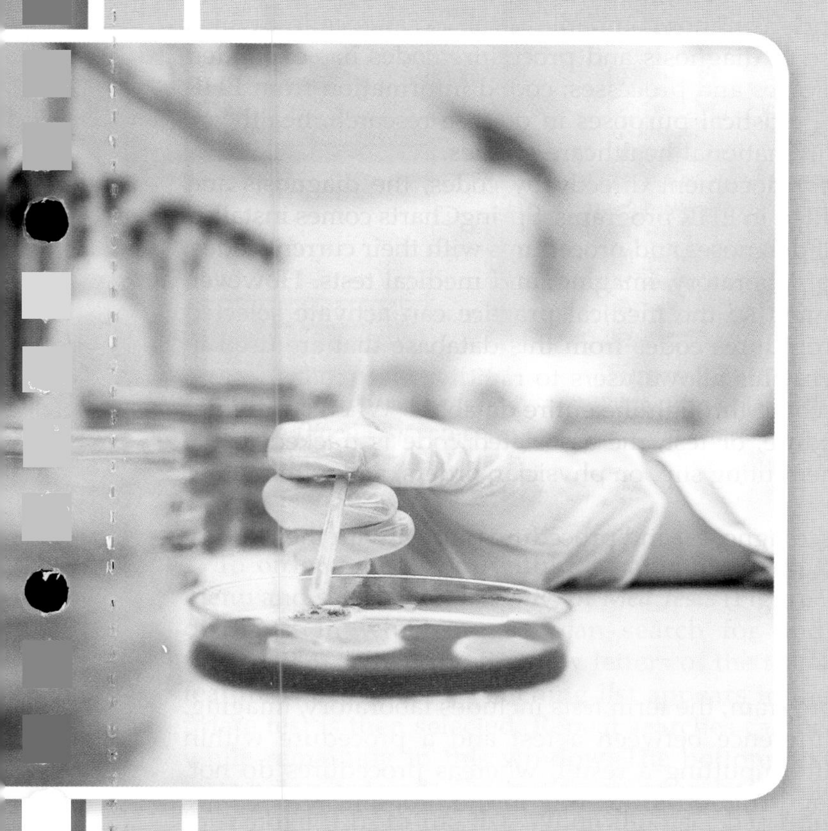

Learning Outcomes

After completing Chapter 9, you will be able to:

- LO 9.1 Describe how to order lab, imaging, and medical tests.
- LO 9.2 Process *Reference Lab* results that are received electronically.
- LO 9.3 Process and chart tests manually.
- LO 9.4 Create a test report.
- LO 9.5 Create, edit, and document procedures.
- LO 9.6 Create, edit, and document diagnoses.

What You Need to Know

To understand Chapter 9 you will need to know:

- How to open an electronic patient chart and navigate within it
- How to open a new and an established office visit note
- How to navigate within the *Office Visit* screen
- How to navigate within the *Practice View* screen
- How to use pop-up text

Key Terms

- American Medical Association (AMA)
- Diagnosis codes
- Lab analyte
- Procedure codes
- Reference lab
- World Health Organization (WHO)

Exercise 9.1 Ordering a Lab Test

1. Open Patti Adams's chart.
2. From the *Actions* menu, select: *Lab > Order New Lab.*
3. Search for a CMP (comprehensive metabolic panel), select the test, and then press [Done]. Close the patient's chart.
4. On the *Practice View* screen, select *Pending Tests* under the *Edit* menu.
5. Locate Patti Adams's CMP test within the *Pending Tests* window.
6. Close the *Pending Tests* window.

Exercise 9.2 Viewing Outstanding Tests

Open a Patient's Chart icon

1. Open Robert Underhagen's chart by using the speed icon in the Toolbar (shown in margin).
2. Locate the two uncharted tests in the face sheet. One pending test and one completed test have not been charted.
3. Write the name of the pending test: ____________________
4. Write the name of the completed test: ____________________
5. Close Robert Underhagen's chart.

9.2 SpringLabs and Reference Lab Results

One of the most convincing reasons for adopting EHRs is the ability to exchange data with other providers and healthcare entities. Through EHRs, physicians can send and receive information about their patients to and from hospitals, labs, imaging companies, and other providers. Through this exchange, relevant clinical information will always be available at the point of care. The ONC requires that eligible professionals (EPs) have a health information exchange (HIE) interface that allows exchanging common clinical data, as part of their EHR system. In Stage 1 of the MU program, EPs were required to perform at least one test using the certified EHR's ability to exchange information electronically (Table 9.1).

Focal Point

SpringLabs

This SpringCharts feature provides the capability to automatically receive lab test results directly from reference laboratories using electronic data interchange (EDI) standards and protocols over a secure Internet connection.

Table 9.1 Meaningful Use Core Measure

Information Exchange	
ONC Stage 1 Objective	**Meaningful Use Measure**
Implement capability to electronically exchange key clinical information for example, diagnostic test results, among providers and 'patient-authorized entities.'	Perform at least one test of EHR's capacity to electronically exchange information.

Notes:

- A physician is allowed to perform the exchange test using data on a fictional patient to qualify.
- 'Patient-authorized entities,' as used in this objective, includes any entity for which the patient has given specific authorization to receive their data. Examples could include other physicians, hospitals, lab companies, or health plans that cover the patient.
- The test can happen before the beginning of the EHR Reporting Period; the physician just has to attest that data exchange has occurred.

SpringLabs is a lab interface that provides medical clinics the capability to electronically receive lab results directly from laboratories such as Quest, Lab Corp, Spectrum, and many others, and record the results as structured data. Lab results are sent directly to the EHR program over a secure Internet connection using electronic data interchange (EDI) standards and protocols. The results can then be reviewed by a physician and placed directly into a patient's chart. Within SpringCharts, once test results are received electronically from the lab, they are automatically imported into a staging area called *Reference Lab* for processing.

Reference Lab is a secured area within SpringCharts accessed only by users with appropriate security permission to view or process the information. Users set up in the server with the *Get Pending Tests* access level are notified of newly received results when a *LAB* icon appears next to the user's log-in name in the upper left corner of the *Practice View* screen (Figure 9.4). Authorized users can access and process the test results by selecting *Reference Lab/Reports* from the main *Edit* menu (Figure 9.5).

The *Imported Reference Lab Tests* screen shows the tests sent directly from the labs in a list that includes the test date, test name, patient name, performing lab, and ordering physician (Figure 9.6). The authorized user can view the test results by clicking on any test. The data sent securely from the lab company includes the patient's name, date of birth, and gender, as well as the lab results (Figure 9.7). For each test item, the results indicate whether they are *In Range* or *Out Of Range* (i.e., within normal limits or outside acceptable limits), and the acceptable range *(Reference Range)*, established by the lab company, is provided.

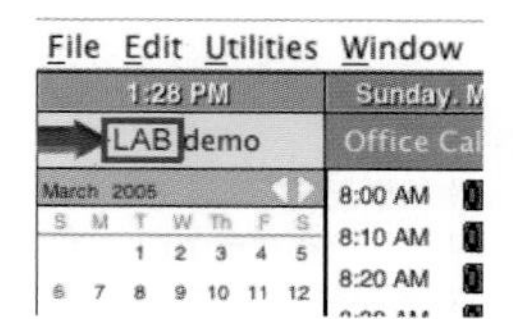

Figure 9.4 Visual indication that lab results have been received from outside labs.

Reference Lab
Reference Lab is a secured area within SpringCharts accessed only by users who have appropriate security permission to view or process the information. When test results are received electronically from specific lab companies, they are automatically imported into the *Reference Lab* for processing.

Access Stored Data

All imported lab results are stored permanently in the lab repository within SpringLabs. By selecting [Access Stored Data] in the *Imported Reference Lab Tests* window, the user can conduct global searches for stored tests by test name,

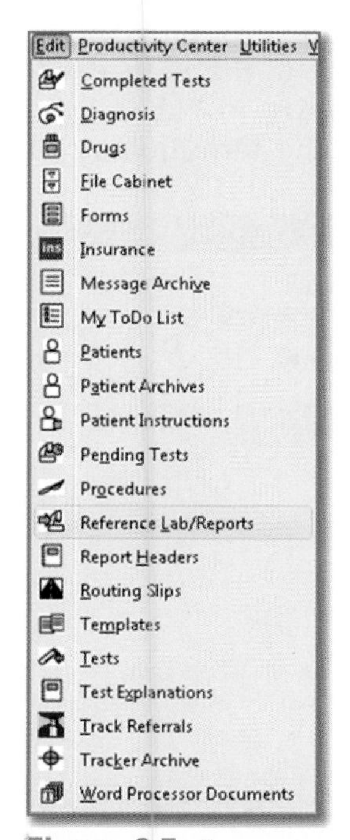

Figure 9.5 Accessing *Reference Lab/Reports* from the *Edit* menu.

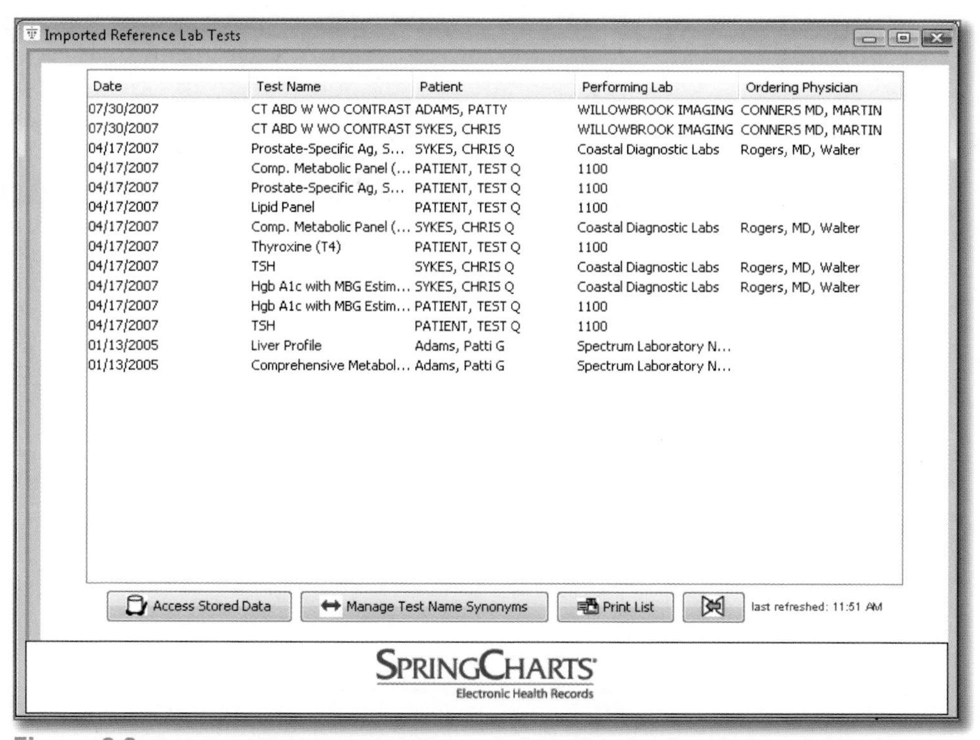

Figure 9.6 *Imported Reference Lab Tests* window, showing list of tests received.

SpringCharts Tip

The *Reference Range* may differ from the acceptable range the clinic has set up for a particular test in the EHR program; however, the imported lab's ranges are used when storing the completed test in the patient's chart so the test results reference the original source's ranges.

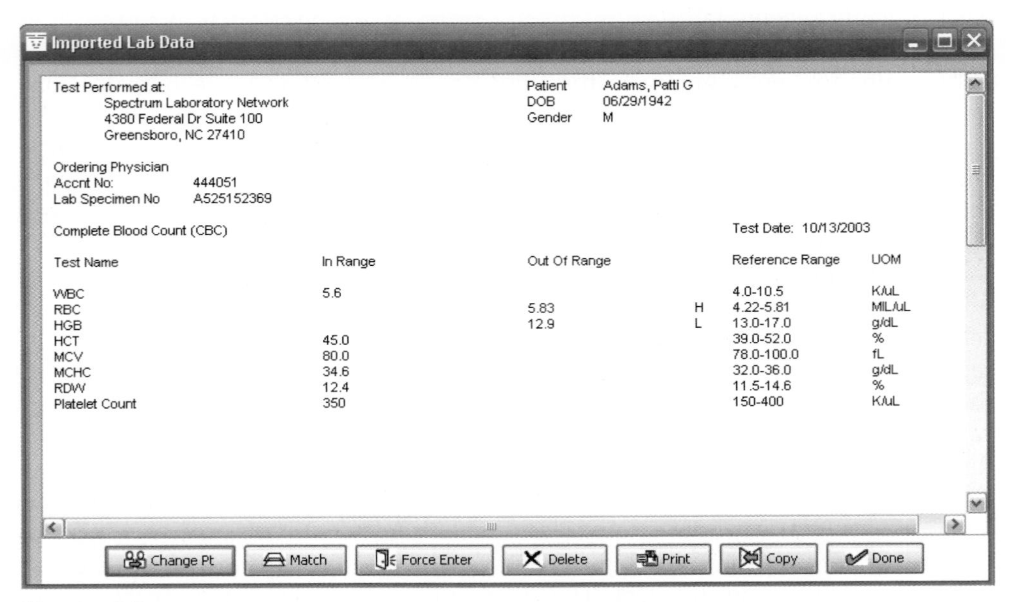

Figure 9.7 *Reference Lab* test results in *Imported Lab Data* window.

date of test, or patient name in the *Searched Stored Reference Lab Tests* screen (Figure 9.8). Although a copy of each imported reference lab test is placed in the patient's chart when the provider links it to the ordered pending test, the original imported lab test is stored in SpringLabs for research purposes.

Manage Test Name Synonyms

At times the terms used in the imported lab results differ from the terms used in the pending test ordered within the EHR program. For example, a lab item in *Pending Tests* may read *Protein, Total,* whereas the imported lab results may read *Total Protein.* Because of this difference, the program cannot match the imported result for this lab item to the lab item in the EHR *Pending Tests* area. A unique feature of SpringLabs is its ability to "learn" the terms that imported labs use and automatically match the terminology of

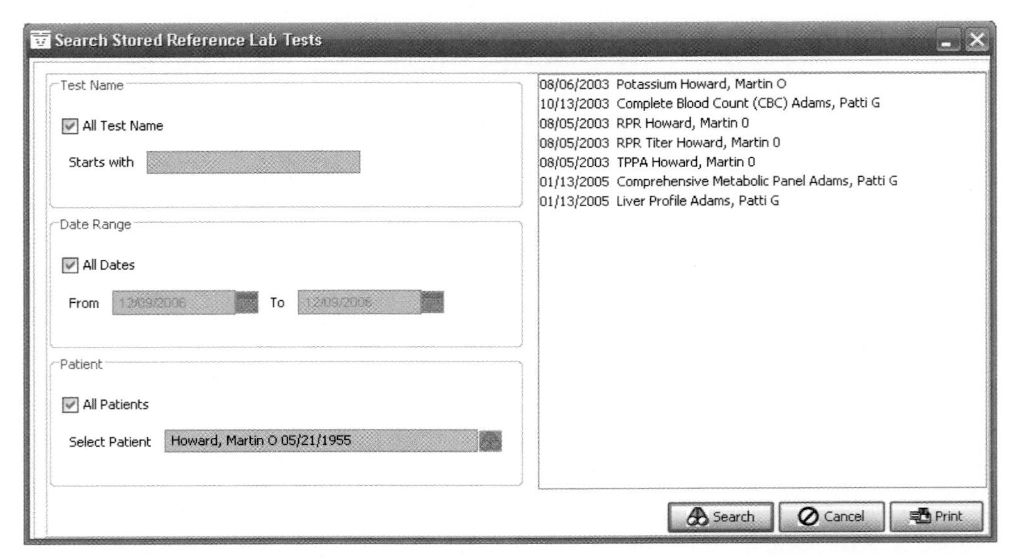

Figure 9.8 *Search Stored Reference Lab Tests* window for performing global searches for reference lab results.

the incoming lab test to the appropriate line item of the test ordered and pending within SpringCharts.

When the lab's test name differs from the name used in SpringCharts, the program asks the user to manually match the imported test item name to a pending test name. The program then remembers these synonyms for subsequent automatic test matching. Users can view and edit the list of test name synonyms by selecting the [Manage Test Name Synonyms] button in the *Imported Reference Lab Tests* window. The *Search Imported Lab Test Synonyms* window then opens (Figure 9.9). If a name match is deleted in this window, SpringLabs prompts for another name match the next time that type of lab is imported into the system.

Search Imported Lab Test Synonyms
Imported Test Name
SpringCharts Test Name
Basos
Basophils
CBC With Differential/Platelet
CBC
Comp. Metabolic Panel (14)
CBC
Complete Blood Count (CBC)
CBC
CT ABD W WO CONTRAST
CT Abdomen w/o Contrast
Eos
Eosinophils
Hematocrit
HCT
Hemoglobin
HGB
LDL Cholesterol Calc
LDL Cholesterol
Lymphs
Lymphocytes
Neutrophils (Absolute)
Neutrophils
Platelets
Platelet
VLDL Cholesterol Cal
Cholesterol
Edit...
Delete
Done
Print

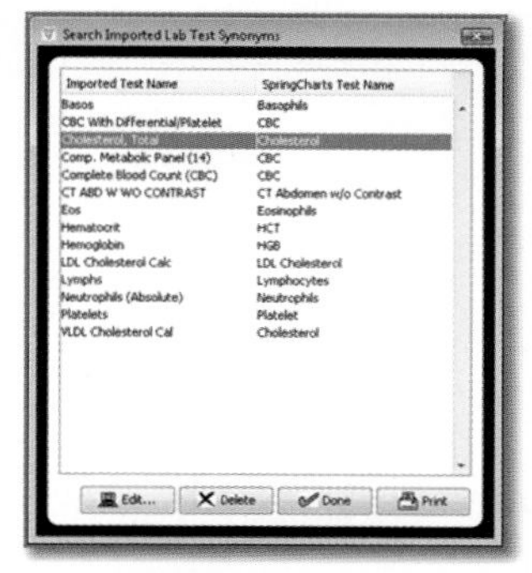

Figure 9.9 *Search Imported Lab Test Synonyms* window.

Matching

Once a test is selected in the *Imported Reference Lab Tests* window, the *Imported Lab Data* window displays, allowing the user to copy the lab test results into SpringCharts (Figure 9.7). This can be done by (1) matching the result with a pending test; (2) force entering; or (3) deleting specific tests.

To reconcile the received lab result with an ordered pending test within the program, the user selects the [Match] button. Matching a lab test result can include one or more of the following tasks:

- ***Identify Patient:*** SpringLabs can automatically match an imported reference lab result with a SpringCharts patient by using multiple data fields, including name and date of birth, so the need to manually identify a patient is a rare occurrence. If the patient is not automatically identified by SpringLabs, the user must search for and identify the matching patient in the *Choose Patient* window (Figure 9.10). After this match is made, SpringLabs will "remember" this link; when this particular lab company sends another lab result for this patient, the match will not need to be made again manually.
- ***Match Test:*** SpringLabs automatically matches an imported lab test with a patient's pending test. If, however, SpringLabs is not able to recognize the name of the lab test, the user must identify the test by selecting from a window that displays a list of pending tests for that specific patient (Figure 9.11). SpringLabs then "remembers" the lab name association, so the user is not required to match the test names again.
- ***Match Test Analyte:*** If the imported lab result is a lab panel with a series of **lab analytes** (i.e., individual test components within a given test

Focal Point

SpringCharts has the unique ability to "learn" terminology used in imported lab results that are matched to pending test items for import to the patient's chart.

Focal Point

Reference Lab results are sent directly to the patient's chart after they are matched to a pending test.

Focal Point

Among other matching criteria, an imported reference lab result may need to be associated with a patient's name or the test item name.

Lab analyte
This blood test compound is the subject of its own specific chemical analysis. A lab panel is composed of multiple analytes that undergo analysis.

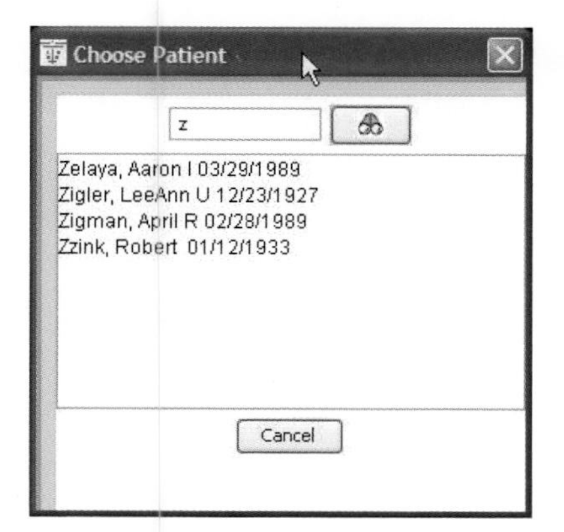

Figure 9.10 Matching a lab result with a SpringCharts patient.

Match Test
Match to the patients pending test:
CBC 20050615
Folic Acid 20050615
Glucose 20050615
PTT 20050615
Done
Cancel

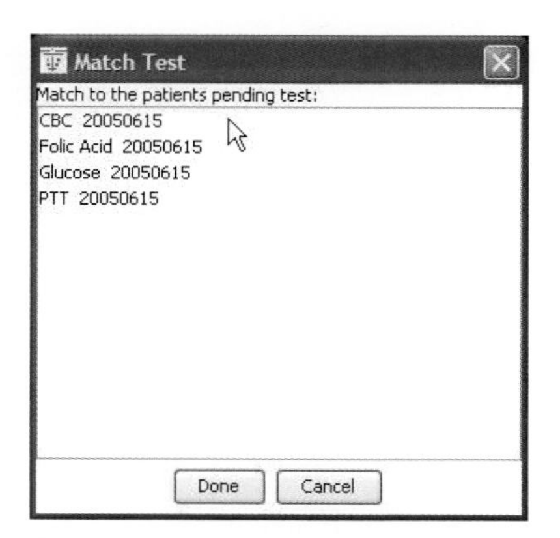

Figure 9.11 Matching a lab result with a patient's pending tests.

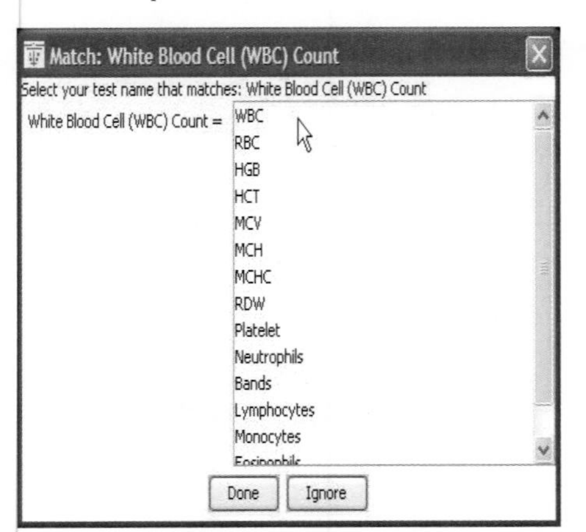

Figure 9.12 Matching lab analytes with pending test analytes.

panel), SpringLabs must match the analytes of the imported test with those of the pending test in the program for the results and ranges to go to the appropriate places. Once the matching process has begun, lab items that appear in grey in the imported test are analytes that cannot be automatically matched to lab items in the pending test. Unmatched test analytes activate a screen requiring the user to manually match a lab's analyte name with one defined within the chosen SpringCharts pending test (Figure 9.12). Each time an analyte is matched, the link is stored in SpringLabs's synonym list, so this process only needs to be conducted the first time SpringLabs receives a result with an unidentified analyte. The reason that some analytes from an imported test won't match up with lab items in the pending test is because lab companies may test for more or fewer items than what the physician has set up in the EHR test bank. They may also be called by different names.

- ***Review Match Results:*** The final matched test data is shown in a window that displays the details of the pending lab side-by-side with the imported lab (Figure 9.13). At this point, the clinician may send a *ToDo/Reminder* to the physician to notify him or her of the new lab results, using the [Make ToDo] button. If the data match is accurate, the user clicks the [Done] button and the imported lab results and their normal ranges are sent immediately into the patient's chart and stored under the *Lab* category in the care tree. The lab test has now been removed from the imported list; however, a permanent copy is stored in the test repository area of SpringLabs.

Force Entering and Deleting

The [Force Enter] button in the *Imported Lab Data* window is used when SpringLabs cannot match an imported test result to a patient or test name in the *Pending Tests* area. Perhaps a test was not ordered through SpringCharts, in which case

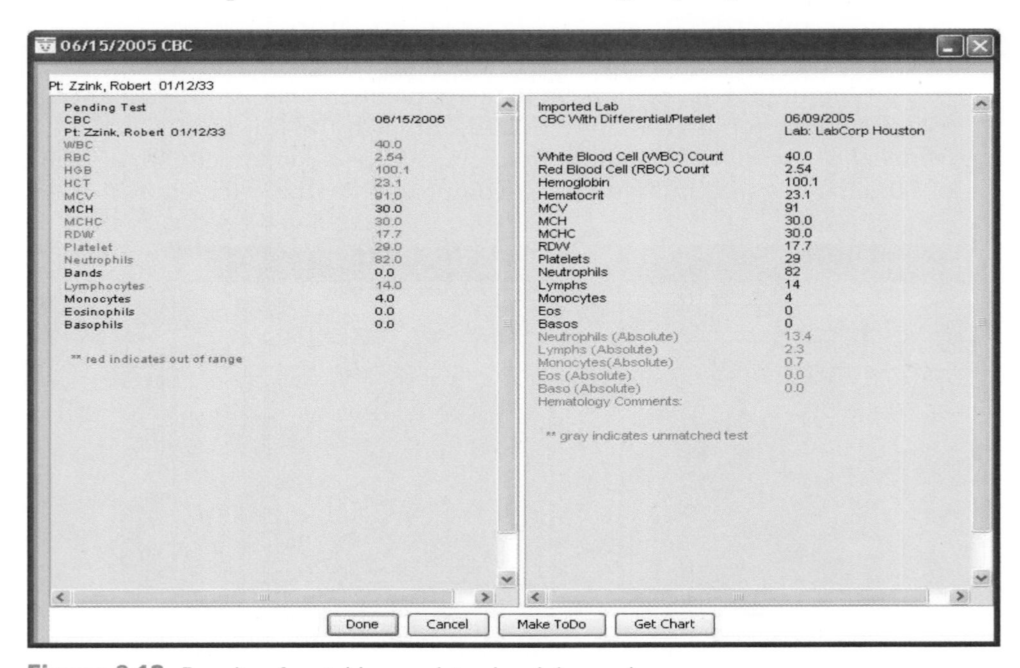

Figure 9.13 Results of matching analytes in a lab panel.

the test will not appear in the *Pending Tests* list. Using the [Force Enter] button requires the user to choose a patient's name and enter a CPT code for the test (or accept the default code of 000). This creates a one-time lab test and places the test results into the care tree of the patient's chart. Force entering does not add the test name or any of the analytes into the list of test name synonyms.

The [Delete] button removes a test from the *Reference Lab* list, but stores a copy in the test repository. This data does not go into a patient's chart, but can be found by searching through the [Access Stored Data] button. There may be times when a lab company inadvertently transmits the wrong patient's test results to the medical clinic. In this case, the reference lab would simply be deleted from the list.

Focal Point

A user may need to "force enter" an imported lab result into a patient's chart if the pending test is not found in SpringCharts.

Concept Checkup 9.2

A. How are lab results entered into the *Reference Lab* area of the EHR program? Select the correct option below.

a) Manually, after the test results arrive in the mail

b) Electronically, over a secure Internet connection

B. Which EHR users are notified that a lab test result has been imported into SpringLabs?

C. For imported lab test results to correspond to the pending tests ordered in the EHR program, what needs to happen to the imported lab test terminology?

D. When an imported lab test is successfully matched with the patient's pending test, where is it sent?

Exercise 9.3 Processing a Lab Test Result

1. Under the *Edit* menu on the *Practice View* screen, choose the *Reference Lab/Reports* option.
2. Within the *Imported Reference Lab Tests* window, select the CMP (comprehensive metabolic panel) lab for Patti Adams.
3. In the *Imported Lab Data* window, locate the patient's results in both the *In Range* and *Out Of Range* columns.
4. Click on the [Match] button to match this test to the EHR patient.
5. Enter Patti's last name, activate the search function, and select her full name.
6. Notice the list of pending tests in the *Match Test* window. Select *CMP* to link the imported lab results to this pending test.
7. Drag the smaller window to the side to view the larger comparison window in which the imported lab results on the right have been matched with the SpringCharts pending tests on the left. The lab items that appear in gray on the right side are unmatched test analytes. The smaller *Match* window prompts the user to match each analyte (in this case, *Potassium*) to an item in the pending test.
8. In the smaller *Match* window, select *Potassium, Serum* to complete the match. Confirm the match by clicking the [Yes] button.
9. Repeat these steps to match *AST/SGOT* with *AST (SGOT)*, *ALT/SGPT* with *ALT (SGPT)*, and *Total Protein* to *Protein, Serum Total,* confirming each match. Many times lab companies test for more or fewer items than what the physician needs, based upon the lab companies' protocols.

(continued)

Exercise 9.3 (Concluded)

10. Click the [Make ToDo] button and send a *ToDo/Reminder* to *Dr. Finchman,* alerting him to *Check Lab* using pop-up text.
11. Click the [Send] button to place the reminder in the physician's *ToDo List.*
12. Click the [Done] button in the CMP match window, and notice that the patient's CMP test has been removed from the list of imported reference lab test results.
13. Close the *Imported Reference Lab Tests* window.
14. Open Patti Adams's chart, expand the *Lab* category in her care tree, and locate the CMP lab dated 1/13/2005, which was added. Click on that item.
15. Use the [Print] button to print out the lab results, write your name on the paper, and submit it to your instructor. Close the patient's chart.

9.3 Processing and Charting Tests

Table 9.2 outlines the meaningful use (MU) criteria regarding clinical lab test results. The Office of the National Coordinator for Health Information Technology (ONC) requires that eligible professionals (EPs) record lab results in certified EHR programs as structured data. Structured data refers to data organized in a certain format, such as numbers, as compared with unstructured data, like free text. In MU Stage 1, ONC-certified EHR programs must have the ability to record results of lab tests and then transmit them to other practitioners or provide them for their patients. This measure does not cover all tests, but is limited to lab test results expressed in a positive/negative format or as a number.

When tests are conducted in the clinic (versus an outside testing facility), the *SpringLab* interface will not be in use, therefore the test results must be manually entered into the *Pending Tests* area of SpringCharts and then sent to the *Completed Tests* area. The test results are then viewed by a physician before they are sent to the patient's chart.

To manually enter test results, the user selects *Pending Tests* from the main *Edit* menu of the *Practice View* screen (Figure 9.14). The *Pending Tests* window appears,

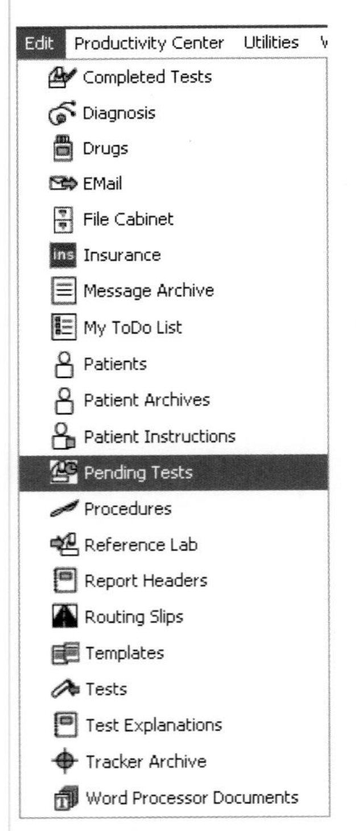

Figure 9.14 Accessing *Pending Tests* through the *Edit* menu.

Table 9.2 Meaningful Use Menu Measure

Clinical Lab Test Results	
ONC Stage 1 Objective	**Meaningful Use Measure**
Incorporate clinical laboratory test results into EHRs as structured data, such as numbers.	More than 40 percent of clinical laboratory test results in positive/negative or numerical format must be incorporated into EHRs as structured data.

Notes:

- This objective does not address how the clinic receives lab results. They may come through an electronic interface, by fax, or by regular mail. The measure simply requires that the physician enter the result into the EHR program as structured data.
- A physician who does not order any lab tests during the EHR reporting period would be excluded from this requirement.

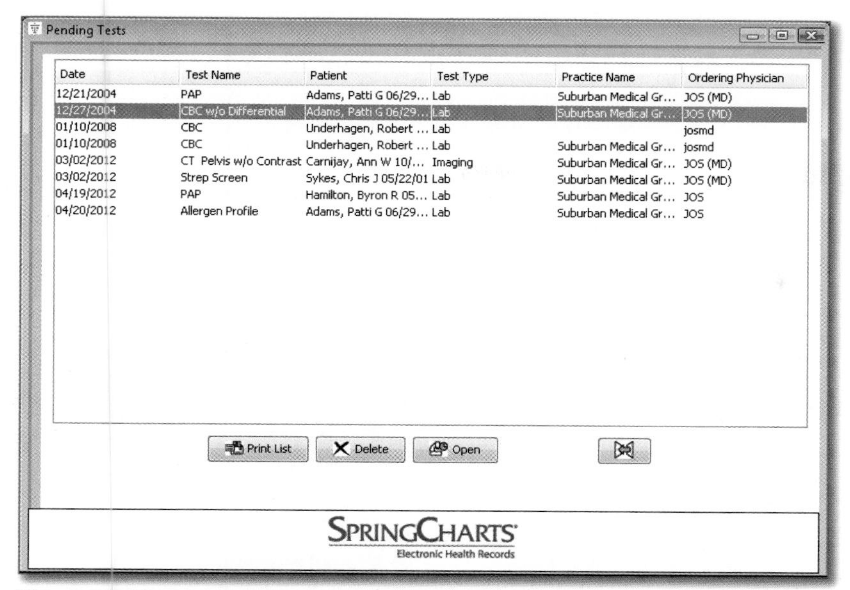

Figure 9.15 *Pending Tests* window.

showing all tests ordered in SpringCharts still waiting for results to be entered (Figure 9.15). The user selects the specific test and clicks on the [Open] button.

Some test results require simply clicking a radio button to enter a *Positive* or *Negative* test result, whereas others require clicking the [Normal Test] button, as seen at the bottom of Figure 9.16. Still other tests may require entering discrete number values, such as for a lab panel, as in the test shown in Figure 9.17. If the pending test is an imaging or medical test, more detailed text may need to be added to define the results. If the clinic receives an extensive evaluation from an outside testing facility in a digital format, the document may be copied and pasted into the *Results* text box of the specific pending test's window. To paste a Word document into the pending test window, the clinic must have received the test evaluation electronically via e-mail or electronic

> **SpringCharts Tip**
>
> By right-clicking the mouse in any text box within SpringCharts, the user is able to *Copy, Cut,* or *Paste* saved text into the text box.

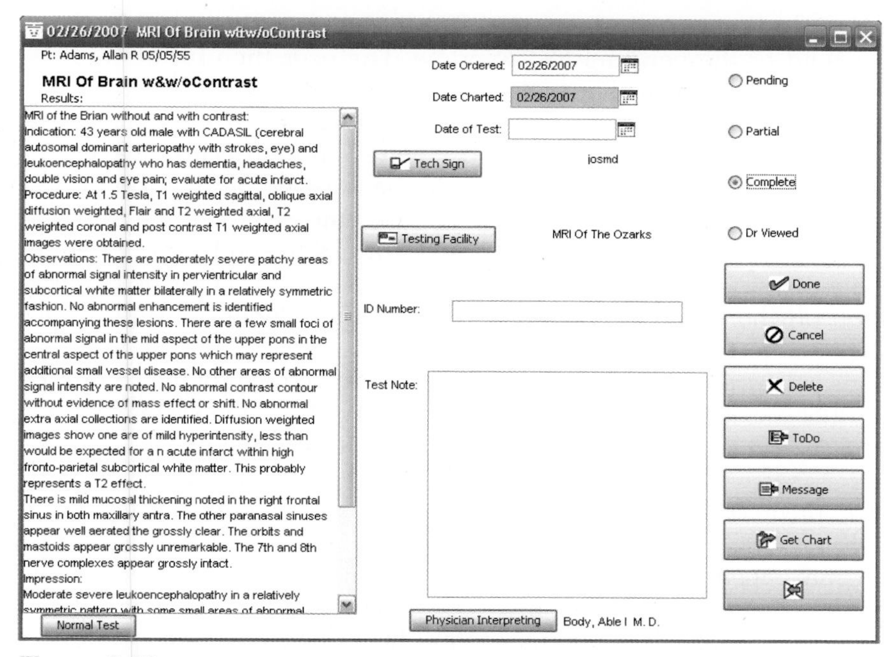

Figure 9.16 Test results in Word format copied and pasted into a pending test.

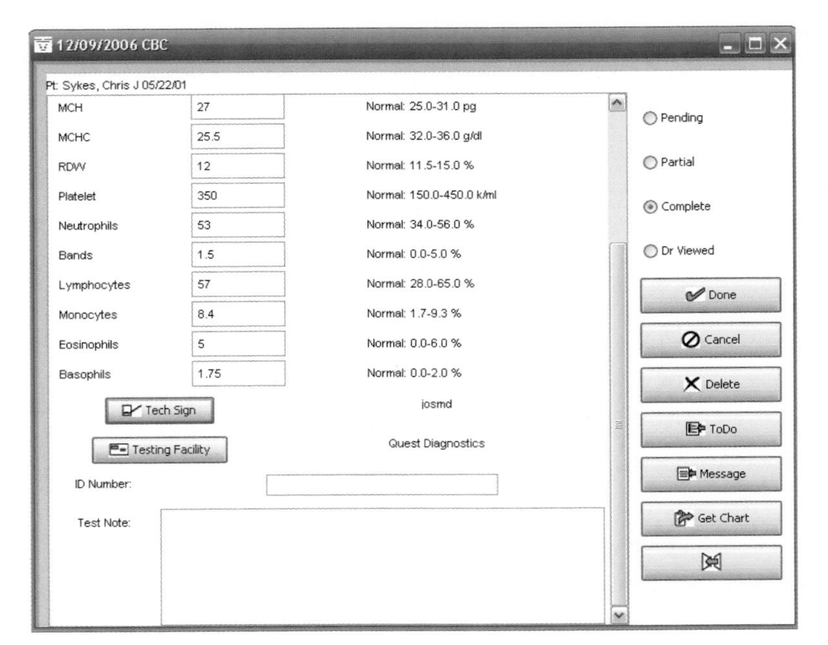

Figure 9.17 Test results being entered into a pending test.

fax. If the test result arrives at the clinic in a paper format, the medical test evaluation must be scanned as an electronic file to be pasted in the *Results* text field of the pending test (Figure 9.16).

If a clinic does not use the SpringLabs electronic interface for outside lab facilities, or the lab was processed internally, the lab results must be entered manually (Figure 9.17). To do so, the user opens a pending test, clicks the [Tech Sign] button to indicate the source of the data entry, and then the [Testing Facility] button to choose the appropriate originating facility (Figures 9.16 and 9.17). If a testing facility is not listed, it must be set up in the address book under the *New* menu or the *Productivity Center* menu. Each test comes with an identification number from the testing facility so that easy reference can be made. The user places this number in the *ID Number* field of the pending test window. The user then inputs the test results. Lab results entered manually need to be double-checked for accuracy. Once the test has entered the patient's chart, the results cannot be altered. If a mistake in data entry is discovered after the test leaves the *Pending Tests* areas, the test will need to be deleted and another test "ordered" for the patient so that results can be entered again correctly.

The user may use the [ToDo] or [Message] buttons to send a *ToDo* item or message to a physician or another clinician. The user then clicks the *Complete* radio button on the right side of the screen and the [Done] button to move the *Pending Tests* to the *Completed Tests* list.

Physicians either receive an internal message notifying them of the completed test results that await their review, or they routinely check the system for any completed tests. When ready to evaluate a completed test, the physician opens the *Completed Tests* window, which is accessed from the *Practice View* screen by selecting *Edit* menu (Figure 9.18). The *Completed Tests* window display all *Pending Tests* to which results have been entered. The list of tests can be organized by date, test name, patient name, test type, practice name, or ordering physician by clicking on the appropriate heading. In a large practice with multiple physicians, this feature enables a physician to quickly find his or her ordered tests.

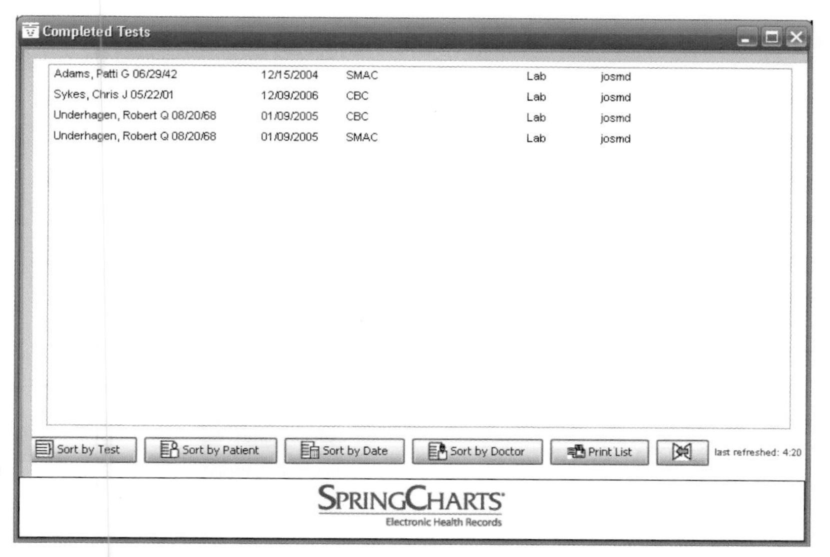

Figure 9.18 List of completed tests.

When a completed test is selected, a window opens to display the test results. Any abnormalities in the results—for example, lab levels outside the normal range—are highlighted in a color bar to alert the physician (Figure 9.19). From this screen, the physician can perform all of the administrative functions necessary to process the test. He or she can open the patient's chart to look for other medical information, send a *ToDo/Reminder* to himself/herself or another user to follow up on a needed assignment, or send a *Message* to another user. Free text can be typed into the *Test Note* field, such as an observation or a plan of care.

When the results have been evaluated and processed, the practitioner selects the *Dr Viewed* radio button on the right side of the screen and clicks the [Done] button. This activity removes the test from the *Completed Tests* window and

Focal Point

Test results outside of the normal range are highlighted in the completed test window to more readily alert the physician.

SpringCharts Tip

The *Dr Viewed* radio button in the *completed test* window is only available if the user is logged on as a doctor. This ensures a test result is not charted until a physician evaluates it.

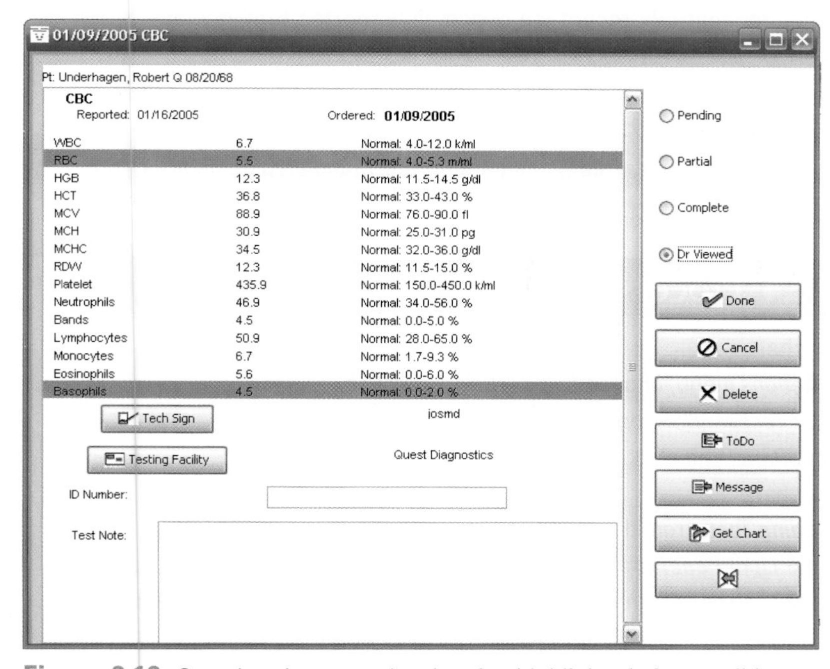

Figure 9.19 Completed test results showing highlighted abnormalities.

9.4 Creating a Test Report

The ONC requires that patients have access to electronic copies of certain health information, such as test reports. As outlined in Table 9.3, under MU Stage 1, EPs were required to supply healthcare information in an electronic format to 50 percent of the patients who requested copies. The remaining 50 percent could receive healthcare information as photocopies from their charts. The measure allows for physicians to withhold medical information if the provider believes the information will be harmful to the patient. The requests must be fulfilled within three business days.

Once a test is entered into a patient chart, it is considered final and cannot be edited. If a test is ordered within the office visit note, the result appears in the *H&P* (history and physical) *Report* and the *Examination Report*, which are both created from within the *Office Visit* screen. Because test results are entered into the pending test area in this manner, rather than imported into the chart as a scanned document, SpringCharts can use the data to create trend analyses and reports and to add test results in letters and e-mails.

Focal Point

If test results are entered into SpringCharts through the *Pending Tests* area, the program is able to create test reports for the patients.

A test report can be created for a patient from within his or her chart. The test report can include any test results saved under the *Lab, Imaging,* or *Medical Tests* categories in the patient's care tree. Test reports are created by accessing the *New Test Report to Pt* option under the *New* menu of the patient's chart and selecting the desired test. A test report is created for the patient and displays the desired test results, along with a description and the purpose of the test (Figure 9.21).

The EHR program comes with simple, customizable explanations for many of the tests. To add new test descriptions or modify existing ones, the user accesses the *Edit* menu on the main *Practice View* screen and selects the *Test Explanations* submenu. In the *Edit Test Explanation* window, the user selects the appropriate test and then adds the explanation in the right-side text box (Figure 9.22). These explanations are universal to the program and available to all users.

Table 9.3 Meaningful Use Core Measure

E-copies of Healthcare Information	
ONC Stage 1 Objective	**Meaningful Use Measure**
On request, provide patients with an electronic copy of their healthcare information (including diagnostic test results, problem lists, medication lists, and information regarding medication allergies).	More than 50 percent of requesting patients receive electronic copies of healthcare information within 3 business days.

Notes:

- If a physician has no requests from patients for their healthcare information during the reporting period, that physician is excluded from this objective.
- Physicians are allowed to withhold information potentially harmful to the patient.
- Physicians are allowed to charge a fee for photocopying information, per HIPAA regulations.
- Patients are allowed to choose the format in which they receive their information.
- Disclosure of the information to a parent, family member, or caretaker is allowed under this objective.

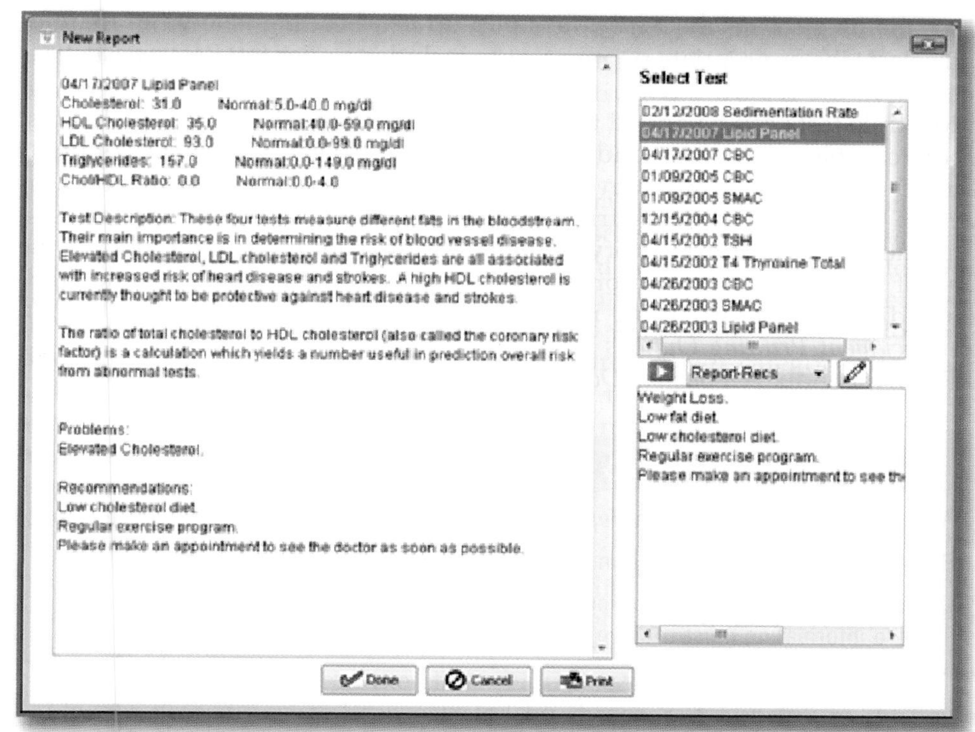

Figure 9.21 *New Report* window.

When the patient's test is selected in the *Test Report* window, the explanation text associated with the test is included in the report. If no explanation has been associated with the test in the program, only the test results appear in the report.

Within the *New Report* window, identified *Problems* and *Recommendations* can be added from the pop-up text in the lower right. The window defaults to the *Report-Probs* pop-up text category; the user places the cursor under the *Problems* heading in the body of the report and selects the appropriate pop-up text.

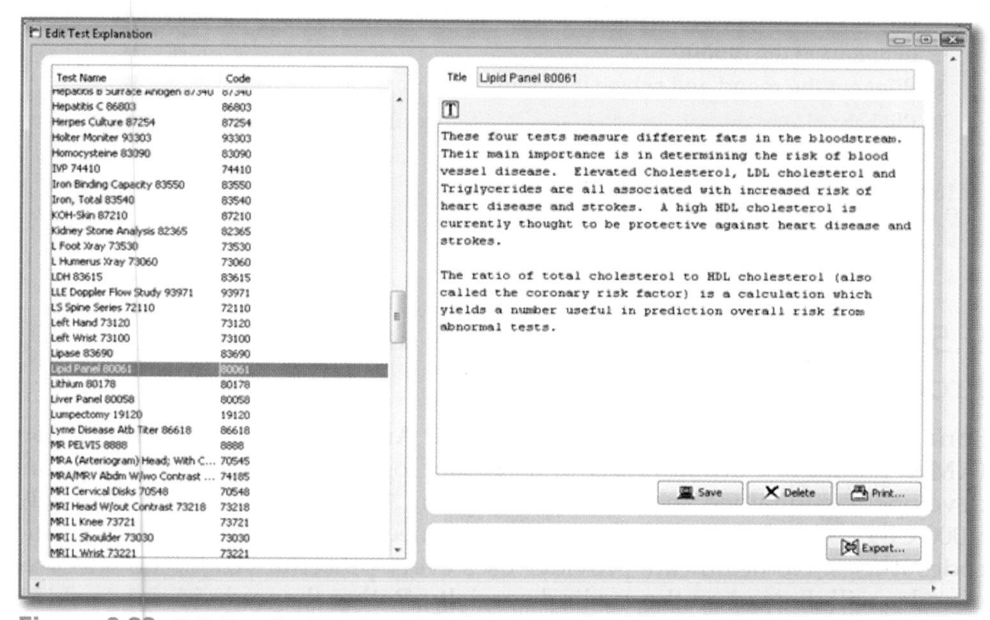

Figure 9.22 *Edit Test Explanation* window.

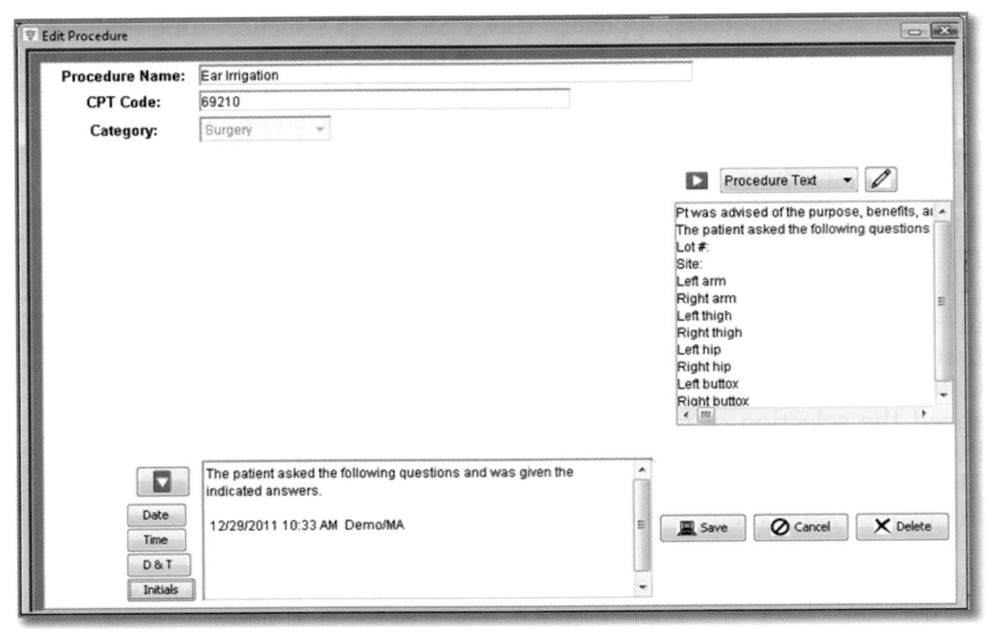

Figure 9.25 *Edit Procedure* window in the *OV* screen.

Focal Point

Procedures are chosen within the *OV* screen under the [Proc] navigation tab by typing the procedure name, selecting from category lists, or selecting from a list of previous procedures for that patient.

screen. In the *New Procedure* window (Figure 9.26), the user completes the *Procedure Name* and *CPT Code* fields, and selects the correct type of procedure from the *Category* drop-down menu. If the user does not know the full name or code for a procedure, the [LookUp] button provides access to the complete procedure code database embedded in the EHR. Although the CPT database is installed with SpringCharts, specific codes need to be manually activated in this manner. This enables only the relevant codes for the clinic to be sorted and processed in the program. Once the code has been selected in the *LookUp* window, the program automatically populates the code and description fields.

Procedural text can be chosen from the pop-up text panel on the right side of the *New Procedure* window. It can also be manually typed into the test text box.

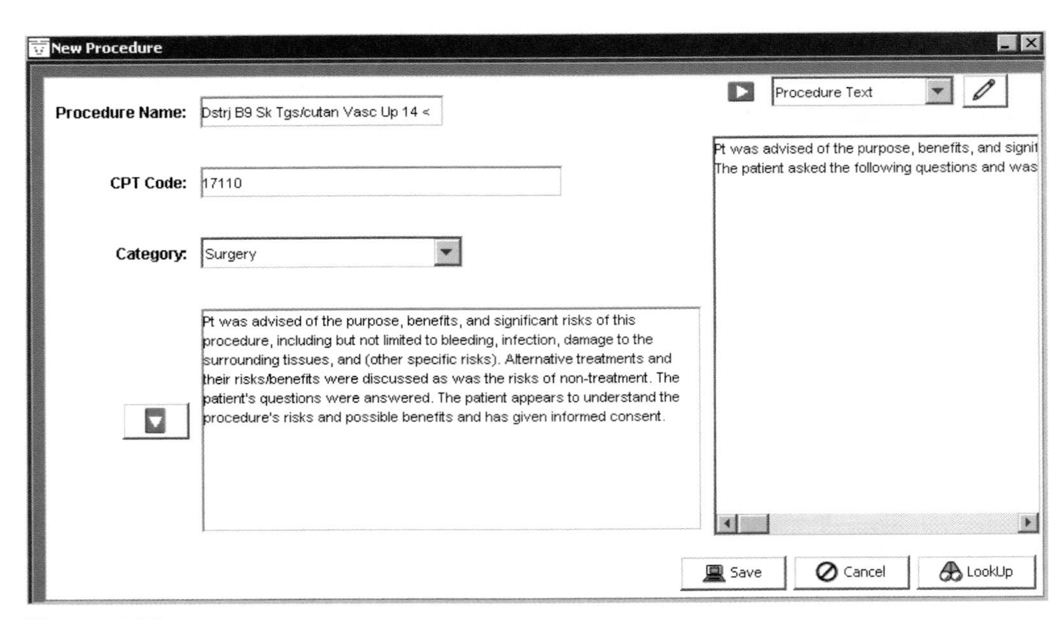

Figure 9.26 Creating a new procedure code.

If the provider consistently uses specific text when administrating a certain procedure, this text should accompany the procedure. As described in Chapter 8, text associated with a procedure functions like a template; any text added to the setup of a new procedure automatically populates the OV note when the procedure is selected under the [Proc] navigation tab in the *OV* screen. Although the procedure text functions as a template, the user can modify text for a specific patient in the OV note by clicking on the selected procedure in the lower middle panel. Procedure text modified within the *OV* screen only affects the note for the current patient; it does not change the original text in the procedure setup.

Focal Point

Mini-templates can be created by adding text when new procedures are set up. When the procedure is selected in the *OV* screen, the predefined text accompanies it to the note.

Creating an Immunization Procedure

EHRs can automate the process of reporting administered immunizations to local and national immunization registries. For this reason, the ONC requires all ONC-certified EHR programs to have the ability to record specific details regarding immunization procedures, such as the vaccine code (CVX), manufacturer code (MVX), lot numbers, expiration dates, and so on. By recording this structured data when setting up a vaccine in the EHR program, a medical facility then ensures that local and national immunization registries can recognize the immunization(s) when the facility transmits electronic reports.

In Stage 1 of MU, the ONC required EPs to at least test the transmission of patients' immunizations in locations where there were functioning health information exchanges (Table 9.4). This measure is not a required core measure. It is one of the 10 menu measures from which an EP must choose 5 to implement and demonstrate during the 90-day testing period. EPs must choose at least one of three public health objectives in the menu set; immunization is one of these three choices.

When the *Immunization* category is chosen in the *New Procedure* window, several additional fields open for the user to complete (Figure 9.27). ONC-certified EHR programs are required to document this detailed information with each vaccine in the database. When immunization reports are sent to local and national registries from EHRs, this information helps providers and families by consolidating immunization information into one reliable source. They also save money by ensuring children get only the vaccines they need and improve office efficiency by reducing the time needed to gather and review immunization records. Public health agencies use immunization registries to

Table 9.4 Meaningful Use Menu Measure

Immunization Registries	
ONC Stage 1 Objective	**Meaningful Use Measure**
Demonstrate capability to submit electronic data to immunization registries or immunization information systems and actual submission in accordance with applicable law and practice.	Perform at least one test of EHR's capacity to submit electronic data to immunization registries and follow up submission if the test is successful.

Notes:

- Physicians are allowed to report that their local immunization registry does not accept electronic submissions.
- A physician who does not administer any immunizations during the EHR reporting period would be excluded from this objective.

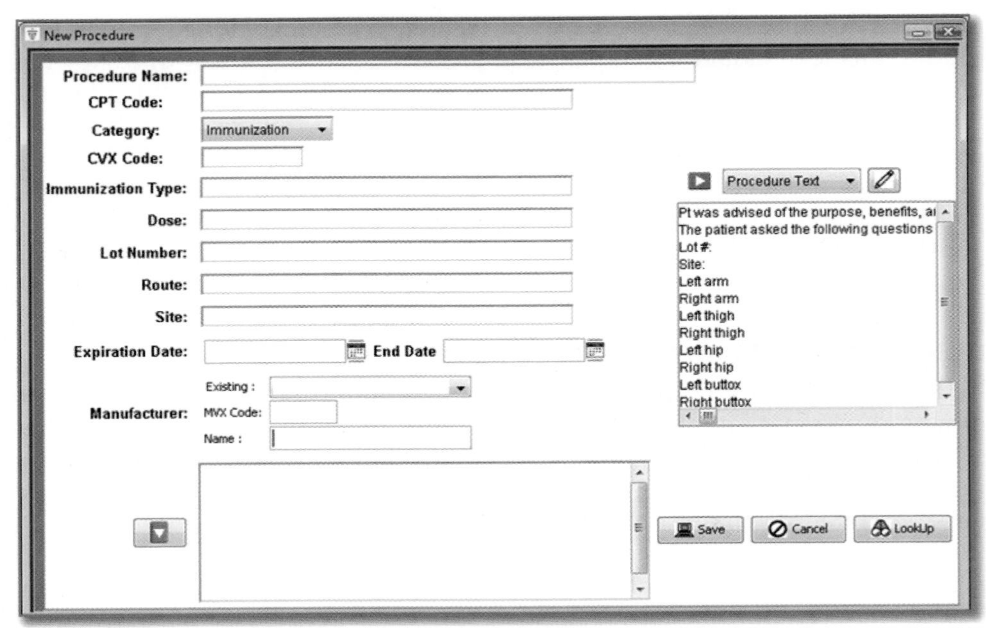

Figure 9.27 *New Procedure* window, showing *Immunization* category.

conduct surveillance, maintain high immunization coverage rates for the population, and manage disease outbreaks and emergency responses.

Editing a Procedure

As the practice of healthcare changes, the American Medical Association (AMA) creates new procedure codes for new services; current codes are revised; and old, obsolete codes are discarded. Thousands of codes are in use and are updated annually. Clinics and providers are kept up-to-date on new and modified codes through the Centers for Medicare & Medicaid Services (CMS) bulletins. Clinic staff members responsible for insurance billing endeavor to keep abreast of any procedure code changes so that practitioners can be reimbursed for their services speedily and accurately.

To edit a procedure name or code, the user selects *Edit > Procedures* from the *Practice View* screen. In the *Edit Procedure* window, activated procedure codes can be selected by *Procedure Name* or *CPT Code* by selecting the appropriate search criteria in the left-side drop-down menu, then typing the term or code in the search field. To view the clinic's complete list of activated codes, the user selects the [Search] key without typing in a term or code. Figure 9.28 shows a list of activated procedure codes. This list can be printed out to compare with the list of common codes the clinic typically uses during the initial setup phase of the program.

To edit the procedure, the user selects the desired procedure from the list, and the details, including the category heading, are displayed in the right-side panel. All displayed fields can be modified. Remember, immunization procedures include more fields than other procedure codes. Lot numbers and expiration dates change from time to time and need to be updated. The *Edit Procedure* window also includes a text field for describing the details of the procedure; this text can be modified as well. When the modifications are complete, the user selects the [Save] button. New procedures can also be activated from the *Edit Procedure* window by selecting either the [New] or [Lookup] buttons.

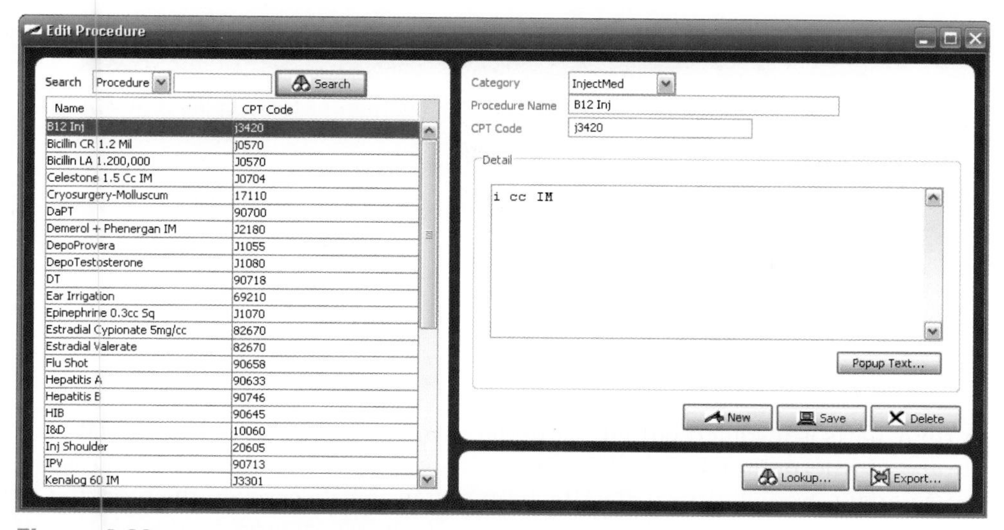

Figure 9.28 Editing a procedure code.

Concept Checkup 9.5

A. From which window in the *OV* screen can a provider reselect existing procedures for the patient?

B. Where are procedure category headings set up?

C. Where does template text added to a new procedure appear when the procedure is selected in the *OV* screen?

D. Why is additional information required when setting up an immunization procedure?

Exercise 9.7 Creating a New Procedure Code

In this exercise, we will create a new procedure code: *Destruction of 15 or more Benign Lesion—17111*. First, we need to make sure the code is not already activated.

1. Open the *Edit* menu in the *Practice View* screen and select *Procedures.*
2. In the *Edit Procedure* window, select *CPT Code* as the search mode and type *17111* in the search field.
3. Click the [Search] button. We know this procedure code has not yet been activated in the EHR program because no procedure is found in the search process.
4. Click the [New] button in the bottom right corner of the window.
5. Look up the code in the CPT dictionary database using the [Lookup] button located in the bottom right corner of the *Edit Procedure* window. In the *Search Procedure Master List* window, select *CPT Code* as the search mode and type *17111* in the search field. Click the [Search] button. When the code has been located, highlight it and click the [Select] button.
6. Complete the *Category* type by choosing *Surgery* from the drop-down menu of the *Edit Procedure* window.
7. To add text to this procedure that will be consistent each time the procedure is conducted, click the [Popup Text] button.

(continued)

Exercise 9.7 (Concluded)

8. In the *PopUp Text Composer* window, select the paragraph that begins with: *Pt was advised of the purpose, benefits . . . etc.* and click the [OK] button. The text is now added to the *Detail* window and will be associated with this code.
9. Save the new procedure code by clicking the [Save] button and close the window.

World Health Organization (WHO) This international organization was established in 1948 for the purpose of coordinating international public health to achieve the highest possible level of global healthcare. A specialized agency of the United Nations (UN), headquartered in Geneva, Switzerland, the WHO has been responsible for developing and modifying ICD codes since 1948.

HIPAA/HITECH Tip

ICD codes are the mandated diagnosis code set for HIPAA transactions. They are required to be current as of the date of service.

9.6 Documenting, Activating, and Editing Diagnosis Codes

SpringCharts is installed with the complete **World Health Organization (WHO)** library of International Classification of Diseases (ICD) codes. The ICD is the most widely used statistical classification system for diseases in the world. ICD codes are alphanumeric designations given to every diagnosis, description of symptoms, and cause of death known. These codes are developed, monitored, and copyrighted by the WHO. In the United States, the Department of Health and Human Services (HHS) maintains the official version for the United States, and the Centers for Medicare & Medicaid Services (CMS) oversees all changes and modifications to the ICD codes, in cooperation with WHO. There are thousands of ICD codes; however, as with CPT codes in SpringCharts EHR, a clinic needs to activate only the specific codes it intends to use. No healthcare provider uses every diagnosis code; the selection of codes depends on the medical specialty. Rather than providers searching through thousands of terms and codes in the database, the process of activating only codes that the clinic uses speeds up selection time and documentation. When SpringCharts is initially installed, a limited set of ICD codes are automatically activated.

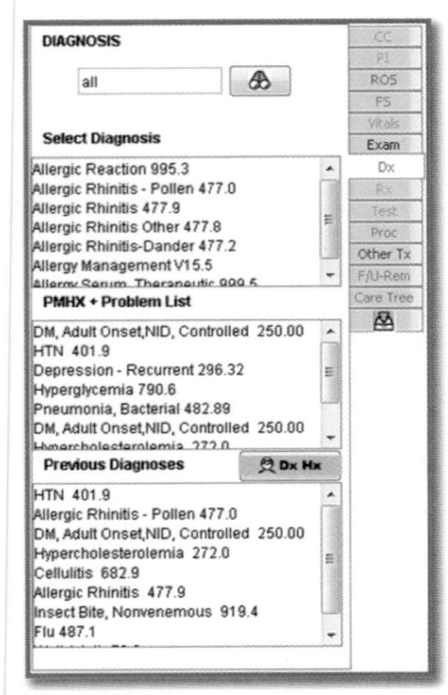

Figure 9.29 Selecting a diagnoses in the *OV* screen.

Documenting a Diagnosis

Diagnoses can only be selected within the OV note by clicking on the [Dx] navigation tab in the *OV* screen. In this window, the practitioner can choose a diagnosis from the *Previous Diagnoses* field in the lower right corner of the screen or from the *PMHX + Problem List* field (Figure 9.29). The *Previous Diagnoses* field displays all of the diagnoses recorded for this patient in all previous OV notes saved in the EHR program. The *PMHX + Problem List* window displays the diagnoses from these two sections of the patient's face sheet. Many times patients are examined by the provider for the same symptoms and chief complaints reported at previous visits; having previous diagnoses available to choose from in the OV note speeds up documentation. If the desired diagnosis is not displayed in either window, the provider can search for a new diagnosis by either the name or code in the EHR database by using the *DIAGNOSIS* search field in the top right corner of the *OV* screen (Figure 9.29).

When a diagnosis is selected, it appears in the lower middle work area. The provider may add notes to the chosen diagnosis specific to this patient by clicking on the diagnosis in the work area, which opens a *Diagnosis* window (Figure 9.30). Because the diagnosis notes can only be added in the OV note window, they only affect the specific note for this specific patient. The diagnosis note does not get added to the diagnosis database, and the associated note does not appear when this diagnosis

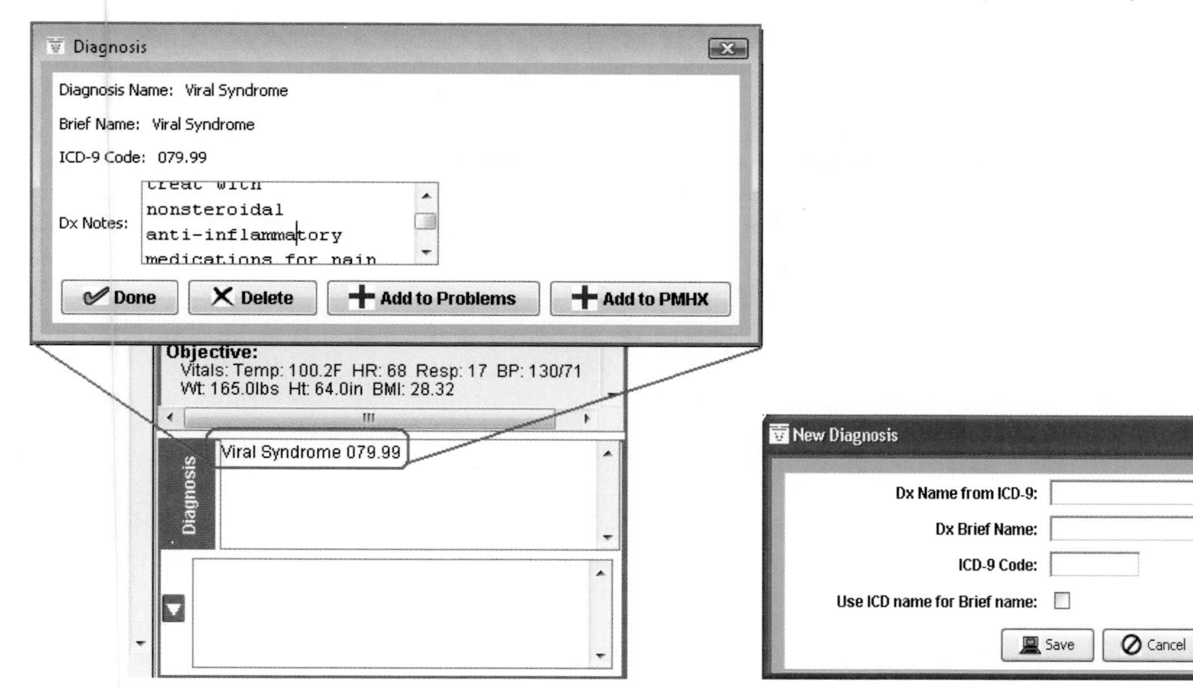

Figure 9.30 Documenting diagnosis notes.

Figure 9.31 Activating a new diagnosis code.

is used for another patient. Also, in the *Diagnosis* window, the provider can select the [Add to Problems] button or the [Add to PMHX] button to add this chosen diagnosis back into one of these two areas of the patient's face sheet (Figure 9.30). Once the provider moves to another area of the OV note, the diagnosis and the note associated with the diagnosis are added to the *Assessment* area of the SOAP note.

Creating a New Diagnosis

As mentioned earlier, SpringCharts is installed with the complete library of ICD codes. However, the clinic staff needs to activate the specific codes they intend to use to make the selection and documentation processes more efficient. When SpringCharts is initially installed, a limited set of diagnosis codes is activated automatically. To activate a new diagnosis, the user selects *New Diagnosis* under the *New* menu on the *Practice View* screen, opening the *New Diagnosis* window (Figure 9.31). A new diagnosis can be added directly into the appropriate text and code fields or by selecting the [Lookup] button. The [Lookup] button provides access to the current ICD-9 database, enabling the user to search for a new diagnosis by either code or description. When the desired ICD code has been selected, the *Dx Brief Name* field needs to be completed. The name entered into this field determines the text the practitioner uses when searching for a diagnosis code in the *OV* screen. If the clinic normally uses the same text as the ICD database, the user simply clicks in the *Use ICD name for Brief name* check box.

The EHR program enables the practitioner to activate a diagnosis while in the *Office Visit* screen. This saves time because the OV note does not need to be closed and a new diagnosis activated under the main *New* menu. If the practitioner needs a particular diagnosis that has not been activated, he or she

Focal Point

Although the entire diagnosis code list comes with the EHR program, only those codes that are activated can be used in the EHR program.

Focal Point

During the initial setup of SpringCharts in a doctor's office, additional CPT and ICD-9 codes are typically added to the activated codes in the program.

Focal Point

Text in the *Dx Brief Name* field of the *Edit Diagnosis* window determines the description by which the code is searched in the *OV* screen.

can choose *New Diagnosis* from the *Database* menu within the *Office Visit* screen, opening the same *New Diagnosis* window there. Again, the diagnosis can be entered manually or the [Lookup] button used to access the ICD-9 database, enabling the user to search for a new diagnosis by code or description. The provider then clicks the [Save] button, and the diagnosis code and description are activated to the EHR diagnosis list and can then be chosen under the [Dx] tab in the *OV* screen.

Editing a Diagnosis

ICD codes are revised periodically; they are currently in the ninth edition, hence the designation ICD-9. Medical facilities and providers are informed of new, modified, and deleted ICD codes through annual publications from CMS. It is crucial that clinical staff responsible for filing medical claims with insurance companies be kept abreast of changes to ICD codes. ICD codes need to be updated in the EHR program so the most up-to-date codes appear on the routing slip and reimbursement to the provider is timely and accurate. Typically, a provider does not choose a diagnosis code in the OV note; rather, he or she chooses the diagnosis name. The EHR program tracks the code associated with the name and displays it on the routing slip for billing purposes.

To edit a diagnosis, the user selects the *Edit* menu on the main *Practice View* screen and chooses *Diagnosis.* The *Edit Diagnosis* window enables the user to search for a diagnosis by either the brief name or the ICD code based on the drop-down selection in the *Search* field. To display all activated ICD codes in the EHR program, the user clicks the [Search] button *without* first selecting a name or code (Figure 9.32). If the code description requires modifying, remember the text placed in the *Brief Name* field is the text by which the code is searched in the *Office Visit* screen, not the *official* ICD name. As with procedure codes, new diagnoses can also be activated from the *Edit Diagnosis* window by selecting the [New] button or the [Lookup] button.

ICD-10 Codes

As described above, the WHO adopted diagnosis codes for the purpose of coordinating international public health. The United States and many other

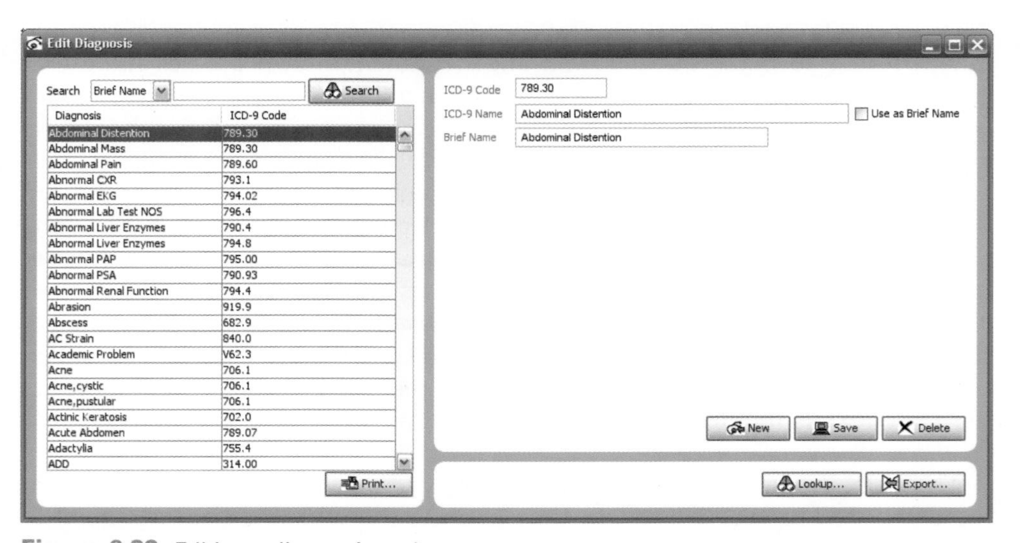

Figure 9.32 Editing a diagnosis code.

Table 9.5 Comparisons of the Diagnosis Code Sets

ICD-9 Codes	ICD-10 Codes
3–5 characters in length	3–7 characters in length
Approximately 13,000 codes	Approximately 68,000 available codes
First digit may be alpha (E or V) or numeric; digits 2–5 are numeric	Digit 1 is alpha; digits 2 and 3 are numeric; digits 4–7 are alpha or numeric
Limited space for adding new codes	Flexible for adding new codes
Lacks detail	Very specific
Lacks laterality	Has laterality (i.e., codes identifying right vs. left)

Source: American Medical Association. *The Differences between ICD-9 and ICD-10, Fact Sheet 2.* June 2, 2010. www.ama-assn.org/ama1/pub/upload/mm/399/icd10-icd9-differences-fact-sheet.pdf (accessed December 29, 2011).

countries use these diagnosis codes to identify illnesses, diseases, and infections. By using these codes, every medical provider in the United States and many other parts of the world can understand the same diagnosis the same way. For example, if a patient is diagnosed with gastroesophageal reflux disease (GERD), or acid reflux, the patient is given the diagnosis code of 530.81. If that patient travels across the country or internationally and is examined by a physician for the same condition, the patient will be given the same diagnosis of 530.81.

In 1977, most WHO member states adopted the ninth edition of the ICD codes. In 1979, the USA adopted the ICD-9 codes for Medicare and Medicaid claims and the national medical insurance industry followed suit. ICD codes are modified periodically by the WHO to incorporate changes in the international medical field. However, the tenth revision (ICD-10) is not a modification; rather, it has undergone a complete restructuring from ICD-9. ICD-10 codes were developed in 1992 and have been implemented globally by most countries. HHS has now adopted the ICD-10 terms and codes, and CMS will require their implementation by U.S. providers on October 1, 2014.

Focal Point

ICD-10 diagnosis codes must be used on and after October 1, 2014, CMS claims using ICD-9 codes after this date will be rejected.

The ICD-10 revision is more robust and descriptive (Table 9.5). The terms and codes differ from the ninth revision in that ICD-10's first digit is always alpha, they have alphanumeric categories rather than just numeric categories, and the ICD-10 classifications have almost twice as many categories as ICD-9 codes. The ICD-10 diagnosis codes are 3–7 characters in length and total 68,000, whereas ICD-9 diagnosis codes are 3–5 digits in length and number approximately 13,000. Moving to ICD-10 codes is expected to affect *all* physicians due to the increased number of codes, the change in the number of characters per code, and increased code specificity.

Although Stage 1 of the ONC's meaningful use criteria did not require the use of ICD-10 codes, it is anticipated that ONC-certified EHR programs will be compliant by Stage 3 of the MU program. CMS published the final rule for adopting ICD-10 as a standard in the United States in January 2009, and a

SpringCharts Tip

SpringCharts EHR versions released after October 2014 will have the official ICD-10 code set.

compliancy date was initially set for October 1, 2013. However, based on input from the provider community regarding concerns about the administrative burden of ICD-10 implementation by 2013, HHS Secretary Kathleen Sebelius announced in April 2012 that HHS began a process to postpone the date by which certain healthcare entities have to meet ICD-10 compliancy and to establish the new compliancy date as October 1, 2014.

Updated information about ICD-10 codes regarding timelines, compliancy, and so on can be found on the CMS website: www.cms.gov/ICD10.

Concept Checkup 9.6

A. A new diagnosis can be activated through the *New Diagnosis* window under the *New* menu on the *Practice View* screen. In what other screen can a new diagnosis code be activated?

B. In an *OV* screen, existing diagnoses can be used from the *Previous Diagnoses* window. From what other window in the *OV* screen can a patient's existing diagnosis be selected?

C. What is the established compliancy date for ICD-10 set by HHS?

Exercise 9.8 Using Diagnosis and Procedure Codes

1. Open your chart and launch a new office visit. *This is a follow-up visit scheduled to conduct a removal procedure for maculopapular skin lesions.*
2. Under the [CC] navigation button, select the pop-up text *Follow-Up Visit.*
3. Open the [Vitals] tab and add several normal vitals.
4. Open the [Exam] navigation tab and choose *(0 Abnormals)* as the pop-up text category. Scroll down and select the text: *SKIN: + maculopapular lesions.*
5. In the [Dx] navigation tab, search for a new diagnosis starting with *lesion.* The pigmented lesion code that appears is not the correct code, so we will need to activate another diagnosis code.
6. In the *Database* menu of the *OV* screen select *New Diagnosis.*
7. To access the ICD dictionary database, click the [Lookup] button. In the *LookUp Dx Code* window, search for the main 102 code. From the list select: *Yaws Unspecified.* The diagnosis description and code will appear in the *New Diagnosis* window.
8. For the *Dx Brief Name,* enter *maculopapular lesions.*
9. Save the newly activated diagnosis.
10. In the diagnosis field of the OV screen, type *mac* and search for the code. From the presenting list, select the new code.
11. Under the [Proc] navigation button, select *Surgery* as the category and choose the newly activated procedure *destruction of benign lesion.*
12. Open the [F/U-Rem] tab. Notice that all text associated with this procedure during its creation is now added into the body of the SOAP note. Choose a follow-up in 1 week.
13. Click on the *Create a Reminder* icon and send a *ToDo/Reminder* to Jan to schedule a follow-up appointment in 1 week, using pop-up text. Send the *ToDo* item.

Exercise 9.8 (Concluded)

14. Click the [Done] button in the *OV* screen and create a routing slip.
15. In the *Routing Slip* window, bill for the surgical tray you find itemized in the *Superbill Form* in the right pane by clicking on the item. You do not need to choose an E&M code because this visit will be billed as a procedure, not an office visit.
16. Print the routing slip and submit it to your instructor.
17. Send the routing slip and close the chart.

Exercise 9.9 Creating and Using an ICD-10 Code

Note: Perhaps your clinic's physician inadvertently used an ICD-9 code after the compliance date for ICD-10 codes; therefore, the claim needs to be re-filed with the correct code. You will need to create the equivalent ICD-10 code, update it in the OV note, and create a new routing slip.

1. On the *Practice View* screen, select the *Edit* menu and the *Diagnosis* submenu.
2. In the *Edit Diagnosis* window, type *diarr* in the *Search* field and click on the *Search* icon.
3. On the right side of the screen, type *(09)* after *Diarrhea, Acute* in the *Brief Name* field. This will signal the physician that this is an ICD-9 code if an attempt is made to use it again. Click the [Save] button. Notice the name of the code has updated on the left-hand side.
4. On the right-hand side, click on the [New] button and answer *Yes* to the question: *Do you want to use the displayed data?*
5. Change the ICD code field to *R19.7*. Change the *Brief Name* field to *Diarrhea, Acute (10)* and click the [Save] button. Close the *Edit Diagnosis* window.
6. Click on *Chris Sykes* on the *Office Calendar* and open his chart by selecting the [Get Chart] button in the *Edit Appointment* window.
7. Expand the *Encounters* category in the care tree and locate the *Office Visit* with the chief complaint of *Acute Diarrhea*. Open the OV note by selecting the [Edit] button.
8. In the *OV* screen, select the [Dx] navigation tab on the right-hand side.
9. Click on the diagnosis: *Diarrhea, Acute 787.91* in the lower middle window. Click on the [Delete] button in the *Diagnosis* window and answer *Yes* to the confirmation question. In the *Note* box below, type *Dx changed from 787.91 to R19.7.*
10. In the *DIAGNOSIS* field in the upper right, type *Diarr* and conduct a search. Select the appropriate code *R19.7*.
11. Click the [Done] button. Click the [Save and Edit Routing Slip] button in the *Save As* window.
12. In the *Routing Slip* window, select the recommended E&M code by clicking on the [Use Code] button. Click on the [Send] button. Close the patient's chart.
13. On the *Practice View* screen select the *Edit* menu and the *Routing Slips* submenu.
14. Scroll to the bottom of the list in the *View Routing Slips* window and select the routing slip created for Chris Sykes.
15. Click on the [Print] button and print the routing slip. Write your name on the routing slip and submit to your instructor. Close the *View Routing Slips* window. Close the patient's chart.

chapter 9 summary

Learning Outcomes	Key Concepts
9.1 Describe how to order lab, imaging, and medical tests. **Pages 238–240**	Tests are classified as lab tests, imaging tests, and medical tests. All ordered tests are stored in the *Pending Tests* area of the EHR program. When data is input to a pending test it is then sent to the *Completed Tests* area of the program for the physician's viewing. Tests are ordered from within the *Office Visit* screen or within the *Patient Chart* screen. The printer icon in the OV note enables printing of an order form for ordered tests.
9.2 Process *Reference Lab* results that are received electronically. **Pages 240–245**	Importing lab results as structured data is an ONC MU criterion. SpringLabs is the electronic data interchange (EDI) that interfaces SpringCharts to lab companies across the Internet. Imported lab results have to be manually matched to the patient, pending test, and lab items (analyte) to ensure accuracy.
9.3 Process and chart tests manually. **Pages 246–252**	Assessment or evaluation text is added to the imaging and medical pending test. Structured data is added to the lab pending test. In the *Pending Tests* and *Completed Tests* windows, the clinician can open the patient's chart, send a message, create a *ToDo Item,* and add a note. The completed lab test highlights results outside the normal range to alert the physician.
9.4 Create a test report. **Pages 252–254**	The ONC requires that patients have access to electronic copies of certain health information like test reports. A test report is created from within the patient's chart. The test report can run utilizing any of the test results saved under the lab, imaging, or medical tests categories in the patient's care tree. A test report displays the test result along with a description of and the purpose for the test.
9.5 Create, edit, and document procedures. **Pages 254–259**	Although the EHR program comes with the entire CPT code dictionary, only codes necessary for the clinic need to be activated for use. Procedures are documented in the OV note where additional notes can be added to the procedure. Procedural text can be added to a new procedure and becomes part of the OV note when the procedure is selected. The ONC requires EHRs to report administered immunization procedures to local and national immunization registries. An immunization procedure has many more fields to complete than a typical procedure code.
9.6 Create, edit, and document diagnoses. **Pages 260–265**	Diagnosis codes are developed, monitored, and copyrighted by the WHO. Diagnoses are documented only in the *OV* screen. Diagnosis notes can be added to the selected diagnosis, affecting only the OV note for this specific patient. A new diagnosis can be activated from the *OV* screen or the main *Practice View* screen. The *Dx Brief Name* field determines the text for which the practitioner will search when selecting a diagnosis in the *OV* screen. In 1977, the United States adopted the ninth edition of the ICD codes and has now adopted the ICD-10 terms and codes. ICD-10 compliance initially meant that all HIPAA-covered entities would successfully conduct healthcare transactions on or after October 1, 2014, using the ICD-10 diagnosis codes. However, this compliancy date has been under review by HHS.

chapter 9 review

Name ______________________ Instructor ______________ Class ______________ Date ______________

Using Terminology

Match the terms on the left with the definitions on the right.

_____ 1. **LO 9.1** SpringLabs
_____ 2. **LO 9.2** Reference labs
_____ 3. **LO 9.2** Lab analyte
_____ 4. **LO 9.2** EDI
_____ 5. **LO 9.5** AMA
_____ 6. **LO 9.6** WHO
_____ 7. **LO 9.5** Procedure codes
_____ 8. **LO 9.6** Diagnosis codes

A. A blood test compound subject to its own specific chemical analysis.
B. Lab results received from lab companies over a secure Internet connection.
C. EDI interface that receives electronic data to SpringCharts using HL7 language and protocols.
D. Electronic data transfer standards and protocols.
E. An international organization established for the purposes of coordinating international public health.
F. Founded in 1847 for the purpose of promoting the art and science of medicine.
G. Collect data according to the International Statistical Classifications of Diseases
H. Collect data according to Current Procedural Terminology

Checking Your Understanding

Choose the best answer and circle the corresponding letter.

9. **LO 9.5, LO 9.6** What complete dictionaries are part of the SpringCharts EHR installed database? Select all that apply.
   a) ICD codes
   b) PMHX codes
   c) CPT codes
   d) Problem list codes

10. **LO 9.1** Tests that have been ordered in the EHR program and are awaiting results will appear as *Uncharted Tests* in what window?
    a) *OV* screen
    b) Patient's face sheet
    c) Pending Tests
    d) Completed Tests

11. **LO 9.2** If the lab items of the imported lab panel differs from that of the pending test in the EHR program, what needs to happen to the imported lab items so the lab interface will 'remember' the association next time?
    a) Reconciled to the database
    b) Deleted from the program
    c) Stored as completed tests
    d) Matched to the pending test items

12. **LO 9.3** Once data has been manually entered into the pending test, what area of the program does the test move to?
    a) Patient Chart
    b) Completed Tests
    c) Pending Tests
    d) Reference Lab

13. **LO 9.1** Tests are stored in certain categories in the care tree. Select all that apply.
    a) Lab
    b) Completed tests
    c) Imaging
    d) Medical tests

14. **LO 9.1** A new imaging test creates:
    a) The report produced after a MRI scan
    b) A new x-ray, MRI, or CT scan
    c) A computer-generated body makeover
    d) A stress test

15. **LO 9.5** The procedure categories are set up in the *Administrator* menu. The administrator can set up to:
    a) 50 categories
    b) 25 categories
    c) 30 categories
    d) No additional categories

16. **LO 9.6** The *Edit Diagnosis* window enables the user to search for a diagnosis by:
    a) Brief name
    b) ICD code
    c) CPT code
    d) Brief name or ICD code

17. **LO 9.6** ICD-9 is a term used for a(n):
    a) Diagnosis code
    b) Medical procedure
    c) Procedure code
    d) EHR software provider

18. **LO 9.2** When test data is received through Spring-Labs, into which area does it go?
    a) Pending Tests
    b) Completed Tests
    c) Patient Chart
    d) Reference Lab

19. **LO 9.2** When a lab company sends test data, the term "out of range" means:
    a) Abnormal level
    b) The patient couldn't be reached by cell phone
    c) The lab results could not be transmitted
    d) Outside the danger level

20. **LO 9.2** Users with the access level of *Get Pending Tests* are notified of newly imported lab results by a:
    a) Red flag in the patient's chart
    b) Lab icon next to the user's log-in name
    c) Pop-up box that appears on the screen when accessing a patient's chart
    d) Message in the user's message center

21. **LO 9.4** Under the MU stipulations, the ONC requires that patients have access to electronic copies of health information like test results. To qualify for financial remuneration during the testing period, EPs must supply electronic copies to:
    a) All patients who request copies within 3 business days
    b) All patients whether they request copies or not
    c) At least 50 percent of requesting patients within 3 business days
    d) All patients who come to the medical facility to obtain the copy

22. **LO 9.6** In 2009, HHS adopted the ICD-10 terms and codes. However, implementation has been postponed to October 1, 2014 because:
    a) Providers were not sure of the reimbursement amount for the new codes.
    b) Many countries around the world have yet to adopt the ICD-10 codes.
    c) Providers have had concerns about the administrative burden of implementation.
    d) Most EHR programs are not designed to take the new ICD-10 codes.

23. **LO 9.3** *Completed Tests* are labs, imaging, and medical tests that have been:
    a) Ordered by the clinician and are awaiting results
    b) Completed at an outside testing facility
    c) Processed and stored in the patient's chart
    d) Processed as *Pending Tests* and are awaiting the physician's viewing

24. **LO 9.4** A *Test Report to Pt* can be created from lab, imaging, or medical tests that are:
    a) Pending tests
    b) Stored in the patient's chart
    c) Completed tests
    d) Sent to outside testing facilities

25. **LO 9.5** The EHR program comes with the entire CPT code file embedded in the database. However:
    a) Physicians need to memorize their most frequently used CPT codes.
    b) The routing slip recommends the most appropriate CPT codes.
    c) Providers need to look up the database list when documenting a CPT code.
    d) CPT codes need to be activated from the database to be seen in the EHR program.

Applying Your Knowledge

Use your critical-thinking skills to answer the following questions.

26. **LO 9.3** As a clinician, explain what you would do and where you would go in the EHR program to process the patient's lab results that the clinic received in the mail.

27. **LO 9.4** During the MU testing period, several patients have received photocopies of test results that came to the clinic from outside testing facilities. To meet the ONC requirement that 50 percent of patients receive test results from the EHR program during the testing period, what do you need to do to make sure the clinic reaches this goal, and how would you do it?

28. **LO 9.5** Why is it important that the clinic record the vaccine code (CVX), the manufacturer code (MVX), lot numbers, expiration dates, and so on of immunizations activated for use in the EHR program?

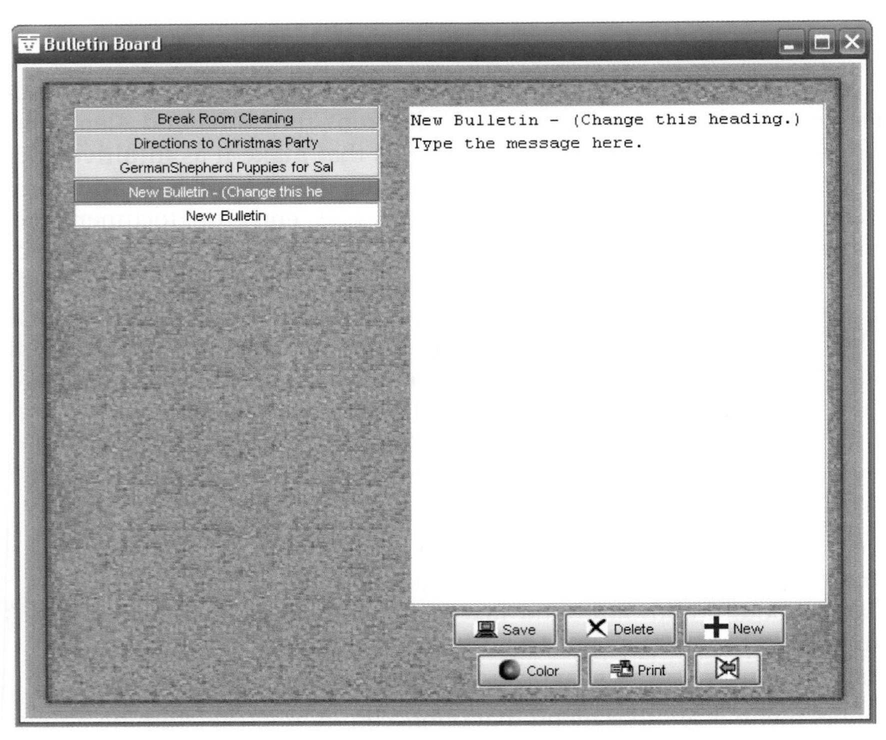

Figure 10.3 *Bulletin Board* feature for posting and retrieving bulletins.

SpringCharts Tip

Shortcut:

Open Bulletin Board

The fourth speed icon from the left on the *Practice Menu* Toolbar enables the user to quickly open the *Bulletin Board* to check for new notices or post a new bulletin without first opening the *Productivity Center.*

Focal Point

The electronic bulletin board in SpringCharts is designed to ensure every user has instant access to bulletins and can easily post messages for everyone to see.

feature can be used. Bulletins can include information about office-wide policies, office gatherings, personal items for sale, and so on.

Once the *Bulletin Board* feature is opened, the user can select any subject heading on the left, which then displays the corresponding bulletins or notes on the right (Figure 10.3). To add a new bulletin to the board, the user clicks the [New] button, replaces the phrase *New Bulletin* with the appropriate subject heading, and types the message under the heading. The user can add colored backgrounds to bulletins by selecting the [Color] button and choosing from a range of colors. Each user must routinely check the *Bulletin Board* for new messages; there is no automatic announcement when items are placed on the board. Posted bulletins may be printed by selecting the [Print] button.

Concept Checkup 10.1

A. Which two menus enable users to access frequently used administrative activities in SpringCharts?

B. What does it mean that the *Bulletin Board* is network-defined?

Exercise 10.1 Creating a New Bulletin Board Post

1. Open the *Bulletin Board* by clicking on the icon on the Toolbar of the main *Practice View* screen.
2. Click on the [New] button to open a new bulletin.
3. Highlight the phrase *New Bulletin* and replace it with the name of a new bulletin: *Inclement Weather Policy.* (Include your name in the heading.)
4. On the next lines of the new bulletin, type a message that encourages employees to call the Inclement Weather Hotline at (800) 694-5289 on snowy mornings to determine whether the office is opening late.
5. Assign a color to your bulletin by accessing the color options under the [Color] button.
6. Click the [Save] button.
7. Repeat steps 2–6 and create another bulletin that announces a fundraising auction to benefit a local family in need.
8. Notice that each new bulletin is added to the list on the left side for other users to view. Select your original 'inclement weather' bulletin.
9. Print a copy of your original bulletin, circle your name, and hand in to your instructor. Close the *Bulletin Board* window.

10.2 Integrated Faxing

SpringCharts interfaces with ***InterFax*** (www.Interfax.net) to allow users to send and receive faxes to and from any SpringCharts client computer over the Internet. Electronic faxing eliminates paper and saves money. SpringCharts faxing requires an Internet connection, but no separate analog phone/fax line is required. InterFax assigns a new fax number to a clinic, when the clinic establishes an account. Once the account is set up and the faxing option activated in SpringCharts, the fax feature is available in the EHR program anywhere the print function is available.

InterFax
InterFax is one of many subscriber-based online fax services that enable users to fax wherever Internet access is available.

Focal Point

SpringCharts allows for Internet faxing through a third-party company, which eliminates the need for a separate fax line and modem.

To fax from SpringCharts, the user selects the [Print] button from any one of multiple print option windows in the program. The user is then presented with the choice to print or fax (Figure 10.4). Selecting the [Fax] button takes the user to the *Fax* dialog window (Figure 10.5). Here the user enters the recipient's name and fax number and the document's subject. The *Lookup/Search* icon can be used to access the SpringCharts *Address Book,* from which the user can select the fax numbers of individuals and businesses on file (Figure 10.6). Once

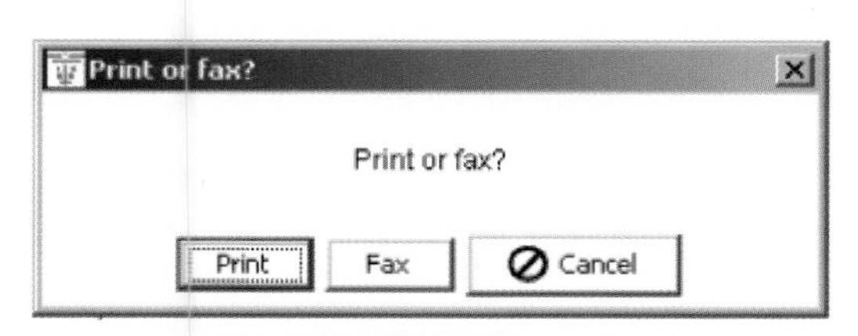

Figure 10.4 Fax option available in print windows.

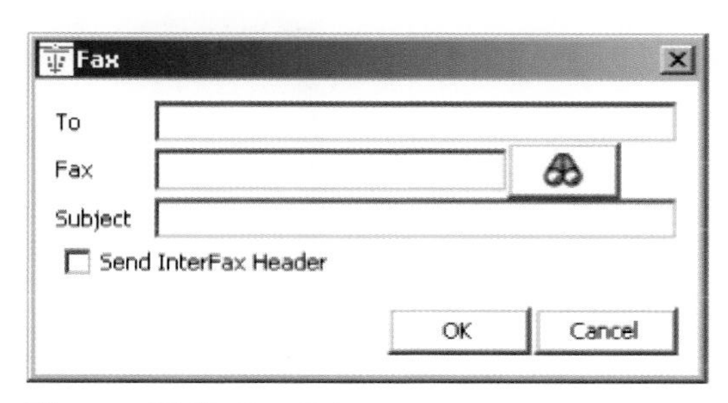

Figure 10.5 *Fax* dialog window.

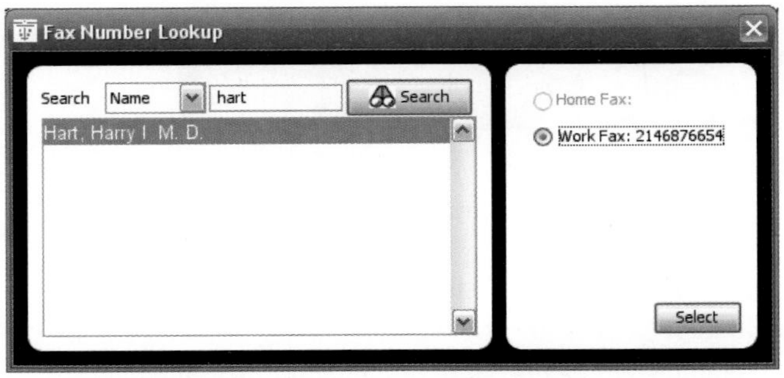

Figure 10.6 Selecting the recipient in the *Fax Number Lookup* window.

a number is selected, the program automatically populates the recipient's name and fax number in the *Fax* dialog window. The user can choose whether to use the page header that resides on the InterFax account screen.

Outbound Fax History

To check the status of faxes sent through the SpringCharts program, the user selects submenu *Outbound Fax History* from the *Productivity Center* menu (Figure 10.7). Figure 10.8 shows the *OutBound Fax History* window, which displays the most recently transmitted faxes. The *Status* column displays pending, completed, and failed transmissions. The remaining columns display the recipient's name *(Contact),* the contact's fax number, subject, the date of original submission, and date of completion. The [Refresh] button enables the user to update the records in the window to include any outbound faxes logged from other users at InterFax while the *Outbound Fax History* window is open.

Inbound Fax List

Users can check for received faxes by accessing the *Inbound Fax List* option from the *Productivity Center* menu. Figure 10.9 shows the *Inbound Fax List* window, which displays the sender's fax number, the time received, and the number of pages. When a fax is received in the clinic's account at Interfax, a corresponding e-mail is sent to the clinic to announce the inbound fax. The SpringCharts user who has the security clearance to receive e-mails receives this notice.

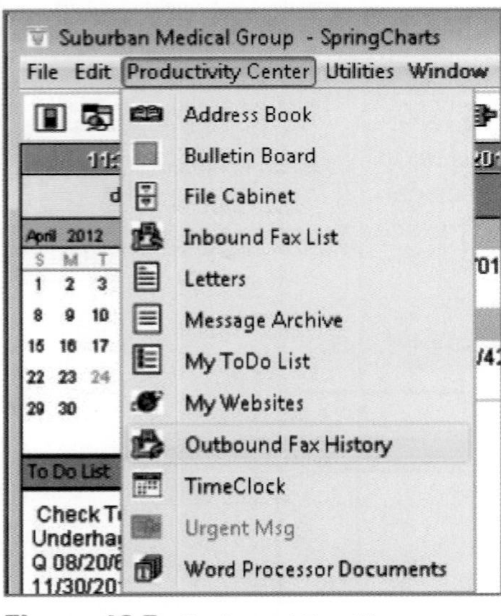

Figure 10.7 *Outbound Fax History* option in the *Productivity Center.*

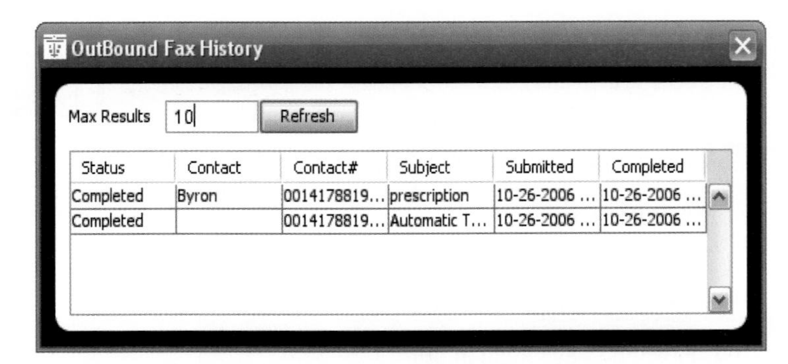

Figure 10.8 *Outbound Fax History* window.

By highlighting a fax in the *Inbound Fax List* window and then selecting the [View] button, the user can view the actual faxed document on the computer screen. The [Refresh] button refreshes the inbound fax list to retrieve any new faxes that may have arrived in the InterFax account while the dialog window was open.

The [Add to File Cabinet] button allows the user to import a selected faxed document directly into a patient's file cabinet category of the care tree in the patient's chart. This feature enables the clinic to electronically capture medical information, evaluations, and consultations faxed from external sources. It bypasses the paper fax, which typically would need to be scanned back into the electronic health record. The [Delete] button deletes the selected fax; however, it is still retrievable through the InterFax website for some time.

Inbound Fax List

Sender	Received	Pages
2107062200	10-4-2006 15:28	1
9037633360	10-9-2006 9:16	1
2107062200	10-9-2006 11:58	1
2813040628	10-9-2006 13:20	3
2814771000	10-10-2006 11:48	2

Refresh | View | Add to File Cabinet... | Delete

Figure 10.9 *Inbound Fax List* window.

Focal Point

Lists of inbound and outbound faxes can be viewed through the SpringCharts *Productivity Center.*

Concept Checkup 10.2

A. What is the name of the Web-based company that enables SpringCharts to send and receive electronic faxes over the Internet?

B. Access to both the *OutBound* and *Inbound Fax History* windows are located under which menu?

C. Which button in the Inbound Fax List window is accessed to add an inbound fax directly to a patient's chart?

Exercise 10.2 Faxing a Prescription Electronically

1. In the *Productivity Center* menu, select the *Address Book* option.
2. Change the search criterion from *Name* to *Category.*
3. In the *Find* field, type *pharmacy* and conduct the search.
4. Select the *Walshop Pharm.*
5. In the *Address* window, add a fictitious fax number to the *Work Fax* field.
6. Click the [Save] button and close the *Address* window.
7. Open your chart.
8. Under the *Encounters* category of the care tree, select the office visit note related to adult allergy symptoms.
9. Click on the [Edit] button to open the *OV* screen.
10. Open the [Rx] navigation tab to display the ordered prescriptions.
11. Click on the *Print Prescriptions* icon in the lower center section of the screen.
12. In the *Prescription Printing Options* window that appears, select *Use Digital Signature* and *Print License No. on Rx.*
13. Click on the [Fax] button.
14. In the *Fax* window, click on the *Search* icon, which opens the *Fax Number Lookup* window.

(continued)

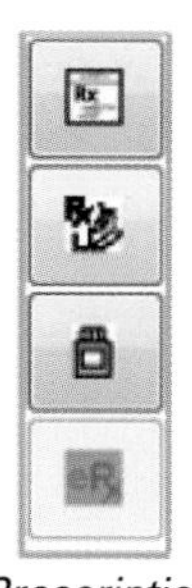

Print Prescription icon

Exercise 10.2 (Concluded)

15. Choose *Category* as the search criterion, type *phar* in the search field, and activate the search.
16. Select *Walshop Pharmacy* and notice the fax number you added appears on the right side.
17. Click the radio button beside the fax number and then click the [Select] button.
18. Back in the *Fax* window, type *Prescription* in the *Subject* field and ensure that the boxes to *Send InterFax Header* and *Send Cover Note* are checked.
19. Click the [Send] button. The fax will now be transmitted to the pharmacy.
20. Close the *OV* note and skip billing. Close the patient's chart.

10.3 Time Clock

In addition to storing patients' healthcare records, EHR programs are designed to enhance productivity in the medical office by streamlining data collection, facilitating routine workflow in an electronic format, integrating many elements of staff tasks, and minimizing the use and storage of paper documents. SpringCharts's **time clock system** feature supports moving the medical office closer to a paperless environment by providing users with a central location for digitally recording their time in and out of the workplace.

Time clock system
Electronic time clock systems replace cumbersome time-tracking paperwork and eliminate manual collection of payroll information. They enable employee work time and attendance to be organized accurately into reports for payroll.

The *Time Clock* feature is not automatically activated in SpringCharts when the EHR is first installed, because some clinics may choose not to utilize this function. Clinics that do want to use the feature "enable" it from the *Administrator* panel on the SpringCharts server by selecting the *Time Clock Setup* option. The user whose name is placed in the setup window becomes the time clock administrator (Figure 10.10) and receives all employees' time clock information. This person is also responsible for approving or disallowing requested time logged changes in the time clock.

Once the feature is enabled on the SpringCharts server, each client version needs to be rebooted to refresh the feature for each workstation. Figure 10.11 shows the *TimeClock* submenu item available from the *Productivity Center* menu in the *Practice View* screen. The *Time Clock* window on the administrator's log-in is slightly different from the *Time Clock* window on other users'

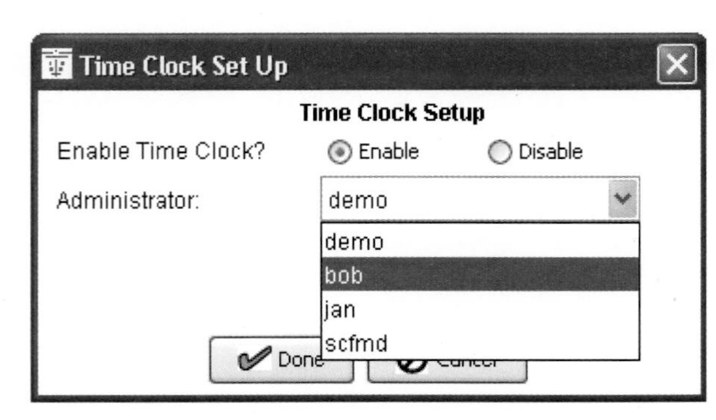

Figure 10.10 *Time Clock Set Up* window.

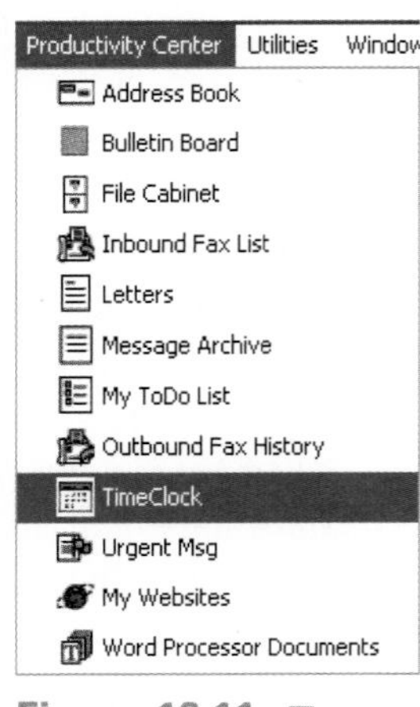

Figure 10.11 *Time Clock* feature in the *Productivity Center* menu.

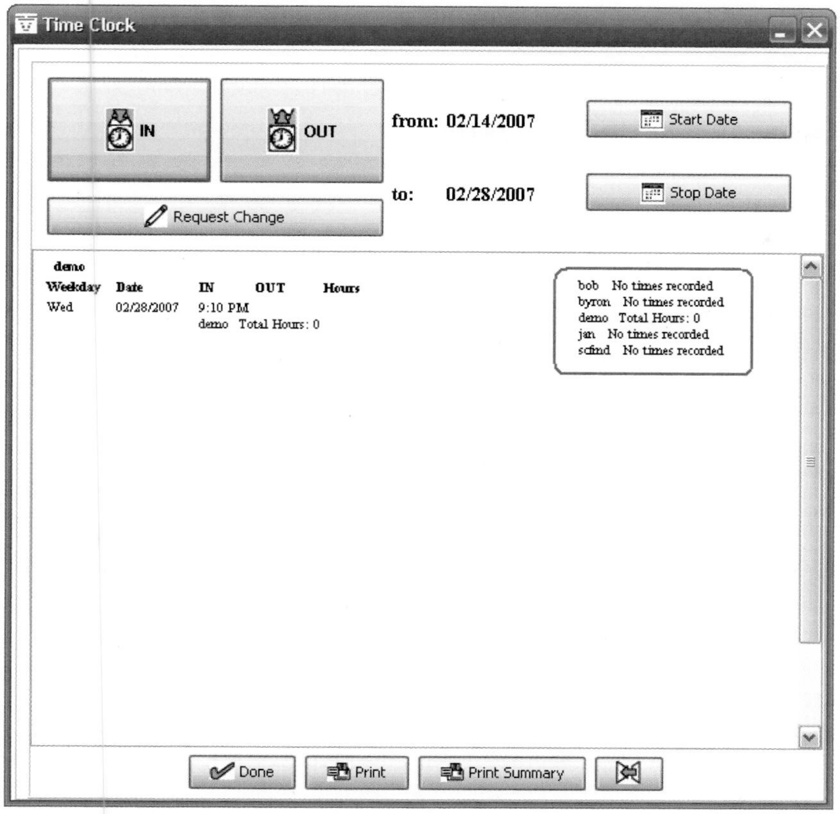

Figure 10.12 Administrator's *Time Clock* window.

screens, in that the administrator's window displays the logged time in and out for *all* users (Figure 10.12). This enables the administrator to run time clock reports over a specific period of time and administer payroll.

Clinic employees use the *Time Clock* feature to record when they arrive at the clinic to work and when they leave. If an employee forgets to log in, he or she can use the [Request Change] button to request a time change from the administrator. This request, when sent, activates a *ToDo/Reminder* item in the administrator's *To Do List* and gives the administrator the opportunity to either approve or deny the request. Once the administrator responds, a message is sent back to the user's *To Do List*, indicating the request was either approved or denied. If the request is approved, SpringCharts automatically updates the user's time clock record to the corrected time. The *Edit Time Clock Item* window and the administrator's response window are seen in Figure 10.13.

Focal Point

The *Time Clock* feature in SpringCharts provides the clinic staff with another means of moving the office toward a paperless environment.

SpringCharts Tip

Shortcut:

Open Time Clock

The eighth speed icon from the left on the *Practice View* screen Toolbar enables users to quickly open the *Time Clock* and record their time in and out of the clinic without opening the *Productivity Center* menu.

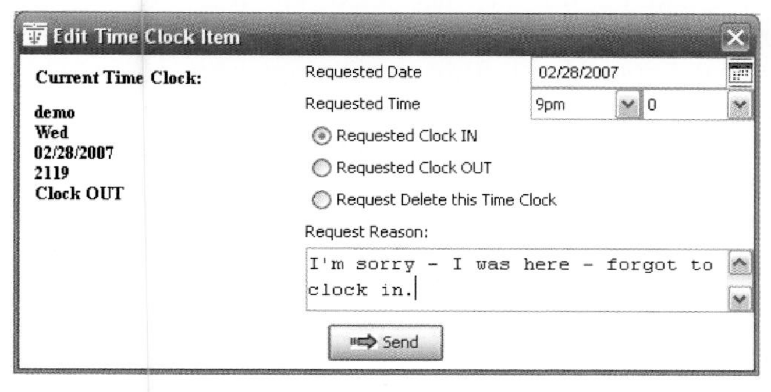

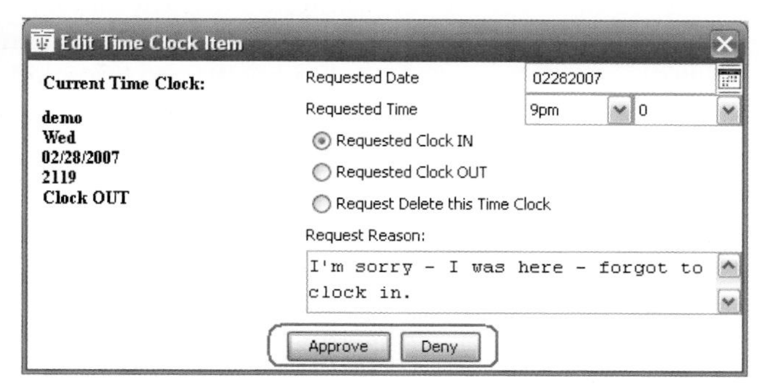

Figure 10.13 *Edit Time Clock Item* windows.

Concept Checkup 10.3

A. Where is the *Time Clock* feature enabled so it becomes available to all users?

B. Requests for time record changes can be sent to the time clock administrator. Where do these change requests appear?

Exercise 10.3 Working with the Time Clock

1. From the *Productivity Center* menu, select *Time Clock.*
2. In the *Time Clock* window, click the [In] button and then confirm the clock-in by selecting [Yes]. Your time-in is stamped into the window.
3. Imagine you were actually in the clinic earlier, but had forgotten to clock in. Click the [Request Change] button and then [Edit] to change your existing time.
4. Highlight the time you clocked in, and the *Edit Time Clock Item* window will open.
5. On the right side of the window, change the time to the top of the hour. In the *Request Reason* text box, type *Was in meeting and then forgot* and then click the [Send] button.
6. The program has now sent your request to the office administrator as an item in the administrator's *To Do List,* marking it with an orange bar. The administrator is able to open the item and either approve or deny the request. If the administrator approves the request, your *Time Clock* will be adjusted to reflect the newly requested time.
7. Close the *Time Clock* window.

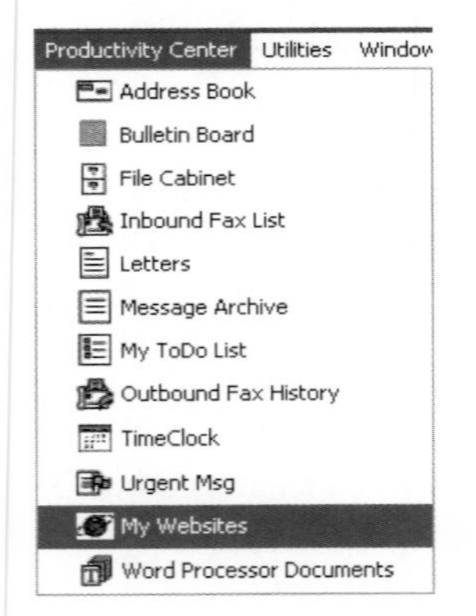

Figure 10.14 Accessing the *My Websites* feature in the *Productivity Center* window.

Focal Point

The *My Websites* feature is a user-defined function of SpringCharts that contains websites commonly accessed by the user.

10.4 My Websites

EHR programs use many Internet databases from which they collect and analyze important and useful data that would be cost-prohibitive to store on computers in medical offices. For this reason, EHR programs allow users to launch important Internet websites from within the program. Many times these features can be customized to meet the individual users' needs.

My Websites is a feature found in SpringCharts's *Productivity Center* menu (Figure 10.14). The *My Websites* window displays a list of websites intended to provide rapid access to Internet-based knowledge systems. For example, patient educational material can be quickly accessed via this means and printed for patients. Figure 10.15 shows the Web addresses of several highly rated healthcare knowledge bases included within the SpringCharts setup. This feature is user-defined, so all users can create their own unique list of website links they access for job-related tasks. The user simply clicks on a website name in the list to activate the browser and go immediately to the website from within SpringCharts.

A user's *My Websites* list can be edited by clicking the [Edit] button, which opens the window shown in Figure 10.16. Here the user enters the website name and address (URL) in the format indicated, and the new website is added to the list.

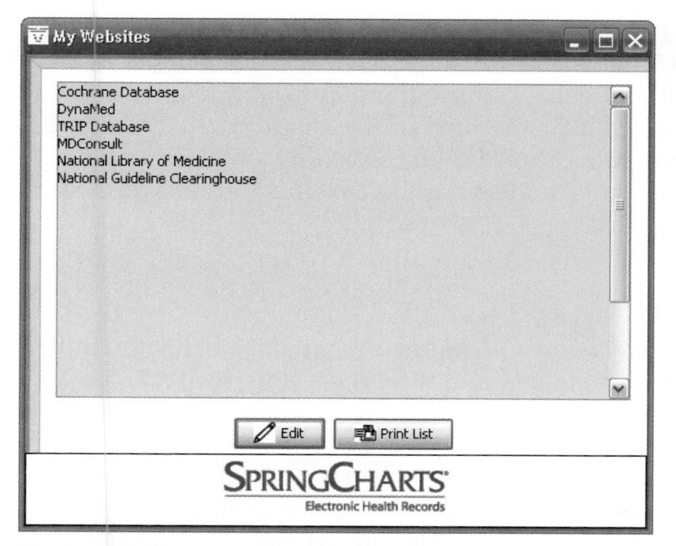

Figure 10.15 List of user-defined websites.

Figure 10.16 *My Websites* setup window.

Concept Checkup 10.4

A. Is the *My Websites* feature user–defined or network-defined?

B. What two items must be added when creating website locations to the *My Websites* feature?

Exercise 10.4 Adding a New Link to *My Websites*

1. Under the *Productivity Center* menu, select the *My Websites* option and click on the [Edit] button.
2. Enter the phrase *Patient Instructions* in the first blank field on the left. Place the cursor as far to the left as possible.
3. In the corresponding field on the right, type in the Web address: *http://www.familydoctor.org* and then click the [Save] button.
4. In the *My Websites* window, click on the newly added *Patient Instructions* link. The Internet browser activates, and you then gain access to the website directly from SpringCharts.
5. Close the Internet browser and the *My Websites* window.

SpringCharts Tip

Shortcut:

Open My Websites

The seventh speed icon from the left on the *Practice View* Toolbar enables the user to quickly access a list of his or her most commonly used Internet sites without first having to open the *Productivity Center.*

10.5 Calculators

Calculators have been used in the medical environment since the 1970s. Many of the healthcare calculations are performed using metric units, and calculators are necessary to convert imperial measurements a patient may give into metric units for uniformity of the healthcare record. In the 1980s, the functionality of hand-held calculators became incorporated into computers, enabling the performance of simple mathematical calculations without leaving the computer. Due to the availability of enhanced programming, computer calculators now permit text editing as well. At the turn of the century, calculators were incorporated into EHR programs to improve the ability of users to convert data from imperial measurements to metric; calculate labor and delivery dates; and conduct simple algorithms.

Focal Point

SpringCharts contains three types of calculators: conversion, delivery date, and simple calculators.

Conversion Calculator

SpringCharts contains a ***Conversion Calculator*** that enables users to convert imperial units to metric measurements and vice versa (Figure 10.17). To activate the *Conversion Calculator,* the user clicks on the *Utilities* menu and selects *Calculator* > *Conversion Calculator*. First, the user types in the measurement in the weight, length, or temperature field, selects the originating units of measure, and then clicks on the [Convert To] button to translate the units to the alternate measurements. The *Conversion Calculator* can convert pounds to kilograms, inches to centimeters, and Fahrenheit to Celsius. It can also convert metric units to imperial measurements.

Conversion Calculator This type of calculator in SpringCharts converts imperial measurements to metric units and converts metric measurements to imperial units in weight, length, and temperature.

Pregnancy EDD Calculator

The ***Pregnancy Estimated Delivery Date (EDD) Calculator*** is useful in determining a pregnant patient's estimated date of delivery (Figure 10.18). The clinician simply selects the first date of the last menstrual period (LMP) using the supplied calendar, and the calculator computes the estimated fetal age and delivery date. This calculator is an essential tool for family physicians and OB/GYNs.

Pregnancy Estimated Delivery Date (EDD) Calculator The EDD calculator has been programmed to add 280 days (9 months and 7 days) to the first day of the patient's last menstrual period (LMP). Use of the LMP date to establish the due date may overestimate the duration of the pregnancy and can be subject to an error of approximately 2 weeks.

Simple Calculator

SpringCharts also provides the user with a basic calculator to process simple calculations, such as addition, subtraction, multiplication, and division.

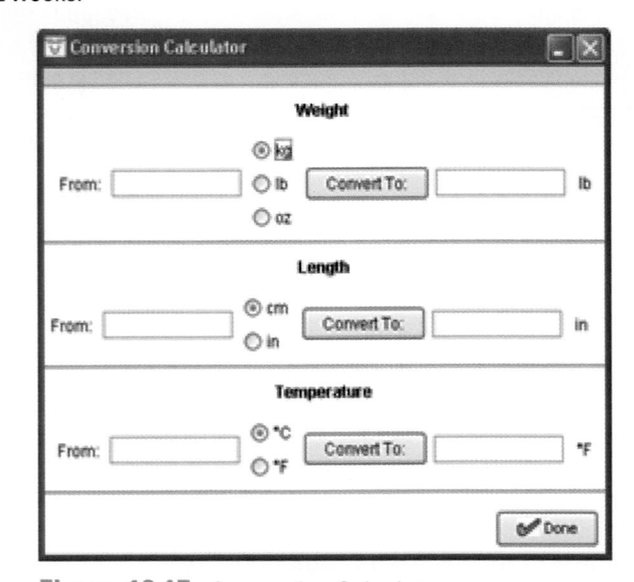

Figure 10.17 *Conversion Calculator.*

Delivery Date Calculator
October
2006
October 2006
Su M T W Th F Sa
First Date of LMP
10/10/2006
Estimated Fetal Age
3 wk(s) and 2 day(s)
Estimated Date of Delivery
07/17/2007
Copy Text
Copy EDD
Done

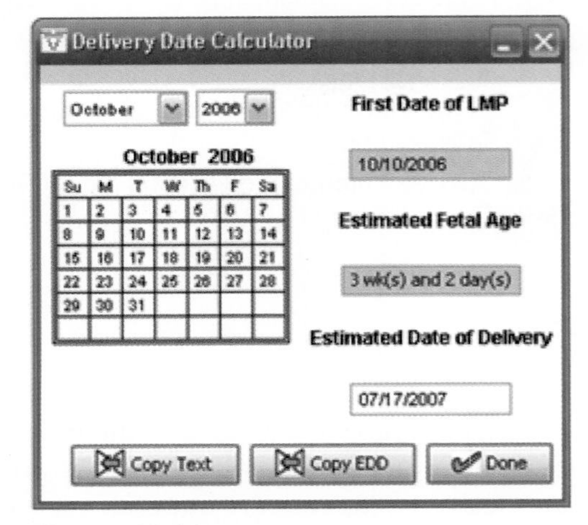

Figure 10.18 *Estimated Delivery Date Calculator.*

Concept Checkup 10.5

A. Which three types of calculators does SpringCharts provide for users?

B. What does the acronym LMP stand for?

Exercise 10.5 Calculating an Estimated Delivery Date

1. Open the *Pregnancy EDD Calculator* under the *Utilities* menu.
2. Assume the first date of the patient's last menstrual period was 6 weeks ago. Select that date from the calendar.
3. Notice that the *First Date of LMP, Estimated Fetal Age,* and *Estimated Date of Delivery* are automatically entered into these fields.
4. Click on the [Copy Text] button and select the [Open in Word Processor] button.
5. Type your name on a new line in the *Notepad* window, print the document by using the *File* menu, and submit to your instructor.
6. Close the word processor window and the calculator window.

10.6 Patient Database Reporting

The ONC has required that all certified EHR programs be able to report on **clinical quality measures (CQMs)** regarding patients' healthcare issues, as outlined in Table 10.1. These reports are submitted to the Centers for Medicare & Medicaid Services (CMS). In 2011, eligible providers (EPs) were required only to attest to the fact that they were able to generate such CQMs. In 2012, EPs qualifying for financial remuneration were required to actually generate the reports and transmit them electronically to CMS. EPs are required to report on 3 mandatory clinical measures (Table 10.2), and then select another 3 CQMs from an alternate list of 41 measures, for a total of 6 clinical measures on which to report. Table 10.3 illustrates an example of

Clinical quality measures (CQMs)
CQMs are measures of processes, experiences, and outcomes of patient care. They encompass observations or treatments that relate to one or more quality aims for healthcare.

Table 10.1 Meaningful Use Core Measure

Clinical Quality Measures	
ONC Stage 1 Objective	**Meaningful Use Measure**
Report on 6 of the patients' clinical quality measures from a list of 41 optional measures.	Report clinical quality measures to CMS or states.

Notes:

- Physicians have the flexibility to select reporting measures most applicable to their practice specialty.
- In 2011, providers needed only to report patient measures by attesting to the fact on the CMS website; for 2012, providers had to electronically submit CQM reports to CMS.

Table 10.2 Mandatory Clinical Quality Measures for Reporting

Measure	Description
Tobacco Use Assessment and Tobacco Cessation Intervention (Preventative Care & Screening pair)	Percentage of patients aged 18 years and older who have been seen for at least 2 office visits and were queried about tobacco use one or more times within 24 months. Percentage of patients aged 18 years and older identified as tobacco users within the past 24 months and seen for at least 2 office visits, who received cessation intervention.
Hypertension: Blood Pressure Measurement	Percentage of patient visits for patients aged 18 years and older with a diagnosis of hypertension who have been seen for at least 2 office visits, with blood pressure (BP) recorded.
Adult Weight Screening and Follow-Up	Percentage of patients aged 18 years and older with a calculated BMI in the past 6 months or during the current visit documented in the medical record *and,* if the most recent BMI is outside parameters, a follow-up plan is documented.

Table 10.3 Examples of Optional Clinical Quality Measures for Reporting

Objective	Description
Weight Assessment and Counseling for Children and Adolescents	Percentage of patients aged 2–17 years who had an outpatient visit with a primary care physician (PCP) or OB/GYN, who had evidence of BMI percentile documentation, and received counseling for nutrition and physical activity during the measurement year.
Diabetes: Blood Pressure Management	Percentage of patients aged 18–75 years with diabetes (type 1 or type 2) who had blood pressure $<$ 140/90 mm Hg.
Asthma Assessment	Percentage of patients aged 5–40 years with a diagnosis of asthma and seen for at least 2 office visits, who were evaluated during at least 1 office visit within 12 months for the frequency (numeric) of daytime and nocturnal asthma symptoms.

3 of the 41 optional clinical measures that an EP will need to report on in order to qualify for financial incentives. All these measures must be recorded in an ONC-certified EHR program from which specific reports are generated. A complete list of optional clinical quality measures are maintained on the CMS website: www.cms.gov.

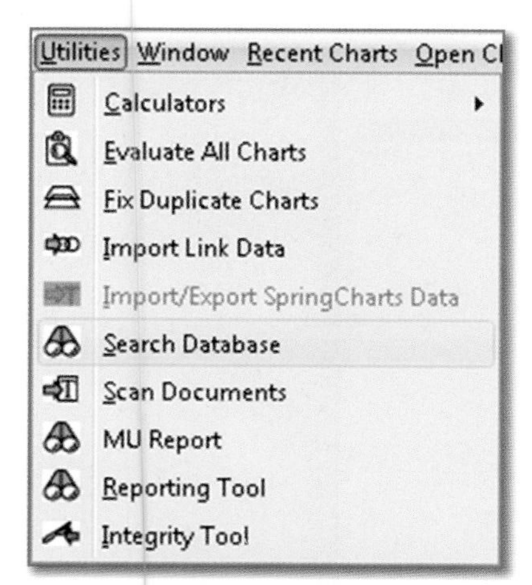

Figure 10.19 Accessing the *Search Database* function.

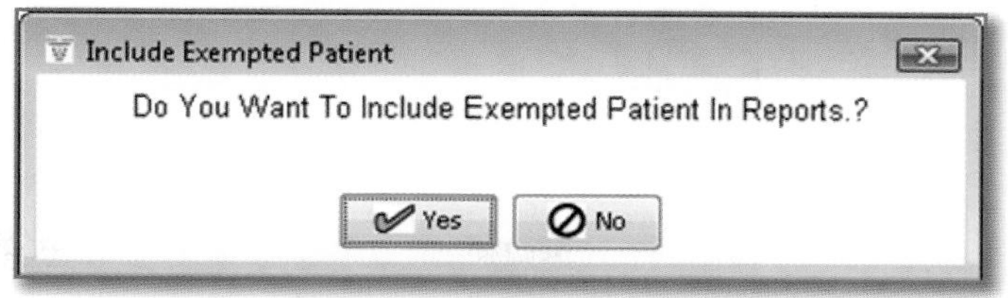

Figure 10.20 Including or excluding exempted patients option.

CQMs are generated by searching patient databases in EHR programs and identifying patients by healthcare issues and diseases. SpringCharts users can conduct database searches via *Utilities > Search Database* (Figure 10.19). A window appears, confirming a database search has been requested. Because the program uses a lot of resources in database searches, other program functions may not operate during the search. For this reason it is best to conduct database searches after working hours. Next, the user is asked if he or she wants to include patients with exempt status in the search (Figure 10.20). Exempt status is given to a patient in the *Edit Patient* window, located under the main *Edit* menu and the *Patients* submenu. After searching for and selecting a patient, the user clicks the [Exempt] button to exclude him or her from database-generated reports. However, the patient will remain active in the EHR program. The [Exempt] button then changes to [UnExempt] in the *Edit Patient* window, enabling the user to include the patient in future database reports. A clinic may exempt patients from reports for several reasons. For example, the physician may be involved in clinical trials using experimental treatments for patients with specific healthcare issues. These patients may be exempted from regular patient reports so the resulting figures are not skewed. The user would do so by clicking the [No] button in this *Include Exempted Patient* window.

SpringCharts Tip

It is best if all users log out of SpringCharts before a database search is conducted.

SpringCharts Tip

An unlocked encounter can still produce a routing slip; i.e., the billing of an office visit note is not held up because the provider has not yet finalized and locked the note.

SpringCharts users can search the entire database of patient charts by diagnosis, drug, procedure, test, insurance company, employer, provider, age, or patient category (Figure 10.21). The *Search Database* function can also be used to locate all encounters that are still open. An open encounter is any office visit, nurse note, or other note stored under the *Encounters* tab in the care tree that has not been signed and permanently locked. Sometimes a provider leaves an office visit note unsigned because he or she needs to return to the note at a later time to complete the documentation. Searching the database for unlocked encounters enables providers to locate incomplete encounter notes, finalize them, sign, and then lock the notes.

In the general *Search Database* option, the clinician can choose only one search criterion from the list of options. Once the criterion has been selected, the *Search Results* window displays a list of qualifying patients (Figure 10.22). If the user wants to review more information on any of these patients, he or she

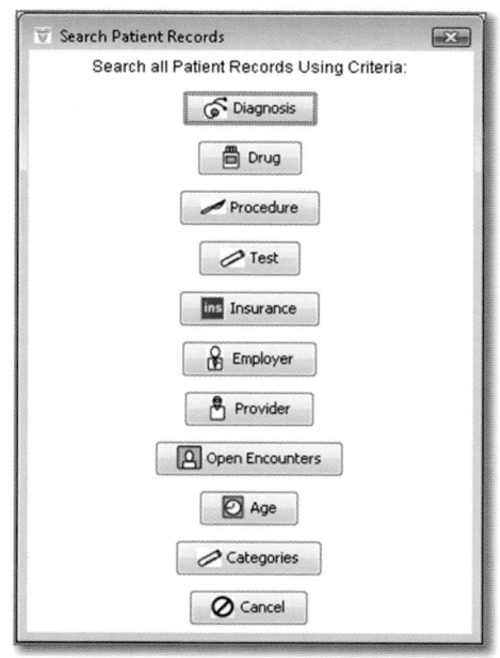

Figure 10.21 Criteria in the *Search Patient Records* window.

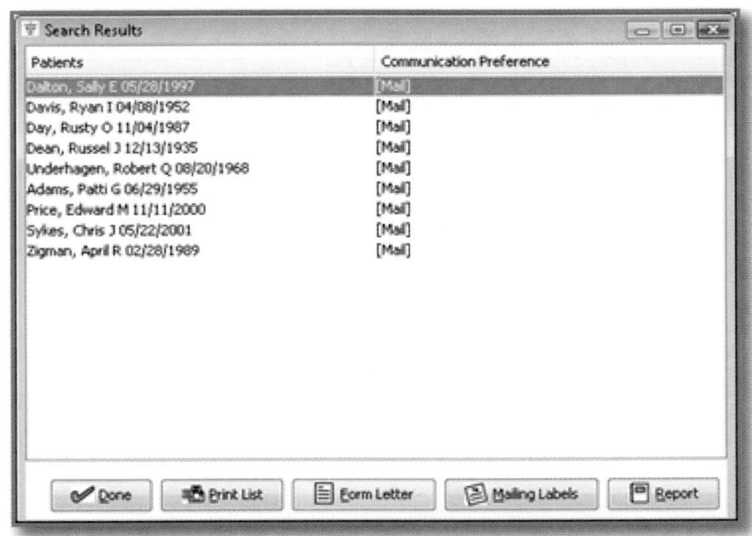

Figure 10.22 *Search Results* window, showing the list of qualifying patients.

highlights the desired patient, and a *Patient Data* window displays. From here, patient demographics can be viewed, edited, and printed, and the user can access the patient's chart. From the *Search Results* window, the user can print the list of qualifying patients, create a form letter, print mailing labels for the qualifying patients, and create reports detailing more specific information about the patients.

Form Letters

To send a form letter to the list of selected patients, the user selects the [Form Letter] button and enters the subject and text of the proposed letter (Figure 10.23). After clicking [Done], the user is given the option to print the newly created template letter for the selected patients. The letter automatically prints the patients' names and addresses in the letter's introductory section. The EHR program prompts the user to choose whether to print the letters with the letterhead and include a copy of the letter in each patient's charts. Physicians who process these letters are given the option to sign the letters electronically.

Mailing labels for the listed patients are created by selecting the [Mailing Labels] button in the *Search Results* window. The labels print in a three-column format to fit commonly used precut, self-adhesive label sheets.

Focal Point

Form letters and reports can be created from patient lists generated through the *Search Database* feature.

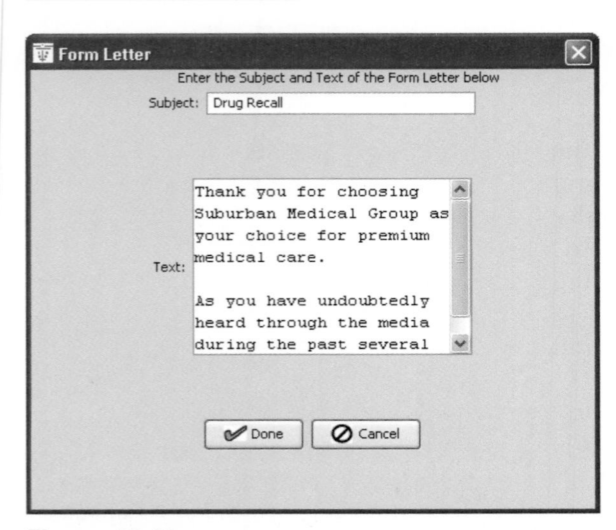

Figure 10.23 Creating a form letter from the *Search Database* results.

Reports

The ONC requires that a certified EHR system must contain the ability to generate lists of patients based specifically on diagnosis (Table 10.4). For example, in Stage 1 of MU qualifications, a physician must be able to generate a list of all patients with diabetes. Lists of patients grouped by diagnosis are useful for research, patient communication and outreach.

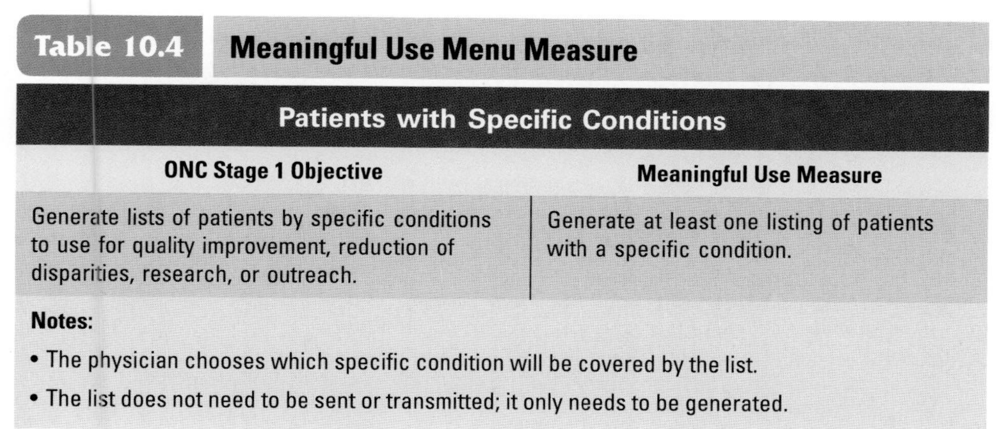

Table 10.4 Meaningful Use Menu Measure

Patients with Specific Conditions	
ONC Stage 1 Objective	**Meaningful Use Measure**
Generate lists of patients by specific conditions to use for quality improvement, reduction of disparities, research, or outreach.	Generate at least one listing of patients with a specific condition.

Notes:

- The physician chooses which specific condition will be covered by the list.
- The list does not need to be sent or transmitted; it only needs to be generated.

Reports can be created in SpringCharts based on the list of patients identified by the *Search Database* criteria. To create a report, the user selects the [Report] button in the *Search Results* window. From the *Include in Report* window (Figure 10.24), the user selects various patient demographics to be included in the report. For more detailed healthcare information the user can cross-reference the list of patients to specific procedures and diagnoses recorded in the patients' charts by selecting the [Add] button in the respective areas. Figure 10.25 illustrates how to cross-reference the list of patients to a procedure. In this case, the report lists the patients who fit the selected demographics and have undergone the selected procedure (Figure 10.26). The report can then be printed out.

In the *Include in Report* window, the user is also given the option to include a list of encounters (date and title only) recorded in the patients' care trees under the *Encounters* category. The user can list all encounters or the most recent one.

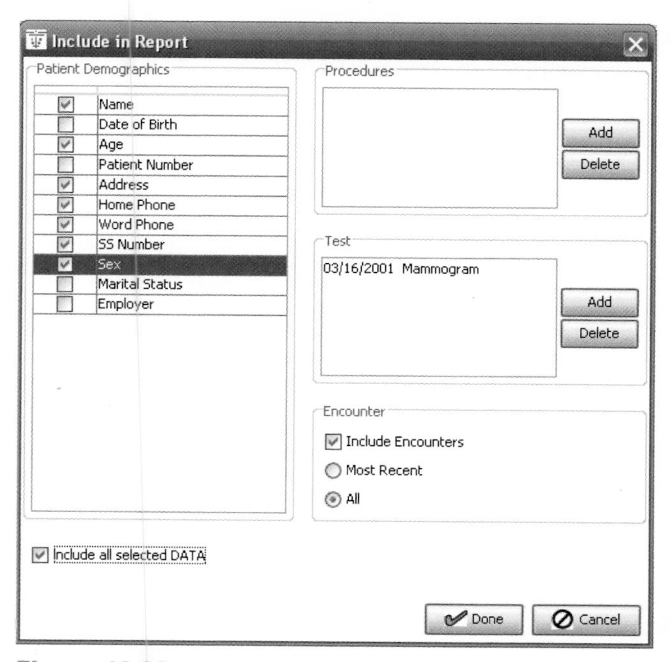

Figure 10.24 Options in the *Include in Report* window.

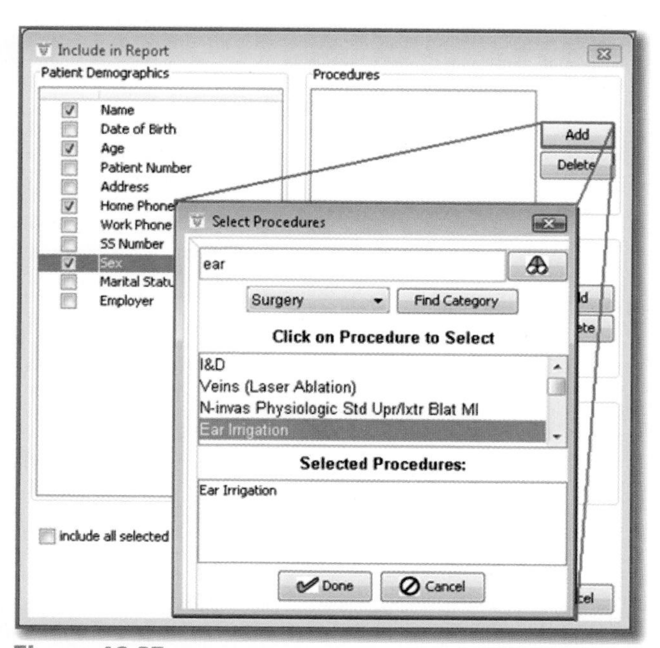

Figure 10.25 Selecting a procedure to cross-reference with the patients in the report.

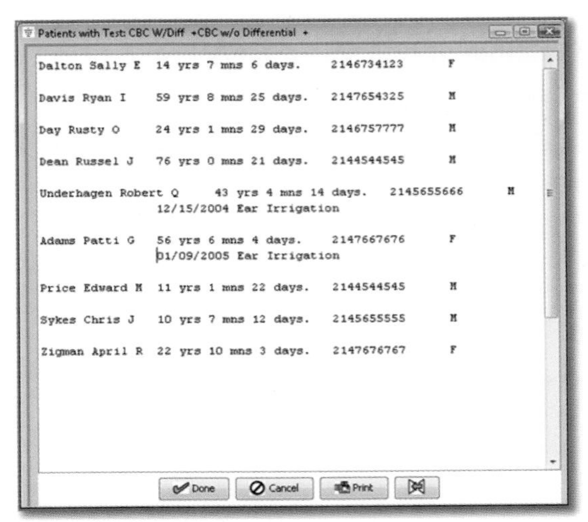

Figure 10.26 Report displaying patients by selected criteria.

Concept Checkup 10.6

A. Name three of the criteria by which patients can be searched in the SpringCharts database.

B. What two options are given to the user once the list of patients has been created?

C. List three items that can be included in the patient report.

Exercise 10.6 Searching the Medical Database

1. Under the *Utilities* menu, select *Search Database.*
2. Click [Yes] to *Search All Patient Records Now?* and *Do You Want To Include Exempted Patients In Reports?* and *You cannot use other functions during a search. Continue?* in the next windows.
3. Select the [Drug] button as the criterion to search by.
4. Type *Lipitor* in the *Find* field and conduct a search. The program displays all strengths of the drug Lipitor.
5. Click on all of the medications to add them to the *Selected Drugs* window.
6. Click the [Done] button, and the program will then begin searching the patient database for patients who have been prescribed the medication Lipitor.
7. In the *Search Results* window, select [Form Letter].
8. In the *Form Letter* window, type in the subject: *Drug Recall.*
9. In the text field, type a letter informing the patients the drug Lipitor has been recalled. Include your name and ask that they contact you to schedule a visit to follow up.
10. When completed, click the [Done] button.
11. In the *Choose Action Below* window, select [Print Letters] and choose *Yes* to chart the letters, print the letterhead, and sign the letters electronically. Print the letters.
12. Close the print window and the search window.
13. Open Russel Dean's chart.
14. Look for the letter you just sent, which has been saved under the *Encounters* category in the patient's care tree. Close the chart.
15. Circle your name on Russel Dean's letter and hand in to your instructor.

10.7 Patient Archive

EHR programs can store millions of patients' healthcare records. It is important, however, that medical clinics keep up-to-date records of the patients currently being seen by the practitioner and who are under medical care. This also allows healthcare reports to be as accurate as possible. The population in the United States is more mobile than at any other time in history. The nature of the computerized workforce and individual transportation enables workers to live almost anywhere in the nation and conduct business. EHR programs have the ability to remove patients from their active lists while still maintaining access to their medical records. When patients move out of the community or when patients are deceased, clinicians can **archive** the patients' charts. When a patient's chart is archived, the patient's name no longer appears in the day-to-day search function; however, his or her medical record has not been removed from the EHR program.

Archive
In electronic terms, this long-term storage folder or device contains records and information of groups of patients no longer used but important to keep for future reference.

The patient archive feature in SpringCharts allows an administrator to move a patient from the current patient list to the archived patient list, while retaining access to the patient's records. To archive a patient, the administrator selects the *Patients* submenu from the main *Edit* menu and searches for the patient who needs to be archived (Figure 10.27). The administrator then clicks on the [Archive] button to remove the patient from active lists within the EHR program.

Once archived, the patient's data can be viewed and the record reactivated if needed. To do so, under the main *Edit* menu, the user selects the *Patient Archives* submenu. The patient can be located by various criteria: last name, first name, middle initial, birth date, address, city, state, zip code, SS number, patient number, date archived, or mother's last name.

Figure 10.28 shows that a patient's chart information can be viewed even when the patient has been archived. This is done by selecting the [View Chart] button in the *Archive Patient* window. The *Archived Patient Chart* window displays a text record of all items within the chart. The information is displayed

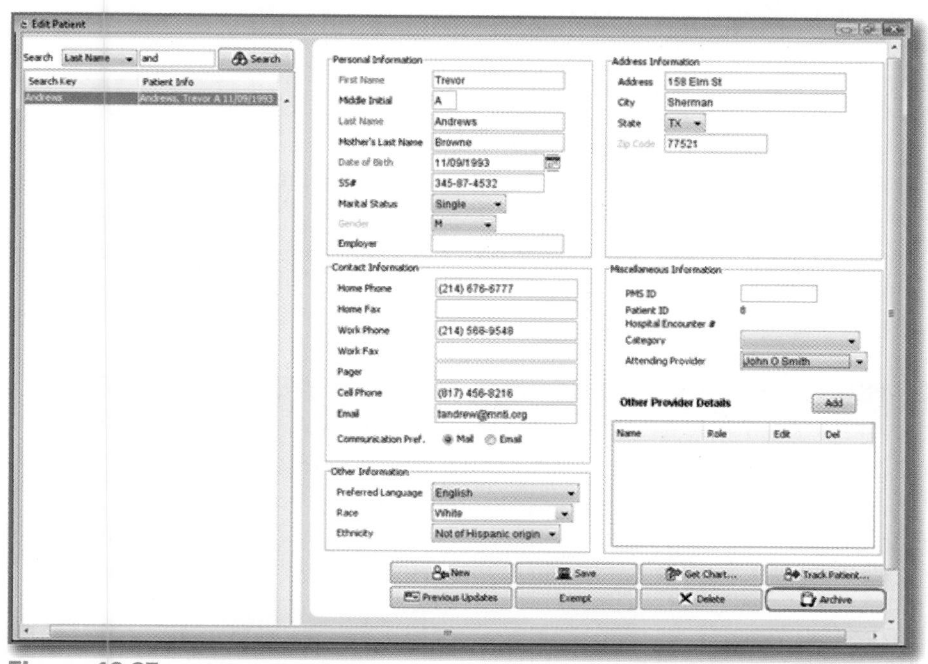

Figure 10.27 *Edit Patient* window

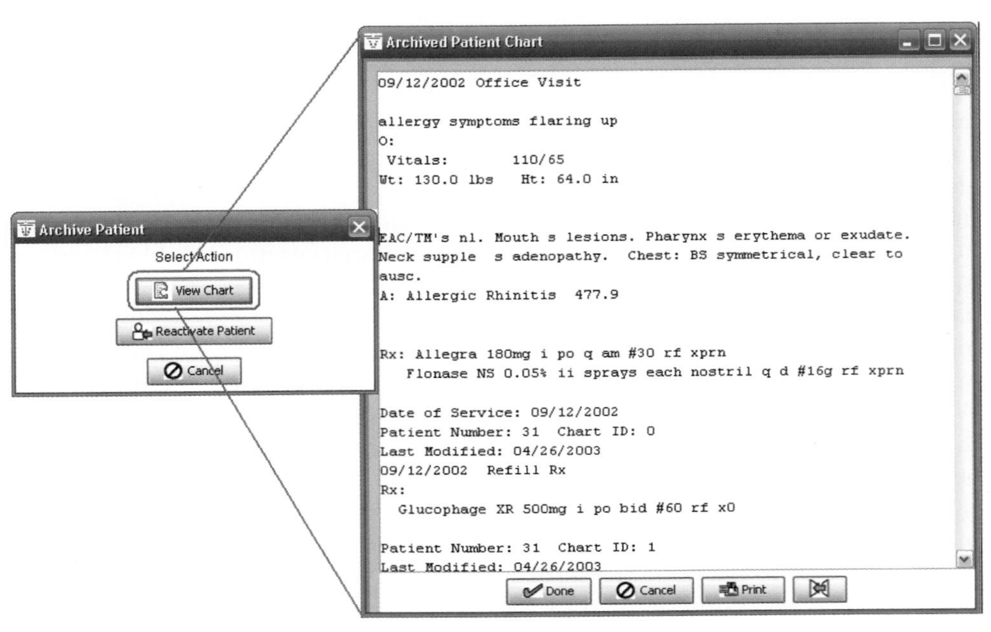

Figure 10.28 [View Chart] option for an archived patient.

by chronological order based on when the item was originally added to the chart. The oldest information appears at the top, and the patient's demographic information appears at the bottom of the documentation. Information in the *Archived Patient Chart* window cannot be altered. It can, however, be printed by using the [Print] button. When the chart record is displayed for an archived patient, the user can export these old records as a .txt file by using the *Export* icon and then opening the file in another program or sending it to a PDA or iPod folder.

Documents stored in the patient's *File Cabinet* prior to archiving the patient's chart are not included in the *Archived Patient Chart* window. However, when the patient is reactivated, the former *File Cabinet* documents are also reactivated in the patient's care tree.

Focal Point

Patients who are no longer active in the clinic may be archived from the main database of SpringCharts. Although the patient can then no longer be viewed in the program, the medical records still can be viewed and reactivated if necessary.

Concept Checkup 10.7

A. The patient archive feature allows the user to remove a patient's name from the day-to-day search in the program. However, what does the user still have access to?

B. Can an archived patient's information be viewed without needing to reactivate the patient?

Exercise 10.7 Archiving a Patient's Record

1. Select the *Edit* menu from the *Practice View* screen and then *Patients*.
2. In the *Edit Patient* window, find the patient *Ann Carnijay*.
3. Archive Ann by pressing the [Archive] button in the lower right and answering *Yes* to the query, *Are you sure you want to archive this patient?* Her name then will disappear from the patient list.

Exercise 10.7 (Concluded)

4. Close the *Edit Patient* window.
5. Open the *Edit* menu once again and select *Patient Archives.*
6. In the *Patient Archive* window, search for Ann Carnijay by last name.
7. Highlight the patient in the list and select the [View Chart] button in the *Patient Archives* window. Notice that the *Patient Archives* window also enables you to reactivate the patient into the active lists in SpringCharts if necessary.
8. Close the *Patient Archives* windows.
9. Now reactivate Ann Carnijay. In the *Edit* menu, open the *Patient Archives* window.
10. Locate the archived patient. This time, select the [Reactivate Patient] button. A progress bar appears, indicating the patient is being placed back into the active list of patients in SpringCharts. Close the *PATIENT ARCHIVES* window.

chapter 10 summary

Learning Outcomes	Key Concepts
10.1 Demonstrate how to post a new item on the EHR's *Bulletin Board.* **Pages 271–273**	The *Productivity Center* and *Utilities* menus bring together in one place some of the most common functions of SpringCharts. The *Bulletin Board* is network-defined and contains general messages for all in the clinic to read and print. Each user needs to routinely check the *Bulletin Board* for new messages; there is no automatic announcement when items are placed on the board.
10.2 List the steps to send and receive electronic faxes. **Pages 273–276**	SpringCharts interfaces with *InterFax* (www.Interfax.net) to allow users to send and receive faxes over the Internet to and from any SpringCharts client computer. The fax feature is available in SpringCharts anywhere the print function is available. The status of outbound faxes is checked in the *Outbound Fax History* feature. Incoming faxes are located in *Inbound Fax List* feature in the *Productivity Center* menu. An internal e-mail is sent to the authorized user notifying the user a fax has been received. Incoming faxes can be stored directly in the patient's *File Cabinet* in the care tree.
10.3 Use the *Time Clock* feature. **Pages 276–278**	The *Time Clock* feature records users' time in and out of the workplace. The administrator whose name appears within the *Time Clock Setup* receives all the employees' time clock information. An employee who fails to log in or out at the appropriate time can electronically request a time change from the administrator. The time clock administrator can run reports to analyze employees' work time.
10.4 Set up and use the *My Websites* feature. **Pages 278–279**	The *My Websites* feature in the *Productivity Center* menu lists websites that provide rapid access to Internet-based knowledge systems. *My Websites* is user-defined so all users can have their own unique list of website links.
10.5 Demonstrate the use of three types of electronic calculators. **Pages 279–281**	SpringCharts contains three types of calculators: conversion, pregnancy, and simple calculators. • A *Conversion Calculator* converts imperial units to metric measurements and vice versa. • A *Pregnancy Calculator* calculates estimated date of delivery. • A *Simple Calculator* processes basic algorithms.

Learning Outcomes	Key Concepts
10.6 Perform a search of the medical database. **Pages 281–286**	The ONC requires all certified EHR programs have the ability to report on clinical quality measures (CQMs) and list patients by diagnoses. EPs are required to report on 3 mandatory clinical measures and then select another 3 CQMs from an alternate list of 41 measures. SpringCharts can exempt specific patients from reports generated from the database. SpringCharts can sort patients by 10 categories and search the database for still-open encounter notes. Users can create and send form letters to the list of selected patients. Mailing labels can be created. Reports can be generated from lists of patients that include demographic information and are cross-referenced to specific procedures and diagnoses recorded in the patients' charts.
10.7 Describe how to archive a patient's records. **Pages 287–289**	A patient's name and record can be archived. The patient then no longer appears in the routine search function; however, the medical record is not removed from the EHR program. Archived patient data can be viewed and printed, and the patient record can be reactivated if needed.

chapter 10 review

Name ______________________ Instructor ______________ Class ______________ Date ______________

Using Terminology

Match the terms on the left with the definitions on the right.

_____ 1. **LO 10.5** Conversion Calculator

_____ 2. **LO 10.5** Pregnancy EDD Calculator

_____ 3. **LO 10.7** Archive

_____ 4. **LO 10.3** Time Clock System

_____ 5. **LO 10.2** InterFax

_____ 6. **LO 10.6** CQMs

A. This SpringCharts feature replaces the need for tracking paperwork and eliminates manual collection of payroll information.

B. This subscriber-based online service enables SpringCharts users to send and receive faxes wherever Internet access is available.

C. Enables clinical staff to change imperial units to metric measurements and vice versa.

D. Allows an administrator to remove a patient from the current list but still retain access to the patient's records.

E. With a selected LMP date, extrapolates the estimated date of delivery.

F. Measures regarding quality of patients' healthcare; EPs required to submit to CMS.

Checking Your Understanding

Choose the best answer and circle the corresponding letter.

7. **LO 10.1** The electronic *Bulletin Board* feature in SpringCharts replaces the typical bulletin board in the break room and is:
   a) User-defined
   b) Network-defined
   c) Accessed only by the administrator
   d) Accessed only by the physicians

8. **LO 10.2** InterFax service allows users to send and receive faxes to and from any company in the world if they have:
   a) Security access in SpringCharts
   b) A paperless environment
   c) Internet access
   d) No office fax machine

9. **LO 10.3** The *Time Clock* feature in SpringCharts is *inactive* by default when the program is first installed because:
   a) The *Time Clock* is an optional feature.
   b) Clinics don't typically track employees' attendance.
   c) The *Time Clock* takes too long to activate.
   d) It is a complex module.

10. **LO 10.3** The administrator's *Time Clock* window displays the logged-in and -out time of all:
    a) Tardy users
    b) Excused users
    c) Administrative users
    d) Users

11. **LO 10.4** The *My Websites* feature lists a user's websites, intended to provide rapid access to:
    a) Internet-based healthcare knowledge systems
    b) Personalized private websites
    c) A user's most popular websites
    d) The clinic's authorized websites

12. **LO 10.5** By using the EDD calculator the clinician can determine the:
    a) Date the patient conceived
    b) Metric conversion from imperial units
    c) Estimated date of delivery
    d) Earliest due date

13. **LO 10.1** In the *Productivity Center* the users have access to one menu where regular administrative activities can be performed such as (select all that apply):
    a) Posting on the *Bulletin Board*
    b) Searching the patient database
    c) Checking inbound and outbound faxes
    d) Accessing favorite websites

14. **LO 10.7** A reason a clinician may archive a patient is:
    a) The patient has moved out of the area.
    b) There are too many patients in the database.
    c) The patient is a family member of the physician.
    d) The patient is above 65 years of age.

15. **LO 10.6** To qualify for MU in 2012, EPs must transmit CQM reports to CMS containing:
    a) Weight assessment, blood pressure management, and asthma assessment
    b) 3 core measures and 3 alternate measures
    c) 6 measures from the 41 alternate measures supplied by the ONC
    d) Patient diagnoses, medications, procedures, and tests

16. **LO 10.6** Data reports can be created based on the list of patients identified by:
    a) Archived patient criteria
    b) The *Encounters* criteria in the care tree
    c) The *Search Database* criteria
    d) Diseased patients

17. **LO 10.2** Because the EHR program uses an Internet service to transmit and receive faxes, the clinic does not need to:
    a) Receive any more mail
    b) Print any more documents
    c) Maintain a separate analog phone/fax line
    d) Receive electronic lab results

18. **LO 10.6** Some of the criteria that a user may select to search the entire database of patients are:
   a) Medications and allergies
   b) Diagnoses and procedures
   c) Archived patients
   d) Medications, allergies, diagnoses, and procedures

19. **LO 10.5** With the simple calculator, users can:
   a) Count simple sugar grams for diabetic patients
   b) Process simple algorithms
   c) Have medication dosages broken down into simple compounds
   d) Convert imperial measurements to metric units

20. **LO 10.3** If employees fail to log in on their time clock at the appropriate time, they can:
   a) Reset their time clock to the appropriate time
   b) Send a note to the administrator requesting a time change
   c) Use the manual time clock and "punch in"
   d) Reboot the computer

21. **LO 10.4** This speed icon enables the user to rapidly access:
   a) *Time Clock*
   b) *My Websites*
   c) *Bulletin Board*
   d) *Report Center*

22. **LO 10.7** When a patient is archived, the patient's chart information:
   a) Can still be viewed
   b) Can no longer be viewed
   c) Is deleted from the system
   d) Can only be printed out

23. **LO 10.4** The *My Website* feature is:
   a) User-defined so each user can have his or her own list of websites
   b) Networked-defined so the clinic can operate off the same websites
   c) Preset with a limited number of activated websites
   d) Not activated when SpringCharts is first installed

24. **LO 10.1** This speed icon enables the user to rapidly access:
   a) *My Websites*
   b) *Time Clock*
   c) *Bulletin Board*
   d) *Received Faxes*

25. **LO 10.5** The *Conversion Calculator* can convert:
   a) 12-hour time to military time
   b) Years to months
   c) Fahrenheit to Celsius
   d) LMP date to the EDD date

Applying Your Knowledge

Use your critical-thinking skills to answer the following questions.

26. **LO 10.2** In a typical medical office, faxes arrive throughout the day and are printed out by the fax machine. If the fax is regarding a patient's healthcare, it is then be scanned and stored in the patient's electronic chart. The hardcopy is then shredded. If the medical office has an EHR that sends and receives faxes via the Internet, how does this process differ and what are the benefits?

27. **LO 10.7** A patient has moved out of the community and has requested a copy of his or her electronic chart be sent to a new primary care provider. The patient has been gone for 5 years; however, the patient has now moved back into the community. What does the clinic need to do instead of creating a new chart for the patient?

28. **LO 10.6** Suppose that the AMA has notified the physician in your clinic that the drug Actos has been recalled because of possible risks of bladder cancer. Your physician wants you to create a letter for all patients taking Actos who have had a urinalysis. How would you go about doing this?

11

Applying Your Knowledge

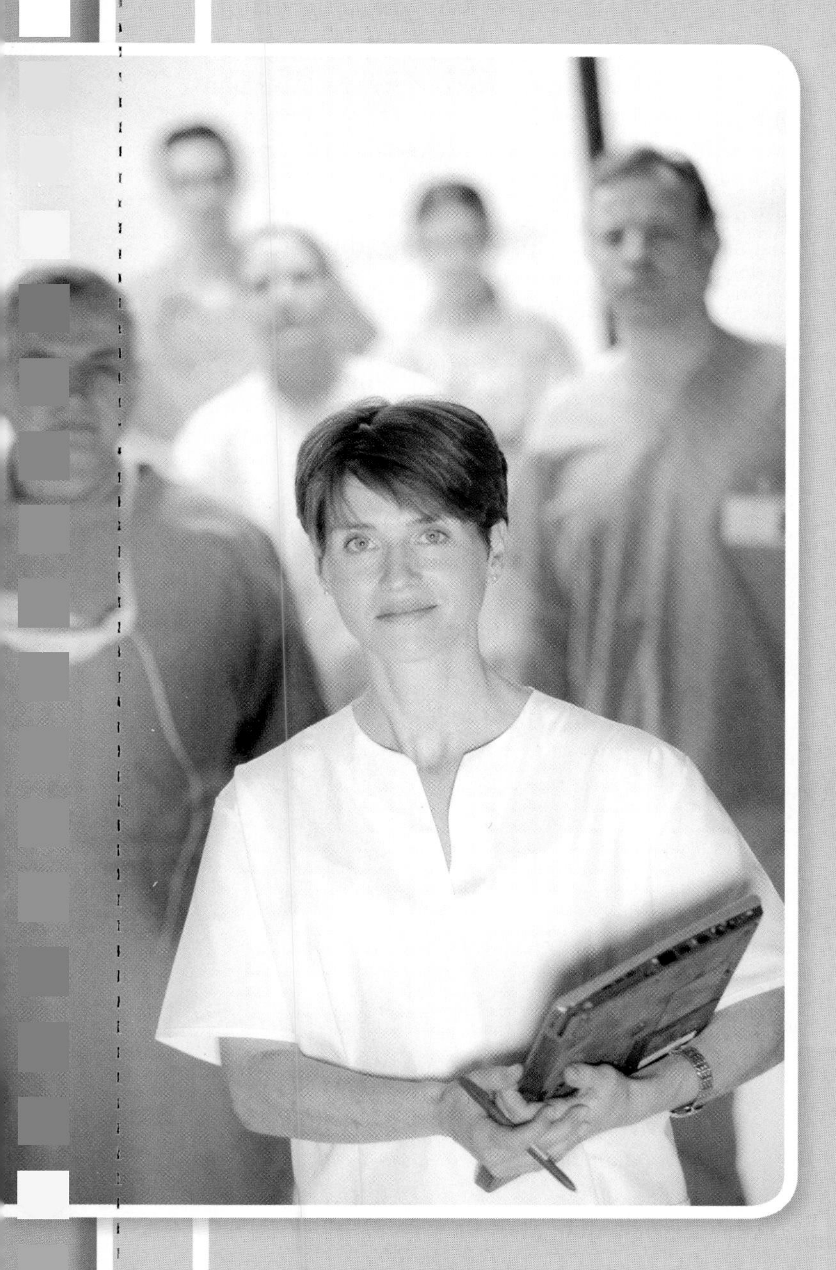

Learning Outcomes

After completing Chapter 11, you will be able to:

LO 11.1 Successfully function in all aspects of the *Practice View* screen.

LO 11.2 Successfully function in all aspects of the *Patient Chart* screen.

LO 11.3 Successfully function in all aspects of the *Office Visit* screen.

What You Need to Know

To understand Chapter 11, you will need to know:

- How to navigate within the *Practice View* screen
- How to navigate within the *Patient Chart* screen
- How to navigate within the *Office Visit* screen

Introduction

EHR programs were initially designed to record patient medical data and provide a central location for all healthcare providers to access the patient's health information. However, they have evolved into much more than a repository of medical records. As demonstrated throughout this book, the EHR program is used by every member of a medical office. Administrative staff members use the EHR program to schedule appointments, process new patients, track patients during their office visits, record phone calls, coordinate communication between staff and patients, and order supplies, among other activities. Clinical staff members use the EHR program to process physician orders, record test results, manage referrals, administer patient requests for medical reports, create excuse notes, maintain immunization records, and so on. Medical assistants can now execute many of their responsibilities through EHR programs, including recording patients' personal healthcare information, family medical history, medications, chief complaints, and vitals, as well as test results and procedures. Coding and billing specialists maintain up-to-date procedure and diagnosis descriptions and codes in the EHR program, ensuring the medical clinic is reimbursed at the maximum rate and with the greatest efficiency.

Patients are also an interactive component of the EHR program. Patients can now request healthcare information, record medical data, print personal records, and communicate with medical staff through the security of patient portals over the Internet.

The advanced exercises presented in this chapter enable you to process many clerical and clinical functions of the medical office through the EHR program. They are designed to bring together many duties of the front office, clinical area, and back office so you can apply the knowledge gained from studying specific elements of the EHR program and incorporate this information into practical tasks. Chapter 11 is designed to be a self-study chapter in preparation for Chapter 12 in which you will be required to navigate to many different sections of the EHR program to input data. Use the figures associated with each exercise in this chapter to check your work. You will not be turning in any work.

11.1 Practice View Screen

Office Schedule

Exercise 11.1 Setting Up New Patients

(Refer to Chapter 3, page 72)

1. Set up a new patient in the *New Patient* window (Figure 11.1) with the following information:

   Dustin J. Eatman

   6021 Hodges Place
   Mansfield, TX 76063
   DOB: 10/5/73 (mmddyyyy)
   SS#: 456-78-2371
   Male
   Home Phone: (817) 473-0328
   Work Phone: (817) 966-2484
   Cell Phone: (817) 504-0903
   E-mail: dustine@nofencedland.net
   Employer: No Fenced Land Company
   Mother's Last Name: Hubbard

   Dustin is a white Caucasian, of non-Hispanic origin, and speaks English. He is married to Carrie and has two children, Dillon and Emma. He carries insurance on the family. His attending provider is Dr. Finchman, the family's primary care physician.
2. Save Dustin's information.
3. To set up a second, related patient (Dustin's son, Dillon), go to the *Edit* menu and select *Patients.*
4. In the search field of the *Edit Patient* window (Figure 11.2), type the name *eatman* and locate Dustin Eatman.
5. Select the [New] button and answer *Yes* to the question, *Do you want to use the displayed data?* Notice

Exercise 11.1 (Concluded)

that much of Dustin Eatman's information is carried across into the new record.

6. Enter the following information about Dillon:

   Dillon B. Eatman was born on October 16, 1998.

   He does not have an e-mail address.

   His Social Security number is: 456-67-9451.

   Dillon's cell phone number is: (682) 559-2611.

   Delete or change any information that is not applicable to Dillon.

7. Save the record and close the *Edit Patient* window.

New Patient
First Name*:
Dustin
MI:
J
Last Name*:
Eatman
Date of Birth*:
10/05/1973
Address:
6021 Hodges Place
City:
Mansfield
State:
TX
Zip+:
76063
Gender+:
Male
Female
Unknown
Marital Status:
Married
Employer:
No Fenced Land Company
EMail:
dustine@nofencedland.net
SS#:
456-78-2371
Category:
Preferred Language#:
English
Race#:
White
Ethnicity#:
Not of Hispanic ori...
Home Phone:
(817) 473-0328
Home Fax:
Work Phone:
(817) 966-2484
Work Fax:
Pager:
Mobile Phone:
(817) 504-0903
PMS ID:
Patient ID:
Mother's Last Name:
Hubbard
Attending Provider#:
Stephen C Finchm...
Other Provider Details
Add
Name
Role
Edit
Del
* Required
+ Required for eRx
# Required for MU
Previous Updates
Exempt
Save

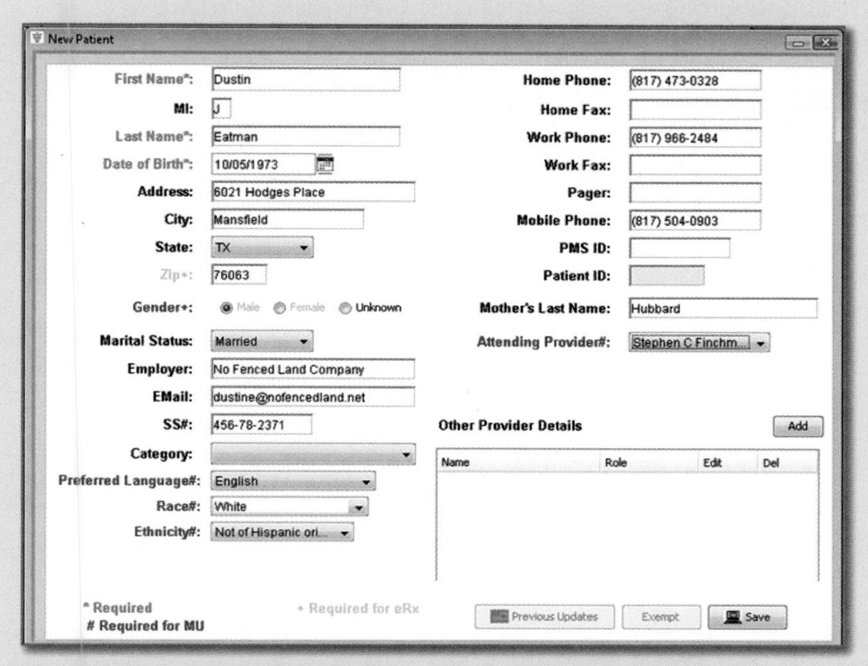

Figure 11.1 *New Patient* window.

Edit Patient
Search
Last Name
Search
Search Key
Patient Info
Personal Information
First Name
Dillon
Middle Initial
B
Last Name
Eatman
Mother's Last Name
Hubbard
Date of Birth
10/16/1998
SS#
456-67-9451
Marital Status
Single
Gender
M
Employer
Address Information
Address
6021 Hodges Place
City
Mansfield
State
TX
Zip Code
76063
Contact Information
Home Phone
(817) 473-0328
Home Fax
Work Phone
Work Fax
Pager
Cell Phone
(682) 559-2611
Email
Communication Pref.
Mail
Email
Miscellaneous Information
PMS ID
Patient ID
Hospital Encounter #
Category
Attending Provider
Stephen C Finchman
Other Provider Details
Add
Name
Role
Edit
Del
Other Information
Preferred Language
English
Race
White
Ethnicity
Not of Hispanic origin
New
Save
Get Chart...
Track Patient...
Previous Updates
UnExempt
Delete
Archive

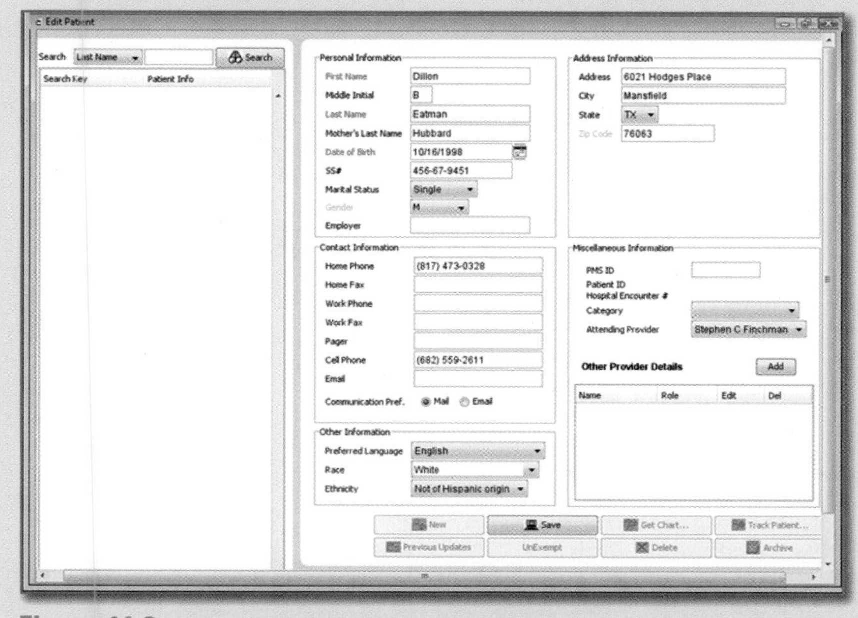

Figure 11.2 *Edit Patient* window for Dillon Eatman.

Exercise 11.2 Scheduling and Updating Patient Information

(Refer to Chapter 4, page 87)

1. If your main screen of SpringCharts is not the patient schedule, click on the *Actions* menu and select the *Change View* submenu. Select the *Calendar* option.
2. From the *Practice View* screen (Figure 11.3), add both Dustin and Dillon to today's schedule. Dustin is presenting for a routine well visit and Dillon is presenting for diarrhea.
3. On today's schedule block out from 4 p.m. to 5 p.m. for a staff meeting.
4. Dustin indicates on the sign-in sheet that his cell phone number has changed to an out-of-state number: (214) 766-8271. Update the patient's record under the *Edit* menu (Figure 11.4).

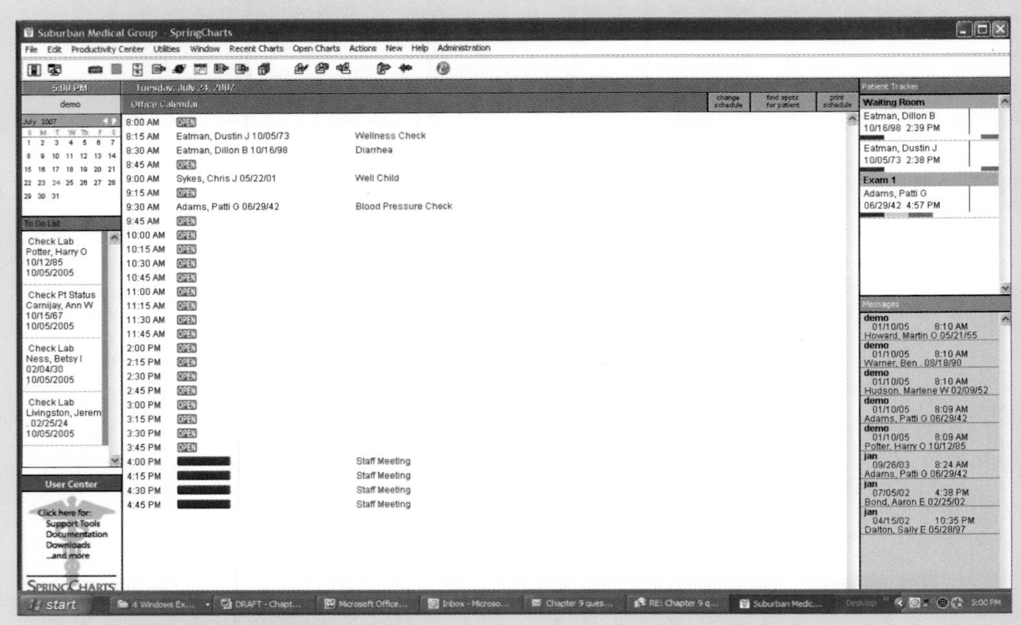

Figure 11.3 *Practice View* screen.

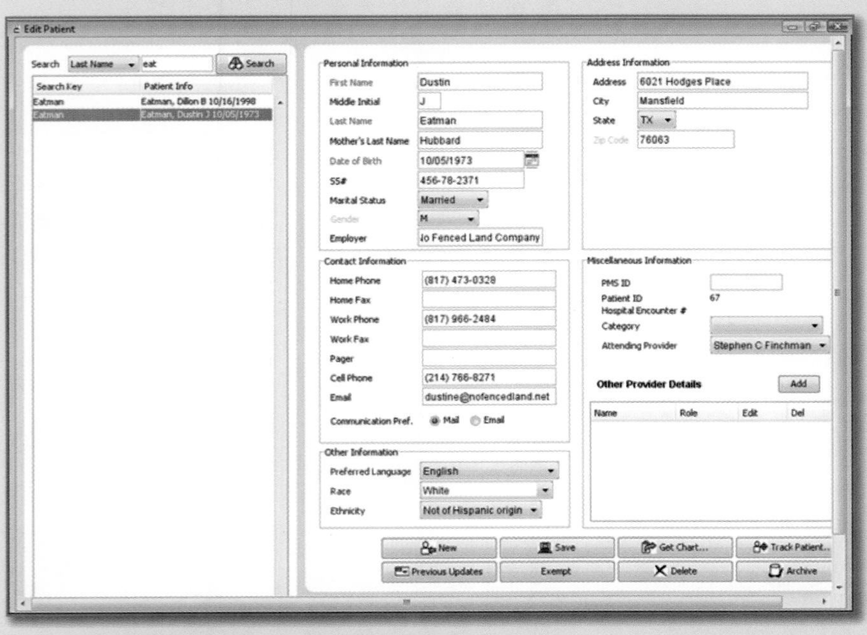

Figure 11.4 *Edit Patient* window for Dustin Eatman.

Patient Tracker

Exercise 11.3 Adding Patients to the Tracker

(Refer to Chapter 4, page 93)

1. Add Dustin and Dillon Eatman to the *Waiting Room* in the *Patient Tracker* by clicking on their name in the schedule and selecting [Track Pt].
2. The clinic has assigned the following *Patient Tracker* colors and their associative usage:
   Blue—Dr. Finchman
   Yellow—Dr. Smith
   Green—Self Pay
   Red—Lab Work
   Black—Procedures
   Fuchsia—Commercial Insurance

   Assign Dustin and Dillon the appropriate colors (Figure 11.5).

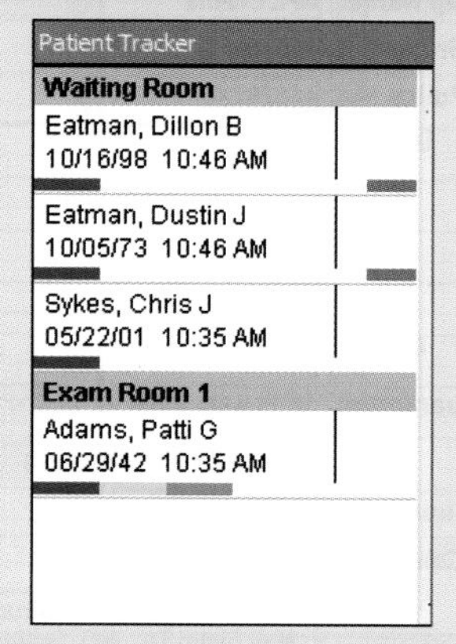

Figure 11.5 *Patient Tracker* window.

Exercise 11.4 Adding Insurance Information

(Refer to Chapter 3, page 78)

1. Add the following insurance information to the program accessed under the main *Edit* menu (Figure 11.6) and then to the face sheet of Dustin's and Dillon's patient charts (Figure 11.7).
   Insurance Company: Prudential Financial Group
   Mail Claim To: NFL Group Claims
   Address: PO Box 18974
   City: Plano
   State: TX
   Zip: 56781
   Phone: (800) 281-9823
   Group Name: NFL Claims
   Group Number: 10978NFL
   Policy Number: 456782371
   OV Co-Pay: $25
   Guarantor: Dustin J. Eatman

   Make a note in the *Details* box of Dillon's *Edit Patient Insurance* window: *Insurance Confirmed.*

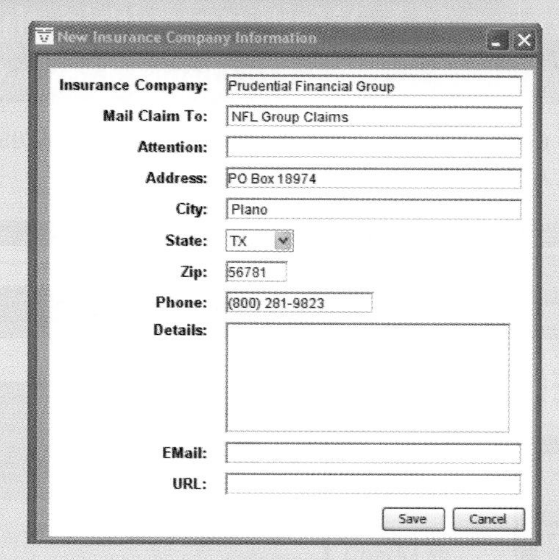

Figure 11.6 *New Insurance Company Information* window.

Note: Insurance will be visible on the face sheet when chart has been closed and reopened.

(continued)

Exercise 11.7 Editing To-Do Pop-Up Text

(Refer to Chapter 4, page 102)

1. Open the *Edit PopUp Text* window under the *File* menu > *Preferences* and add the sentence, *Remind patient about scheduled labs*, within the *ToDo/Reminders* category (Figure 11.12).
2. Create a *ToDo* message for yourself to call a patient and remind the patient about scheduled labs. Select the patient *Taylor Jones*.
3. Send the *ToDo* item to yourself in two weeks.
4. Check *My ToDo List* under the *Edit* menu and find the future item in the *Edit ToDo* window (Figure 11.13).

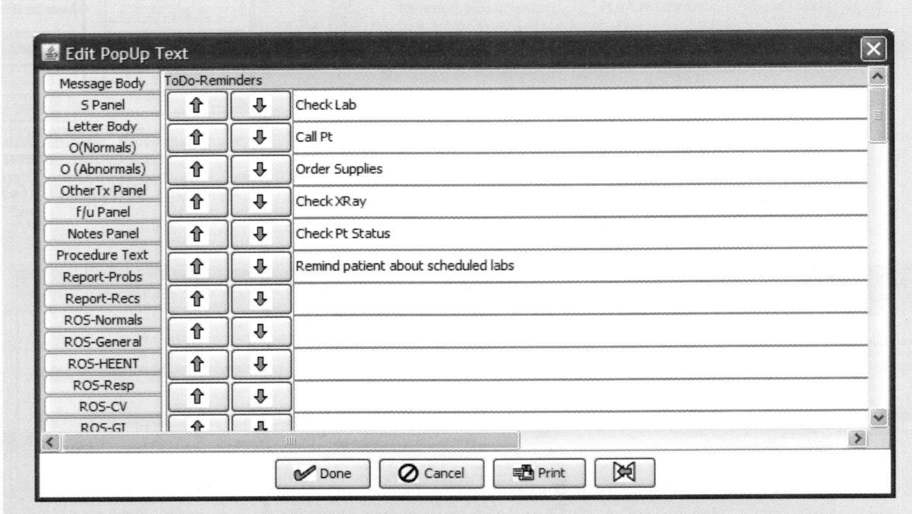

Figure 11.12 *Edit PopUp Text* window.

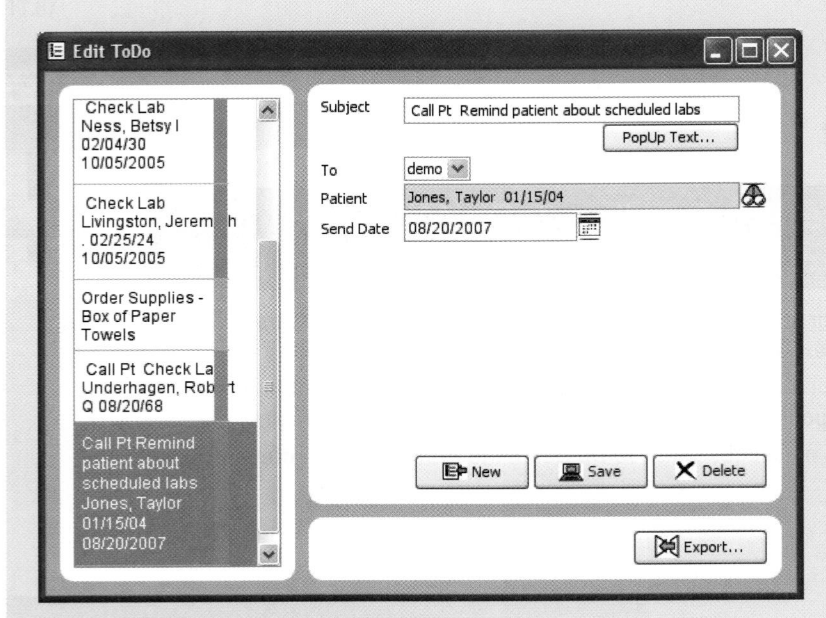

Figure 11.13 *Edit ToDo* window.

Messages

Exercise 11.8 Creating a Message
(Refer to Chapter 4, page 105)

Mr. Dean has called the doctor's office to request some samples of the medicatioLipitor. The medical staff is not available, so a message is created at the front desk.

1. Open a *New Message* window linked to the patient *Russel Dean.*
2. Create new pop-up text stating the patient called to request medication samples.
3. Use the new pop-up text in the body of the message.
4. From the [Rx] button in the *New Message* window, select *Lipitor* from the *Previous Prescription* list. Save the medication to the note.
5. While you have Mr. Dean on the phone, you notice you do not have a work phone number or a cell phone number for him. Mr. Dean informs you he is retired, but gives you a mobile phone number: (214) 766-8272 and an e-mail address: russeldean201@aol.com. Update his demographics by selecting the [Pt Info] button.
6. While in the *Edit Patient* window, update the patient records to show Dr. Finchman as his attending provider.
7. Since you can't log in as the doctor, send the message to *Demo.*

Exercise 11.9 Answering and Returning a Message
(Refer to Chapter 4, page 105)

1. Locate and open the message regarding Russel Dean in the *Messages* area of the *Practice View* screen.
2. In the message window, change the number of refills on the medication to *0* and the quantity to *15.*
3. Add new pop-up text to the *Message Body* category: *OK to give patient sample medication.*
4. Add the newly created text to the message, making sure the doctor's response goes on a new line in the message window.
5. On a new line in the *Message Body,* time-stamp and initial the note.
6. Click on the [Send Back] button to send the message back to the sender.

Exercise 11.10 Charting a Message
(Refer to Chapter 4, page 105)

1. Select the message in the *Messages* center recently sent back to you from Dr. Smith (Demo).
2. Add the following pop-up text to the *Message Body* pop-up text category: *Called patient and advised to pick up sample medication.*
3. Using the up and down arrows in the *Edit PopUp Text* window, position the new text above the line: *Let Pt know that we are out of samples.*
4. Add the new pop-up text on a new line in the text area of the message.
5. Time-stamp and initial your note on a new line in the message text panel (Figure 11.14).
6. Using the printer icon below the *Rx* section of the message window, print a copy of the prescription (Figure 11.15). Because this prescription is not being sent to the pharmacy, it does not require the doctor's license and DEA number.
7. Chart the message in the patient's chart, adding *Lipitor Samples* to the message heading.

(continued)

Exercise 11.11 (Continued)

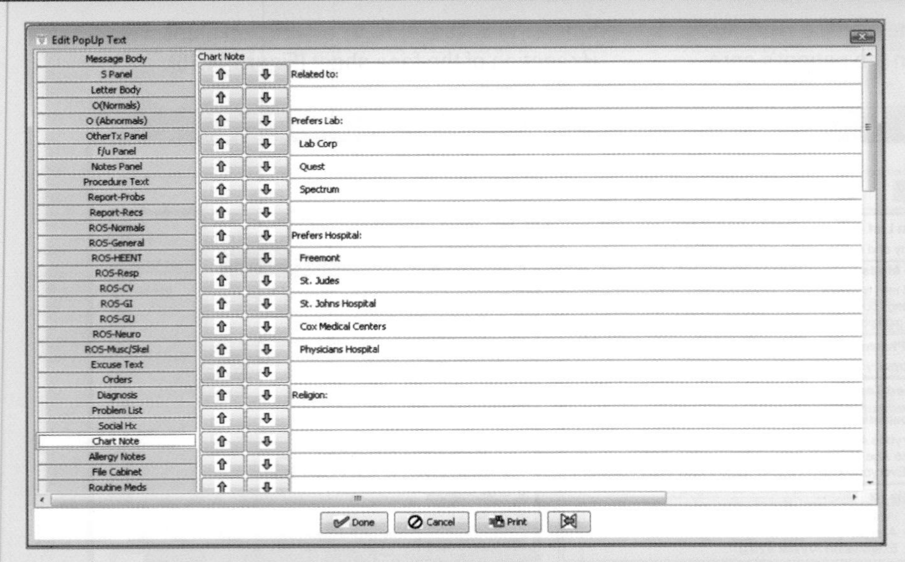

Figure 11.17 Adding hospital preferences in *Edit PopUp Text* window.

e) Referred By: *This patient was referred by Dr. Able Body.*

f) Chart Note: Click on the *Edit* icon for the pop-up text (Figure 11.17). In the *Edit PopUp Text* window, add the following hospitals: *St. Johns Hospital, Cox Medical Centers,* and *Physicians Hospital,* indenting each line three spaces. Using the up and down arrows, position the new text under the *Prefers Hospital* line. Now move an empty line between the list of hospitals and the line *Religion.* Click the space bar to add an invisible character on the empty line to create a space between the text lines. Save the material in the *Edit PopUp Text* window. In the face sheet window, check your results with Figure 11.18.
Select the text *Prefers Hospital:*
St. Johns Hospital

g) Routine Meds: Select the following medications:
Aleve—275 mg
Lipitor—20 mg
Aspirin—81 mg
Edit the Lipitor entry to change the number of refills to *0.* In the *Notes and OTC Meds* window, select *Omega-3*

h) Problem List: Select *Allergic Rhinitis 477.9, Bronchitis 466.0,* and *Abdominal Pain 789.60* from the upper *Dx* field.

i) Chart Alert: In the *Edit PopUp Text* window, add the following sentence: *Insurance approval needed for elective surgery.* Save and select the new text. Click on the [Back] button and check your work with Figure 11.19.

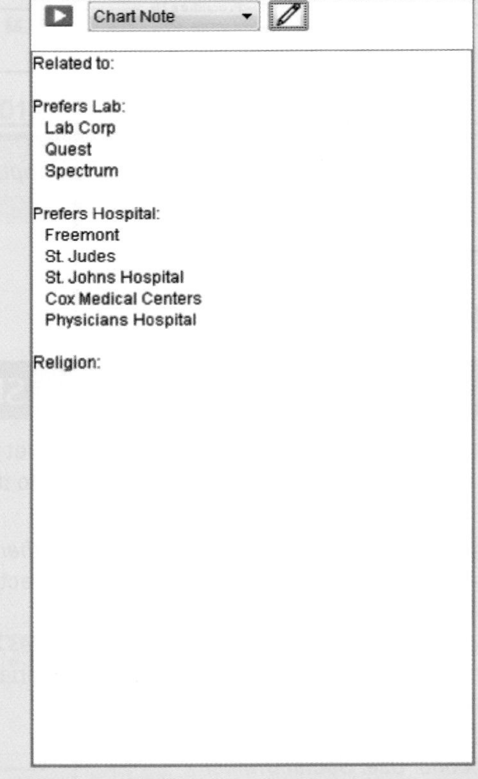

Figure 11.18 *Chart Note* section of face sheet window.

Exercise 11.11 (Concluded)

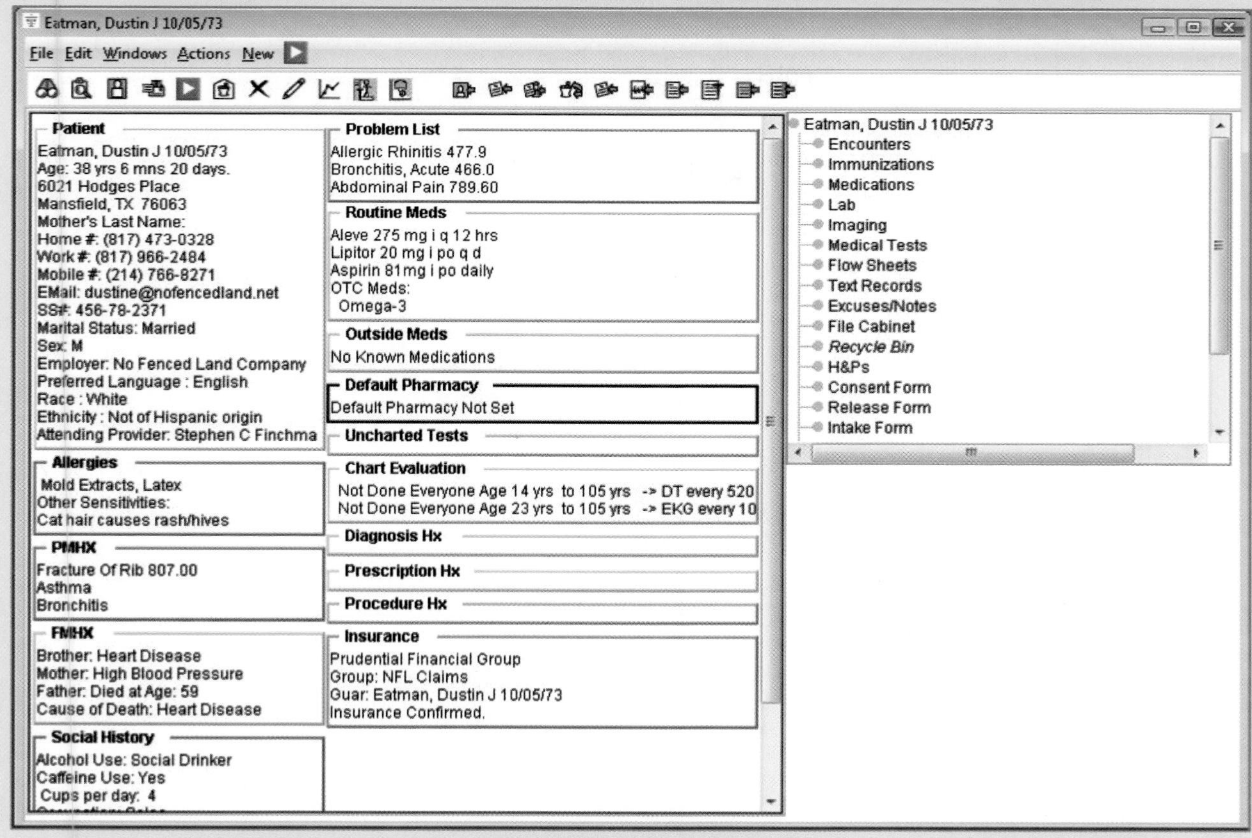

Figure 11.19 Completed face sheet windows in patient's chart.

Patient Chart Activities

Exercise 11.12 Running a Chart Evaluation (Refer to Chapter 7, page 190)

1. In the *Patient Tracker* move Dustin Eatman into Exam Room 3 and change his status to *Nurse Check*.
2. Open the chart and run a Chart Evaluation of Dustin Eatman's chart by accessing the *Evaluate Chart* icon.
3. Record Mr. Eatman's response that he will get a DT shot today and mark the recommendation as *Completed.* You will not be recommending the EKG today so you will *not* check the radio button *Mark this 'Completed.'* Save the evaluation.
4. Check your results under the *Encounters* tab in the patient's care tree (Figure 11.20).

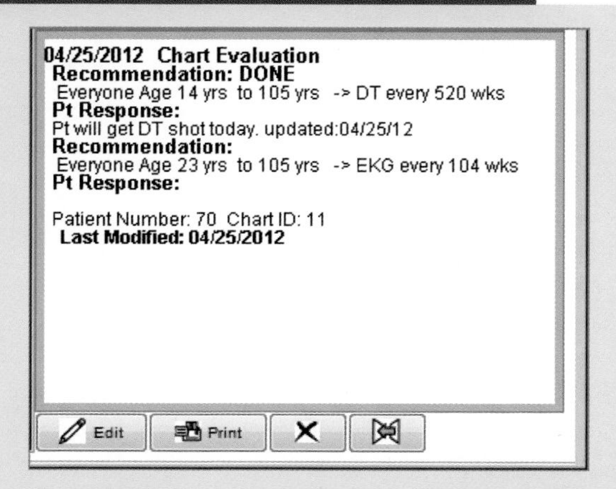

Figure 11.20 *Saved Chart Evaluation* in care tree.

Exercise 11.13 Printing a Patient's Face Sheet

(Refer to Chapter 5, page 123)

1. Open Dustin's chart. Select the File menu and the Print Face Sheet submenu.
2. Click the [Print] button in the *Document Printing Options* window and print the patient's face sheet information.
3. Compare the patient's face sheet with Figure 11.21.

Suburban Medical Group
101 Elm Street Sherman, TX 77521
(214) 674-2000

Name: Dustin J Eatman 10/05/73
Age: 38 yrs 5 mns 3 days.
Mother's Last Name:
Address: 6021 Hodges Place Mansfield, TX 76063
Home Phone: (817) 473-0328
Home Fax:
Work Phone: (817) 966-2484
Work Fax:
Pager:
Mobile Phone: (817) 504-0903
EMail: dustine@nofencedland.net
SS#: 456-78-2371
Marital Status:
Sex: M
Pt ID #: 67
Employer:
Preferred Language :
Race :
Ethnicity :
PMS ID:
Provider:
This Patient's Chart is Included In Searches
Date Entered: 03/08/2012
Last Modified: 03/08/2012
Allergies:
Mold Extracts entered 03/08/2012 4:00 PM by demo note:
Latex entered 03/08/2012 4:00 PM by demo note:
Patient Number: 67 Chart ID: 0
Last Modified On: 03/08/2012
Last Modified By : demo
Note: Allergy Reviewed Pending
Other Sensitivities
Cat hair causes rash/hives
Patient Number: 67 Chart ID: 2
Last Modified: 03/08/2012
Social History
Tobacco Use: Social Drinker
Caffeine Use: Yes Cups per day: 4
Occupation: Sales
Education: College
Smoking Status :4-Never Smoker

Patient Number: 67 Chart ID: 3

Patient: Eatman, Dustin J 10/05/73 — Page 1 of 3
Prepared by SpringChartsEMR — Suburban Medical Group

Last Modified: 03/08/2012
PMHX
Fracture Of Rib 807.00
Asthma
Broncjitis
Patient Number: 67 Chart ID: 5
Last Modified: 03/08/2012
FMHX
Brother: Heart Disease
Mother: Hypercholesterolemia
Father: Died at Age: 59
Cause of Death: Heart Disease
Patient Number: 67 Chart ID: 4
Last Modified: 03/08/2012
Patient Annotation : none listed
Problem List
Dx:
Allergic Rhinitis 477.9
Bronchitis, Acute 466.0
Abdominal Pain 789.60

Patient Number: 67 Chart ID: 9
Last Modified: 03/08/2012
Last Modified By : demo
Routine Meds
Aleve 275 mg i q 12 hrs
Lipitor 20 mg i po q d Updated by demo on 3/8/12 4:13 PM
Aspirin 81mg i po daily
OTC Meds:
Omega-3
Patient Number: 67 Chart ID: 8
Last Modified: 03/08/2012
Referral Details:
No Details Found
Patient Number: 67 Chart ID: 6

Last Modified: not defined
Last Refer To : not defined
Last Refer By : not defined
Chart Notes
Prefers Hospital:
St. Johns Hospital
Patient Number: 67 Chart ID: 7
Last Modified: 03/08/2012
Insurance Company Info
Insurance Company: Prudential Financial Group

Patient: Eatman, Dustin J 10/05/73 — Page 2 of 3
Prepared by SpringChartsEMR — Suburban Medical Group

Mail Claim To: NFL Group Claims
Attention:
Address: PO Box 18974
City: Plano
State: TX
Zip: 56781
Phone: 8002819823
Details:
EMail:
URL:
Patient Insurance Info
Group Name: NFL Claims
Group No: 1097NFL
Certif No: 456782371
Insured's relation to patient: Insured
CoPay: $25.00
Insurance Comfirmed

Patient: Eatman, Dustin J 10/05/73 — Page 3 of 3
Prepared by SpringChartsEMR — Suburban Medical Group

Figure 11.21 Patient's printed face sheet.

Exercise 11.14 Adding a Default Pharmacy

(Refer to Chapter 3, page 66)

1. Locate the following pharmacy, which Dustin typically uses, in SpringCharts's address book and complete the information.

    Walgreens Pharmacy
    10 Campbell Ave.
    Mansfield, TX 76063
    Ph: (817) 786-3654
    Fx: (817) 786-9785

2. Under the *Edit* menu in Dustin's chart, add *Walgreens Pharmacy* as the patient's default pharmacy.
3. Check to make sure the patient's preferred pharmacy is displayed in the patient's face sheet (Figure 11.22).

Default Pharmacy
Walgreens
8177863654

Figure 11.22 Default pharmacy window in face sheet.

Exercise 11.15 Adding a Photo

1. Add Dustin's photo to his chart by accessing the *Pt Photo* feature under the *Edit* menu.
2. Select the [Edit] button in the *Photo* window and click the [OK] button in the *Picture Size* window.
3. Direct your research in the *Open* dialog box through the *Desktop* access to locate the folder titled: *EHR Material,* (or follow your instructor's directions to locate the *EHR Materials* folder). Double-click on this folder to open it.
4. Highlight *Dustin's Photo* and select the [Open] button.
5. Select the [Done] button back in the *Photo* window.
6. Click on the *Pt Photo* category in the patient's care tree to view Dustin's photo (Figure 11.23).

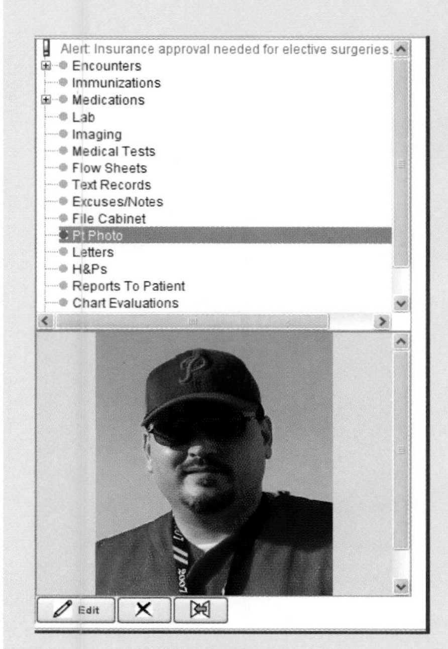

Figure 11.23 Patient's photo in care tree.

Exercise 11.16 Creating a New TC Note

(Refer to Chapter 5, page 140)

Mr. Russel Dean calls the office and requests a list of medications prescribed for him at your office.

1. Using both pop-up text and typing, record the details of the conversation in a *New TC Note,* under the *New* menu in Mr. Dean's chart.
2. Initial- and time-stamp the note by using the [Sign] button, and then select [Done].
3. Save the telephone note and skip billing. Notice the call has been documented on the patient's care tree (Figure 11.24).
4. Print out the list of all medications prescribed to Mr. Dean by accessing the *Medications List* under the *Actions* menu (Figure 11.25).

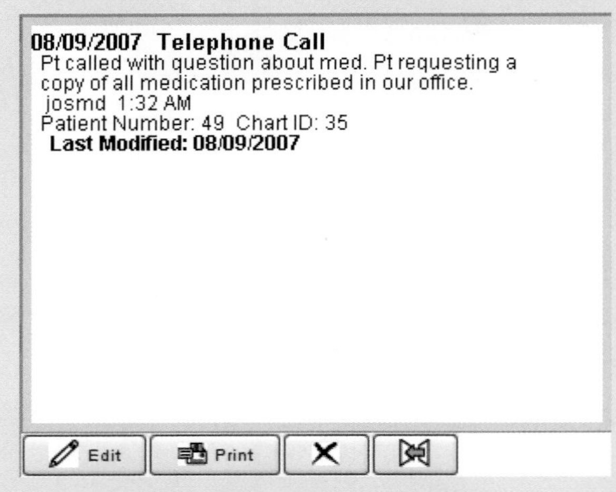

Figure 11.24 Telephone Call note in care tree.

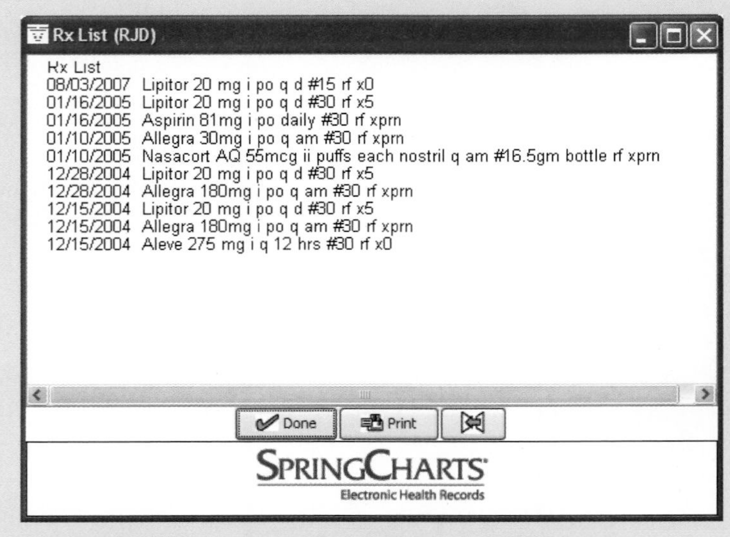

Figure 11.25 Patient's medication list in patient's chart.

Exercise 11.17 Creating a Nurse Note

1. Open a *New Nurse Note* in Mr. Eatman's chart.
2. Choose the *Well Adult V70.0* diagnosis and, within the [Proc] tab, record the administration of a DT shot. (Select the *Immunization* category under the *Choose Procedure* window to locate the DT procedure.)
3. Once selected, click on the DT procedure and add the procedure detail of lot number 2695A, expiration date of 11/1/2015, route of intramuscular, and a site of left deltoid. Use the appropriate popup text.
4. Add your initials and time by selecting the appropriate buttons.
5. Save the nurse note under the *Encounters* tab and send a routing slip.
6. In the *Routing Slip* window, select *Immunization 90471* from the *Superbill Form* for the administration of the injection.
7. Send the routing slip, and check the details of the *Nurse Note* in the patient's chart (Figure 11.26). Note that the *Patient Tracker* shows that the routing slip has been sent.

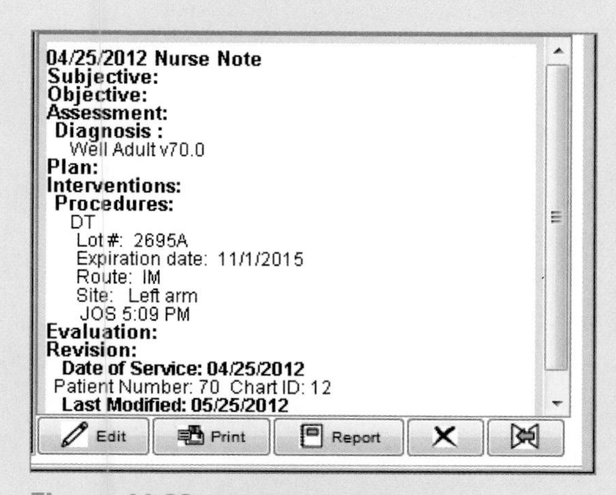

Figure 11.26 *Nurse Note* in care tree.

Exercise 11.18 Adding a Vitals Check

(Refer to Chapter 5, page 140)

1. Open Patti Adams's chart.
2. Because she has diabetes, Patti comes into the clinic on a regular basis to have her vitals taken. Under the *New* menu, select *New Vitals Only.*
3. Add fictitious vitals, as well as the fact that Mrs. Adams is 5 ft 4 inches and weighs 156 pounds. Remember BMI is calculated automatically from the height and weight, and head circumference (HC) is only used for pediatric patients.
4. By using pop-up text found under the *Notes* tab, specify that Mrs. Adams's blood pressure was taken on her right arm. Time- and initial-stamp the note.

(continued)

Exercise 11.18 (Concluded)

5. Save the new vitals under the *Encounters* tab and skip billing. Notice the Vitals Check information in the patient's care tree (Figure 11.27).

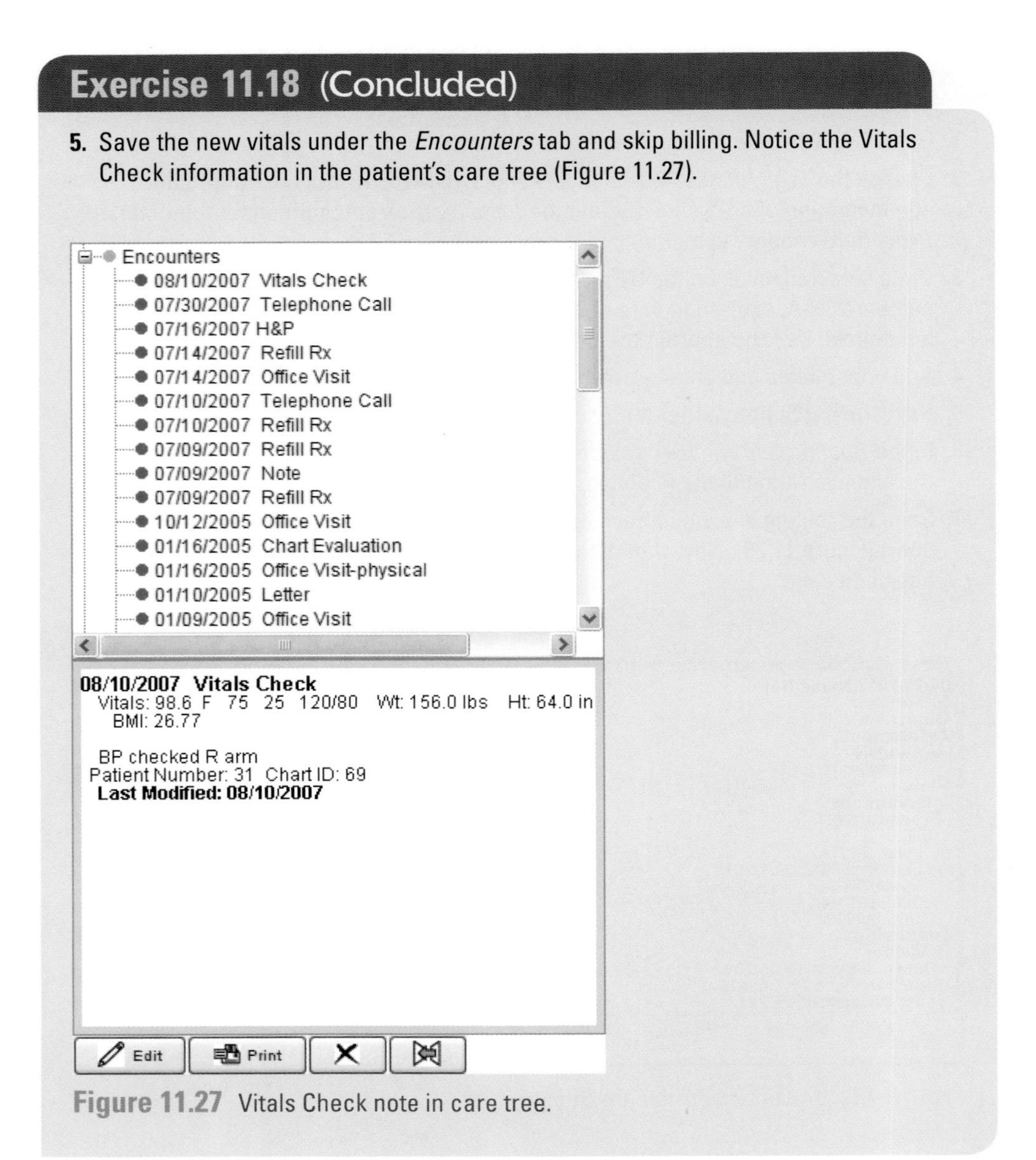

Figure 11.27 Vitals Check note in care tree.

11.3 Office Visit Screen

Office Visit Note

Exercise 11.19 Starting a New Office Visit Note (Refer to Chapter 6, page 156)

1. In Dustin Eatman's chart, open a *New OV.*
2. Mr. Eatman has come to the doctor's office for an annual well checkup. Under the chief complaint [CC] navigation button select *Well Visit.*
3. Stamp the time and initial the note.
4. Under the [Vitals] tab, add fictitious well vitals for Mr. Eatman.
5. Save the office visit under the *Encounters* tab and skip billing.

Exercise 11.19 (Concluded)

6. Close Mr. Eatman's chart and update his location and status on the *Patient Tracker* to *Exam Room 2* and *Doctor Ready.* Notice the new information in the office visit in the patient's care tree (Figure 11.28).

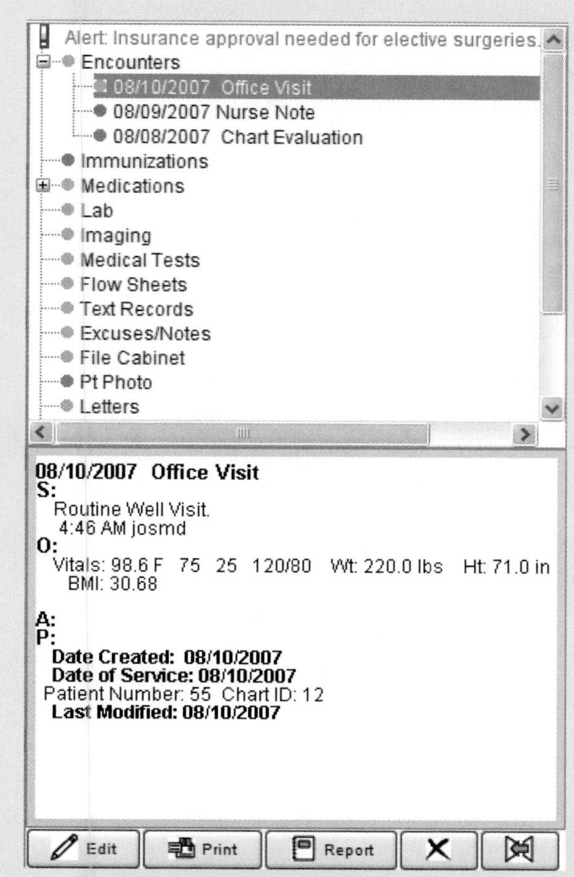

Figure 11.28 Beginning of OV note.

Exercise 11.20 Completing an Office Visit Note (Refer to Chapter 6, page 156)

1. Open Mr. Eatman's chart and highlight the partially completed office visit note.
2. Click on the [Edit] button to open the *Office Visit* screen.
3. Under the [ROS] tab, select the following pop-up text under the *ROS-Normals* category (remember to start a new line for each system):
   a) *GENERAL: No weight change, fever, chills, night sweats, generalized weakness.*
   b) *HEENT: No headache, dizziness, lightheadedness, diplopia, tearing, eye pain, blind spots, excessive blinking, tinnitus, ear pain or discharge, nose bleeding, nasal obstruction, nasal discharge, gingival bleeding, dental problem, sore throat, hoarseness, difficulty swallowing, neck stiffness, neck pain.*

(continued)

Exercise 11.20 (Continued)

c) *PULMONARY: No wheezing, cough, congestion, hemoptysis, respiratory infections, tuberculosis, chest wall pain.*
d) *CV: No chest pain, arrhythmia, syncope, dyspnea, exertional dyspnea, orthopnea, paroxysmal nocturnal dyspnea, intermittent claudication, dependent edema, varicose vein, phlebitis, heart murmur, hypertension.*
e) *GI: No change in appetite, difficulty swallowing, indigestion, heartburn, belching, nausea, vomiting, hematemesis, hematochezia, abdomen pain, flatulence, changes in bowel habits, constipation, diarrhea, abnormal stools, incontinence, hemorrhoids, jaundice.*

4. Under the [Exam] button, select the following pop-up text:
a) *GENERAL: Well developed. Well nourished. Alert. Oriented to person, place, and time. In no apparent distress.*
b) *HEAD: Normocephalic. Atraumatic.*
c) *EYES: Eyes and lids appear symmetrical. No exudate. Sclera clear. PERRLA, EOMI. Discs sharp.*
d) *EARS: External auditory canals and TMs normal. Hearing normal as tested by whisper and Rinne/Weber.*
e) *MOUTH/THROAT: Dentition good. Normal mucosa, tongue, gingiva, and oropharynx. Palate elevates in midline. No thrush, erythema, or exudate.*
f) *CV: RRR, normal S1 S2, no S3/S4, murmur, gallop, rub, arrhythmia, or heave. PMI normal in location and character.*
g) *ABDOMEN: Bowel sounds are normal. No evidence of scarring or past surgical procedures. Abdomen is flat, soft, and nontender, without rebound or guarding. No evidence of masses, organomegaly, or abdominal aneurysm. Normal to percussion.*
h) *MUSCULOSKELETAL: Posture normal. Pulses normal and symmetrical. Motor strength normal. Sensory normal and symmetrical to soft touch and pinprick. Joints show normal range of motion and are without erythema or effusions. Nails: Normal capillary filling and appearance w/o clubbing or pitting. No masses or dependent edema noted.*
i) *RECTAL: No mass palpable. Prostate normal in size, shape, and consistency for age. Guaiac negative.*

5. Under the [Dx] tab, choose the *Well Adult* v70.0 code.
6. Order a CBC with differential and a SMAC under the [Test] tab.
7. Add the patient's primary insurance to the order form.
8. Because these tests will be conducted at an outside testing facility, print a physician's order form.
9. Compare the order form to that shown in Figure 11.29.
10. Save a copy in the patient's chart under the *Encounters* category in the care tree.
11. The doctor decides to give Mr. Eatman a flu shot during the office visit because of the upcoming flu season. Under the [Proc] tab, search for and select *flu shot.*
12. Highlight the flu shot procedure and change the Aventis Pasteur number to *U0701BA,* and the vaccine date to today's date, for example, *30 JUNE 12.*
13. Date-, time-, and initial-stamp the procedure note before saving it.
14. Under the [Other Tx] button select the counseling notes: *Discussed weight loss strategies. Encouraged pt to exercise 30 minutes 5 times a week.*
15. Plan a follow-up for 1 year. Select the *Create a Reminder* icon and send a *ToDo/Reminder* note to Jan to call the patient and check the lab work (use pop-up text). Send it to her so she will receive it in 3 business days (Figure 11.30).

Exercise 11.20 (Continued)

Suburban Medical Group
101 Elm Street
Sherman, TX 77521
(214) 674-2000 Fax (214) 674-2100

Date: 08/10/07
Pt: Eatman, Dustin J 10/05/73
Address: 6021 Hodges Place Mansfield, TX 76063

Physician Order

Orders:
CBC 85025
SMAC 80054

Diagnosis:
Well Adult v70.0

Patient Insurance Info
Group Name: NFL Claims
Group/Policy No: 10978NFL
Guarantor: Eatman, Dustin J 10/05/73
Certif No: 456782371
Insured
CoPay: 25.0

Insurance Company: Prudential Financial Group
Mail Claim To: NFL Group Claims
Attention:
Address: PO Box 18974
City: Plano
State: TX
Zip: 56781
Phone: 8002819823
Details:
EMail:
URL:

Prepared by SpringChartsEMR

Suburban Medical Group

Figure 11.29 Physician order form.

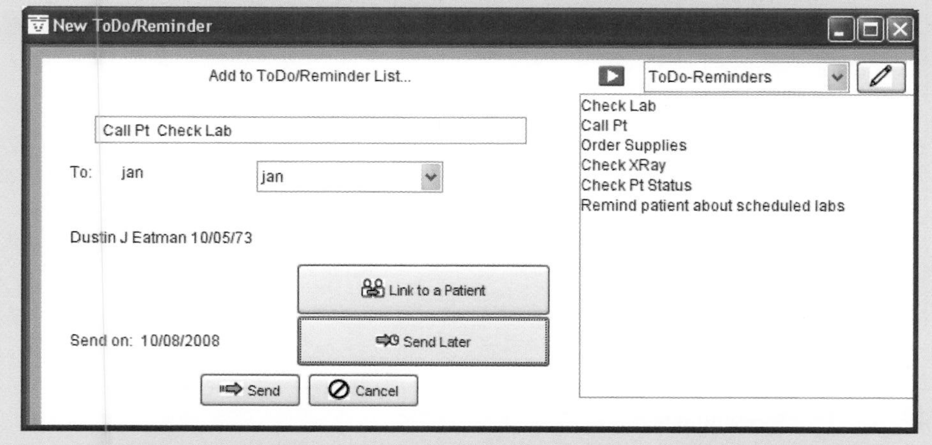

Figure 11.30 *New ToDo/Reminder* window.

(continued)

Exercise 11.20 (Concluded)

16. Save the office visit note and create a routing slip.
17. From the *Superbill* form, select the *Injections CPT code 90472* because of the additional inoculation that was done.
18. Click in the *New Patient Type* radio button and choose the displayed E&M code for a new patient by selecting the [Use Code] button.
19. Send the routing slip.
20. Under the main *Edit* menu, locate and print the routing slip that you just generated. Compare your results to Figure 11.31.

Suburban Medical Group
101 Elm Street
Sherman, TX 77521
(214) 674-2000 Fax (281) 537-0184

Eatman, Dustin J 10/05/73
6021 Hodges Place
Mansfield, TX 76063
Mother's Last Name:
Home #: (817) 473-0328
Work #: (817) 966-2484
Pager:
EMail: dustine@nofencedland.net
SS#: 456-78-2371
Sex: M
Employer: No Fenced Land Company

Home Fax:
Work Fax:
Mobile #: (214) 766-8271

Marital Status: Married
Pt ID #: 70
PMS ID #:

Date of Service: 04/25/2012

Doctor: John O. Smith, M.D. NPI: 1256984

E&M Code Recommended: 99201

Diagnosis:
Well Adult v70.0

Other Diagnosis:

Tests:
CBC W/Diff 85025
SMAC 80054

Other Procedures:
additional Immunization 90472

Flu Shot 90658
Discussed weight loss strategies. Encouraged pt to exercise 30 minutes 5 times a week.

Followup:
1 year

Patient Insurance Info
Group Name: NFL Claims
Group No: 10978NFL
Guarantor: Eatman, Dustin J 10/05/73
Certif No: 456782371
Insured
CoPay: 25.0
Insurance Confirmed.

Insurance Company: Prudential Financial Group
Mail Claim To: NFL Group Claims
Attention:
Address: PO Box 18974
City: Plano
State: TX
Zip: 56781
Phone: 8002819823
Details:
EMail:
URL:

Prepared by
SpringChartsEMR

Figure 11.31 Routing slip.

Office Visit Activities

Exercise 11.21 Printing an Office Visit Note

(Refer to Chapter 6, page 181)

1. From Mr. Eatman's chart, print a copy of the recent office visit note and compare it to Figure 11.32.

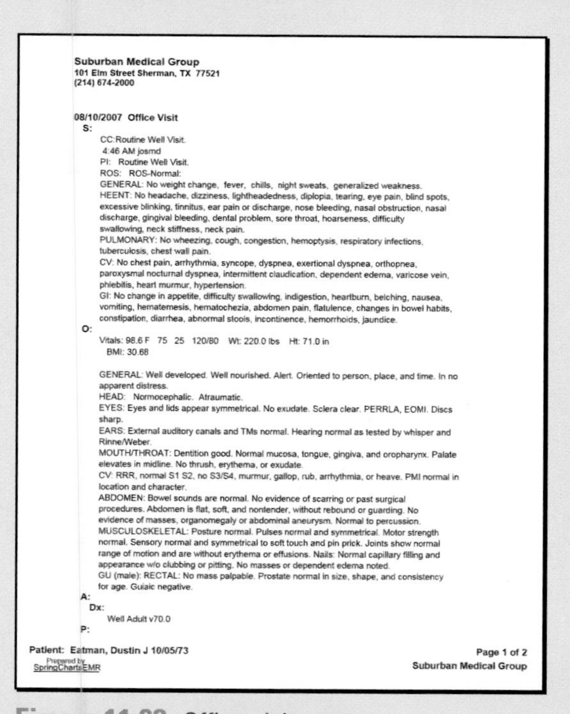

Suburban Medical Group
101 Elm Street Sherman, TX 77521
(214) 674-2000

08/10/2007 Office Visit
S:
CC:Routine Well Visit.
4:46 AM josmd
PI: Routine Well Visit.
ROS: ROS-Normal:
GENERAL: No weight change, fever, chills, night sweats, generalized weakness.
HEENT: No headache, dizziness, lightheadedness, diplopia, tearing, eye pain, blind spots, excessive blinking, tinnitus, ear pain or discharge, nose bleeding, nasal obstruction, nasal discharge, gingival bleeding, dental problem, sore throat, hoarseness, difficulty swallowing, neck stiffness, neck pain.
PULMONARY: No wheezing, cough, congestion, hemoptysis, respiratory infections, tuberculosis, chest wall pain.
CV: No chest pain, arrhythmia, syncope, dyspnea, exertional dyspnea, orthopnea, paroxysmal nocturnal dyspnea, intermittent claudication, dependent edema, varicose vein, phlebitis, heart murmur, hypertension.
GI: No change in appetite, difficulty swallowing, indigestion, heartburn, belching, nausea, vomiting, hematemesis, hematochezia, abdomen pain, flatulence, changes in bowel habits, constipation, diarrhea, abnormal stools, incontinence, hemorrhoids, jaundice.
O:
Vitals: 98.6 F 75 25 120/80 Wt: 220.0 lbs Ht: 71.0 in
BMI: 30.68

GENERAL: Well developed. Well nourished. Alert. Oriented to person, place, and time. In no apparent distress.
HEAD: Normocephalic. Atraumatic.
EYES: Eyes and lids appear symmetrical. No exudate. Sclera clear. PERRLA, EOMI. Discs sharp.
EARS: External auditory canals and TMs normal. Hearing normal as tested by whisper and Rinne/Weber.
MOUTH/THROAT: Dentition good. Normal mucosa, tongue, gingiva, and oropharynx. Palate elevates in midline. No thrush, erythema, or exudate.
CV: RRR, normal S1 S2, no S3/S4, murmur, gallop, rub, arrhythmia, or heave. PMI normal in location and character.
ABDOMEN: Bowel sounds are normal. No evidence of scarring or past surgical procedures. Abdomen is flat, soft, and nontender, without rebound or guarding. No evidence of masses, organomegaly or abdominal aneurysm. Normal to percussion.
MUSCULOSKELETAL: Posture normal. Pulses normal and symmetrical. Motor strength normal. Sensory normal and symmetrical to soft touch and pin prick. Joints show normal range of motion and are without erythema or effusions. Nails: Normal capillary filling and appearance w/o clubbing or pitting. No masses or dependent edema noted.
GU (male): RECTAL: No mass palpable. Prostate normal in size, shape, and consistency for age. Guiaic negative.
A:
Dx:
Well Adult v70.0
P:

Patient: Eatman, Dustin J 10/05/73 **Page 1 of 2**
Prepared by SpringChartsEMR **Suburban Medical Group**

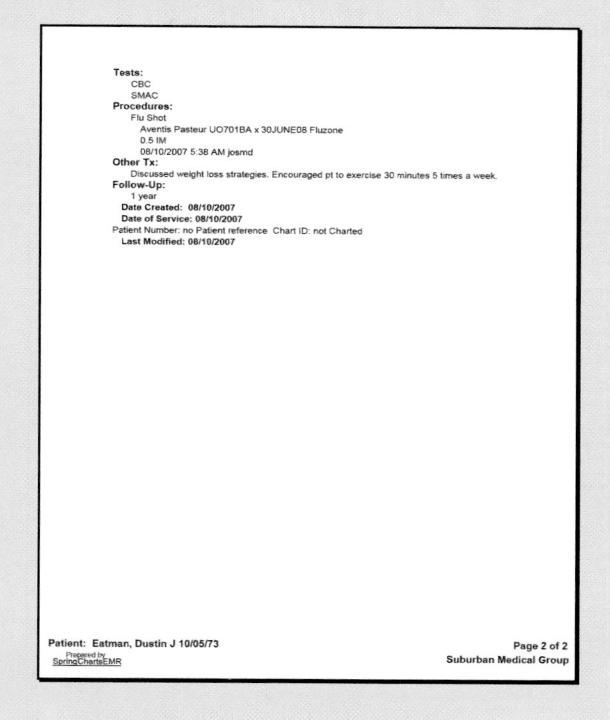

Tests:
CBC
SMAC
Procedures:
Flu Shot
Aventis Pasteur UO701BA x 30JUNE08 Fluzone
0.5 IM
08/10/2007 5:38 AM josmd
Other Tx:
Discussed weight loss strategies. Encouraged pt to exercise 30 minutes 5 times a week.
Follow-Up:
1 year
Date Created: 08/10/2007
Date of Service: 08/10/2007
Patient Number: no Patient reference Chart ID: not Charted
Last Modified: 08/10/2007

Patient: Eatman, Dustin J 10/05/73 **Page 2 of 2**
Prepared by SpringChartsEMR **Suburban Medical Group**

Figure 11.32 Office visit note.

Exercise 11.22 Printing an H&P Report (Refer to Chapter 6, page 182)

1. Mr. Eatman requests a copy of the history and physical report of his medical encounter. Open the current office visit note and select the *H&P Report* from the *Tools* menu.
2. Print the report. Compare it to Figure 11.33.
3. Save the *H&P Report* under the *H&Ps* category in the care tree, and close the *Office Visit* screen and the patient's chart.
4. Update the *Patient Tracker* to reflect Mr. Eatman being sent to the *Checkout Desk* with a status of *Ready*. Click [Done].
5. Reopen the *Edit Tracker* window and click on the [CheckOut] button.
6. The *Patient Tracker* shows Dustin Eatman as *Done* with the *Routing Slip* stamp (Figure 11.34).

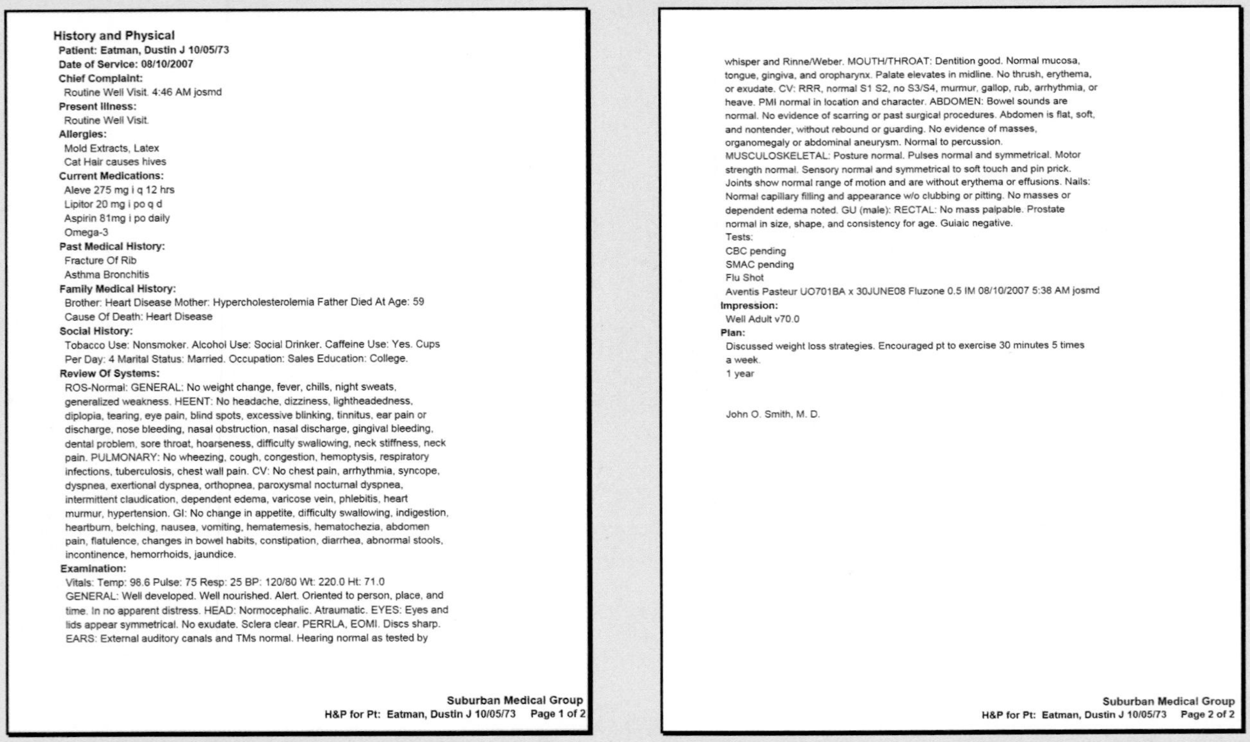

History and Physical
Patient: Eatman, Dustin J 10/05/73
Date of Service: 08/10/2007
Chief Complaint:
Routine Well Visit. 4:46 AM josmd
Present Illness:
Routine Well Visit.
Allergies:
Mold Extracts, Latex
Cat Hair causes hives
Current Medications:
Aleve 275 mg i q 12 hrs
Lipitor 20 mg i po q d
Aspirin 81mg i po daily
Omega-3
Past Medical History:
Fracture Of Rib
Asthma Bronchitis
Family Medical History:
Brother: Heart Disease Mother: Hypercholesterolemia Father Died At Age: 59 Cause Of Death: Heart Disease
Social History:
Tobacco Use: Nonsmoker. Alcohol Use: Social Drinker. Caffeine Use: Yes. Cups Per Day: 4 Marital Status: Married. Occupation: Sales Education: College.
Review Of Systems:
ROS-Normal: GENERAL: No weight change, fever, chills, night sweats, generalized weakness. HEENT: No headache, dizziness, lightheadedness, diplopia, tearing, eye pain, blind spots, excessive blinking, tinnitus, ear pain or discharge, nose bleeding, nasal obstruction, nasal discharge, gingival bleeding, dental problem, sore throat, hoarseness, difficulty swallowing, neck stiffness, neck pain. PULMONARY: No wheezing, cough, congestion, hemoptysis, respiratory infections, tuberculosis, chest wall pain. CV: No chest pain, arrhythmia, syncope, dyspnea, exertional dyspnea, orthopnea, paroxysmal nocturnal dyspnea, intermittent claudication, dependent edema, varicose vein, phlebitis, heart murmur, hypertension. GI: No change in appetite, difficulty swallowing, indigestion, heartburn, belching, nausea, vomiting, hematemesis, hematochezia, abdomen pain, flatulence, changes in bowel habits, constipation, diarrhea, abnormal stools, incontinence, hemorrhoids, jaundice.
Examination:
Vitals: Temp: 98.6 Pulse: 75 Resp: 25 BP: 120/80 Wt: 220.0 Ht: 71.0
GENERAL: Well developed. Well nourished. Alert. Oriented to person, place, and time. In no apparent distress. HEAD: Normocephalic. Atraumatic. EYES: Eyes and lids appear symmetrical. No exudate. Sclera clear. PERRLA, EOMI. Discs sharp. EARS: External auditory canals and TMs normal. Hearing normal as tested by

Suburban Medical Group
H&P for Pt: Eatman, Dustin J 10/05/73 Page 1 of 2

whisper and Rinne/Weber. MOUTH/THROAT: Dentition good. Normal mucosa, tongue, gingiva, and oropharynx. Palate elevates in midline. No thrush, erythema, or exudate. CV: RRR, normal S1 S2, no S3/S4, murmur, gallop, rub, arrhythmia, or heave. PMI normal in location and character. ABDOMEN: Bowel sounds are normal. No evidence of scarring or past surgical procedures. Abdomen is flat, soft, and nontender, without rebound or guarding. No evidence of masses, organomegaly or abdominal aneurysm. Normal to percussion. MUSCULOSKELETAL: Posture normal. Pulses normal and symmetrical. Motor strength normal. Sensory normal and symmetrical to soft touch and pin prick. Joints show normal range of motion and are without erythema or effusions. Nails: Normal capillary filling and appearance w/o clubbing or pitting. No masses or dependent edema noted. GU (male): RECTAL: No mass palpable. Prostate normal in size, shape, and consistency for age. Guiaic negative.
Tests:
CBC pending
SMAC pending
Flu Shot
Aventis Pasteur UO701BA x 30JUNE08 Fluzone 0.5 IM 08/10/2007 5:38 AM josmd
Impression:
Well Adult v70.0
Plan:
Discussed weight loss strategies. Encouraged pt to exercise 30 minutes 5 times a week.
1 year

John O. Smith, M. D.

Suburban Medical Group
H&P for Pt: Eatman, Dustin J 10/05/73 Page 2 of 2

Figure 11.33 *History & Physical Report.*

Done	
Eatman, Dustin J 10/05/73 6:58 AM √ Routing Slip	Done

Figure 11.34 Updated *Patient Tracker* window.

12

EHR Practicum

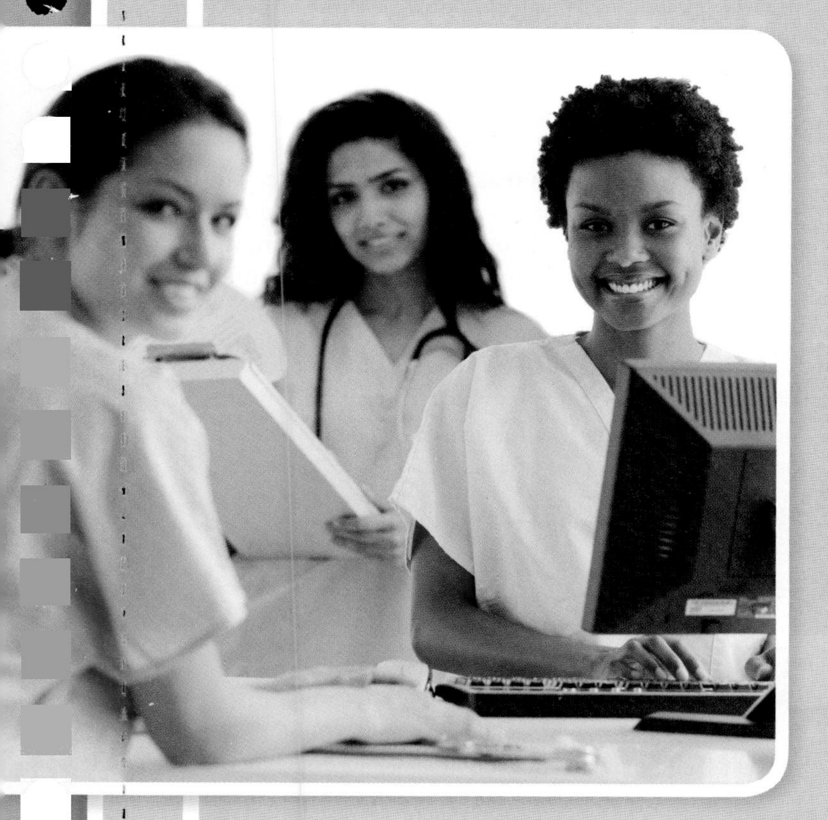

Learning Outcome

After completing Chapter 12, you will be able to:

LO 12.1 Successfully use all of the major features of the SpringCharts EHR program.

What You Need to Know

To understand Chapter 12 you will need to know:

- How to navigate within the *Practice View* screen
- How to navigate within the *Patient Chart* screen
- How to navigate within the *Office Visit* screen

Introduction

The U.S. Department of Health and Human Services (HHS), through the Office of the National Coordinator for Health Information Technology (ONC), is focused on encouraging physicians and other healthcare providers to adopt EHR programs. The majority of providers in the United States now use electronic health records for their staff and patients, and over the next several years, EHRs will become mainstream. However, graduating medical assistants and other health professionals and health information technology students may find employment in medical offices that have not yet transitioned to electronic records. They may find themselves employed in medical offices that need to make use of their EHR training and skills to implement electronic medical records.

This chapter incorporates healthcare documents used in medical offices that have not converted to the electronic medium. It is important to be able to locate the data on these documents and know where to store this information in an EHR program. In this chapter, you will examine the source documents contained in Appendix B and record the information in the appropriate areas of the SpringCharts EHR program.

Note: Before printing any documents from the following exercises, check with your instructor to determine whether you should turn in the printed documents after each exercise or wait to turn in *all* your documents at the completion of *all* exercises.

12.1 Recording Information from Paper Source Documents

Exercise 12.1 Adding a New Patient (Refer to Chapter 3, page 77)

1. Using *Source Document 1—Patient Information Sheet (See Appendix B)*, add a new patient to the EHR program and save the information.
2. Go to the *Edit Patient* window, locate the patient.
3. Click on the *Copy or Export This Data* (universal export) icon (lower right) and *Open in Word Processor.*
4. Type your name at the top of the document. Print the patient's information, circle your name, and submit it to your instructor.

Exercise 12.2 Scheduling a New Patient (Refer to Chapter 4, page 88)

1. Using *Source Document 1—Patient Information Sheet (See Appendix B)*, add the patient to the appropriate time slot on the schedule. The patient has scheduled a doctor's appointment for allergies.
2. Add yourself to the schedule. The reason for your visit is an annual physical.
3. Print today's schedule, circle your name on the document, and turn in to your instructor.

Exercise 12.3 Adding a New Insurance Company (Refer to Chapter 3, page 79)

1. Using appropriate information from *Source Document 2—Primary Insurance Card Information (See Appendix B)*, set up a new insurance company in SpringCharts.
2. Click on the *Export* icon button and *Open in Word Processor.*
3. Type your name at the top of the document. Print the insurance information, circle your name, and submit it to your instructor.

Exercise 12.4 Adding a Patient's Insurance Information

(Refer to Chapter 5, page 139)

1. Using *Source Document 2—Primary Insurance Card Information (See Appendix B)*, add the primary insurance details to the face sheet of the patient you added in Exercise 12.1 *(Chloe Hill)*. Use the employer name from the *Patient Information Sheet* as the Group Name.
2. Print out the patient's primary insurance information, write your name on the document, and submit it to your instructor.

Exercise 12.5 Adding a Physician's Address

(Refer to Chapter 3, page 68)

1. Using *Source Document 3—Patient Intake Sheet (See Appendix B)*, add the patient's primary care physician as a new entry in SpringCharts' address book.
2. Print the address card, write your name on the document, and submit it to your instructor.

Exercise 12.6 Completing a Face Sheet (Refer to Chapter 5, page 134)

1. *Using Source Document 3—Patient Intake Sheet (See Appendix B)*, complete Chloe Hill's face sheet.
2. Print the face sheet, write your name on the document, and submit it to your instructor.

Exercise 12.7 Adding a New Pharmacy (Refer to Chapter 3, page 69)

1. *Using Source Document 4—Default Pharmacy Information (See Appendix B)*, add a new entry to the *Address Book* in SpringCharts.
2. Click the [Print Card] button, write your name on the document, and submit it to your instructor.

Exercise 12.8 Identifying a Patient's Default Pharmacy

Using *Source Document 4—Default Pharmacy Information (See Appendix B)*, record this pharmacy as Chloe Hill's default pharmacy in the face sheet.

Exercise 12.9 Importing a Patient Photo

Import Choe Hill's photo into her chart through the *Edit* menu (access the file from the *EHR Material* folder).

Exercise 12.10 Updating a Patient's Immunization Record

(Refer to Chapter 5, page 137)

1. *Using Source Document 5—Immunization Record Card (See Appendix B)*, update the immunization archive in Chloe Hill's chart. Use the same start and end date for the immunizations.
2. Click on the *Date* heading and organize the immunizations with the oldest at the top and print the immunization record. Write your name on the document and submit it to your instructor.

Exercise 12.11 Conducting a Chart Evaluation

(Refer to Chapter 7, page 190)

1. Perform a *Chart Evaluation* of Chloe Hill's chart.
2. Record that the patient did **not** agree to have the indicated items conducted.
3. Print the Chart Evaluation summary. Write your name on the document and submit it to your instructor.

Exercise 12.12 Documenting a New Office Visit

(Refer to Chapter 6, page 155)

Using *Source Document 6—Office Visit Notes (See Appendix B)*, record the information into a *New OV* window in the patient's chart. Complete Exercises 12.12 through 12.15 from within the newly created OV note.

Exercise 12.13 Creating an Electronic Prescription

(Refer to Chapter 6, page 159)

1. Using *Source Document 6—Office Visit Notes (See Appendix B)*, create three *Prescription Forms* within the OV note for the medication prescribed to the patient. Include the physician' license and NPI numbers.
2. Print the prescription, write your name on the document, and submit it to your instructor.

Exercise 12.14 Creating an Order Form (Refer to Chapter 7, page 197)

1. Using *Source Document 6—Office Visit Notes (See Appendix B)*, create an *Order Form* within the OV note for the ordered test. Add the patient's insurance.
2. Type your name at the top of the document. Print the order form, chart it, circle your name on the printed document and submit it to your instructor.

Exercise 12.15 Creating a Procedure Note

(Refer to Chapter 6, page 164)

1. *Using Source Document 6—Office Visit Notes (See Appendix B)*, create a *Procedure Note* by clicking on the selected procedure.
2. On a new line add the *PopUp Text* that begins with *The patient's questions were answered. . . .*
3. On a new line use the time and initials stamp.

Exercise 12.16 Creating a Routing Slip (Refer to Chapter 6, page 179)

1. Create a *Routing Slip*. Type your name on the document at the top of the *Routing Slip* window.
2. From the *Edit* menu, locate the *Routing Slip* and print it. Circle your name on the document and submit it to your instructor.

Exercise 12.17 Creating an Excuse Note (Refer to Chapter 5, page 147)

1. Using *Source Document 7—Patient Excuse Note (See Appendix B)*, create an excuse note for Chloe Hill within her chart. Type your name at the top of the document.
2. Print the excuse note, use the digital signature, circle your name on the document, and submit it to your instructor.

Exercise 12.18 Creating a Letter About a Patient

(Refer to Chapter 5, page 144)

1. Using *Source Document 8—Letter to Primary Care Physician (See Appendix B)*, create a letter in Chloe Hill's chart to her primary care physician. Include the recent office visit notes. Type your name at the bottom of the letter.
2. Save the letter under the *Letters* category in her care tree.
3. Print the letter, circle your name on the document, and submit it to your instructor.

Exercise 12.19 Processing Test Results (Refer to Chapter 9, page 245)

1. Using *Source Document 9—Patient Lab Results (See Appendix B)*, record the lab results into Chloe Hill's chart under *Pending Tests*. Type your name into the *Test Note* area.
2. Process the test results into the *Completed Tests* area. Indicate that the doctor has viewed the test.
3. Save the results in the patient's chart.
4. From the patient's chart, print the lab results, circle your name on the document, and submit it to your instructor.

Exercise 12.20 Documenting a Telephone Call Message

(Refer to Chapter 4, page 107)

1. Using *Source Document 10—Telephone Call Message (See Appendix B)*, create a message from Chloe Hill requesting a letter regarding the negative lab results from the recent strep test. Use appropriate popup text and free text.
2. Send the message to yourself (Demo).
3. Open the message from the *Message Center* as the recipient and document that you have sent the patient a letter. Initial- and time-stamp the message. Type your name at the bottom of the message.
4. Chart the message into the patient's chart under the *Encounter* tab.
5. Open the patient's chart and print a copy of the message. Circle your name and turn in to your instructor.

Exercise 12.21 Creating a Letter to a Patient

(Refer to Chapter 5, page 143)

1. Using *Source Document 11—Letter to Patient (See Appendix B)*, create a letter to Chloe Hill within her chart. Include a copy of recent lab results. Type your name at the bottom of the letter.
2. Save the letter under the *Letters* category in her care tree.
3. Print the letter, circle your name on the document, and submit it to your instructor.

Exercise 12.22 Creating a Test Report (Refer to Chapter 5, page 149)

1. Create a *New Test Report* for a strep screen within Chloe Hill's chart.
2. Remove the *Problems* and *Recommendations* headings from the report. Type your name at the bottom of the report.
3. Print the test report, add the signature, circle your name on the document, and submit it to your instructor.

appendix A

Sample Documents

Document 1 Prescription Forms

Suburban Medical Group
101 Elm Street
Sherman, TX 77521
Office:(214) 674-2000 Fax:(214) 674-2100
EMail:doc@sfischermd.com

John O. Smith, M. D.
Lic: J87877 DEA: AJ3434343
11/27/11

Pt: Patti G Adams
198 Elm St
Sherman, TX 77521
DOB: 06/29/1942

℞ Allegra 180mg
disp: 30 thirty
sig: i po q am
Refill: prn

John O. Smith, M. D.
**** Electronic Signature Verified ****

John O. Smith, M. D.

A generically equivalent drug product may be dispensed unless the practitioner hand writes the words 'BRAND NECESSARY' or 'BRAND MEDICALLY NECESSARY' on the prescription face

Suburban Medical Group
101 Elm Street
Sherman, TX 77521
Office:(214) 674-2000 Fax:(214) 674-2100
EMail:doc@sfischermd.com

John O. Smith, M. D.
Lic: J87877 DEA: AJ3434343
11/27/11

Pt: Patti G Adams
198 Elm St
Sherman, TX 77521
DOB: 06/29/1942

℞ Tamiflu 75mg
disp: 10 ten
sig: i po bid
Refill: 0 zero

John O. Smith, M. D.
**** Electronic Signature Verified ****

John O. Smith, M. D.

A generically equivalent drug product may be dispensed unless the practitioner hand writes the words 'BRAND NECESSARY' or 'BRAND MEDICALLY NECESSARY' on the prescription face

Suburban Medical Group
101 Elm Street
Sherman, TX 77521
Office:(214) 674-2000 Fax:(214) 674-2100
EMail:doc@sfischermd.com

John O. Smith, M. D.
Lic: J87877 DEA: AJ3434343
11/27/11

Pt: Patti G Adams
198 Elm St
Sherman, TX 77521
DOB: 06/29/1942

℞ Ibuprofen 400mg
disp: 120 one hundred twenty
sig: i po q 6 hr
Refill: 5 five

John O. Smith, M. D.
**** Electronic Signature Verified ****

John O. Smith, M. D.

A generically equivalent drug product may be dispensed unless the practitioner hand writes the words 'BRAND NECESSARY' or 'BRAND MEDICALLY NECESSARY' on the prescription face

Document 2 Patient's Face Sheet

Suburban Medical Group
101 Elm Street Sherman, TX 77521
(214) 674-2000

Name: Patti G Adams 06/29/55
Age: 56 yrs 8 mns 21 days.

Mother's Last Name: Rucker
Address: 198 Elm St Sherman, TX 77521
Home Phone: (214) 766-7676
Home Fax:
Work Phone:
Work Fax:
Pager:
Mobile Phone: (214) 777-7987
EMail: mom5645566@aol.com
SS#: 876-45-6676
Marital Status: Married
Sex: F
Pt ID #: 31
Employer: Home Engineer
Preferred Language : English
Race : White
Ethnicity : Not of Hispanic origin
PMS ID:
Provider:
This Patient's Chart is Included In Searches
Date Entered: 04/02/2002
Last Modified: 03/20/2012

Allergies:

Demerol entered 08/30/2007 2:29 PM by psy note:
Patient Number: 31 Chart ID: 3
Last Modified On:
Last Modified By :
Note: Allergy Reviewed Pending

Other Sensitivities

Nausea
Headache
Patient Number: 31 Chart ID: 4
Last Modified: 02/05/2008

Social History

Alcohol: Occassionally
Wears seat belt 100%
Coffee: 5 cups per day

Patient: Adams, Patti G 06/29/55
Prepared by SpringChartsEMR

Page 1 of 3
Suburban Medical Group

Document 2 ***(continued)***

Smoking Status :4-Never Smoker

Patient Number: 31 Chart ID: 11
Last Modified: 03/20/2012

PMHX

DM, Adult Onset,NID, Controlled 250.00
HTN 401.9
Depression - Recurrent 296.32
Hyperglycemia 790.6
Pneumonia, Bacterial 482.89
Type 2 diabetes for 10 years
Hospitalized March 2006 Hyperglycemia
Hospitalized once for Pneumonia
Last Tetanus 2004
Influenza Vaccine 10/05
Patient Number: 31 Chart ID: 5
Last Modified: 09/23/2007

FMHX

Lung CA 162.9
Father CA of the Lung (contributing factor)
Patient Number: 31 Chart ID: 6
Last Modified: 03/20/2012
Patient Annotation : none listed

Problem List

Dx:

DM, Adult Onset,NID, Controlled 250.00
Hypercholesterolemia 272.0
Depression - Recurrent 296.32
HTN 401.9
Migraine 346.90

Patient Number: 31 Chart ID: 7
Last Modified: 03/20/2012
Last Modified By : demo

Routine Meds

Lipitor 10mg i po q am
Aleve 275 mg i q 12 hrs
Aspirin 325mg ii po qid prn
HCTZ 12.5mg i q am
Lopressor 100 mg i po bid
Wellbutrin XL 300mg i po q am
Glyburide 2.5 mg i po bid Stopped :02/07/2008 Reason: Causes Dizziness Stopped by : demo o
11/17/11 3:10 PM
HCTZ 12.5mg i q am
Lipitor 10mg i po q am Updated by demo on 11/17/11 3:28 PM (Dispensed In-house)
Nexium 40mg i po daily

Patient: Adams, Patti G 06/29/55 — Page 2 of 3
Prepared by SpringChartsEMR — Suburban Medical Group

Document 2 *(continued)*

OTC Meds:
fish oil, glucosamine
Patient Number: 31 Chart ID: 8
Last Modified: 03/06/2012

Referral Details:
Referred To : Hart, Harry I M. D. By : demo On : 11/17/2011 02:18:54 PM Reason : Chest Pain
Patient Number: 31 Chart ID: 9

Last Modified: 11/17/2011 02:18:54 PM
Last Refer To : Hart, Harry I M. D.
Last Refer By : demo

Chart Notes
Friend of Mrs Bibi.

Received informational letter on Naproxen.
Patient Number: 31 Chart ID: 10
Last Modified: 01/16/2005

Insurance Company Info
Insurance Company: United Healthcare
Mail Claim To: Claims
Attention:
Address: 19900 Molson Dr.
City: San Antonio
State: TX
Zip: 77890
Phone: 8008880404
Details:
EMail:
URL:

Patient Insurance Info
Group Name: Retired Teachers Association
Group No: 78329
Certif No: 876456676
Insured's relation to patient: Insured
CoPay: $10.00

Patient: Adams, Patti G 06/29/55
Prepared by SpringChartsEMR

Page 3 of 3
Suburban Medical Group

Document 3 Printed Immunization Record

Suburban Medical Group
101 Elm Street
Sherman, TX 77521
(214) 674-2000 Fax (214) 674-2100

Immunizations for Sykes, Chris J 05/22/01
DPT 04/08/2002
MMR 04/08/2002
HepatitisB 02/15/2002
HepatitisB 04/17/2002
DaPT 03/15/2002
HFlu 03/15/2002
IPV 03/15/2002
Pneumococcus 05/18/2002
HFlu 05/18/2002
IPV 05/18/2002
DaPT 07/16/2002
HFlu 07/16/2002
Pneumococcus 07/16/2002
Varicella 01/08/2003
MMR 01/08/2003
Flu Shot 12/21/2004
date printed: 11/27/11

Prepared by
SpringChartsEMR

Suburban Medical Group

Document 4 Letter to a Patient

Suburban Medical Group
101 Elm Street
Sherman, TX 77521
(214) 674-2000 Fax (214) 674-2100

November 30, 2011

Patti G Adams
198 Elm St
Sherman, TX 77521

Re: New Appointment

Dear Ms. Adams:

An appointment has been scheduled for you on 12/15/11. Please contact our office as soon as possible if you need to change this appointment.

Please arrive at your appointment 10 minutes early in order to complete your new patient forms. You will need to bring all medications that you are currently taking with you.

If you have any questions regarding this appointment, please call our office at (214) 881-3516.

Sincerely,

Document 5 Letter About a Patient

Suburban Medical Group
101 Elm Street
Sherman, TX 77521
(214) 674-2000 Fax (214) 674-2100

November 27, 2011

Harry I Hart M. D.
220 Elm St
Sherman, TX 77521

Re: Chris J Sykes 05/22/01

Dear Dr. Hart;

Thank you for allowing me to participate in this patient's care. If you have any questions or observations for me, please do not hesitate to call.

I will update you on this patient's progress after our next appointment.

Below please find a copy of the patient's recent lab results.

11/13/2011 Strep Screen

Strep Screen negative Normal: negative

ID:
Note:
Tech: josmd
Test Facility: Quest Diagnostics
Reported: 11/13/2011 Last Modified: 11/13/2011
ID#:
Note:

Sincerely,

Document 8 Test Order Form

Suburban Medical Group
101 Elm Street
Sherman, TX 77521
(214) 674-2000 Fax (214) 674-2100

Date: 11/27/11
Pt: Adams, Patti G 06/29/42
Address: 198 Elm St Sherman, TX 77521

Physician Order

Orders:
CBC 85025
SMAC 80054

Diagnosis:
HTN 401.9

Patient Insurance Info
Group Name: Retired Teachers Association
Group/Policy No: 78329
Guarantor: Adams, Patti G 06/29/42
Certif No: 876456676
Insured
CoPay: 10.0

Insurance Company: United Healthcare
Mail Claim To: Claims
Attention:
Address: 19900 Molson Dr.
City: San Antonio
State: TX
Zip: 77890
Phone: 8008880404
Details:
EMail:
URL:

Prepared by SpringChartsEMR

Suburban Medical Group

Document 9 Routing Slip

Suburban Medical Group
101 Elm Street
Sherman, TX 77521
(214) 674-2000 Fax (214) 674-2100

Adams, Patti G 06/29/42
198 Elm St
Sherman, TX 77521
Home #: (214) 766-7676
Work #:
Pager:
EMail: mom5645566@aol.com
SS#: 876-45-6676
Sex: F
Employer: Home Engineer

Home Fax:
Work Fax:
Mobile #: (214) 777-7987

Marital Status: Married
Pt ID #: 31

Date of Service: 04/28/2012
Doctor: John O. Smith, M. D.
E&M Code Recommended: 99214
Diagnosis:
HTN 401.9
DM, Adult Onset,NID, Controlled 250.00
Hypercholesterolemia 272.0
Tests:
CBC 85025
SMAC 80054
Lipid Panel 80061
HGBA1C 83036
Other Procedures:
Ear Irrigation 69210
ref to ophth for yearly checkup
Followup:
3 months.

Patient Insurance Info
Group Name: Retired Teachers Association
Group/Policy No: 78329
Guarantor: Adams, Patti G 06/29/42
Certif No: 876456676
Insured
CoPay: 10.0

Insurance Company: United Healthcare
Mail Claim To: Claims
Attention:
Address: 19900 Molson Dr.
City: San Antonio
State: TX
Zip: 77890
Phone: 8008880404
Details:
EMail:
URL:

Prepared by
SpringChartsEMR

Document 12 History & Physical Report

History and Physical

Patient: Sykes, Chris J 05/22/01

Date of Service: 11/27/2011

Chief Complaint:

Acute Diarrhea.

Present Illness:

Pt c/o watery diarrhea which began 2 days ago. Notes the diarrhea is moderate. Comes on suddenly. - Pt denies nausea, vomiting, pain. - Pt has not noted stools floating or food particles within stool. - History of sick contacts, antibiotic use, foreign travel, bad food exposure. Past Hx of similar episodes: Negative. Family Hx of similar episodes: Negative.

Allergies:

Penicillin

pollen

Current Medications:

Allegra 30mg i po q am

Nasacort AQ 55mcg ii puffs each nostril q am

Children's aspirin, benedryl

Past Medical History:

Chickenpox

Family Medical History:

HTN, Mother, father and sister have had consistent problems with allergies.

Social History:

Review Of Systems:

GENERAL: + - no weight change, fever, chills, night sweats, generalized weakness Gastrointestinal: + -Appetite is normal. No dysphagia, dyspepsia, abd. pain, heartburn, nausea, vomiting, vomiting blood or coffee ground material, jaundice, constipation, melena, blood in or on stools, hemorrhoids.

Examination:

Vitals: Temp: 98.6 Wt: 42.0 Ht: 41.0

GENERAL: + - Well developed. Well nourished. In no distress / evident discomfort / Appears ill. ABDOMEN: + - Bowel sounds present and normal. - No evidence of scarring or past surgical procedures. - Flat, soft, nontender, without rebound or guarding. No fluid wave elicited. - No evidence of masses, organomegaly or abdominal aneurysm. - Normal to percussion. RECTAL: + - No abnormality. No masses, hemorrhoids, no fissures. - Hemoccult: Negative.

Impression:

Diarrhea, Acute 787.91

Plan:

Flagyl 500mg i po bid #10 rf x0

Discussed keeping up hydration and eating crackers until diarrhea remits. Once better add complex carbohydrates to diet (cereals, rice, potatoes, bread). Avoid fatty foods until well. Watch for lactose intolerance. Pt Instr: Diarrhea given

Suburban Medical Group

H&P for Pt: Sykes, Chris J 05/22/01 Page 1 of 1

appendix B

Source Documents for SpringCharts Single-User Version

Source Document 1 Patient Information Sheet

Suburban Medical Group

101 Elm Street
Sherman, TX 77521

PH: (214) 674-2000
FX: (214) 674-2100

Appointment: Time 10:00 AM Date Today's Date

Physician: Dr. Smith

PATIENT INFORMATION SHEET

Patient Name: Hill, CALOE, ELIZABETH
Last, First, Middle

Date of Birth: 10/8/89

Address: 78 RICHARDS ST.
LOGANLEA, MO 65807

Social Security #: 048-69-4281

E-mail Address: ceh89@hotmail.com

Home Phone: 417-881-3968

Cell Phone:

Gender (Circle one): Male, Female (circled: Female)

Marital Status (Circle one): Married, Single, Divorced, Widowed, Separated (circled: Single)

Preferred Language: ENGLISH

Race (Circle one): American Indian, Asian, Black, White, Hispanic, Native Hawaiian, Unknown, Other (circled: White)

Ethnicity (Circle one): Hispanic, Non-Hispanic (circled: Non-Hispanic)

Mother's Maiden Name:

Emplyoyer: LOGAN CITY

Work Phone: 417-969-4123

Work Fax: 417-969-7821

Signature of Patient or Patient-Guardian: CE Hill

Source Document 2 Primary Insurance Card Information

Physician Visit & Hospital Program

Universal Health Network

National Provider Network

Office Visit Co-Pay: $35.00

Name of Insured: CHLOE ELIZABETH HILL

Member Number: 041020102

Group Number: 76022

Members: In an Emergency Seek Medical Attention First

For questions or to locate a provider visit www.uhnbenefits.com

Or call 800-275-1258.

Before seeking hospital services you must register for CAP benefits

To register call 800-975-2589

Members Are Responsible For Network Contracted Rates Incurred.

Members are required to register for referral authorization before seeking hospital services.

PROVIDERS:

Send bills to: UHN; PO Box 221458; Dallas, TX 75225

For questions call: 866-404-5489

For lab work use Lab Diagnostics or call 800-975-1452.

In emergency please admit the patient and call 800-975-1452 by the next business day.

All members have limited inpatient and outpatient benefits.

Underwritten by various insurance companies.

This program is administered by UHN

6732 DownUnder Blvd., Mackay, CO 80922

Source Document 3 Patient Intake Sheet

Suburban Medical Group

101 Elm Street
Sherman, TX 77521

PH: (214) 674-2000
FX: (214) 674-2100

Primary Care Physician
Name: Jon Clark, MD
Address: 1800 E WOODHURST ST
WATERFORD, MO 65804
Phone: 417-890-6777
Family Practice

Patient Name: CHLOE E. HILL

Date of Birth: 10/8/89   SS #: 048-69-4281

PERSONAL HEALTH INFORMATION

Allergies:
Drugs & Medications? Please list.
CODEINE

Foods? Please list with adverse reactions.
PEANUT PRODUCTS - RASH
SHELLFISH - HIVES

Personal Medical History:	Yes	No
Asthma	✓	
Bronchitis	✓	
Cancer		✓
Diabetes		✓
Gout		✓
Heart Disease		✓
Hernia		✓
High Cholesterol		✓
HIV Positive		✓
Kidney Disease		✓
Liver Disease		✓
Migraines		✓
Pneumonia	✓	
Thyroid Problems		
Other:		
Other:		

Social History: (Check the appropriate line)

Tobacco Use: (Choose one)
- Current - Every day? ____
- Current - Some days? ____
- Former Smoker? ____
- Never Smoked? ✓

Alcohol Use:
- Non Drinker? ____
- Social Drinker? ✓
- Heavy Drinker? ____

Caffeine Use:
- Yes ✓
- No ____
- Cups per Day? 2

Living Arrangements:
- Lives with Family/Parents ✓
- Lives with Spouse/Partner ____

Education:
- Highschool ____
- College ✓
- Post-Graduate ____

Occupation: Receptionist

Family Medical History: (List chronic health problems)
Father: ASTHMA
Mother:
Brother(s): 1 BROTHER - ASTHMA.
Sister(s):

Has your physical activity been restricted during the past 5 years? NO
Have you been hosptialized during the past 5 years? Explain: APPENDECTOMY - 2004
Have you lived or travelled outside the US in the past 5 years? NO

Current Medical Problems:	Yes	No	Details:
Asthma/Hay Fever	✓		TWICE PER YR.
Back Problems		✓	
Blood Pressure Problems		✓	
Cholesterol Problems		✓	
Colds and chronic coughs		✓	
Diarrhea/Constipation		✓	
Eating Problems		✓	
Female Problems		✓	
Gall Bladder Problems		✓	
Hernias		✓	
Jaundice/Hepatitis		✓	
Kidney Problems		✓	
Liver Problems		✓	
Pains		✓	
Other:			

Routine Medications:
ALEVE - 275mg
CLARITIN D-24

Over-The-Counter Meds:
CALCIUM SUPPLEMENTS
MULTI-VITAMINS

Personal Preferences:
Hospital: ST. JOHNS
Lab Company: LAB CORP

Additional Concerns:
ENGLISH - SECOND LANGUAGE.

HIPAA Notice of Privacy Practices Acknowledges
I acknowledge receipt of and have read the **Suburban Medical Group Notice of Privacy Practices.**

Patient's Signature: C E Hill   Date: 11/15/2012

Source Document 4 Default Pharmacy Information

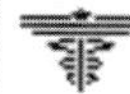

Walgreens

Crn Campell Ave. & Battlefield St.
Loganlea, MO 68504

Office:(417) 887-8546
Fax:(417) 887-5623

Category: Pharmacy

Source Document 5 Immunization Record Card

VACCINE ADMINISTRATION RECORD
FOR CHILDREN & TEENS
LOGANLEA, MO 56801
PH: (417) 889-2222 FX: (417) 889-2224

Immunizations for Hill, Chloe E 10/08/89
Flu Shot 2/5/1990
Varicella 4/10/1990
MMR 4/10/1990
IPV 8/15/1990
Hepatitis A 10/15/1990
IPV 4/15/1991
DaPT 10/5/1991
IPV 4/15/1994
DaPT 4/15/1994
MMR 10/15/2001
DaPT 10/15/2001
Hepatitis B 6/2/2002
Meningitis 8/19/2005
Flu Shot 5/5/2007
Date printed: 04/26/12

Source Document 8 **Letter to Primary Care Physician**

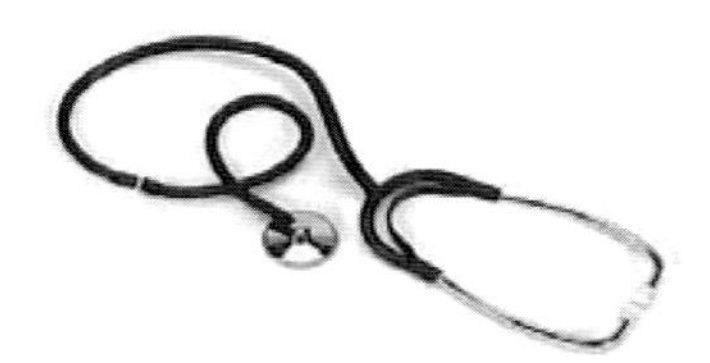

Suburban Medical Group

101 Elm Street
Sherman, TX 77521

PH: (214) 674-2000
FX: (214) 674-2100

Today's Date

Jon D. Clark
Clark Family Medicine
1200 E. Woodhurst St.
Waterford, MO 65804

Re: Chloe E. Hill 10/8/89

Dear Dr. Clark:

Thank you for allowing me to participate in this pt's care. If you have any questions or observations for me, please do not hesitate to call.

Below please find a copy of the recent examination

Sincerely,
J.O. Smith MD

Source Document 9 Patient Lab Results

TEST PERFORMED AT:
Lab Corp
4380 Federal Dr. Suite 100
Marsdon, MO 65803

PATIENT:
Hill, Chloe Elizabeth
DOB: 10/08/1989
Gender: F

Ordering Physician: John O. Smith MD
Accnt No: 444051
Lab Specimen: No N321850003

Test Name	In Range	Out Of Range	Reference Range
Strep Screen	Normal		Normal

Test Date: 08/05/2011

Source Document 10 Telephone Call Message

Suburban Medical Group
PH: (214) 674-2000
FX: (214) 674-2100

Telephone Call Message

To: Demo

Date: Today's Date Time: 10:35 (A.M.) P.M.

From: Chloe Hill

Phone Number: 417-881-3968

[X] Telephoned [ ] Returned Your Call [ ] Please Call [ ] Will Call Again [X] Please Rush Request [ ] Special Attention

Message:
Pt called and requested letter regarding her recent lab work results.
She needs to show her employer that the strep results were negative.

Name: User Demo Signed: [signature]

Exercise 3.2(N) Adding New Addresses—Physician

1. Access the *New* menu at the top of the main screen and select *New Address.*
2. Enter the name and demographics of your primary care physician (PCP) or general practitioner (GP). (If you do not have a PCP or GP, you may make up the information.)
3. In the *Category* field, select *Physician* from the drop-down menu.
4. Choose the appropriate medical specialty from the drop-down menu in the *Specialty* field.
5. Complete the remaining fields except *Account#*, and leave *Notes* blank. (Again, you may make up any information, such as telephone numbers, that you do not have.)
6. Save the information by clicking on the [Save] button.

SpringCharts Tip

Although SpringCharts users are set up as *Users* in the *Administration* panel of SpringCharts server, they also need to be entered into the *Address Book* as employees, to capture their addresses and other demographic information.

Exercise 3.3(N) Adding New Addresses—Employee

1. Access the *New* menu at the top of the main screen and select *New Address.*
2. Enter your name and demographics.
3. In the *Category* field, select *Employee* from the drop-down menu. (You do not need to complete the *Company* or *Specialty* fields when creating an address file for an individual.)
4. Complete all of the appropriate remaining fields except *Account#*, and leave *Notes* blank.
5. Save the information by clicking on the [Save] button.

SpringCharts Tip

The *Specialty* field is only completed if a practitioner is being set up in the *Address Book* within SpringCharts.

Exercise 3.4(N) Adding New Addresses—Pharmacy

1. Access the *New* menu at the top of the main screen and select *New Address.*
2. Set up a pharmacy of your choice, starting with entering information in the *Company* field. (You do not need to complete the *Name* information.)
3. Select *Pharmacy* in the *Category* field.
4. Complete all the appropriate remaining fields except *Account#*, and leave *Notes* blank. (Remember the *Specialty* field is only used to designate the medical specialty when setting up a provider.)
5. Save the information by clicking on the [Save] button.

Exercise 3.5(N) Adding New Addresses—Testing Facility

1. Access the *New* menu at the top of the main screen and select *New Address.*
2. Set up a *Testing Facility.* This could be a lab, imaging, or any medical testing company. (As with the pharmacy, you do not need to complete the name information or choose a *Specialty.*
3. Select *Testing Facility* in the *Category* field.
4. Complete the remaining fields except *Account #,* and leave *Notes* blank. (You may make up information, such as telephone numbers.)
5. Save the information.

Exercise 3.6(N) Adding New Addresses—Medical Supplier

1. Access the *New* menu at the top of the main screen and select *New Address* (shown in margin).
2. Set up a medical supplier, starting with entering information in the *Company* field.
3. Select one of the following medical supply companies: *Johnson & Johnson, GE Healthcare, Baxter, Philips Medical, B. Braun, 3M Healthcare, Alcon, Biomet, Invacare,* or *St. Jude Medical.*
4. Create a local address and phone and fax number for your company.
5. Select *Medical Supplies* in the *Category* field.
6. Save the information by clicking on the [Save] button.

SpringCharts Tip

Shortcut:

Open Address Book

The third speed icon located on the Spring-Charts Toolbar enables the user to open the *Address Bbook,* where nonpatient addresses can be added and edited.

Exercise 3.7(N) Printing Addresses

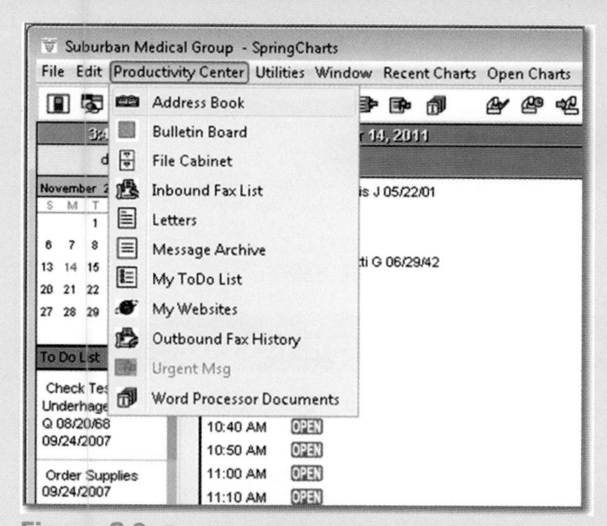

Figure C.2 *Productivity Center > Address Book* menu.

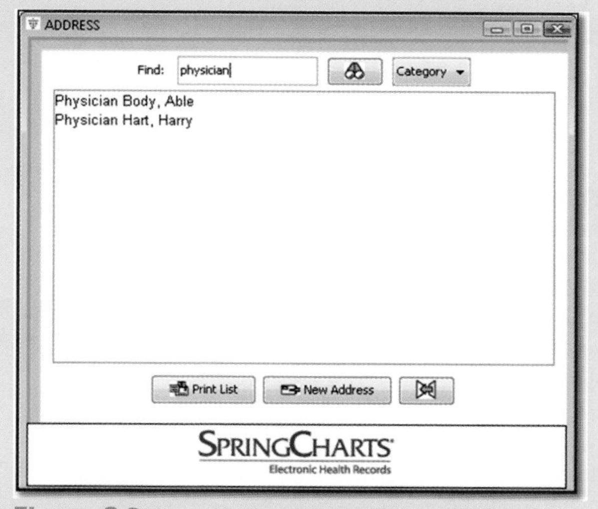

Figure C.3 Searching for a physician in the *Address Book.*

1. Access the *Productivity Center* menu at the top of the main screen and select the *Address Book* (Figure C.2).
2. Locate each of your new addresses (physician, employee, pharmacy, and testing facility) by selecting the appropriate option (*Name, Company, Specialty,* or *Category*) in the drop-down menu and then entering the type of category or the name in the *Find* field. (Figure C.3 shows an example.)
3. In each category, click on the *New Address* entry you added to open the address details.
4. Print out each of your addresses by selecting the [Print Card] button, choosing the printer, and then clicking [OK]. A sample of the printed address cards appear in Figure C.4.

Print Card

[Print Card] button

5. Close the *Address* window by clicking the red [X] in the upper right corner.
6. Write your name on each page and submit them to your instructor.

(continued)

Exercise 3.7(N) (Concluded)

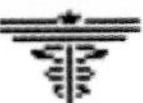
Clarke, Jason M.D
123 Main St.
Springfield, MO 65807
Office:(417) 239-0856
Fax:(214) 456-7890
Category: Physician Specialty: Family Practice

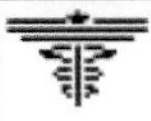
Burnich, Steve M.A.
Sherman, TX 77521
Office:(214) 567-8765
Fax:(214) 123-9876
Category: Employee

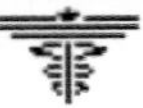
PharmWorld
345 Davis Dr
Sherman, TX 77521
Office:(214) 567-8765
Fax:(214) 234-5678
Category: Pharmacy

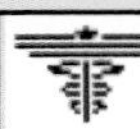
MRI Of The Ozarks
103 E. Battlefield St.
Springfield, MO 65807
Office:(214) 567-9087
Fax:(214) 342-7896
Category: TestingFacility

Figure C.4 Sample of printed address cards.

SpringCharts Tip

When entering a patient's name in Spring-Charts, the first name is entered first, and then the last name. If you enter the last name first, you will not be able to locate the patient's chart later, because the program searches for the patient by the last name field.

Exercise 3.8(N) Adding a New Patient Record

1. Select the *New* menu at the top of the main *Practice View* screen.
2. Select the *New Patient* submenu.
3. Enter yourself as a patient. Complete as much information as possible. Please use the zip code: 77521. For security reasons, do not use your actual Social Security number for your profile. For the purpose of exercises later in the text, make yourself a female patient with an age somewhere between 21 and 30.
4. Save the information by clicking on the [Save] button.

SpringCharts Tip

Reminder: Telephone numbers and Social Security numbers can be typed into the appropriate fields without punctuation. Once the user tabs off the field, punctuation is automatically inserted.

Exercise 3.9(N) Editing a Patient Record

1. Select the main *Edit* menu at the top of the main *Practice View* screen.
2. Choose the *Patients* submenu.
3. Locate your chart by last name in the *Search* field.
4. Click the [Search] button and select your chart.
5. Add or change the *Work Phone* to your demographics.
6. Click the [Save] button, but do not exit the *Edit Patient* window.

Exercise 3.10(N) Exporting a Patient List

1. Within the *Edit Patient* window, which still shows a list of patients with the zip code of 77521, click the [Export] button in the bottom right corner.

> **Note:** Depending on the size of your screen, you may have to use your scroll bars to locate the [Export] button.

2. Select *Export List.*
3. Choose the [Open in Word Processor] option from the *Export Patient List* window. SpringCharts will recreate the list of patients with a zip code of 77521 in your computer's default word processing program. In most cases, this will be Notepad. From here, the list can be printed out or saved on the computer. Notice that the date of birth is in the *yyyymmdd* format. Also, Notepad defaults to the font size last used on the computer. You may change the text size by selecting *Format* > *Font* in Notepad.
4. Print out the list of patients with the zip code of 77521, circle your name on the paper, and submit to your instructor.

Exercise 3.11(N) Adding a New Insurance Company

1. Access the *Edit* menu at the top of the main *Practice View* screen and select *Insurance.*
2. Click the [New Insurance Company] button.
3. Add a new insurance company to SpringCharts, using your insurance information if you have your own insurance card, or create a fictitious insurance company and all the contact information.
4. In the *Details* box add the name and number of a contact person at the insurance company.
5. Save the new insurance company.
6. Highlight the newly added insurance company and select the *Copy or Export This Data* (or *Export*) button (shown in margin) in the lower right corner.
7. Select the [Open in Word Processor] button.
8. In the word processing program, type your name at the top of the insurance information.
9. Print the document and submit it to your instructor.

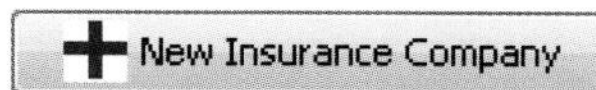

[New Insurance Company] button

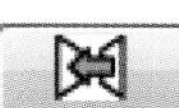
Copy or Export This Data button

Exercise 3.12(N) Editing Insurance Information

1. Access the *Edit* menu at the top of the main *Practice View* screen.
2. Select the *Insurance* submenu.
3. Click on the insurance company you added.
4. Click the [Edit] button.
5. Change the name and number of the contact person in the *Attention* field.
6. Add an e-mail address to the *Email* field.
7. Save this information by selecting the [Save] button.

Chapter 4 The Clinic Administration

Exercise 4.1(N) Becoming Familiar with the Toolbar

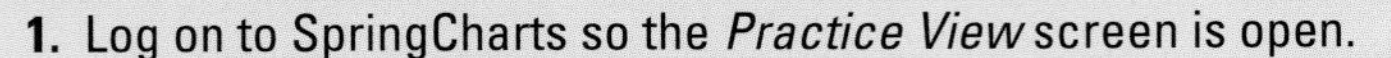

New ToDo Item icon

New Message icon

New Urgent Message icon

1. Log on to SpringCharts so the *Practice View* screen is open.
2. Click on the *New ToDo item* icon (shown in margin). A *New ToDo/Reminder* box displays.
3. Examine the *New To Do/Reminder* window, and then close it.
4. Click on the *Open New Message* icon (shown in margin). A *Link Message to Patient* window opens.
5. Click the [No] button in the *Link Message to Patient* window.
6. Examine the *New Message* window, and then close it.
7. Click on the *New Urgent Message* icon (shown in margin). A *Send Urgent Message* window displays.
8. Examine the *Send Urgent Message* window, and then close it.

Note: It is important to complete Exercises 4.2 through 4.9 in one day. Because SpringCharts EHR is an industry-standard program, patients placed on today's schedule will not appear on the schedule when you log in the next day.

Note: For Exercises 4.2 through 4.9, your instructor will assign you a different calendar day than the other students to work with.

Exercise 4.2(N) Adding an Existing Patient to the Schedule

1. Log on to SpringCharts.
2. Click on any *OPEN* icon on the appointment schedule.
3. When the *Edit Appointment* window displays, click on the [Choose Patient] button.
4. With the *Choose Patient* window open, type the first few letters of your last name, and then press the [Search] button.
5. Select your name from the list.
6. Enter a fictitious reason for your visit in the *Note* field of the *Edit Appointment* window.
7. Add your initials after the note.
8. Click the [Done] button.

Exercise 4.3(N) Blocking Out Time on the Schedule

Note: Ask your instructor to assign you a unique date on the calendar (upper left corner) to work the following Exercise 4.3 through Exercise 4.9. If you do not work these exercises during the same session, you will need to remember your assigned date the next time you log into SpringCharts.

1. Click on the *OPEN* time slot for the beginning of the last hour of the work day, where you will block out time on the schedule for a staff meeting. Depending on the day, you may have to use the scroll bar to slide down to the last hour on the Appointment Schedule.
2. Type *Staff Meeting* in the *Note* field of the *Edit Appointment* window.
3. Click on the [Block This Time] button.
4. Repeat this exercise for each 10-minute increment until the entire hour is blocked.

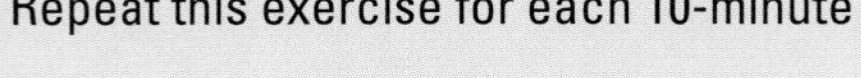

Exercise 4.4(N) Adding a New Patient to the Schedule

1. Click on an *OPEN* time slot on the appointment schedule.
2. Type a new patient's name in the *Patient* field.
3. Type in *Physical* for the visit reason in the *Note* field.
4. Add your initials after the note.
5. Click the [Done] button.

> **Note:** You will notice that this patient's appointment will be scheduled with the *New* icon in the time slot because he is not currently in the database; this indicates that he is a new patient to the practice.

Exercise 4.5(N) Adding a Note to the Schedule

1. Add two established patients, *Sally Dalton* and *Robert Underhagen,* to the appointment schedule.

> **Note:** Refer back to Exercise 4.2 if you need help adding existing patients to the schedule.

2. Add the reason note *UTI* (urinary tract infection) to Sally's appointment and the reason note *Lab* to Robert's.
3. After you add the notes to your schedule, also add your initials.

Exercise 4.6(N) Adding Additional Patients to the Schedule

1. Add two new patients to the appointment schedule, along with the appropriate reason notes. You may make up the names of your patients and the reasons for their visits.

> **Note:** Remember, these are *New/Unregistered* patients, so you cannot search for them in the database.

Exercise 4.7(N) Scheduling a Meeting on a Future Schedule

1. Open the calendar schedule exactly one month from the day you are currently working.
2. In the appointment window for that date, click on the 4:30 p.m. *OPEN* time slot.
3. When the *Edit Appointment* window displays, type *Staff Meeting* in the *Note* field.
4. Click on the [Block This Time] button.
5. Repeat this exercise for each 10-minute increment until the one-half hour is blocked for the staff meeting. (You do not need to repeat *Staff Meeting* for subsequent time slots.)
6. Block out time in the schedule for a half-hour staff meeting on the last Friday of each month for the next 3 months. Close the additional appointment windows by clicking the red [X] in the upper right corner of each window.

Exercise 4.16(N) Moving a Patient from One Location to Another

1. Click on your name in the tracker.
2. In the *Edit Tracker* window, change the status of the patient to *Nurse Check.*
3. Move your patient into one of the *Exam Rooms.*

Note: Ask your instructor to assign you a unique exam room; however, due to the number of students doing this exercise, more than one patient may be in an exam room. This would not normally happen in a medical office.

4. Open your patient's chart by clicking on the [Get Chart] button.
5. Close the patient's chart.

Exercise 4.17(N) Communicating to Co-Workers through the *Patient Tracker*

The nurse assigned to your patient has finished recording the patient's chief complaints and taking his or her vital signs. During the initial evaluation you determine that the patient needs to be seen by the physician, so you will need to change the status and the color coding.

1. Update the *Patient Tracker* by changing the status of your patient to *Doctor Check.* Dr. Smith will see the update on his *Patient Tracker* and know the location of the patient who now requires his attention.
2. Change the color code to indicate that the patient will now be seen by Dr. Finchman. (Refer to Exercise 4.12 for color coding instructions).

Exercise 4.18(N) Changing the Tracker Location and Status

Assume you are the doctor and have finished the patient examination in the *Exam Room.*

1. Click on your patient's name in the tracker.
2. In the *Edit Tracker* window, change the patient's location to *Checkout Desk.*
3. Change the patient's status to *Ready.*
4. Click the [Done] button.

Exercise 4.19(N) Checking Out a Patient in the *Tracker*

Your patient has been processed at the front desk, setting another appointment and paying his or her co-pay.

1. Click on your patient's name in the tracker.
2. Click on the [Check Out] button in the *Edit Tracker* window. Notice the program changes the patient's location and status to *Done* and removes the color flags from the patient. The window automatically closes.

Exercise 4.20(N) Changing the Patient's Location, Status, and Color Code

1. Click on your walk-in patient in the *Waiting Room.*
2. Change the Location to the same exam room that you just moved your first patient out of. Change the Status to *Nurse Check.* Assign the color coding to indicate that this patient does not have healthcare insurance and is a self-pay. The patient is coming in just to do lab work. (Refer to Exercise 4.12 for color coding instructions).
3. Click the [Done] button.

Exercise 4.21(N) Working with the *Tracker Archive*

1. Click on the *Edit* menu on the main *Practice View* screen.
2. Click on the *Tracker Archive* submenu. The *Edit Tracker Archive* window displays the patients processed through the *Patient Tracker* today.
3. Click on your patient and notice the *Time In* and *Time Out* stamps on the right-side panel.
4. Click on the [Export] button.
5. Select the *Export List* option.
6. Select the [Open in Word Processor] button in the *Export Tracker List* window.
7. Select the *File* menu and then the *Print* option.
8. Print out the list of patients, circle your name, and submit the list to your instructor.
9. Close the word processor window.
10. Close the *Edit Tracker Archive* window.

Exercise 4.22(N) Setting a Reminder

1. Click on the *To Do List* title bar.
2. In the *New ToDo/Reminder* window, type *Schedule Staff Meeting* in the empty item field.
3. Click on the [Send] button. Notice the new *ToDo* item has been added to your *To Do List* with a green bar.
4. Assume you have completed the task, and click the *Schedule Staff Meeting ToDo* item. The program adds a checked box to the item, indicating it has been completed. The next time you log on to SpringCharts, this item will have been removed from your *To Do List.*

Exercise 4.23(N) Setting a Patient Reminder

1. Click on the *To Do List* title bar.
2. In the *New ToDo/Reminder* window, select *Call Pt* and *Check Lab* from the pop-up text panel.
3. Click the [Link to a Patient] button.
4. In the *Choose Patient* window, type *under* and conduct a search.

(continued)

Exercise 4.28(N) (Concluded)

12. Click *No* when the program asks if you want to update the patient's chart to reflect this as the patient's default pharmacy. The selected pharmacy is added to the body of the message note.
13. Typically, the user would send this message to the practitioner. However, since we are in a classroom environment, send the message to yourself by selecting your user name from the drop-down list of names in the *To:* field.
14. Click on the [Send] button. The message should appear at the top of your *Messages* panel.

Note: Notice that the EHR program automatically records the date, time, and sender in the header.

Exercise 4.29(N) Sending an Urgent Message

New Urgent Message icon

1. Click on the *New Urgent Message* icon on the Toolbar of the *Practice View* screen.
2. Select the log-in name of the student sitting beside you, and give your neighbor your SpringCharts's log-in name.
3. Select *Urgent call from* in the pop-up text list. Add *Dr. Smith* after the phrase *Urgent call from* in the *Message* box.
4. Click the [Send] button. The urgent message is sent to your neighbor's computer and appears on his or her screen.

Exercise 4.30(N) Responding to an Urgent Message

Assume you are the practitioner who has received an urgent message on your computer screen.

1. In the pop-up text window, select the following phrases: *OK. Thanks. Tell them I will call back later. Send me this info in a message.*
2. Click the [Send] button. The urgent message is sent back to your neighbor's computer.

Exercise 4.31(N) Creating a Regular Message from an Urgent Message

The practitioner has indicated he or she cannot take the call now and wants the urgent message sent to him or her as a reminder to call Dr. Smith.

1. In the *Open Urgent Message* window, click on the [Message] button.
2. Answer [No] to the question in the prompt window, *Does this message concern a Patient?*
3. In the subject line (*Re:*) on the *New Message* window, type *Urgent Message.*
4. Select your neighbor's log-in name in the drop-down *To* field.
5. Click the [Send] button in the middle panel.
6. You have received a similar message in your *Messages* center from your neighbor. Open the message by clicking on it.
7. Click in the body of the message under the phrase *Urgent call from Dr. Smith.*
8. Type your name in full.
9. Click on the [Print] button in the middle panel.
10. Click the [Print] button in the *Document Printing Options* window.
11. Print out the message, circle your name, and turn the page into your instructor.
12. Click on the red [X] in the upper right corner of the *Messages* window.

Exercise 5.1(N) Building Category Preferences

EHR programs can be customized for specific medical specialties. The major portion of customization occurs on the server.

1. Open your own chart by selecting the *Open a Patient Chart* icon on the main menu. Type in the first few letters of your last name in the *Choose Patient* window. Select your name. Your chart should be empty except for your demographic information.
2. Within your chart, click on the *Show Chart/Face Sheet* icon to open your face sheet *Edit* window.
3. Click on the [Social Hx] navigation button on the left-hand side and locate the list of *Preferences* beginning with *Alcohol Use:* in the lower right panel. This list of *social history preferences* was created on the SpringCharts server and provides the user with a rapid way to enter data into the patient's face sheet. Retype this list into the appropriate heading of Table C.1 below. This activity is similar to how the administrator of SpringCharts created this list on the server. Because the list appears as category headings in the *Face Sheet* window, you can place a colon (:) after each group heading.
4. Similarly, locate the *Preferences* list under the [PMHX] and [FMHX] navigation buttons of the face sheet and record the lists in the respective columns in Table C.1 below.

Table C.1 ***Category Preferences* List.**

Social Hx	Past Hx	Family Hx

Exercise 5.2(N) Building a New Patient's Face Sheet

1. Open your own chart by selecting the *Open a Patient Chart* icon (shown in margin) on the main menu. Type the first few letters of your last name into the window and click on the *Search* icon.
2. Select your name and your chart opens, empty except for your demographic information.
3. Within your chart, click on the *Show Chart/Face Sheet* icon (shown in margin) located at the far right of the menu bar, to open the *Edit Face Sheet* window.

(continued)

SpringCharts Tip

Shortcut:
Open a Chart
The third speed icon from the right on the Toolbar enables the user to quickly open a patient's chart and bypass the *Actions* menu.

Hamilton, Byron R 05/05/58
File Edit Windows Actions New

Show Chart/Face Sheet icon

Exercise 5.2(N) (Continued)

SpringCharts Tip

Remember you only need to type the first few letters of the word to conduct a search. The more letters you type, the more likely you are to make a mistake, and the system will not be able to locate the term.

SpringCharts Tip

Place your cursor after the *Preferences* category item you selected and then click on the pop-up text item. The placement of the cursor determines where the pop-up text is inserted.

Allergies

4. The window opens to the *Allergies* section.
5. In the *Allergy* field on the right side, type *peni* and press the search button.
6. Select *Penicillins* from the list. The program adds this drug to your allergy list on the left side.
7. Repeat these steps to add the drug *Codeine* and the allergen *Peanut-Containing Prod.*
8. In the *Other Sensitivities* window, in the lower section of the window, type the medication *Erythromycin.* Then select *causes nausea* from the *Allergy Notes* pop-up text.

Social History

9. Click on the [Social Hx] navigation button to open the *Social History* window.
10. In the *Preferences* window in the lower right, select the *Alcohol Use:* category.
11. Select the appropriate item from the *Social Hx* pop-up text section in the upper window, for example, *Alcohol Use: Non-Drinker.*
12. Repeat these steps to add information in the *Caffeine Use* and *Living Arrangements* categories, using the pop-up text of your choice.

Past Medical History

13. Click on the [PMHX] navigation button to open the *Past Medical History* window.
14. Select several items of your choice from the *Preferences* list to build your past medical history.
15. Add a medical condition not in the *Preferences* list by searching for a diagnosis in the *Dx* field in the upper right. Type *HTN* for hypertension, hit the search icon and select the diagnosis.

Family Medical History

16. Click on the [FMHX] navigation button to open the *Family History* window.
17. Select several medical conditions of your choice from the *Preferences* list to build your family medical history.
18. Select Father: Died At Age: and Cause of Death: from the *Preferences* list. Place your cursor at the end of the *Father* and *Died at Age:* phrase in the *Other FMHX* window and then type a fictitious age. Hit the [Enter] key.
19. Place your cursor at the end of *Cause of Death:* phrase and select a medical condition from the list.
20. In the *Parents Information* section in the lower left, check the box to indicate that the father is deceased. Select the date from the calendar icon: 6/9/1969.

Chart Note

21. Click on the [Chart Note] navigation button to open the *Chart Note* window.
22. Click in the *Chart Note* section on the left side of the window. Hit the [Enter] key to move your cursor to a new line.
23. Select *Prefers Hospital* in the pop-up text on the right side. Then select *St. Judes* from the right side.
24. Select *Religion* in the pop-up text on the right side. Place your cursor at the end of this word and type a specific religion (can be fictitious).

Exercise 5.2(N) (Concluded)

Routine Medications

25. Click on the [Routine Meds] navigation button to open the *Routine Medications* window.
26. In the upper right quadrant, search for and select each of the following medications: *Diovan, Glucophage,* and *Lipitor.* You can select the strength of your choice. All three medications then appear on the left side of the window.
27. In the *Notes and OTC Meds* section, select several OTC (over-the-counter) items from the *Routine Meds* pop-up text in the lower-right quadrant.

Problem List

28. Click on the [Problem List] navigation button to open the *Problem List* window.
29. In the *Dx* field in the upper right, type in *htn* and conduct a search. Select *HTN 401.9* for hypertension.
30. In the same field, type the code *250* and conduct a search. Select *Diabetes.*
31. In the *Dx* field, type *hypercholest* and conduct a search. Select *Hypercholesterolemia272.0.*
32. Search for and select *Allergic Rhinitis—Pollen 477.0.*

Chart Alert

33. Click on the [Chart Alert] navigation button to open the *Chart Alert* window.
34. Click on the pop-up text edit icon on the far right. Place your [Caps Lock] key on and type *SPANISH—ENGLISH IS SECOND LANGUAGE* on the next empty line in the *Edit PopUp Text* window. Click the [Done] button.
35. Select *SPANISH—ENGLISH IS SECOND LANGUAGE* from the available pop-up text.

Printing the Face Sheet

36. Click on the [Print FS] button in the lower left corner of the *Edit Face Sheet* window.
37. Click the [Print] button in the *Document Printing Options* window. Select the printer and print your documents.
38. Click on the [Back] button in the *Edit Face Sheet* window. All the data selected is now positioned in the various face sheet categories within your chart.
39. Collect your printed face sheet document and turn it in to your instructor.

Exercise 5.3(N) Adding the Patient's Primary Insurance

1. Open your chart by clicking on the *Open a Patient Chart* icon on the main Toolbar, entering your last name in the *Choose Patient* window, conducting a search, and selecting your name.
2. Right-click in the *Insurance* section of your face sheet and select the *Edit* option.
3. Enter the following information:
   - *Group Name: Springfield School System*
   - *Group No.: SSS24589*
   - *Policy No.: 4578954*
   - *Details: Deductible for procedures and tests—$250.00*
   - *Co-pay: $25.00*
   - *Insured (Guarantor):* Click in the *Pt is the guarantor* check box
   - *Insurance Company: Principal Financial Group*

(continued)

Exercise 5.3(N) (Concluded)

4. Save the primary insurance information by clicking the [Save] button.

Note: The primary insurance information will not appear on your face sheet until the chart has been closed and reopened.

5. Close the chart.
6. Click on the *Recent Charts* heading on the main menu bar. Select your name. You should see the primary insurance information on your face sheet. Close your chart.

Exercise 5.4(N) Accessing an Immunization Record

1. Open the patient chart for Chris Sykes.
2. Click on the *Immunization* category in the patient's care tree and view the list of past immunizations.
3. Click on the *Immunization* header in the window to sort the list by vaccination. Click on the *Date* header to sort the list by date.
4. Click on the [Print] button, opening the *Document Printing Options* window. Click on the [Print] button again to print a copy of Chris Sykes's immunizations.
5. Write your name on the printed document and turn it in to your instructor. Close Chris Sykes's chart.

Exercise 5.5(N) Recording and Reviewing Vitals

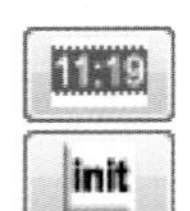

Time and initial buttons

1. Open your chart. Click on the *Create a New Vitals Only Note* speed icon.
2. Record the following vitals: *Temperature 98.6, Respiration 17, Pulse 69, Blood Pressure 129/70, Height 64 inches,* and *Weight 163 pounds.*
3. Click on the [Notes] tab in the upper right and select any verbiage from the pop-up text. Add the time and your initials by clicking on the time and initial icon buttons (shown in margin).
4. Click the [Done] button and [Save and Skip Billing].
5. Close and reopen your chart by selecting the patient's name from the *Recent Charts* menu on the main menu bar.
6. Open the *Actions* menu within the patient's chart. Select *Graph Vital Signs* and view the various graphed vitals.
7. Open the *BP/BMI* entry and print a copy. Submit it to your instructor. Close all open windows.

SpringCharts Tip

Shortcut: ***Create New Letter About Patient***
The fourth speed icon from the right on the tool-bar within the patient's chart enables the user to access the *New Letter ABOUT Patient* window without needing to use the *New* menu drop-down window.

Exercise 5.6(N) Creating a Letter About a Patient

1. Open your chart. Click on the *New Letter ABOUT Patient* icon.
2. Select the referring physician, *Dr. Harry Hart,* from the [Get Address Book] button.
3. Choose the pop-up text that begins with *Thank you for allowing me to participate . . .*
4. Click on the *Edit PopUp Text* icon (shown in margin). Add the following sentence on an empty line: *Below please find detail of the patient's demographics.* Click on the [Done] button.

Edit PopUp Text icon

Exercise 5.6(N) (Concluded)

5. Place the cursor in the letter body on a new line and select the newly added pop-up text sentence.
6. Click on the sentence: *I will update you on this patient's progress after our next appointment* to add this phrase to the letter as well.
7. Click on the [Add Chart Notes] button and select the patient's name from the *Choose Chart Entry* window. The demographics are then added to the body of the letter.
8. Select the *Change signature of letter* icon button (shown in margin) and select a signature.
9. Print the letter on the clinic's letterhead and submit to your instructor.
10. Click on the [Done] button and select *Letters* as the category where the letter will be stored in the patient's care tree. Click the [Save] button.
11. On the patient's chart, click on the "+" expand symbol beside the *Letter* category in the care tree to see the saved copy of the letter.
12. Close the patient's chart.

[Change signature of letter] button

Exercise 5.7(N) Creating a Test Report for a Patient

1. Open Patti Adams's chart. Under the *New* menu select *New Test Report to Pt.*
2. Highlight the lipid panel in the *Select Test* window. The program automatically adds the test description to the bottom of the test results.
3. Place your cursor in the body of the report under the section heading *Problems.* Select *Elevated Cholesterol* from the pop-up text in the lower right panel.
4. Click on the down arrow in the pop-up text category window to reveal the list of pop-up text categories. Select *Report-Recs.*
5. Place your cursor under the section heading *Recommendations.* Now select the following pop-up text line items: *Low cholesterol diet. Regular exercise program. Please make an appointment to see the doctor as soon as possible.*
6. Print the test report and submit it to your instructor.
7. Click on the [Done] button and store a copy of the report under the *Reports to Patient* category in the care tree. A "+" expand symbol is then placed beside the *Report to Patients* header in the care tree. Click the "+" symbol to see the saved report.

Chapter 6 The Office Visit

Exercise 6.1(N) Building an OV Note (Part 1—MA)

Note: For this exercise, you will use your own chart but also assume you are the medical assistant.

1. Open your own patient chart and select the *Create New Office Visit Note* icon from the *Chart* menu. In the *Office Visit* screen notice the face sheet information on the left side of the window, which was pulled from the chart. Also note that the [CC] (chief complaint) navigation tab is already highlighted on the right.

Create New Office Visit Note icon

(continued)

Exercise 6.1(N) (Concluded)

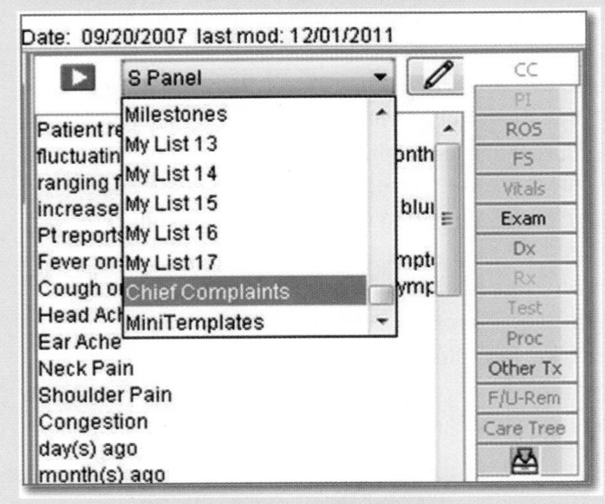

Figure C.5 Pop-up text category list.

2. Click on the down arrow of the pop-up text header and scroll down until you find the pop-up text heading, *Chief Complaints* (Figure C.5).
3. In the *Chief Complaints* pop-up text list, click on *Allergies, Itchy eyes,* and *Runny nose.* The words are added to the lower middle Chief Complaint text box.
4. Click in the Chief Complaint text box and hit [Enter] to start a new line. Click on the time and initial buttons in the lower right section to add the time and your initials to the note.
5. Select the [Vitals] navigation tab on the right. Notice that all previously created text is now added to the *SOAP* format. Add fictitious vital sign information for the patient, including a normal temperature using the SpringCharts Tip in the margin.
6. Click on the [Done] and then the [Save and Skip Billing] buttons. You will come back later, finish the note, and create a routing slip for this office visit. The OV note has been added to the list of encounters in the care tree of your chart.
7. Close the chart.

SpringCharts Tip

Normal Vital Ranges
Temp: 98.6
Resp: 12-20
Pulse: 66-100
BP: Systolic: 100-140
Diastolic: 60-90

Exercise 6.2(N) Building an OV Note (Part 2—Provider)

Note: Now that a medical assistant has completed the initial assessment, the *Office Visit* is handed over to the physician or another healthcare provider. Rather than start a new office visit note, the provider edits the existing note.

1. Open your chart.
2. Click on the "+" sign beside the *Encounters* heading in the care tree and select the office visit entry you started in Exercise 6.1.
3. Click on the [Edit] button at the bottom of the window (shown in margin).
4. Click on the [Template] button (shown in margin) in the bottom right corner of the *Office Visit* screen and, from the displayed list, select *Allergic Rhinitis.* Notice the entire note has been built very quickly into a *SOAP* note.
5. Click on the [PI] navigation tab. The text from the template appears in the lower middle work text box.

SpringCharts Tip

HC stands for head circumference and is used by pediatricians to record head measurements for developing infants. *BMI* (body mass index) is grayed out because the program calculates this item from the height and weight measurements.

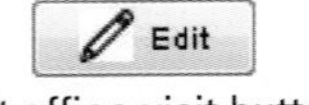

Edit office visit button

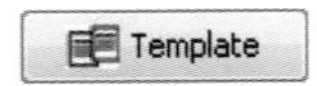

[Template] button in the *OV* screen

Exercise 6.2(N) (Concluded)

6. Move the scroll bar to the top of this window and complete the following sentence: *Pt c/o red, itchy eyes, congested, itchy and runny nose (clear fluid), post-nasal drip, sneezing, itchy ears, scratchy throat and occasional cough for the past_ weeks.* Place your cursor in front of the word *weeks*, highlight the underscore mark, and enter *3*.

> **Note:** The physician would continue this way through the entire note, making changes and additions where necessary to reflect this specific patient's condition.

7. To add a diagnosis, click on the [Dx] navigation tab.
8. Look in the *Previous Diagnoses* window at the bottom to determine if the patient has been in the clinic for this diagnosis in the past. Select *Allergic Rhinitis 477.0* from the *PMHX + Problem List* window.
9. To prescribe a medication, click on the [Rx] navigation tab.
10. In the *Prescription* field, search for *Allegra 180 mg*. Click on the medication to add it to the text box in the bottom middle of the screen.
11. Search for and select *Flonase 50 mcg* to add it to the text box as well.

> **Note:** Always refer to potential allergies at the top on the *Prescription* panel before prescribing medication and shots.

12. The physician asks you to come back into the exam room to administer a subcutaneous allergy shot. To order the injection, select the [Proc] navigation tab.
13. Click on the *Procedure Category* drop-down menu (shown in margin) and select the category *InjectMed*. Choose *Allergy Injection—1*.
14. Click on the [Done] button in the *OV* screen, and choose the [Save and Skip Billing] button in the *Save As* window. (*Later, the medical assistant will re-open this office visit note to document the administration of the allergy injection. The OV note has been added to the list of encounters in the care tree of your chart.*)
15. Close the chart.

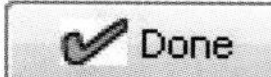

Procedure category headings

[Done] button in the *OV* screen

Exercise 6.3(N) Building an OV Note (Part 3—MA)

> **Note:** The physician communicates with the medical assistant regarding administrating the allergy shot. This may be done via the *Patient Tracker* by changing the *Tracker Status*. As the medical assistant, you administer the injection.

1. Open your chart. Click on the "+" sign beside the *Encounters* heading in the care tree and select the office visit entry you amended in Exercise 6.2(N).
2. Click on the [Edit] button at the bottom of the window.
3. Click on the [Proc] navigation tab and select *Allergy Injection—1* in the lower middle text box.
4. In the *Edit Procedure* window, document the administration of the injection. Choose the pop-up text *Lot#* and type in the lot number *65894*. Select the Expiration date pop-up text and add the date: 9/15/2015.
5. Hit [Enter] to move your cursor to the next line and choose the pop-up text *Site: Left arm*. Scroll down in the pop-up text window and select Route and add the appropriate route for the injection.

(continued)

Exercise 6.3(N) (Concluded)

6. Place your cursor on the next line and click on the [D & T] button and the [Initials] button to add the date and time and your initials to the notation.
7. Click on the [Save] button.
8. Click on the [Done] button in the *OV* screen, followed by [Save and Skip Billing]. The physician can now complete the routing slip and bill for the encounter. The OV note has been added to the list of *Encounters* in the care tree of your chart.

Exercise 6.4(N) Creating an Excuse Note

1. Open your chart and select the most recent office visit note.
2. Select the *Tools* menu, *New Excuse/Note/Order,* and then *New Excuse/Note.*
3. In the *To* field, type the name of your college.
4. In the *Note* window, select pop-up text from the *Excuse Text* category to excuse your absence from college for the time period you were at the doctor's office, for example, 10:00am to 12:00pm.
5. Add your initials to the note by using the [Sign] button.
6. Print the excuse note and submit it to your instructor.
7. Click the [Done] button in the *OV* screen.
8. In the care tree, click on the "+" sign to the left of the *Excuses/Notes* category, to see the saved note. The note is also displayed in the lower right window.

Exercise 6.5(N) Adding an Immunization

Note: While reviewing the face sheet information with your patient, he/she informs you that they received a DT (Diphtheria and Tetanus Toxoids) shot about this time last year.

1. Open your chart and select the most recent office visit note under the *Encounters* category in the care tree.
2. Click on the [Edit] button to open the office visit note.
3. Under the *Edit* menu, select *Immunization* and then the *Add/Edit Immunization Archives* option.
4. Click the [Add Immunization To List] button to display a window in which you will add the past vaccination to the patient's chart.
5. Select *DT* from the *Select Immunization* drop-down menu.
6. Click on the calendar beside the *Enter Immunization Date* field and select a date approximately one year ago (month, year, and day).
7. Enter the same date in the *Enter Immunization End Date* field.
8. Click the [Done] button to add the immunization to the patient's chart, and select [Done] again in the *Add/Edit Immunizations* window.
9. Close the *OV* screen by clicking on the [Done] button and selecting [Save and Skip Billing] in the *Save As* window.
10. Return to the patient's care tree and click on the *Immunization* category.
11. Click on the [Print] button in the *Immunizations* window. Click on the [Print] button to open the *Document Printing Options* window and print the record.
12. Submit the immunization record to your instructor.

NEW Add Immunization To List

[Add Immunization To List] button

Exercise 6.6(N) Creating a Routing Slip

1. Open your patient chart and select the most recent office visit note from the care tree. Open the office visit by using the [Edit] button.
2. Click on the *Tools* menu and select *Resend Routing Slip/Transaction.* Notice in the *Routing Slip* window the diagnoses and follow-up information recorded from the OV note. The *E&M Coder* in the middle section recommends the E&M code of *99215.*
3. Click on [Details] at the bottom of the *Routing Slip* window and read the factors the E&M coder considered to choose the appropriate code about the body systems and areas reviewed during the office visit.
4. Click [OK] and then [Use Code] to use the recommended E&M code.
5. Print the *Routing Slip* and submit it to your instructor.
6. Click on the [Send] button and close the chart.
7. In the main *Practice View* screen, select the *Edit* menu and choose the *Routing Slips* option. In the *View Routing Slip* window, notice the routing slip you just created. This is where billing personnel retrieve the routing slips each day in order to bill the insurance companies or other responsible parties. In a linked environment to a PMS program, this routing slip information would be sent to the PMS interface.

Exercise 6.7(N) Creating an Addendum

1. Open Robert Underhagen's chart by using the *Open a Patient Chart* speed icon on the main screen.
2. In the *Encounters* category of the patient's care tree, highlight the office visit note that has a lock icon associated with it and click on the [Edit] button.
3. Answer [Yes] to the question, *Do you want to add an addendum?*
4. In the *Office Visit Addendum* window, type the following: *Patient developed allergic reaction of hives to the allergy injection. Allergy noted in patient's chart.*
5. Click the [Done] button in the *Office Visit Addendum* window and again in the OV note.
6. Scroll to the bottom of the OV note in the patient's chart and view the addendum you just added. Also notice addendums from other students because they are doing the same exercise in a network environment.

Exercise 6.8(N) Creating an Exam Report

1. Open your chart and highlight the most recent office visit note.
2. Click on the [Report] button at the bottom of the screen.
3. Print the report by clicking on the [Print] button in the report window, and submit it to your instructor. Notice that the clinic letterhead, patient's name and address, greeting, and report introduction are automatically included in the report.
4. Close the report window.

Exercise 6.9(N) Creating an H&P Report

1. In the *OV* window, click on the *Tools* menu and select *H&P.* The *History & Physical Report* is then automatically created.
2. Print the report and submit it to your instructor.
3. Click the [Done] button and save the *H&P* under the *H&P* category in the care tree.

Exercise 7.4(N) Adding Items to the *Superbill*

The screen shot displayed below is a copy of the *Superbill* setup window on the SpringCharts server. Because we cannot access the server, we will complete the screen shot below.

1. In the *Section Titles* field of Figure C.7 below, print *Preventive E&M Codes.* In the two columns below, print the following list of new patient (NP) and established patient (EP) codes in the first column and the description in the next column.

   99381 NP < 1 yr old
   99382 NP 1–4 yrs old
   99383 NP 5–11 yrs old
   99384 NP 12–17 yrs old
   99385 NP 18–39 yrs old
   99386 NP 40–64 yrs old
   99387 NP 65+ yrs old
   99391 EP < 1 yr old
   99392 EP 1–4 yrs old
   99393 EP 5–11 yrs old
   99394 EP 12–17 yrs old
   99395 EP 18–39 yrs old
   99396 EP 40–64 yrs old
   99397 EP 65+ yrs old

   Under the *Supplies* heading, type the following codes and descriptions:

   A4550 Surgical Tray
   D5982 Surgical Stent
   D5988 Surgical Splint

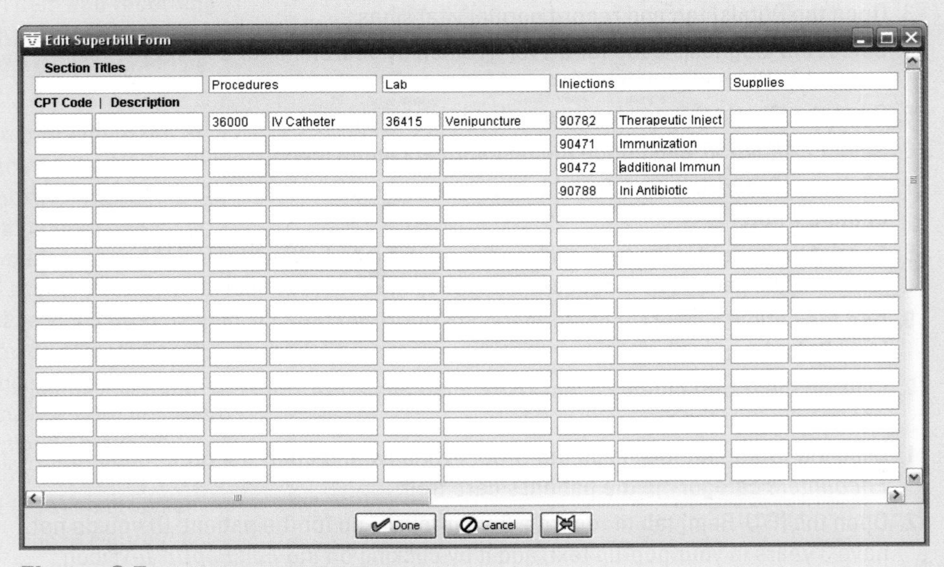

Figure C.7 *Edit Superbill Form* window.

Exercise 7.5(N) Creating a New Patient Information Sheet

1. Click on the *New* menu in the main *Practice View* screen and select the *New Patient Instruction.*
2. Click [OK] in the information window and select the [Write your own] button.

Exercise 7.5(N) (Concluded)

3. Open your Web browser and type in the URL address *www.familydoctor.org.*
4. In the *Disease & Conditions* section click *By Name* to locate an instruction sheet.
5. Select any article by letter.
6. Click on the *Print: Whole Article* option in the *Summary* window.
7. To highlight the article, press the [Ctrl] key and hold it down while pressing the [A] key. Release both keys.
8. Right-click on any highlighted area and choose *Copy.*
9. Close the Web page and return to the SpringCharts program.
10. Click in the *Patient Instruction* window.
11. Using your keypad, press the [Ctrl] + [V] keys to paste the article into the window.
12. At the end of the article add the following phrase: *For more information, contact our office at (214) 674–2000.*
13. At the top of the article, delete the statement, familydoctor.org—health information for the whole family—Return to Web version.
14. Change the *Patient Instruction Name* to the appropriate name for your article and click the [Save] button.
15. To view all of the patient instructions in the program, select the *Edit* menu and choose *Patient Instructions*. Notice your instruction sheet listed here. In this window, instruction sheets can be modified, exported, and deleted, and new ones can be created. Close the window.

Exercise 7.6(N) Administering a Patient Instruction Sheet

1. Open your chart.
2. Locate the office visit note in the *Encounters* category of the care tree that included the well adult visit created in Exercise 7.2(N). Highlight the OV note and click [Edit] in the lower window.
3. In the *OV* screen, select *Tools* and then *Patient Instructions.*
4. Click on the *Pap Smears* instruction sheet in the *Choose Patient Instruction* window.
5. At the top of the Patient Instruction window, type your name on the first line. Print the instruction sheet and submit it to your instructor.
6. Close the OV note and [Save and Skip Billing].
7. Notice the phrase, *Pt Instr: Pap Smears given,* recorded at the bottom of the OV note. This now becomes a permanent record in the patient's chart.

Exercise 7.7(N) Adding a Patient's Care Plan

1. Open your *Patient Chart.*
2. Select the OV note in the care tree that addresses allergy symptoms, and click on [Edit].
3. In the *OV* screen, select *Tools* and *Care Plan.*
4. In the *Care Plan/Guideline* window, click on the [NGC] button.
5. On the NGC website, enter *seasonal allergies* in the *Search* field and search for the care plan. Locate and open the *Allergic Rhinitis* plan. In the *Jump To* section, locate and click *Recommendations.* Highlight and copy sections titled: *Major Recommendations*, *Diagnosis*, and *Therapy.* Close the web browser. Paste the material into the *Care Plan/ Guideline* window by using the [Ctrl]+[V] keys.

(continued)

Exercise 7.7(N) (Concluded)

6. Click the [Done] button, close the *OV* screen, and [Save and Skip Billing]. Notice the care plan has been added to the bottom of the OV note.
7. Print the OV note and submit it to your instructor.
8. Close the patient chart.

Exercise 7.8(N) Importing a Document

1. Open your chart and select *Import Items* from the *New* menu.
2. Select the *Import File Cabinet Document* option.
3. In the *Document Name* field, type *insurance card.*
4. Select the chart tab *Insurance Card.*
5. In the description box, type *Galaxy Health Network—Primary Ins.*
6. Click the [Sign] button and add your initials only.
7. Click on the [Attach] button and choose the *Existing* option.
8. Within the *Open* dialog box, find your *EHR Material* folder. Your instructor will inform you where the *EHR Material* folder is located. Open the folder and select the *Ins Card* file. Make sure the file name shows in the *File name* field.
9. Click the [Open] button to attach the file. If you were successful, the file name should appear in blue in the *File Cabinet Document* window.
10. Click the [Done] button. The newly imported file displays under the *Insurance Card* tab in the care tree.
11. Click on the [Doc] button in the lower right of your patient's chart to view the document. You may have to expand the window to see the entire image.
12. Print the document, write your name on it, and submit it to your instructor.

Chapter 8 Creating Templates

Exercise 8.1(N) Creating and Editing an Office Visit Template

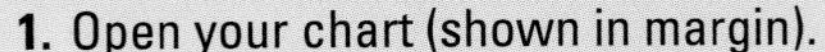

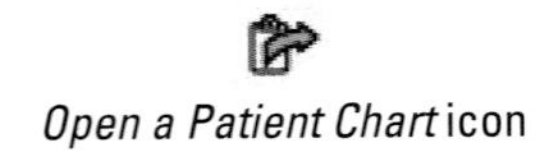

Open a Patient Chart icon

1. Open your chart (shown in margin).
2. Open the office visit note created for the complaints of allergies, runny nose, and itchy eyes (in Chapter 6), by selecting the [Edit] button.
3. Select the *Database* menu and choose *Copy OV To Template.*
4. Name the new template *Adult Allergies + (Your log-in name),* and [Save] it.
5. Close the *Office Visit* screen, save and skip billing, and close the chart.
6. Click on the main *Edit* menu of the main *Practice View* screen and select *Templates.*
7. Select the [Office Visit Templates] button.
8. Choose the *Adult Allergies + (Your log-in name)* template in the *Templates* window.
9. Remove all of the chief complaints (allergies, runny nose, etc.) in the *Chief Complaint* section.
10. Click on the [F/U-Rem] navigation tab. Remove the verbiage in the *F/U-Reminders* field asking the patient to return to the clinic as needed.
11. Save the edited template.

Exercise 8.2(N) Activating an Office Visit Template

1. Open your chart.
2. Open a new *OV* screen from the *New* menu.
3. Click on the [CC] navigation button. Your patient mentions he or she has a runny nose and congestion. The patient believes it is allergies again. You notice in the lower right-hand window that the patient was in your office on a prior date with the same complaints. With your mouse, highlight *Allergies, runny nose, congestion.* (Do not highlight the date.)
4. Click on the *Copy Highlighted Text to Note* button to add the previous chief complaints into the new OV note.
5. Open the [Vitals] tab and enter fictitious vital signs for your patient, including a normal temperature.
6. Click on the [Template] button at the bottom of the window and choose *Allergic Rhinitis + (Your user name).* The template content is added into the OV note to augment the chief complaints and vitals you have already added.
7. *Your patient mentions that a cough started about 7 days ago and the patient tells you she does not have a headache.* Click on the [PI] tab, and notice the content in the *Present Illness* field. Change the statement, *and occasional cough for the past _ weeks* to *7 days.*

Note: Remember to use the [Delete] key on your keyboard, not the [Delete] button in the *OV* screen.

8. Click on the [Dx] navigation tab. In the upper right *Diagnosis* field, type: *allergic* and conduct a search.
9. Select *Allergic Rhinitis 477.9.*
10. In the *Information Available* window, select the *Allergies* patient instruction sheet.
11. Type your name at the top of the instruction sheet. Print a copy of the instruction sheet for the patient and hand in to your instructor.
12. Close the *Information Available* window.
13. The doctor prescribes Flonase. Open the [Rx] tab.
14. Scroll down to the bottom of the *Previous Prescription* field in the lower right corner of the *OV* window, and select *Flonase.*
15. Print the prescription and submit it to your instructor.
16. Save the office visit and edit the routing slip.
17. Use the recommended *E&M code* and [Send] the *Routing Slip.*
18. Notice the completed OV note saved under the *Encounter* category in the care tree of the patient's chart. Close the chart.

Copy Highlighted Text to Note button

Exercise 8.3(N) Using an Order Template

1. Open your patient's chart, and expand the *Encounters* category in the care tree.
2. Highlight the recent OV entry that contains the allergy template, and click the [Edit] button to open the *OV* screen.
3. Open the [Test] navigation tab on the right side.
4. In the *Test* field, type *all* and conduct a search.
5. Click on the *Allergen Profile* to move the test to the lower window.

(continued)

Exercise 8.3(N) (Concluded)

Order Selected Tests

[Order Selected Tests] button

6. Click on [Order Selected Tests] button to move the test to the lower middle window.
7. Click on the print icon in the lower middle window. Notice that the EHR program has automatically added the ordered test and the diagnosis from the patient's OV note.
8. Click on the [Add Pt Ins] button in the *Orders* window to add the patient's primary insurance to the order form.
9. Type your name at the top of the order form. Click on the [Print] button and turn in to your instructor.
10. Click the [Done] button and answer [Yes] button to the question, *Do you want to chart this order?*
11. Save the order under the *Encounters* category of the patient's care tree.
12. Close the patient's chart by clicking on the [Done] button of the *OV* window.
13. Choose the [Save and Skip Billing] option and close the chart.

Exercise 8.4(N) Creating and Using a Letter Template

1. Create a new letter template by accessing the *New* menu in the *Practice View* screen and choosing *New Template > New Letter Template.*
2. In the *Letter Template* window, type the subject (*Re*): *Welcome.*
3. In the body of the letter (*Text*), create a brief letter that welcomes new patients to the clinic and includes the following names and telephone numbers of the *Office Manager: Donna Baird (417) 880-1327* and *Nurse Supervisor: Lissa Raines (417) 866-0062.* The program automatically adds a "close" to the letter.
4. Name the letter template *New Patient Letter + (Your user name)* and click the [Save] button.
5. Open your patient chart.
6. Click on the *New* menu and select *New Letter to Pt.* Notice that the letter is already addressed to the patient and is complete with greetings and closure.
7. Click on the [Template] button at the bottom of the screen and select *New Patient Letter.* Notice that the letter you just created has been added into the body of the letter.
8. To add a signature to the bottom of the letter, click the *Change Signature of Letter* icon at the bottom of the letter and select a signature line. You have the option of providing your default doctor (this was set up initially under *User Preferences*) or your name. Because you are logged in as John Smith in the demo program, you see the name twice.
9. If you used your proper e-mail address when setting up this patient, e-mail the letter to the patient by clicking the [EMail Letter] button to the right of the letter.
10. Print the letter by selecting the [Print] button at the bottom and checking the *Print Letterhead* and *Use Digital Signature boxes.* Submit the letter to your instructor.
11. Click the [Done] button and save the letter under the *Letters* tab in the care tree. Save the letter as *New Patient Letter.* The letter displays in the lower right window of the *Patient Chart* and stored under the *Letter* category.

Exercise 8.5(N) Modifying an OV Template

1. In the main *Practice View* screen, click on the *Edit* menu and select the *Templates* submenu.
2. In the *Templates* window select the [Office Visit Templates] button.

Exercise 8.5(N) (Concluded)

3. In the displayed list of OV templates, locate your *Adult Allergies + (Your log-in name)* template.
4. In the *Office Visit Template* window, select the [PI] navigation tab.
5. In the *Present Illness* text box located in the lower left corner, move the scroll bar to the top of the window.
6. Change the text by deleting or modifying the variable text in this section. For example: *Experiences these Sx: At this time every year. / All the time* can be modified to: *Experiences these Sx: At this time every year.*
7. Click on the [Save] button and close the *Templates* window.

Exercise 8.6(N) Adding a Procedure Template

1. From the main *Practice View* screen, select the *Edit* menu and then *Procedures.*
2. In the *Edit Procedure* window click the [Search] button without typing anything in the search field. All the activated procedure codes will display. Your instructor will assign you a specific code to highlight.
3. Click on the [Popup Text] button in the lower corner to open the *Popup Text Composer* window.
4. Select the pop-up text that begins with: *The patient's questions were answered.* The text will populate the *Body* area to become part of the template. Click the [OK] button. The text will now appear in the *Detail* field of the *Edit Procedure* window.
5. Click the [Save] button and close the *Edit Procedure* window. The next time you use this procedure in the OV note, the associated template text will become part of the OV note.

Chapter 9 Tests, Procedures, and Codes

Exercise 9.1(N) Ordering a Lab Test and an Imaging Test

1. Open your chart.
2. From the *Actions* menu, select *Lab > Order New Lab.*
3. Search for a *CMP,* select the test, and then press [Done].
4. Go to the *Practice View* screen.
5. Under the *Edit* menu, select *Pending Tests.*
6. Locate your patient's CMP test within the *Pending Tests* window.
7. Close the *Pending Tests* window and the patient's chart.

Exercise 9.2(N) Viewing Outstanding Tests

1. Open Robert Underhagen's chart by using the speed icon in the Toolbar (shown in margin).
2. Locate the two uncharted tests in the face sheet. One pending test and one completed test have not been charted.
3. Write the name of the pending test: ______________________________
4. Write the name of the completed test: ______________________________

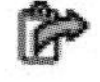

Open a Patient Chart icon

Exercise 9.3(N) Processing an Imported Lab Test Result

1. Under the *Edit* menu on the *Practice View* screen, locate the *Reference Lab* option.
2. Open the *Imported Reference Lab Tests* window and locate the *Comprehensive Metabolic Panel* for Patti Adams. Highlight the test to open the *Imported Lab Data* window. The imported lab shows the patient's results both in range and out of range.
3. In a networked environment of a medical facility, typically a medical technician would select the [Match] button of this imported lab and match it to a pending test ordered for this patient. The data would be placed into the pending test automatically and the test saved into the patient's chart. Because all students are working with the same test, we will not be able to do this. Instead we will input the data manually.
4. Leave the *Imported Lab Data* window for Patti Adams open and also open the pending CMP test you ordered for your patient in the *Pending Tests* submenu of the *Edit* menu. With your mouse, maneuver the two windows so you see them side by side. Now begin copying the lab results from the imported lab and typing them into the pending lab. Notice you have more analytes on the imported test than are listed on the pending test.
5. Click the [Tech Sign] button in the *Pending Tests* window and select the appropriate testing facility from the address list.
6. Click the [ToDo] button and send a *ToDo/Reminder* to the physician alerting him or her that the completed test is now available. Use your pop-up text. Notice the *ToDo* item is already linked to your patient.
7. Click on the *Complete* radio button and then the [Done] button. Close the *Reference Lab* windows.

Exercise 9.4(N) Ordering and Processing a Manual Lab Test Result

1. Open your chart.
2. From the *Actions* menu, choose *Lab* > *Order New Lab.*
3. In the *Order Test* window, type *lip* and activate a search.
4. Select *Lipid Panel* and click the [Done] button.
5. Close your chart.
6. Select *Pending Tests* from the *Edit* menu of the *Practice View* screen.
7. Highlight the *Lipid Panel* just ordered for your chart and click the [Open] button.
8. Enter fictitious lab results in the five fields, with some results falling within normal range, and others out of range (normal ranges are on the right).
9. Click on the [Tech Sign] button and then select an appropriate [Testing facility].
10. Enter a fictitious ID number for the incoming lab.
11. Send a *ToDo* to Dr. Finchman to *Check Lab.* Click [Send].
12. Click the *Complete* radio button and then [Done].
13. Close the *Pending Tests* window.

Let us now assume you are Dr. Finchman.

14. Under the *Edit* menu on the *Practice View* screen, select *Completed Tests.*
15. Select the *Lipid Panel* test just completed for your chart. Find the lab items that are outside the normal ranges.

Exercise 9.4(N) (Concluded)

16. Leaving the *Test Result* window open, open your chart and find the *Routine Meds* section of the face sheet. Note the cholesterol-lowering drug Lipitor.
17. Close the chart.
18. Within the *Test Result* window, click on the [Message] button (shown in margin).
19. Using pop-up text, send a message to Jan, requesting that she *call the patient today to schedule an appointment ASAP*.
20. Place your cursor in the body of the message and start a new line by pressing the [Enter] key.
21. Add the pop-up text: *Call Pt and arrange an appt with Dr. _ for _*. Complete the sentence informing Jan to call the patient and set an appointment with Dr. *Finchman* for *one week*.
22. Initial the message by clicking the [Init] button and hit [Send].
23. Within the *Completed Test* window, check the *Dr Viewed* radio button and then [Done].
24. Close the *Completed Test* window.
25. Open your chart and expand the *Lab* category of the care tree.
26. Click on the expand ("+") sign and locate the recently completed lab panel.
27. Highlight the entry, and notice the results in the lower right quadrant of the chart.
28. Click on the [Print] button at the bottom, write your name on the paper, and submit it to your instructor.

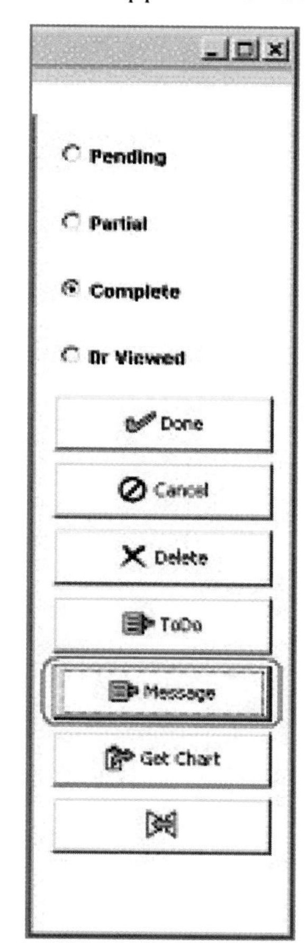

[Message] button inside the *Completed Test* window.

Exercise 9.5(N) Processing a Lab Result Manually

1. From the *Edit* menu of the *Practice View* screen, locate your pending test for a Pap smear.
2. Highlight the pending test and click the [Open] button.
3. In the results window in the upper left, type *Normal*.
4. Click the [Tech Sign] button and then [Testing Facility]. Choose a facility.
5. Click the *Complete* radio button and then [Done]. Close the *Pending Tests* window.
6. Open the same test in the *Completed Tests* area from the *Edit* menu.
7. Notice the result *Normal* appears after the test name. Assuming you are the doctor in this case, check the *Dr Viewed* button and then click [Done].
8. Close the *Completed Tests* window.
9. Open your patient chart. Expand the *Lab* category in the care tree and notice the addition of the Pap test.
10. Print out the lab result and submit it to your instructor.

Exercise 9.6(N) Creating a Test Report

1. Inside your patient chart open a *New Test Report to Pt* under the *New* menu.
2. Select the Pap lab test in the upper right panel. Because this is a "normal" result, we can delete the *Problems* and *Recommendations* headings in the report.
3. Print out the report and submit to your instructor.

Exercise 9.7(N) Creating a New Procedure Code

1. First, we need to make sure the code is not already activated. Open the *Edit* menu in the *Practice View* screen and select *Procedures.*
2. In the *Edit Procedure* window, select *CPT Code* as the search mode and type *17111* in the search field.
3. Click the [Search] button. We know this procedure code has not yet been activated in the EHR program because no procedure is found in the search process.
4. Click the [New] button in the bottom right corner of the window. Look up the code in the CPT dictionary database by using the [Lookup] button. (Depending on the size of your monitor, you may have to scroll to the bottom of the page to see the [Lookup] button).

Note: Because all students are working from the same database, we will not all activate the same procedure code.

5. In the *Search Procedure Master List* window, select *CPT Code* as the search mode and type *17* in the search field. Click the [Search] button. All the procedure codes in the database beginning with *17* will be displayed. Ask your instructor to assign you a specific code. Click the [Select] button.
6. Complete the *Category* type by choosing *Surgery* from the drop-down menu.
7. To add consistent text to this procedure each time it is conducted, click the [PopUp Text] button.
8. In the *PopUp Text Composer* window, select the paragraph that begins with *Pt was advised of the purpose, benefits . . . etc.* and click the [OK] button. The text is now added to the *Detail* window and associated with this code.
9. Save the new procedure code by clicking the [Save] button and close the window.

Exercise 9.8(N) Using Diagnosis and Procedure Codes

1. Open your chart and launch a new office visit. This is a follow-up visit scheduled to conduct a removal procedure for maculopapular skin lesions.
2. Under the [CC] navigation tab, select the pop-up text *Follow-Up Visit.*
3. Open the [Vitals] tab and add several normal vitals.
4. Open the [Exam] navigation tab and choose *(0 Abnormals)* as the pop-up text category. Scroll down and select the text, *SKIN: + maculopapular lesions.*
5. In the [Dx] navigation tab, search for a diagnosis starting with *lesion*. The pigmented lesion code that appears is not the correct code, so you need to activate another diagnosis code.
6. In the *Database* menu of the *OV* screen, select *New Diagnosis.*
7. To access the ICD dictionary database, click the [Lookup] button. In the *LookUp Dx Code* window, search for the main 102 code.

Exercise 9.8(N) (Concluded)

Note: Because all students are working from the same database, each will activate different codes. There are 11 codes beginning with 102. The first 11 students should activate one of these codes each. The next set of students will search for a *Dx* code beginning with 103, then 104, until all students have selected a distinct code. Select your assigned code. The diagnosis description and code appears in the *New Diagnosis* window.

8. For the *Dx Brief Name,* check the box *Use ICD name for Brief name.*
9. Save the newly activated diagnosis.
10. In the diagnosis field of the *OV* screen, type *yaws* and search for the diagnosis *Yaws Unspecified.* Select the diagnosis.
11. Under the [Proc] navigation button, select *Surgery* as the category and choose the newly activated procedure *Destruction Benign Lesions 15/>.*
12. Open the [F/U-Rem] tab. Notice all text associated with this procedure during its creation is now added into the body of the *SOAP* note. Choose a follow-up in 1 week.
13. Click on the *Create a Reminder* icon and send a *ToDo/Reminder* to Jan to schedule a follow-up appointment in 1 week using pop-up text.
14. Send the *ToDo* item, click the [Done] button, and create a *Routing Slip.*
15. In the *Routing Slip* window, bill for the surgical tray you find itemized in the *Superbill Form* in the right panel. You do not need to choose an E&M code because this visit is billed as a procedure, not an office visit.
16. Print the routing slip and submit it to your instructor.
17. Send the routing slip and close the chart.

Exercise 9.9(N) Creating and Using ICD-10 Codes

Note: Perhaps your clinic's physician inadvertently used an ICD-9 code after the compliance date for ICD-10 codes; therefore, the claim needs to be refiled with the correct code. You need to create the equivalent ICD-10 code, update it in the OV note, and create a new routing slip.

1. On the *Practice View* screen, select the *Edit* menu and the *Diagnosis* submenu.
2. On the right-hand side, click on the [New] button.
3. Your instructor will assign you one of the ICD-10 codes from Table C.2.
4. Place the ICD-10 code in the code field. Type in the description. Check the box: *Use as Brief Name* and click the [Save] button. Close the Edit Diagnosis window.
5. Open your chart by selecting the *Open a Patient Chart* icon.
6. Expand the *Encounters* category in the care tree and locate the *Office Visit.* Open the OV note by selecting the [Edit] button.
7. In the *OV* screen, select the [Dx] navigation tab on the right-hand side.
8. Click on the diagnosis in the lower window. Click on the [Delete] button in the *Diagnosis* window and answer *Yes* to the confirmation question. In the *Note* box below, type the following: *Dx changed to ICD-10 code.*
9. In the DIAGNOSIS field in the upper right, type the first few letters of the ICD-10 code you activated. Select the code.
10. Click the [Done] button. Click the [Save and Edit Routing Slip] button in the *Save As* window.
11. In the *Routing Slip* window, select the recommended E&M code by clicking on the [Use Code] button. Click on the [Send] button. Close the patient's chart.
12. In the *Practice View* screen, select the *Edit* menu and the *Routing Slips* submenu.

(continued)

Exercise 9.9(N) (Continued)

Table C.2 ICD-10 Codes *(Sample)*

Symptoms and signs involving the digestive system and abdomen (R10-R19)

R10 Abdominal and pelvic pain

R10.0 Acute abdomen pain

R10.1 Pain localized to upper abdomen

- R10.10 Upper abdominal pain, unspecified
- R10.11 Right upper quadrant pain
- R10.12 Left upper quadrant pain
- R10.13 Epigastric pain

R10.2 Pelvic and perineal pain

R10.3 Pain localized to other parts of lower abdomen

- R10.30 Lower abdominal pain, unspecified
- R10.31 Right lower quadrant pain
- R10.32 Left lower quadrant pain
- R10.33 Periumbilical pain

R10.8 Other abdominal pain

- R10.81 Abdominal tenderness
  - R10.811 Right upper quadrant abdominal tenderness
  - R10.812 Left upper quadrant abdominal tenderness
  - R10.813 Right lower quadrant abdominal tenderness
  - R10.814 Left lower quadrant abdominal tenderness
  - R10.815 Periumbilic abdominal tenderness
  - R10.816 Epigastric abdominal tenderness
  - R10.817 Generalized abdominal tenderness
  - R10.819 Abdominal tenderness, unspecified site
- R10.82 Rebound abdominal tenderness
  - R10.821 Right upper quadrant rebound abdominal tenderness
  - R10.822 Left upper quadrant rebound abdominal tenderness
  - R10.823 Right lower quadrant rebound abdominal tenderness
  - R10.824 Left lower quadrant rebound abdominal tenderness
  - R10.825 Periumbilic rebound abdominal tenderness
  - R10.826 Epigastric rebound abdominal tenderness
  - R10.827 Generalized rebound abdominal tenderness
  - R10.829 Rebound abdominal tenderness, unspecified site
- R10.83 Colic
- R10.84 Generalized abdominal pain

R11 Nausea and vomiting

R11.0 Nausea

R11.1 Vomiting

- R11.10 Vomiting, unspecified
- R11.11 Vomiting without nausea
- R11.12 Projectile vomiting
- R11.13 Vomiting of fecal matter
- R11.14 Bilious vomiting

R11.2 Nausea with vomiting, unspecified

R12 Heartburn

R13 Aphagia and dysphagia

R13.0 Aphagia (inability to swallow)

R13.1 Dysphagia

- R13.10 Dysphagia, unspecified
- R13.11 Dysphagia, oral phase
- R13.12 Dysphagia, oropharyngeal phase
- R13.13 Dysphagia, pharyngeal phase
- R13.14 Dysphagia, pharyngoesophageal phase
- R13.19 Other dysphagia

R14 Flatulence and related conditions

R14.0 Abdominal distension (gaseous)

R14.1 Gas pain

R14.2 Eructation

R14.3 Flatulence

R15 Fecal incontinence

R15.0 Incomplete defecation

Exercise 9.9(N) (Concluded)

13. Scroll to the bottom of the list in the *View Routing Slips* window and select the routing slip created for your patient.
14. Click on the [Print] button and print the routing slip. Submit to your instructor. Close the *View Routing Slips* window.

Chapter 10 Productivity Center and Utilities

Exercise 10.1(N) Creating a New Bulletin Post

1. Open the *Bulletin Board* by clicking on the icon on the Toolbar of the main *Practice View* screen.
2. Click on the [New] button to open a new bulletin.
3. Highlight the phrase *New Bulletin* and replace it with the name of a new bulletin: *Inclement Weather Policy + (Your user name).*
4. On the next lines of the *New Bulletin,* type a message that encourages employees to call the Inclement Weather Hotline at (800) 694-5289 on snowy mornings to determine whether the office is opening late.
5. Assign a color to your bulletin by accessing the color options under the [Color] button.
6. Click the [Save] button.
7. Repeat steps 2–6 and create another bulletin that announces a fundraising auction to benefit a local family in need.
8. Notice each new bulletin is added to the list on the left side for other users to view. Because the *Bulletin Board* is a universal feature, all students will be posting to the same bulletin board. Select your original 'inclement weather' bulletin.
9. Print a copy of your original bulletin, circle your name, and turn in to your instructor.

Exercise 10.2(N) Faxing a Prescription Electronically

1. Open your patient's chart.
2. Select the office visit note under the *Encounters* category of the care tree related to adult allergy symptoms.
3. Click on the [Edit] button to open the *OV* screen.
4. Open the [Rx] navigation tab to display the three ordered prescriptions.
5. Click on the *Print Prescriptions* icon (shown in margin) in the lower center section of the screen.
6. In the *Prescription Printing Options* window, select *Use Digital Signature* and *Print License No on Rx.*
7. Click on the [Fax] button.
8. In the *Fax* window, click on the search icon, which opens the *Fax Number Lookup* window.
9. Choose *Category* as the search criterion, type *phar* in the search field, and activate the search.
10. Select *Walshop Pharmacy* and notice the fax number you added appears on the right side.

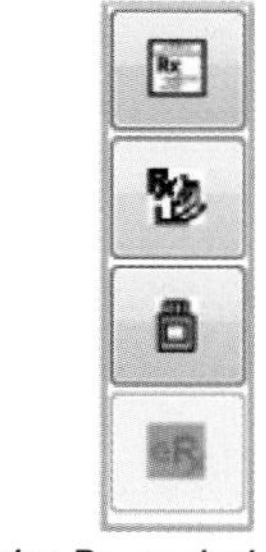

Print Prescription icon

(continued)

Exercise 10.2(N) (Concluded)

11. Click the radio button beside the fax number and then [Select].
12. Back in the *Fax* window, type *Prescription* in the *Subject* field and check the boxes to *Send InterFax Header* and *Send Cover Note*.
13. Click the [Send] button. The fax will now transmit to the pharmacy.

Exercise 10.3(N) Working with the *Time Clock*

1. From the *Productivity Center* menu, select *Time Clock.*
2. In the *Time Clock* window, click the [In] button and then confirm the clock-in by selecting [Yes]. Your time-in is stamped into the window.
3. Imagine you were actually in the clinic earlier, but had forgotten to clock in. Click the [Request Change] button and then [Edit] to change your existing time.
4. Highlight the time you clocked in, and the *Edit Time Clock Item* window opens.
5. On the right side of the window, change the time to the top of the hour. In the *Request Reason* text box, type *Was in meeting and then forgot* and then click the [Send] button.
6. The program has now sent your request to the office administrator as an item in the administrator's *To Do List,* marking it with an orange bar. The administrator is able to open the item and either approve or deny the request. If the administrator approves the request, your *Time Clock* will adjust to reflect the newly requested time.
7. Close the *Time Clock* window.

Exercise 10.4(N) Adding a New Link to *My Websites*

1. Under the *Productivity Center* menu, select the *My Websites* option (shown in margin) and click on the [Edit] button.
2. Enter the phrase *Patient Instructions* in the first blank field on the left. Place the cursor as far left as possible.
3. In the corresponding field on the right, type in the URL: *www.familydoctor.org* and then click the [Save] button.
4. In the *My Websites* window, click on the newly added *Patient Instruction* link. The Internet browser is then activated, and you will receive access to the website directly from SpringCharts.

SpringCharts Tip

Shortcut:

Open My Websites
The seventh speed icon from the left on the *Practice View* Toolbar enables the user to quickly access a list of his or her most commonly used Internet sites.

Exercise 10.5(N) Calculating an Estimated Delivery Date

1. Open the *Pregnancy EDD Calculator* under the *Utilities* menu.
2. Assume the first date of the patient's last menstrual period was 6 weeks ago. Select that date from the calendar.
3. Notice the first date of LMP, estimated fetal age, and estimated date of delivery are automatically entered into these fields.
4. Click on the [Copy Text] button and select the [Open in Word Processor] button.
5. Type your name on a new line in the *Notepad* window, print the document by using the *File* menu, and submit to your instructor.
6. Close the word processor window and the calculator window.

Exercise 10.6(N) Searching the Medical Database

1. Under the *Utilities* menu, select *Search Database.*
2. Click [Yes] to *Search all patient records now?* and *Do You Want To Include Exempted Patients in Reports?* and *You cannot use other functions during a search. Continue?* in the next windows.
3. Select the [Drug] button as the criterion to search by.
4. Type *Lipitor* in the *Find* field and conduct a search. The program displays all strengths of the drug Lipitor.
5. Click on all of the medications to add them to the *Selected Drugs* window.
6. Click the [Done] button, and the program begins searching the patient database for patients who have been prescribed the medication Lipitor.
7. In the *Search Results* window, select [Form Letter].
8. In the *Form Letter* window, type in the subject: *Drug Recall.*
9. In the text field, type a letter informing patients the drug Lipitor has been recalled. Include your name and ask that they contact you to schedule a visit to follow up.
10. When completed, click the [Done] button.
11. In the *Choose Action Below* window, select [Print Letters] and choose *Yes* to chart the letters, print the letterhead, and sign the letters electronically. Print the letters.
12. Open your chart.
13. Look for the letter you just sent, saved under the *Encounters* category in the patient's care tree. Close the chart.
14. Print the letter, circle your name, and submit it to your instructor.

Exercise 10.7(N) Archiving a Patient's Record

1. Select the *Edit* menu from the *Practice View* screen and then *Patients.*
2. In the *Edit Patient* window, find your patient.
3. Archive your patient by pressing the [Archive] button in the lower right and answering *Yes* to the query, *Are you sure you want to archive this patient?* Her name disappears from the patient list.
4. Close the *Edit Patient* window.
5. Open the *Edit* menu once again and select *Patient Archives.*
6. In the *Patient Archive* window, search for your chart by last name.
7. Highlight the patient in the list and select the [View Chart] button in the *Patient Archives* window. Notice the *Patient Archives* window also enables you to reactivate the patient into the active lists in SpringCharts if necessary.
8. Close the *Patient Archives* window.
9. Let's reactivate your patient. In the *Edit* menu, open the *Patient Archives* window.
10. Locate the archived patient. This time, select the [Reactivate Patient] button. A progress bar indicates the patient is being placed back into the active list of patients in SpringCharts.

Exercise 11.2(N) (Concluded)

Edit Patient
Search Last Name eat Search
Search Key Patient Info
Eatman Eatman, Dillon B 10/16/1998
Eatman Eatman, Dustin J 10/05/1973
Personal Information
First Name Dustin
Middle Initial J
Last Name Eatman
Mother's Last Name Hubbard
Date of Birth 10/05/1973
SS# 456-78-2371
Marital Status Married
Gender M
Employer No Fenced Land Company
Address Information
Address 6021 Hodges Place
City Mansfield
State TX
Zip Code 76063
Contact Information
Home Phone (817) 473-0328
Home Fax
Work Phone (817) 966-2484
Work Fax
Pager
Cell Phone (214) 766-8271
Email dustine@nofencedland.net
Communication Pref. Mail Email
Miscellaneous Information
PMS ID
Patient ID 67
Hospital Encounter #
Category
Attending Provider Stephen C Finchman
Other Provider Details Add
Name Role Edit Del
Other Information
Preferred Language English
Race White
Ethnicity Not of Hispanic origin
New Save Get Chart... Track Patient...
Previous Updates Exempt Delete Archive

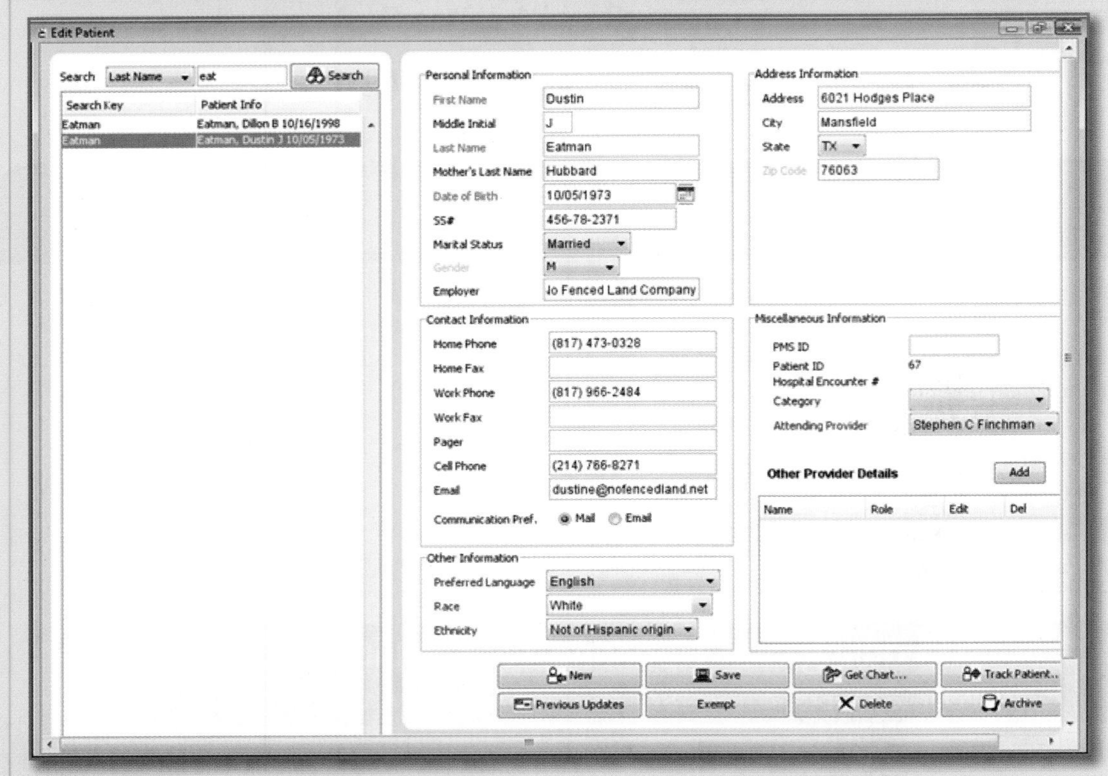

Figure C.11 Updating in the *Edit Patient* window.

2. *Patient Tracker*

Exercise 11.3(N) Adding Patients to the Tracker

(Refer to Chapter 4, page 93)

1. Add your cousin to the *Waiting Room* in the *Patient Tracker* by clicking on his name in the schedule and selecting [Track Pt].
2. The clinic has assigned the following *Patient Tracker* colors and their associative usage:

   Blue—Dr. Finchman
   Yellow—Dr. Smith
   Green—Self Pay
   Red—Lab Work
   Black—Procedures
   Fuchsia—Commercial Insurance

Assign your cousin the appropriate colors (Figure C.12).

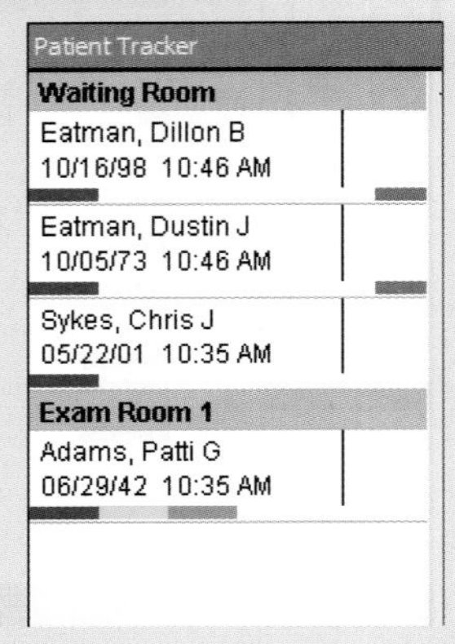

Figure C.12 *Patient Tracker* window.

Exercise 11.4(N) Adding Insurance Information

(Refer to Chapter 3, page 78)

1. Add the following insurance information to the program (Figure C.13) and to your cousin's and Dillon's patient charts (Figure C.14).

   Insurance Company: Make up your own insurance company name.
   Mail Claim To: NFL Group Claims
   Address: PO Box 18974
   City: Plano
   State: TX
   Zip: 56781
   Phone: (800) 281-9823
   Group Name: NFL Claims
   Group Number: 10978NFL
   Policy Number: 456782371
   OV Co-Pay: $25
   Guarantor: your cousin's name

Make a note in the *Details* box of Dillon's *Edit Patient Insurance* window: *Insurance Confirmed.*

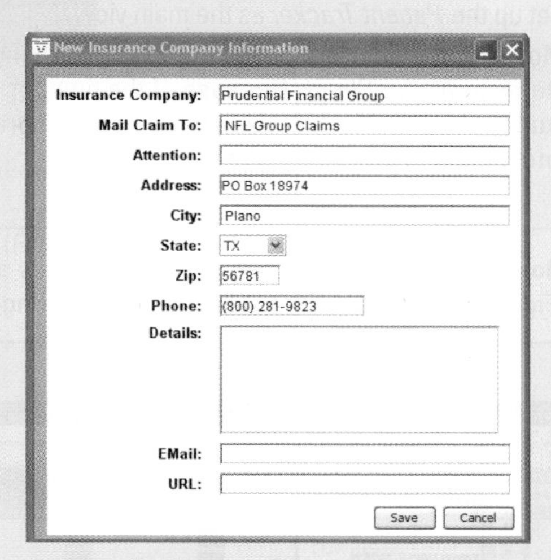

Figure C.13 *New Insurance Company Information* window.

Note: Insurance will be visible on the face sheet when chart has been closed and reopened.

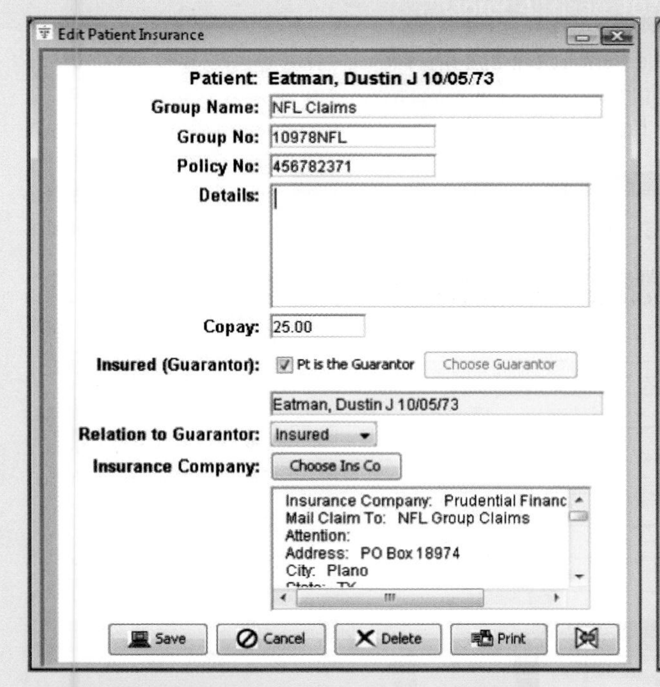

Figure C.14 (a) *Edit Patient Insurance* window.

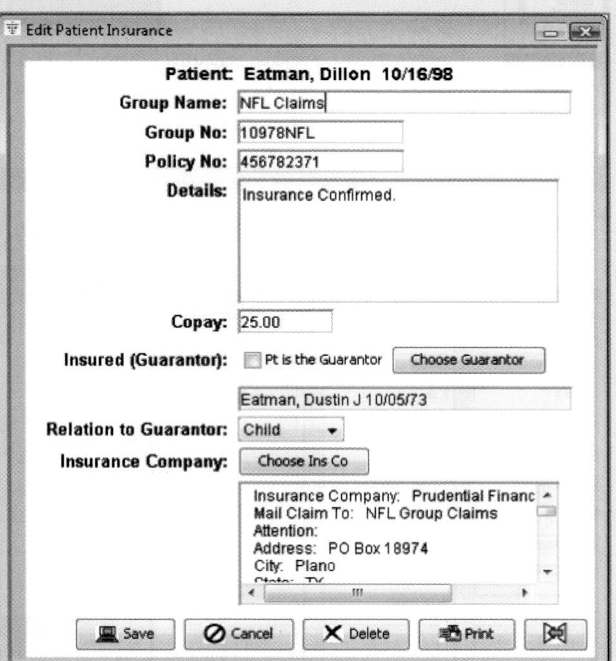

Figure C.14 (b) *Edit Patient Insurance* window.

Exercise 11.7(N) (Concluded)

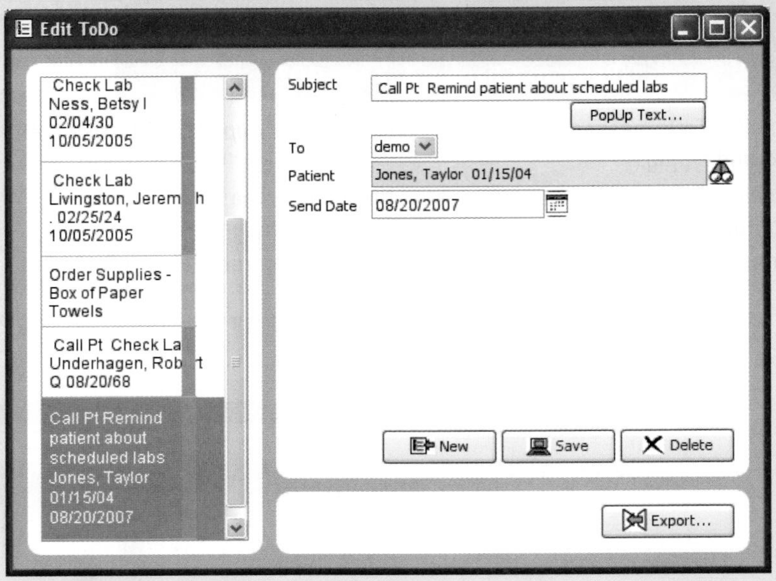

Figure C.20 *Edit ToDo* window.

4. Messages

Exercise 11.8(N) Creating a Message

(Refer to Chapter 4, page 105)

Your patient has called the doctor's office to request some samples of the medication Lipitor. The medical staff is not available, so a message is created at the front desk.

1. Open a *New Message* window linked to your patient chart.
2. Create new pop-up text stating the patient called to request medication samples.
3. Use the new pop-up text in the body of the message.
4. From the [Rx] button in the *New Message* window, select *Lipitor* from the *Previous Prescription* list. Save the medication to the note.
5. While you have your patient on the phone, you notice you do not have a work phone number or a cell phone number for him. Your patient informs you he is retired, but he gives you a mobile phone number, *(214) 766-8272,* and an e-mail address, *urname201@aol.com.* Update his demographics by selecting the [Pt Info] button.
6. While in the *Edit Patient* window, update the patient records to show *Dr. Finchman* as his attending provider.
7. Since you can't log in as the doctor, send the message to yourself.

Exercise 11.9(N) Answering and Returning a Message (Refer to Chapter 4, page 105)

You will now function as Dr. Finchman.

1. Locate and open the message regarding your patient in the *Messages* area of the *Practice View* screen.
2. In the *Message* window, change the number of refills on the medication to *0* and the quantity to *15*.
3. Add new pop-up text to the *Message Body* category: *OK to give patient sample medication.*
4. Add the newly created text to the message, making sure the doctor's response goes on a new line in the message field.
5. On a new line in the message body, time-stamp and initial the note.
6. Click on the [Send Back] button to send the message back to the sender.

Exercise 11.10(N) Charting a Message (Refer to Chapter 4, page 105)

You will now function as the clinician.

1. Select the message in the *Messages* center recently sent back to you from Dr. Smith.
2. Add the following pop-up text to the message body category, *Called patient and advised to pick up sample medication.*
3. Using the up and down arrows in the *Edit PopUp Text* window, position the new text above the line, *Let Pt know that we are out of samples.*
4. Add the new pop-up text on a new line in the message body.
5. Time-stamp and initial your note on a new line in the message body (Figure C.21).
6. Using the printer icon below the [Rx] section of the message window, print a copy of the prescription (Figure C.22). Because this prescription is not being sent to the pharmacy, it does not require the doctor's license and DEA number.
7. Chart the message in the patient's chart, adding *Lipitor Sample* to the message heading.
8. Open your patient's chart. Locate the charted message under the *Encounters* category in the patient's care tree, as well as the new prescription in the *Prescription History* section of the face sheet (Figure C.23).

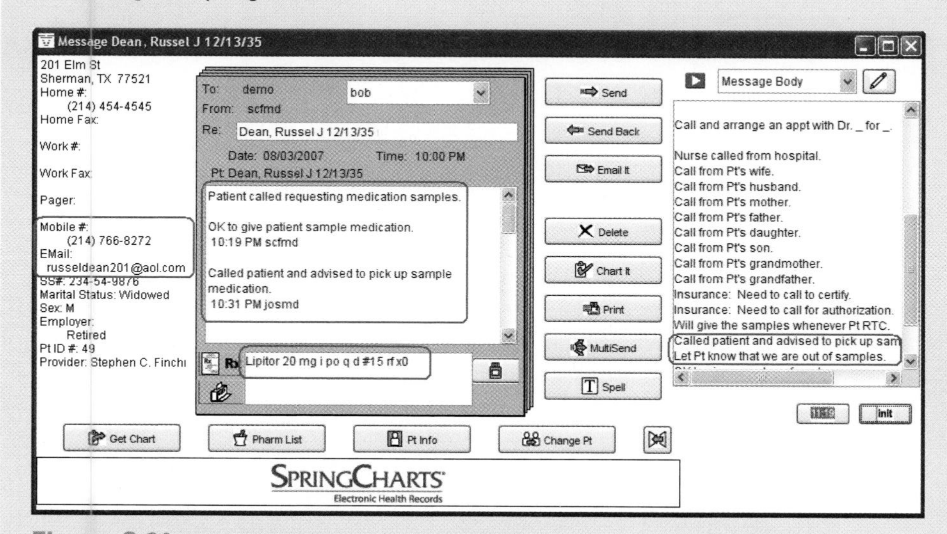

Figure C.21 *New Message to Patient* window.

(continued)

Exercise 11.10(N) (Continued)

Suburban Medical Group
101 Elm Street
Sherman, TX 77521
Office:(214) 674-2000 Fax:(281) 537-0184
EMail:yourname@yourisp.com

Stephen C. Finchman, M.D. John O. Smith, M.D.

April 25, 2012

Pt: Russel J Dean
201 Elm St
Sherman, TX 77521
DOB: 12/13/1935

℞ Lipitor 20 mg
disp: 15 fifteen
sig: i po q d
Refill: 0 zero

John O. Smith, M.D.

A generically equivalent drug product may be dispensed unless the practitioner hand writes the words 'BRAND NECESSARY' or 'BRAND MEDICALLY NECESSARY' on the prescription face

Figure C.22 Printed prescription.

Exercise 11.10(N) (Concluded)

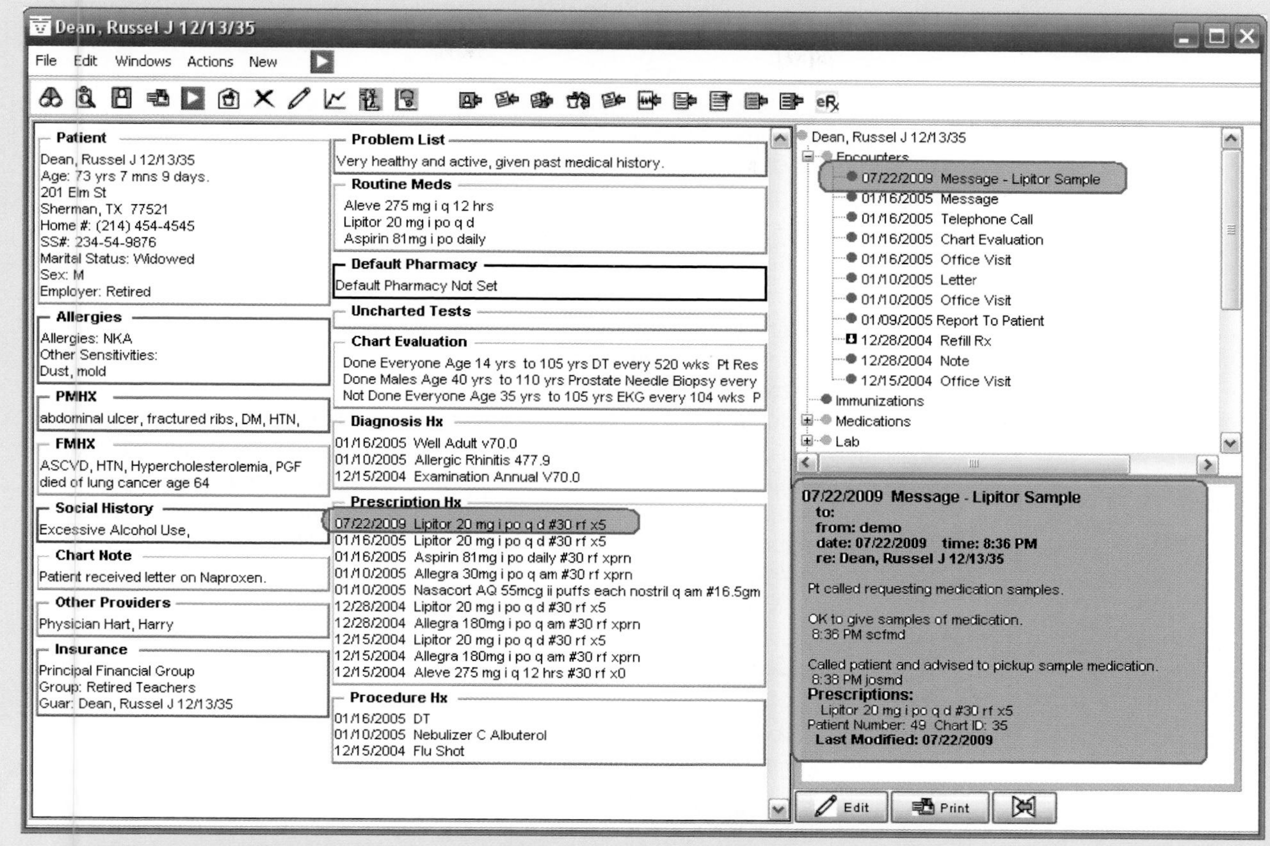

Figure C.23 *Prescription Hx* section of face sheet.

B. *Patient Chart* Screen

1. Face Sheet

Exercise 11.11(N) Building a Face Sheet

(Refer to Chapter 5, page 123)

1. Open your cousin's chart. Open the face sheet window of the chart. Build the following entries into the face sheet:
   a. Allergies: *Mold extracts and latex.* In the *Other Sensitivities* window type: *Cat hair,* then select: *causes hives* from the pop-up text list.
   b. Social History: Using the existing *Preferences* list and the *Social Hx* PopUp Text where appropriate, create the following social history:

   Smoking Status: Never Smoker
   Alcohol Use: Social Drinker.
   Caffeine Use: Yes. Cups Per Day: 4.
   Occupation: Sales.
   Education: College.

(continued)

Exercise 11.11(N) (Continued)

c. Past Medical History: Choose *asthma* and *bronchitis* from the *Preferences* list. Search for and select *Fracture of Rib* in the *Dx* search window.

d. Family Medical History: Using the *Preferences* list, build the following family medical history data:

   Brother: Heart Disease
   Mother: Hypercholesterolemia
   Father: Died At Age: 59
   Cause of Death: Heart Disease
   Check the *Deceased* box below for the father.

e. Referred By: This patient was referred by Dr. Able Body.

f. Chart Note: Click on the edit icon for the pop-up text (Figure C.24). In the *Edit PopUp Text* window, add the following hospitals: *St. Johns Hospital, Cox Medical Centers,* and *Physicians Hospital,* indent each line three spaces. Using the up and down arrows, position the new text under the *Prefers Hospital* line. Now move an empty line between the list of hospitals and the line *Religion.* Click the space bar to add an invisible character on the empty line to create a space between the text lines. Save the material in the *Edit PopUp Text* window. In the face sheet window check your results with Figure C.25. Select the text *Prefers Hospital: St. Johns Hospital.*

g. Routine Meds: Select the following medications:

   Aleve—275 mg
   Lipitor—20 mg
   Aspirin—81 mg
   Edit the Lipitor entry to change the number of refills to *0.* In the *Notes and OTC Meds* window, select: *Omega-3*

h. Problem List: Select *Allergic Rhinitis 477.9, Bronchitis 466.0,* and *Abdominal Pain 789.60* from the upper *Dx* field.

i. Chart Alert: In the *Edit PopUp Text* window, add the following sentence: *Insurance approval needed for elective surgery.* Save and select the new text.

2. Click on the [Back] button and check your work with Figure C.26.

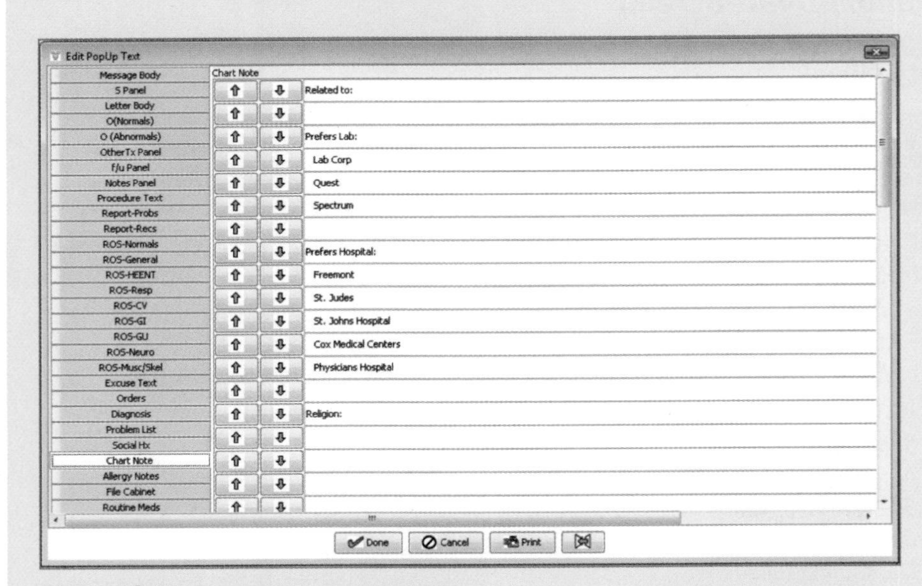

Figure C.24 *Edit PopUp Text* window.

Exercise 11.11(N) (Concluded)

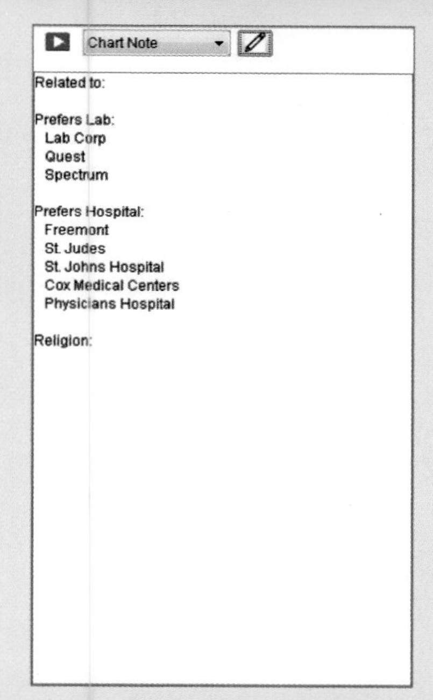

Figure C.25 *Chart Note* section of face sheet.

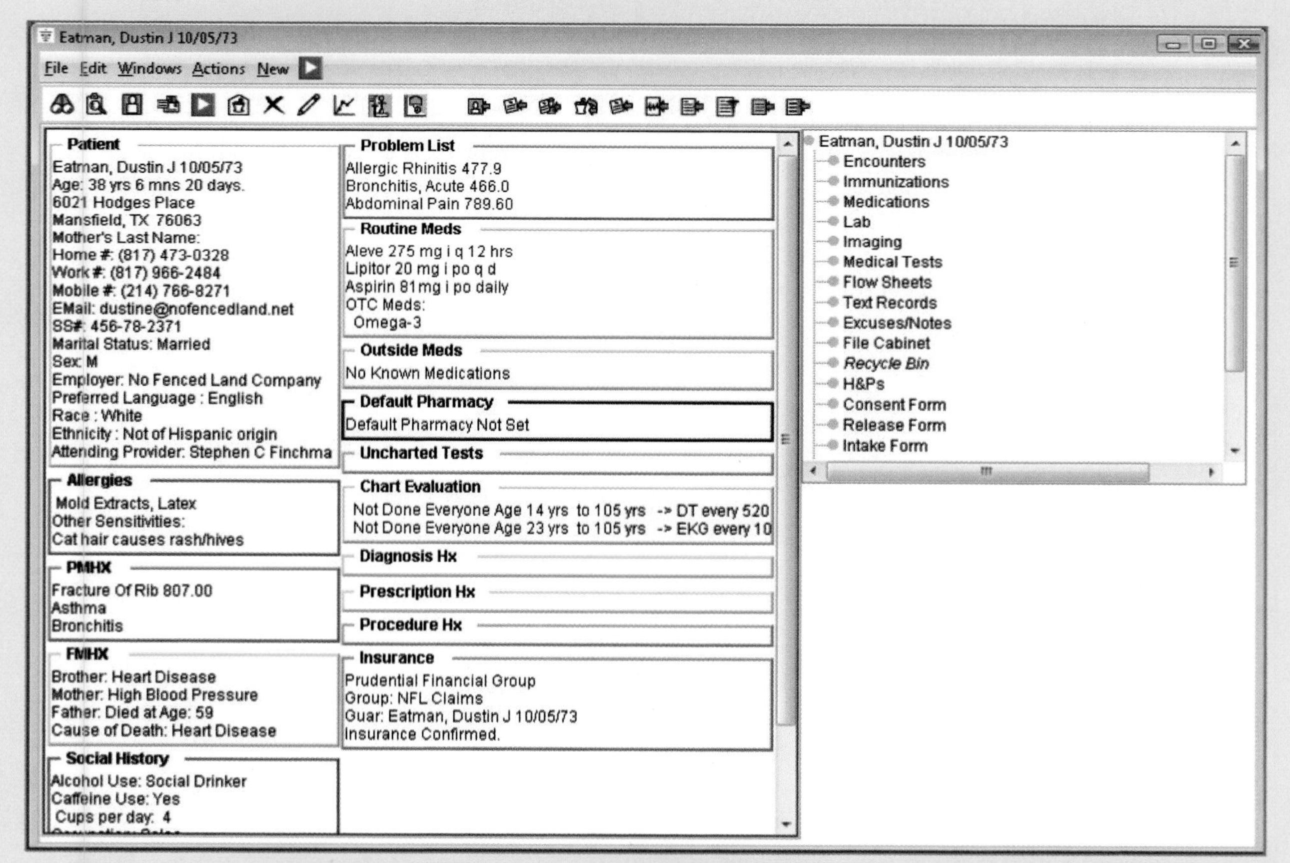

Figure C.26 Completed face sheet.

2. Patient Chart Activities

Exercise 11.12(N) Running a Chart Evaluation

(Refer to Chapter 7, page 190)

1. Run a *Chart Evaluation* of your cousin's chart by accessing the *Evaluate Chart* feature.
2. Record your cousin's response that he will get a DT shot today and mark the recommendation as *Completed.* You are not recommending the EKG today so you will *not* check the radio button *Mark this 'Completed.'* Save the evaluation.
3. Check your results under the *Encounters tab* in the patient's care tree (Figure C.27).

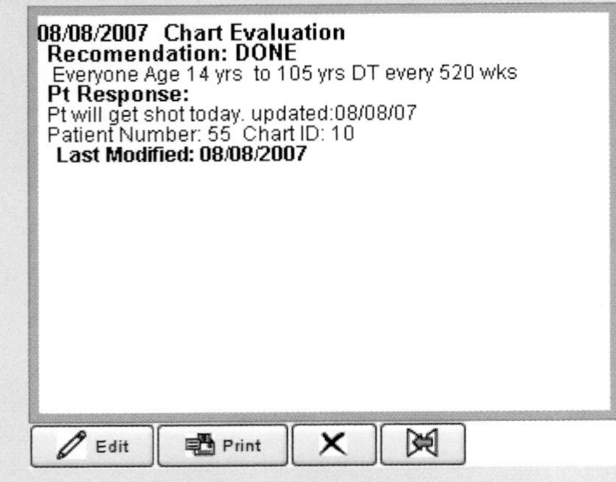

Figure C.27 Saved *Chart Evaluation* in care tree.

Exercise 11.13(N) Printing a Patient's Face Sheet

(Refer to Chapter 5, page 123)

1. Open your cousin's chart. Select the *File* menu and the *Print Face Sheet* submenu.
2. Click the [Print] button in the *Document Printing Options* window and print the patient's face sheet information.
3. Compare the patient's face sheet with Figure C.28.

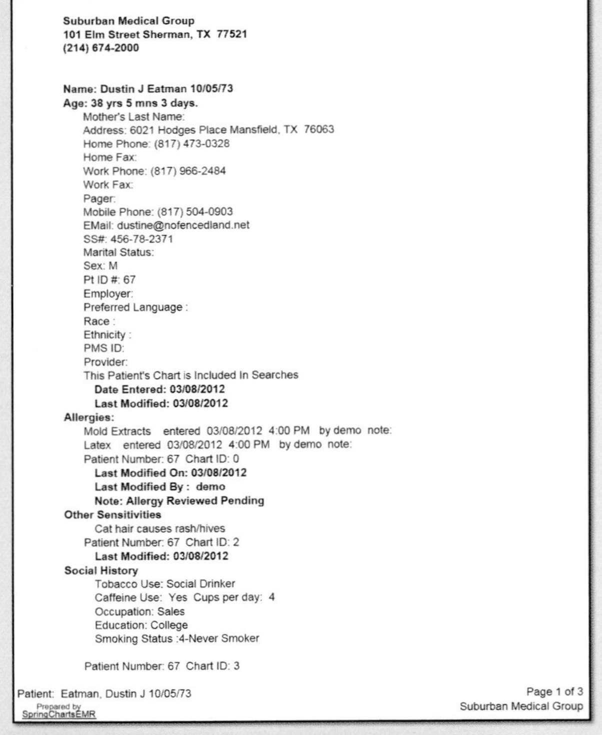

Suburban Medical Group
101 Elm Street Sherman, TX 77521
(214) 674-2000

Name: Dustin J Eatman 10/05/73
Age: 38 yrs 5 mns 3 days.
Mother's Last Name:
Address: 6021 Hodges Place Mansfield, TX 76063
Home Phone: (817) 473-0328
Home Fax:
Work Phone: (817) 966-2484
Work Fax:
Pager:
Mobile Phone: (817) 504-0903
EMail: dustine@nofencedland.net
SS#: 456-78-2371
Marital Status:
Sex: M
Pt ID #: 67
Employer:
Preferred Language :
Race :
Ethnicity :
PMS ID:
Provider:
This Patient's Chart is Included In Searches
Date Entered: 03/08/2012
Last Modified: 03/08/2012
Allergies:
Mold Extracts entered 03/08/2012 4:00 PM by demo note:
Latex entered 03/08/2012 4:00 PM by demo note:
Patient Number: 67 Chart ID: 0
Last Modified On: 03/08/2012
Last Modified By : demo
Note: Allergy Reviewed Pending
Other Sensitivities
Cat hair causes rash/hives
Patient Number: 67 Chart ID: 2
Last Modified: 03/08/2012
Social History
Tobacco Use: Social Drinker
Caffeine Use: Yes Cups per day: 4
Occupation: Sales
Education: College
Smoking Status :4-Never Smoker

Patient Number: 67 Chart ID: 3

Patient: Eatman, Dustin J 10/05/73
Prepared by SpringChartsEMR
Page 1 of 3
Suburban Medical Group

Figure C.28 Printed face sheet information.

Exercise 11.13(N) (Concluded)

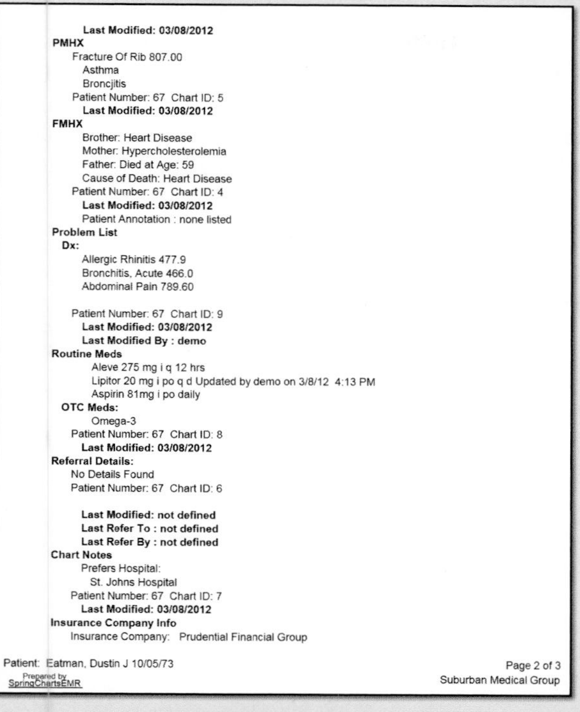

Last Modified: 03/08/2012
PMHX
Fracture Of Rib 807.00
Asthma
Broncjitis
Patient Number: 67 Chart ID: 5
Last Modified: 03/08/2012
FMHX
Brother: Heart Disease
Mother: Hypercholesterolemia
Father: Died at Age: 59
Cause of Death: Heart Disease
Patient Number: 67 Chart ID: 4
Last Modified: 03/08/2012
Patient Annotation : none listed
Problem List
Dx:
Allergic Rhinitis 477.9
Bronchitis, Acute 466.0
Abdominal Pain 789.60

Patient Number: 67 Chart ID: 9
Last Modified: 03/08/2012
Last Modified By : demo
Routine Meds
Aleve 275 mg i q 12 hrs
Lipitor 20 mg i po q d Updated by demo on 3/8/12 4:13 PM
Aspirin 81mg i po daily
OTC Meds:
Omega-3
Patient Number: 67 Chart ID: 8
Last Modified: 03/08/2012
Referral Details:
No Details Found
Patient Number: 67 Chart ID: 6

Last Modified: not defined
Last Refer To : not defined
Last Refer By : not defined
Chart Notes
Prefers Hospital:
St. Johns Hospital
Patient Number: 67 Chart ID: 7
Last Modified: 03/08/2012
Insurance Company Info
Insurance Company: Prudential Financial Group

Patient: Eatman, Dustin J 10/05/73
Prepared by SpringChartsEMR
Page 2 of 3
Suburban Medical Group

Mail Claim To: NFL Group Claims
Attention:
Address: PO Box 18974
City: Plano
State: TX
Zip: 56781
Phone: 8002819823
Details:
EMail:
URL:
Patient Insurance Info
Group Name: NFL Claims
Group No: 1097NFL
Certif No: 456782371
Insured's relation to patient: Insured
CoPay: $25.00
Insurance Comfirmed

Patient: Eatman, Dustin J 10/05/73
Prepared by SpringChartsEMR
Page 3 of 3
Suburban Medical Group

Figure C.28 Printed face sheet information.

Exercise 11.14(N) Adding a Default Pharmacy

(Refer to Chapter 3, page 66)

1. The following pharmacy supplied by the father needs to be added to the Spring-Charts *Address Book*. Because you are working in a network environment, you need to create a unique address for the pharmacy below.

> **Note:** Be sure to add the street name in parentheses after the company's name so you can distinguish it on the list.

Walgreens (____________)
Crn __________ Av. & __________ St.
______________, TX 76063
Ph: (817) ___-______
Fx: (817) ___-______

2. Under the *Edit* menu in the father's chart, add this new pharmacy as the patient default pharmacy.
3. Check to make sure the patient's preferred pharmacy is displayed in the patient's face sheet (Figure C.29).

Default Pharmacy
Walgreens
8177863654

Figure C.29 *Default Pharmacy* section of face sheet.

Exercise 11.15(N) Adding a Photo

1. Add your cousin's photo to his chart by accessing the *Pt Photo* feature under the *Edit* menu.
2. Select the [Edit] button in the *Photo* window and click the [OK] button in the *Picture Size* window.
3. Direct your search in the *Open* dialog box through the *Desktop* access to locate the folder titled: *EHR Material,* (or follow your instructor's directions to locate the *EHR Materials* folder). Double-click on this folder to open it.
4. Highlight the *Dustin Eatman* photo and select the [Open] button.
5. Select the [Done] button back in the *Photo* window.
6. Click on the *Pt Photo* category in the patient's care tree to view the father's photo (Figure C.30).

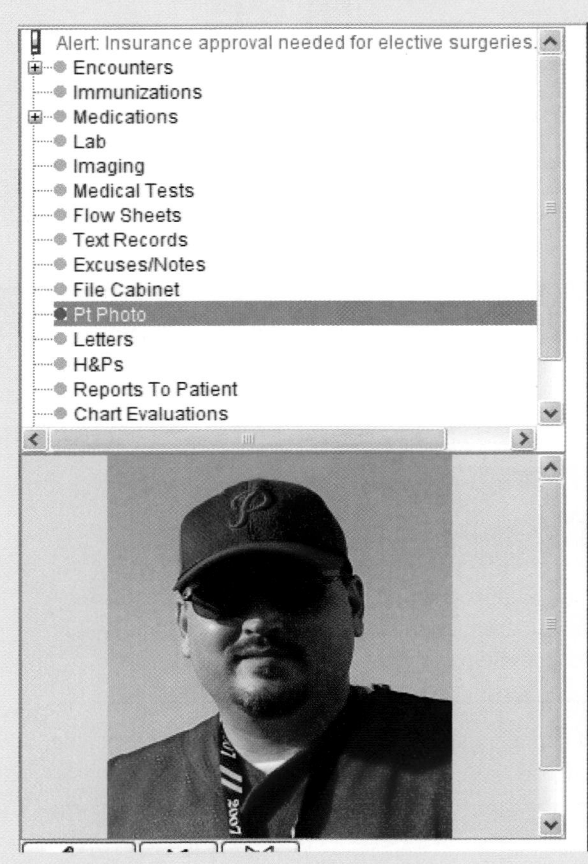

Figure C.30 Patient's photo in patient's chart.

Exercise 11.16(N) Creating a New *TC Note*

(Refer to Chapter 5, page 140)

Your cousin calls the office and requests a list of medications prescribed for him at your office.

1. Using both pop-up text and typing, record the details of the conversation in a *New TC Note,* under the *New* menu in your patient's chart.
2. Initial- and time-stamp the note by using the [Sign] button, and then select [Done].
3. Save the telephone note and skip billing. Notice the call has been documented on the patient's care tree (Figure C.31).
4. Print out the list of all medications prescribed to your patient by accessing the *Medications List* under the *Actions* menu (Figure C.32).

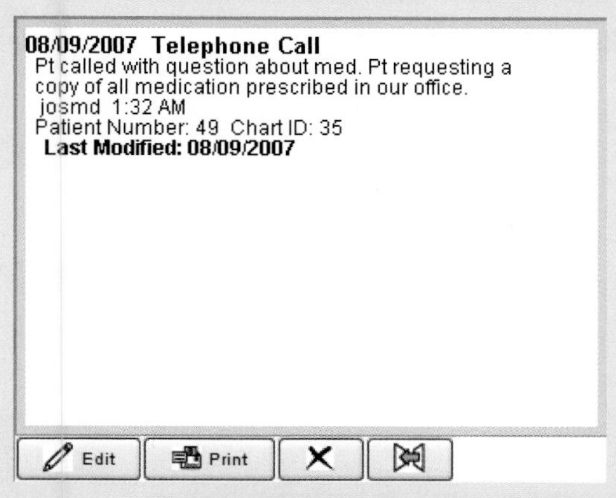

Figure C.31 *Telephone Call* note in care tree.

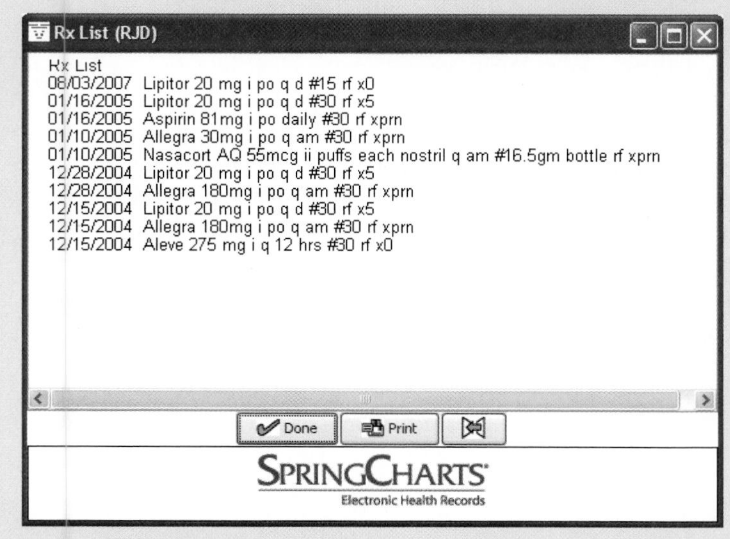

Figure C.32 Patient's *Rx List* in patient's chart.

Exercise 11.17(N) Creating a Nurse Note

1. Open a *New Nurse Note* in your cousin's chart.
2. Choose the *Well Adult V70.0* diagnosis and, within the [Proc] tab, record the administration of a DT shot. (You need to select the *Immunization* category under the *Choose Procedure* window to locate the DT procedure.)
3. Once selected, click on the DT procedure and change the procedure detail to lot number *2695A,* expiration date of 11/1/2015, route of intramuscular, and a site of left deltoid. Use the appropriate popup text.
4. Add your initials and time by selecting the appropriate buttons.
5. Save the nurse note under the *Encounters* tab and send a routing slip.
6. In the *Routing Slip* window, select *Immunization 90471* from the *Superbill Form* for the administration of the injection.
7. Send the routing slip, and check the details of the *Nurse Note* in the patient's chart (Figure C.33). Note that the *Patient Tracker* shows that the routing slip has been sent.

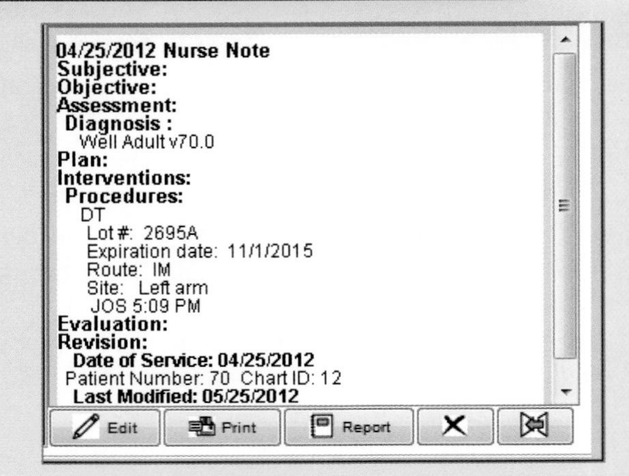

Figure C.33 *Nurse Note* in care tree.

Exercise 11.18(N) Adding a Vitals Check

(Refer to Chapter 5, page 140)

1. Open your patient's chart.
2. Because she has diabetes, your patient comes into the clinic on a regular basis to have her vitals taken. Under the *New* menu, select *New Vitals Only.*
3. Add fictitious vitals, as well as the fact that your patient is 5 ft. 4 inches and weighs 156 pounds. Remember BMI is calculated automatically from the height and weight, and head circumference (HC) is only used for pediatric patients.
4. By using pop-up text found under the [Notes] tab, specify that your patient's blood pressure was taken on his right arm. Time- and initial-stamp the note.
5. Save the new vitals under the *Encounters tab* and skip billing. Notice the *Vitals Check* information in the patient's care tree (Figure C.34).

Exercise 11.18(N) (Concluded)

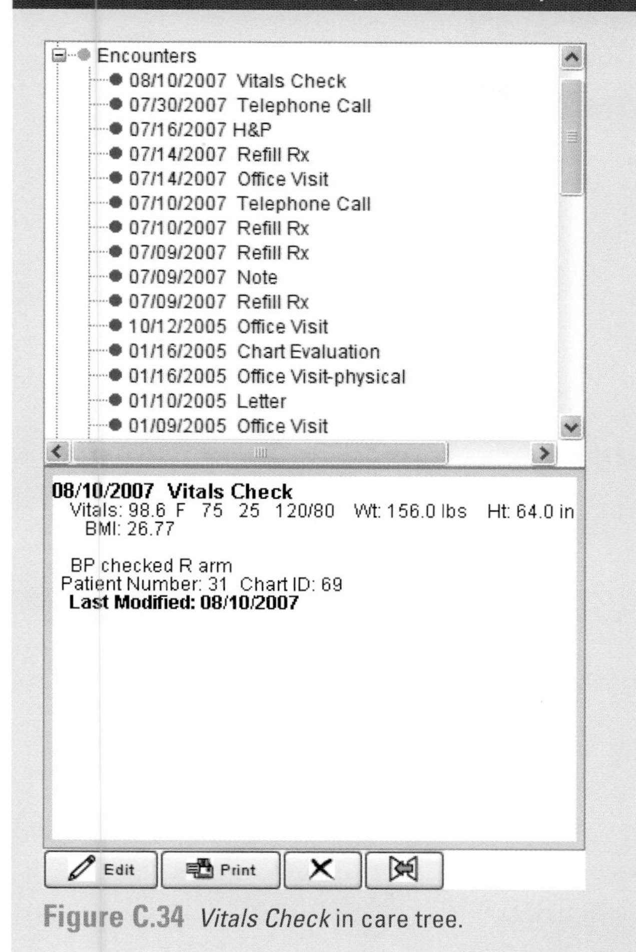

Figure C.34 *Vitals Check* in care tree.

C. *Office Visit* Screen

1. Office Visit Note

Exercise 11.19(N) Starting a New Office Visit Note (Refer to Chapter 6, page 156)

1. In your cousin's chart, open a *New OV.*
2. Your cousin has come to the doctor's office for an annual well checkup. Under the chief complaint (CC) navigation button select *Well Visit.*
3. Stamp the time and initial the note.
4. Under the [Vitals] tab, add fictitious well vitals for your cousin.
5. Save the *Office Visit* under the Encounters tab and skip billing.
6. Close your cousin's chart and update his status in the *Patient Tracker* to *Doctor Ready.* Notice the new information on the *Office Visit* in the patient's care tree (Figure C.35).

(continued)

Exercise 11.19(N) (Concluded)

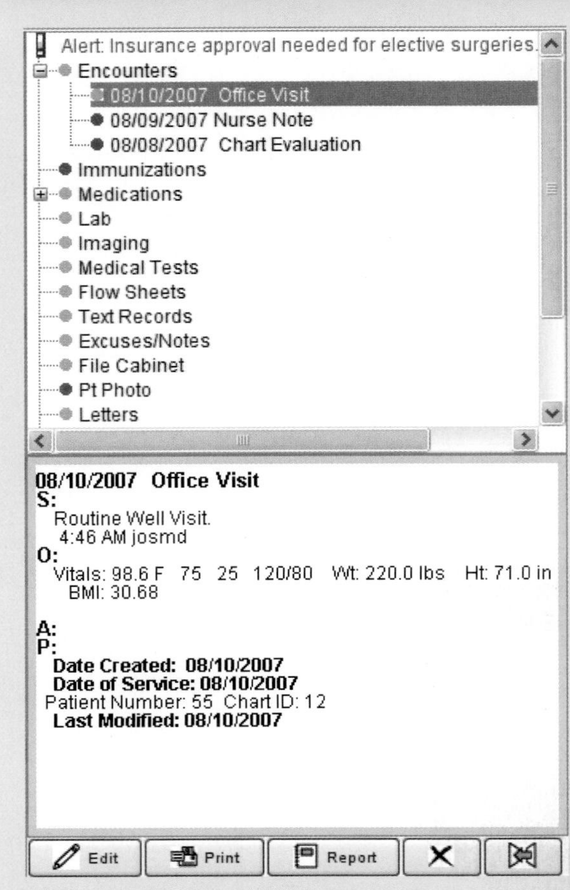

Figure C.35 *Office Visit* note in care tree.

Exercise 11.20(N) Completing an Office Visit Note (Refer to Chapter 6, page 156)

1. Open your cousin's chart and highlight the partially completed office visit note.
2. Click on the [Edit] button to open the *Office Visit* screen.
3. Under the [ROS] tab, select the following pop-up text under the *ROS-Normals* category (remember to start a new line for each system):
   a. *GENERAL: No weight change, fever, chills, night sweats, generalized weakness.*
   b. *HEENT: No headache, dizziness, lightheadedness, diplopia, tearing, eye pain, blind spots, excessive blinking, tinnitus, ear pain or discharge, nose bleeding, nasal obstruction, nasal discharge, gingival bleeding, dental problem, sore throat, hoarseness, difficulty swallowing, neck stiffness, neck pain.*
   c. *PULMONARY: No wheezing, cough, congestion, hemoptysis, respiratory infections, tuberculosis, chest wall pain.*

Exercise 11.20(N) (Continued)

d. *CV: No chest pain, arrhythmia, syncope, dyspnea, exertional dyspnea, orthopnea, paroxysmal nocturnal dyspnea, intermittent claudication, dependent edema, varicose veins, phlebitis, heart murmur, hypertension.*
e. *GI: No change in appetite, difficulty swallowing, indigestion, heartburn, belching, nausea, vomiting, hematemesis, hematochezia, abdomen pain, flatulence, changes in bowel habits, constipation, diarrhea, abnormal stools, incontinence, hemorrhoids, jaundice.*

4. Under the [Exam] button, select the following pop-up text:
a. *GENERAL: Well developed. Well nourished. Alert. Oriented to person, place, and time. In no apparent distress.*
b. *HEAD: Normocephalic. Atraumatic.*
c. *EYES: Eyes and lids appear symmetrical. No exudate. Sclera clear. PERRLA, EOMI. Discs sharp.*
d. *EARS: External auditory canals and TMs normal. Hearing normal as tested by whisper and Rinne/Weber.*
e. *MOUTH/THROAT: Dentition good. Normal mucosa, tongue, gingiva, and oropharynx. Palate elevates in midline. No thrush, erythema, or exudate.*
f. *CV: RRR, normal S1 S2, no S3/S4, murmur, gallop, rub, arrhythmia, or heave. PMI normal in location and character.*
g. *ABDOMEN: Bowel sounds are normal. No evidence of scarring or past surgical procedures. Abdomen is flat, soft, and nontender, without rebound or guarding. No evidence of masses, organomegaly, or abdominal aneurysm. Normal to percussion.*
h. *MUSCULOSKELETAL: Posture normal. Pulses normal and symmetrical. Motor strength normal. Sensory normal and symmetrical to soft touch and pinprick. Joints show normal range of motion and are without erythema or effusions. Nails: Normal capillary filling and appearance w/o clubbing or pitting. No masses or dependent edema noted.*
i. *RECTAL: No mass palpable. Prostate normal in size, shape, and consistency for age. Guaiac negative.*

5. Under the [Dx] tab, choose the *Well Adult v70.0* code.
6. Order a CBC with differential and a SMAC under the [Test] tab.
7. Add the patient's primary insurance to the order form.
8. Because these tests will be conducted at an outside testing facility, print a physician's order form.
9. Compare the order form to that shown in Figure C.36.
10. Save a copy in the patient's chart under the *Encounters* category in the care tree.
11. The doctor decides to give your cousin a flu shot during the office visit because of the upcoming flu season. Under the [Proc] tab, search for and select flu shot.
12. Highlight the flu shot procedure and change the Aventis Pasteur number to *UO701BA*, and the vaccine date to today's date, for example, *30 JUNE 12.*
13. Date-, time-, and initial-stamp the procedure note before saving it.
14. Under the [Other Tx] button select the counseling notes: *Discussed weight loss strategies. Encouraged pt to exercise 30 minutes 5 times a week.*

(continued)

2. *Office Visit* Activities

Exercise 11.21(N) Printing an Office Visit Note

(Refer to Chapter 6, page 181)

1. From your cousin's chart, print a copy of the recent office visit note and compare it to Figure C.39 (a).

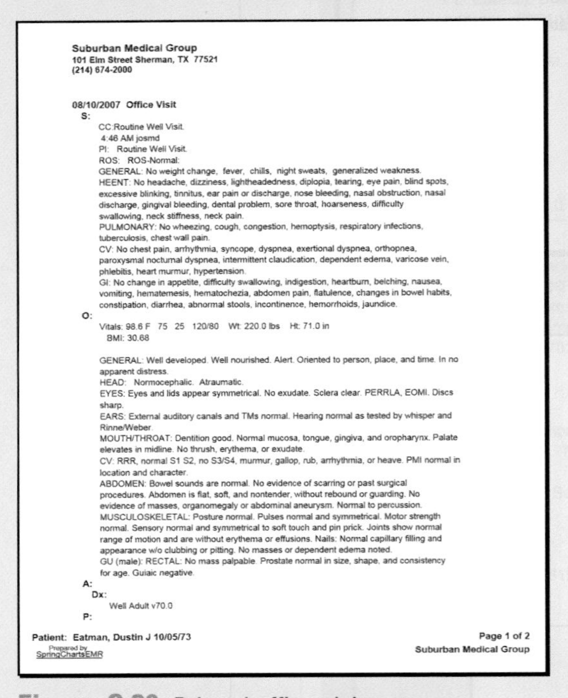

Suburban Medical Group
101 Elm Street Sherman, TX 77521
(214) 674-2000

08/10/2007 Office Visit

S:

CC:Routine Well Visit.
4:46 AM josmd
PI: Routine Well Visit.
ROS: ROS-Normal:
GENERAL: No weight change, fever, chills, night sweats, generalized weakness.
HEENT: No headache, dizziness, lightheadedness, diplopia, tearing, eye pain, blind spots, excessive blinking, tinnitus, ear pain or discharge, nose bleeding, nasal obstruction, nasal discharge, gingival bleeding, dental problem, sore throat, hoarseness, difficulty swallowing, neck stiffness, neck pain.
PULMONARY: No wheezing, cough, congestion, hemoptysis, respiratory infections, tuberculosis, chest wall pain.
CV: No chest pain, arrhythmia, syncope, dyspnea, exertional dyspnea, orthopnea, paroxysmal nocturnal dyspnea, intermittent claudication, dependent edema, varicose vein, phlebitis, heart murmur, hypertension.
GI: No change in appetite, difficulty swallowing, indigestion, heartburn, belching, nausea, vomiting, hematemesis, hematochezia, abdomen pain, flatulence, changes in bowel habits, constipation, diarrhea, abnormal stools, incontinence, hemorrhoids, jaundice.

O:

Vitals: 98.6 F 75 25 120/80 Wt: 220.0 lbs Ht: 71.0 in
BMI: 30.68

GENERAL: Well developed. Well nourished. Alert. Oriented to person, place, and time. In no apparent distress.
HEAD: Normocephalic. Atraumatic.
EYES: Eyes and lids appear symmetrical. No exudate. Sclera clear. PERRLA, EOMI. Discs sharp.
EARS: External auditory canals and TMs normal. Hearing normal as tested by whisper and Rinne/Weber.
MOUTH/THROAT: Dentition good. Normal mucosa, tongue, gingiva, and oropharynx. Palate elevates in midline. No thrush, erythema, or exudate.
CV: RRR, normal S1 S2, no S3/S4, murmur, gallop, rub, arrhythmia, or heave. PMI normal in location and character.
ABDOMEN: Bowel sounds are normal. No evidence of scarring or past surgical procedures. Abdomen is flat, soft, and nontender, without rebound or guarding. No evidence of masses, organomegaly or abdominal aneurysm. Normal to percussion.
MUSCULOSKELETAL: Posture normal. Pulses normal and symmetrical. Motor strength normal. Sensory normal and symmetrical to soft touch and pin prick. Joints show normal range of motion and are without erythema or effusions. Nails: Normal capillary filling and appearance w/o clubbing or pitting. No masses or dependent edema noted.
GU (male): RECTAL: No mass palpable. Prostate normal in size, shape, and consistency for age. Guiaic negative.

A:

Dx:

Well Adult v70.0

P:

Patient: Eatman, Dustin J 10/05/73 **Page 1 of 2**
Prepared by SpringChartsEMR **Suburban Medical Group**

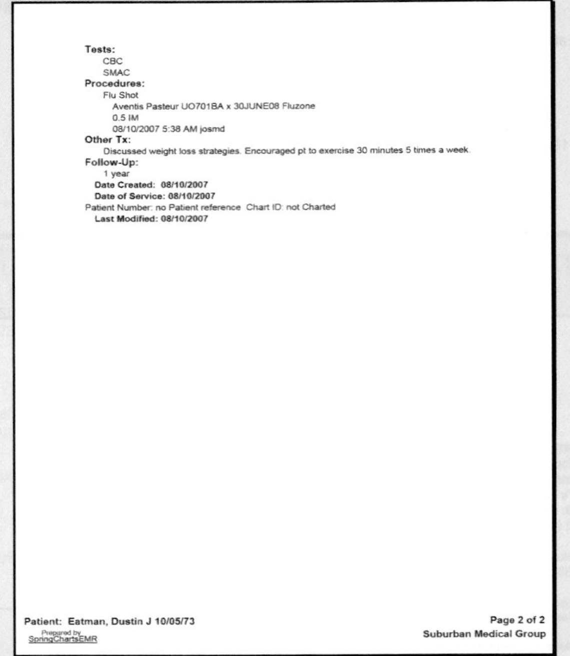

Tests:
CBC
SMAC
Procedures:
Flu Shot
Aventis Pasteur UO701BA x 30JUNE08 Fluzone
0.5 IM
08/10/2007 5:38 AM josmd
Other Tx:
Discussed weight loss strategies. Encouraged pt to exercise 30 minutes 5 times a week.
Follow-Up:
1 year
Date Created: 08/10/2007
Date of Service: 08/10/2007
Patient Number: no Patient reference Chart ID: not Charted
Last Modified: 08/10/2007

Patient: Eatman, Dustin J 10/05/73 **Page 2 of 2**
Prepared by SpringChartsEMR **Suburban Medical Group**

Figure C.39 Printed office visit note.

Exercise 11.22(N) Printing an *H&P Report*

(Refer to Chapter 6, page 182)

1. Your cousin requests a copy of the history and physical report of his medical encounter. Open the current office visit note and select the *H&P Report* from the *Tools* menu.
2. Print the report. Compare it to Figure C.40.
3. Save the *H&P Report* under the *H&Ps* category in the care tree, and close the *Office Visit* screen and the patient's chart.
4. Update the *Patient Tracker* to reflect your cousin being sent to the *Checkout Desk* with a status of *Ready*. Click [Done].
5. Reopen the *Edit Tracker* window and click on the [CheckOut] button.
6. The *Patient Tracker* shows your cousin as *Done* with the *Routing Slip* stamp (Figure C.41).

Exercise 11.22(N) (Concluded)

History and Physical
Patient: Eatman, Dustin J 10/05/73
Date of Service: 08/10/2007
Chief Complaint:
Routine Well Visit. 4:46 AM josmd
Present Illness:
Routine Well Visit.
Allergies:
Mold Extracts, Latex
Cat Hair causes hives
Current Medications:
Aleve 275 mg i q 12 hrs
Lipitor 20 mg i po q d
Aspirin 81mg i po daily
Omega-3
Past Medical History:
Fracture Of Rib
Asthma Bronchitis
Family Medical History:
Brother: Heart Disease Mother: Hypercholesterolemia Father Died At Age: 59
Cause Of Death: Heart Disease
Social History:
Tobacco Use: Nonsmoker. Alcohol Use: Social Drinker. Caffeine Use: Yes. Cups Per Day: 4 Marital Status: Married. Occupation: Sales Education: College.
Review Of Systems:
ROS-Normal: GENERAL: No weight change, fever, chills, night sweats, generalized weakness. HEENT: No headache, dizziness, lightheadedness, diplopia, tearing, eye pain, blind spots, excessive blinking, tinnitus, ear pain or discharge, nose bleeding, nasal obstruction, nasal discharge, gingival bleeding, dental problem, sore throat, hoarseness, difficulty swallowing, neck stiffness, neck pain. PULMONARY: No wheezing, cough, congestion, hemoptysis, respiratory infections, tuberculosis, chest wall pain. CV: No chest pain, arrhythmia, syncope, dyspnea, exertional dyspnea, orthopnea, paroxysmal nocturnal dyspnea, intermittent claudication, dependent edema, varicose vein, phlebitis, heart murmur, hypertension. GI: No change in appetite, difficulty swallowing, indigestion, heartburn, belching, nausea, vomiting, hematemesis, hematochezia, abdomen pain, flatulence, changes in bowel habits, constipation, diarrhea, abnormal stools, incontinence, hemorrhoids, jaundice.
Examination:
Vitals: Temp: 98.6 Pulse: 75 Resp: 25 BP: 120/80 Wt: 220.0 Ht: 71.0
GENERAL: Well developed. Well nourished. Alert. Oriented to person, place, and time. In no apparent distress. HEAD: Normocephalic. Atraumatic. EYES: Eyes and lids appear symmetrical. No exudate. Sclera clear. PERRLA, EOMI. Discs sharp. EARS: External auditory canals and TMs normal. Hearing normal as tested by

Suburban Medical Group
H&P for Pt: Eatman, Dustin J 10/05/73 Page 1 of 2

whisper and Rinne/Weber. MOUTH/THROAT: Dentition good. Normal mucosa, tongue, gingiva, and oropharynx. Palate elevates in midline. No thrush, erythema, or exudate. CV: RRR, normal S1 S2, no S3/S4, murmur, gallop, rub, arrhythmia, or heave. PMI normal in location and character. ABDOMEN: Bowel sounds are normal. No evidence of scarring or past surgical procedures. Abdomen is flat, soft, and nontender, without rebound or guarding. No evidence of masses, organomegaly or abdominal aneurysm. Normal to percussion. MUSCULOSKELETAL: Posture normal. Pulses normal and symmetrical. Motor strength normal. Sensory normal and symmetrical to soft touch and pin prick. Joints show normal range of motion and are without erythema or effusions. Nails: Normal capillary filling and appearance w/o clubbing or pitting. No masses or dependent edema noted. GU (male): RECTAL: No mass palpable. Prostate normal in size, shape, and consistency for age. Guiaic negative.
Tests:
CBC pending
SMAC pending
Flu Shot
Aventis Pasteur UO701BA x 30JUNE08 Fluzone 0.5 IM 08/10/2007 5:38 AM josmd
Impression:
Well Adult v70.0
Plan:
Discussed weight loss strategies. Encouraged pt to exercise 30 minutes 5 times a week.
1 year

John O. Smith, M. D.

Suburban Medical Group
H&P for Pt: Eatman, Dustin J 10/05/73 Page 2 of 2

Figure C.40 Printed H&P report

Done	
Eatman, Dustin J 10/05/73 6:58 AM √ Routing Slip	Done

Figure C.41 Stamped *Routing Slip* in *Patient Tracker.*

Chapter 12 Electronic Recording

In this chapter, you will examine the source documents contained in Appendix D and record the information in the appropriate areas of the SpringCharts EHR program.

Exercise 12.1(N) Adding a New Patient

(Refer to Chapter 3, page 77)

1. Using *Source Document 1—Patient Information Sheet (See Appendix D)*, add a new female patient to the EHR program and save the information. Make up the patient's name.
2. Go to the *Edit Patient* window, locate the patient.
3. Click on the *Copy or Export This Data* (universal export) button (lower right) and *Open in Word Processor.*
4. Type your name at the top of the document. Print the patient's information, circle your name, and submit it to your instructor.

Exercise 12.2(N) Scheduling a New Patient

(Refer to Chapter 4, page 88)

1. Using *Source Document 1—Patient Information Sheet (See Appendix D),* add the patient to a unique time slot designated by your instructor. The patient has scheduled a doctor's appointment for allergies.
2. Add yourself to the schedule. The reason for your visit is an annual physical.
3. Print today's schedule, circle your name on the document, and turn in to your instructor.

Exercise 12.3(N) Adding a New Insurance Company

(Refer to Chapter 3, page 79)

1. Using *Source Document 2—Primary Insurance Card Information (See Appendix D),* set up a new insurance company in SpringCharts.
2. Click on the *Export* button and *Open in Word Processor.*
3. Type your name at the top of the document. Print the insurance information, circle your name, and submit it to your instructor.

Exercise 12.4(N) Adding a Patient's Insurance Information

(Refer to Chapter 5, page 139)

1. Using *Source Document 2—Primary Insurance Card Information (See Appendix D),* add the primary insurance details to the face sheet of the patient you added in Exercise 12.1(N). Use the employer name from the *Patient Information Sheet* as the Group Name.
2. Print out the patient's primary insurance information, write your name on the document, and submit it to your instructor.

Exercise 12.5(N) Adding a Physician's Address

(Refer to Chapter 3, page 68)

1. Using *Source Document 3—Patient Intake Sheet (See Appendix D),* add the patient's primary care physician as a new entry in SpringCharts's *Address Book.* Create the last name for the physician.
2. Print the address card, write your name on the document, and submit it to your instructor.

Exercise 12.6(N) Completing a Face Sheet

(Refer to Chapter 5, page 134)

1. Using *Source Document 3—Patient Intake Sheet (See Appendix D),* complete the patient's face sheet.
2. Print the face sheet, write your name on the document, and submit it to your instructor.

Exercise 12.7(N) Adding a New Pharmacy

(Refer to Chapter 3, page 69)

1. Using *Source Document 4—Default Pharmacy Information (See Appendix D),* add a new entry to the *Address Book* in SpringCharts.
2. Click the [Print Card] button, write your name on the document, and submit it to your instructor.

Exercise 12.8(N) Identifying a Patient's Default Pharmacy

1. Using *Source Document 4—Default Pharmacy Information (See Appendix D),* record this pharmacy as the patient's default pharmacy in the face sheet.

Exercise 12.9(N) Importing a Patient Photo

1. Import the patient's photo into the chart through the *Edit* menu. Access the file from within the *EHR Material* folder. Locate the photo titled *Chloe Hill.*
2. Using the [Print Screen] button on your keyboard, copy the *Patient Chart* screen and paste into a word processor document. You may have to resize the picture to fit the page. Write your name on the document and submit to your instructor.

Exercise 12.10(N) Updating a Patient's Immunization Record

(Refer to Chapter 5, page 137)

1. Using *Source Document 5—Past Immunization Record Card (See Appendix D),* update the immunization archive in the patient's chart. Use the same start and end date for the immunizations.
2. Click on the *Date* heading and organize the immunizations with the oldest at the top and print the immunization record. Write your name on the document and submit it to your instructor.

Exercise 12.11(N) Conducting a *Chart Evaluation*

(Refer to Chapter 7, page 190)

1. Perform a *Chart Evaluation* of your patient's chart.
2. Record that the patient did **not** agree to have the indicated items conducted.
3. Print the *Chart Evaluation.* Record your name on the document and submit to your instructor.

Exercise 12.12(N) Documenting a New Office Visit

(Refer to Chapter 6, page 155)

1. Using *Source Document 6—Office Visit Notes (See Appendix D),* record the information in a *New OV* window in the patient's chart. Complete Exercises 12.12(N) through 12.15(N) from within the *OV* screen.

Exercise 12.13(N) Creating an Electronic Prescription

(Refer to Chapter 6, page 159)

1. Using *Source Document 6—Office Visit Notes (See Appendix D),* create three *Prescription Forms* within the OV note for the medication prescribed to the patient. Include the physician' license and NPI numbers.
2. Print the prescription, write your name on the document, and submit it to your instructor.

Exercise 12.14(N) Creating an *Order Form*

(Refer to Chapter 7, page 197)

1. Using *Source Document 6—Office Visit Notes (See Appendix D),* create an *Order Form* within the OV note for the ordered test. Add the patient's insurance.
2. Type your name at the top of the document. Print the *Order Form,* chart it, circle your name on the printed document, and submit it to your instructor.

Exercise 12.15(N) Creating a Procedure Note

(Refer to Chapter 6, page 164)

1. Using *Source Document 6—Office Visit Notes (See Appendix D),* create a procedure note by clicking on the selected procedure.
2. On a new line, add the pop-up text that begins with *The patient's questions were answered . . .*
3. On a new line, use the time and initials stamp.

Exercise 12.16(N) Creating a *Routing Slip*

(Refer to Chapter 6, page 179)

1. Create a *Routing Slip.* Type your name on the document at the top of the *Routing Slip* window.
2. From the *Edit* menu, locate the *Routing Slip* and print it. Circle your name on the document and submit it to your instructor.

Exercise 12.17(N) Creating an *Excuse Note*

(Refer to Chapter 5, page 147)

1. Using *Source Document 7—Patient Excuse Note (See Appendix D),* create an excuse note for your patient within the chart. Type your name at the top of the document.
2. Print the excuse note, use the digital signature, circle your name on the document, and submit it to your instructor.

Exercise 12.18(N) Creating a Letter About a Patient

(Refer to Chapter 5, page 144)

1. Using *Source Document 8—Letter to Primary Care Physician (See Appendix D),* create a letter in the patient's chart to her primary care physician. Include the recent office visit notes. Type your name at the bottom of the letter.
2. Save the letter under the *Letter* category in her care tree.
3. Print the letter, circle your name on the document, and submit it to your instructor.

Exercise 12.19(N) Processing Test Results

(Refer to Chapter 9, page 245)

1. Using *Source Document 9—Patient Lab Results (See Appendix D),* record the lab results into the patient's chart under *Pending Tests.* Type your name into the *Test Note* area.
2. Process the test results into the *Completed Tests* area. Indicate that the doctor has viewed the test.
3. Save the results in the patient's chart.
4. From the patient's chart, print the lab results, circle your name on the document, and submit it to your instructor.

Exercise 12.20(N) Documenting a Telephone Call Message

(Refer to Chapter 4, page 107)

1. Using *Source Document 10—Telephone Call Message (See Appendix D),* create a message from the patient requesting a letter regarding the negative lab results from the recent strep test. Use appropriate popup text and free text.
2. Send the message to yourself.
3. Open the message from the *Message Center* as the recipient and document that you have sent the patient a letter. Initial- and time-stamp the message. Type your name at the bottom of the message.
4. Chart the message into the patient's chart under the *Encounter* tab.
5. Open the patient's chart and print a copy of the message. Circle your name and turn in to your instructor.

Exercise 12.21(N) Creating a Letter to a Patient

(Refer to Chapter 5, page 143)

1. Using *Source Document 11—Letter to Patient (See Appendix D),* create a letter to the patient within her chart. Include a copy of recent lab results. Type your name at the bottom of the letter.
2. Save the letter under the *Letter* category in her care tree.
3. Print the letter, circle your name on the document, and submit it to your instructor.

Exercise 12.22(N) Creating a Test Report

(Refer to Chapter 5, page 149)

1. Create a *New Test Report* for a strep screen within the patient's chart.
2. Remove the *Problems* and *Recommendations* headings from the report. Type your name at the bottom of the report.
3. Print the test report, add the signature, circle your name on the document, and submit it to your instructor.

appendix D

Source Documents for SpringCharts Network Version

Source Document 1 Patient Information Sheet

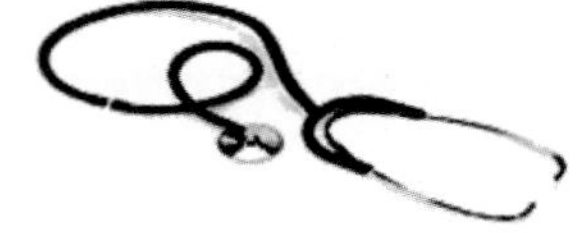

Suburban Medical Group

101 Elm Street
Sherman, TX 77521

PH: (214) 674-2000
FX: (214) 674-2100

Appointment: Time 10:00 AM Date Today's Date

Physician: Dr. Smith

PATIENT INFORMATION SHEET

Patient Name: ______ , ______ , ______
Last, First, Middle

Date of Birth: 10/8/89
Address: 78 RICHARDS ST.
LOGANLEA, MO 65807
Social Security #: 048-69-4281
E-mail Address: ceh89@hotmail.com
Home Phone: 417-881-3968
Cell Phone: ______
Gender (Circle one): Male, (Female)
Marital Status (Circle one): Married, (Single), Divorced, Widowed, Separated
Preferred Language: ENGLISH
Race (Circle one): American Indian, Asian, Black, (White), Hispanic, Native Hawaiian, Unknown, Other ______
Ethnicity (Circle one): Hispanic, (Non-Hispanic)
Mother's Maiden Name: ______
Emplyoyer: LOGAN CITY
Work Phone: 417-969-4123
Work Fax: 417-969-7821

Signature of Patient or Patient-Guardian: CEHill

Source Document 2 Primary Insurance Card Information

Physician Visit & Hospital Program
(Name of Insurance Company)
National Provider Network
Office Visit Co-Pay: $35.00
(Patient Name)
Member Number: 041020102
Group Number: 76022

Members: In an Emergency Seek Medical Attention First
For questions or to locate a provider visit www.uhnbenefits.com
Or call 800-275-1258.
Before seeking hospital services you must register for CAP benefits
To register call 800-975-2589
Members Are Responsible For Network Contracted Rates Incurred.
Members are required to register for referral authorization before seeking hospital services.
PROVIDERS:
Send bills to: UHN; PO Box 221458; Dallas, TX 75225
For questions call: 866-404-5489
For lab work use Lab Diagnostics or call 800-975-1452.
In emergency please admit the patient and call 800-975-1452 by the next business day.
All members have limited inpatient and outpatient benefits.
Underwritten by various insurance companies.
This program is administered by UHN
6732 DownUnder Blvd., Mackay, CO 80922

Source Document 3 Patient Intake Sheet

Suburban Medical Group

101 Elm Street
Sherman, TX 77521

PH: (214) 674-2000
FX: (214) 674-2100

Primary Care Physician
Name: Jow MD
Address: 1300 E WOODHURST ST
WATERFORD, MC 65804
Phone: 417-890-6777
Family Practice

Patient Name: ______

Date of Birth: 10/8/89 SS #: 048-69-4281

PERSONAL HEALTH INFORMATION

Allergies:
Drugs & Medications? Please list.
CODEINE

Foods? Please list with adverse reactions.
PEANUT PRODUCTS - RASH
SHELLFISH - HIVES

Personal Medical History:	Yes	No
Asthma	✓	
Bronchitis	✓	
Cancer		✓
Diabetes		✓
Gout		✓
Heart Disease		✓
Hernia		✓
High Cholesterol		✓
HIV Positive		✓
Kidney Disease		✓
Liver Disease		✓
Migraines		✓
Pneumonia	✓	
Thyroid Problems		
Other:		
Other:		

Social History: (Check the appropriate line)

Tobacco Use: (Choose one)
- Current - Every day? ___
- Current - Some days? ___
- Former Smoker? ___
- Never Smoked? ✓

Alcohol Use:
- Non Drinker? ___
- Social Drinker? ✓
- Heavy Drinker? ___

Caffeine Use:
- Yes ✓
- No ___
- Cups per Day? 2

Living Arrangements:
- Lives with Family/Parents ✓
- Lives with Spouse/Partner ___

Education:
- Highschool ___
- College ✓
- Post-Graduate ___

Occupation: Receptionist

Family Medical History: (List chronic health problems)
Father: ASTHMA
Mother:
Brother(s): 1 BROTHER - ASTHMA
Sister(s):

Has your physical activity been restricted during the past 5 years? NO
Have you been hosptialized during the past 5 years? Explain: APPENDECTOMY - 2004
Have you lived or travelled outside the US in the past 5 years? NO

Current Medical Problems:	Yes	No	Details:
Asthma/Hay Fever	✓		TWICE PER YR.
Back Problems		✓	
Blood Pressure Problems		✓	
Cholesterol Problems		✓	
Colds and chronic coughs		✓	
Diarrhea/Constipation		✓	
Eating Problems		✓	
Female Problems		✓	
Gall Bladder Problems		✓	
Hernias		✓	
Jaundice/Hepatitis		✓	
Kidney Problems		✓	
Liver Problems		✓	
Pains		✓	
Other:			

Routine Medications:
ALEVE - 275 mg
CLARITIN D-24

Over-The-Counter Meds:
CALCIUM SUPPLEMENTS
MULTI-VITAMINS

Personal Preferences:
Hospital: ST. JOHNS
Lab Company: LAB CORP

Additional Concerns:
ENGLISH - SECOND LANGUAGE.

HIPAA Notice of Privacy Practices Acknowledges
I acknowledge receipt of and have read the Suburban Medical Group Notice of Privacy Practices.

Patient's Signature: C. Hill Date: 11/15/2012

Source Document 7 Patient Excuse Note

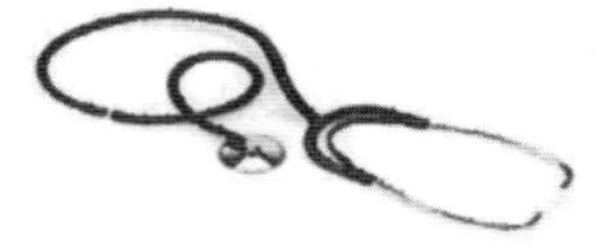

Suburban Medical Group

101 Elm Street
Sherman, TX 77521

PH: (214) 674-2000
FX: (214) 674-2100

EXPLAINED ABSENCE

Date: Today's Date

To: Springs Community College

Please excuse this student's/employee's absence today due to our office visit from:

10:00 Am to 12:00 am/pm

Sincerely,

John O. Smith, M.D.

By: Jan Barton

Source Document 8 Letter to Primary Care Physician

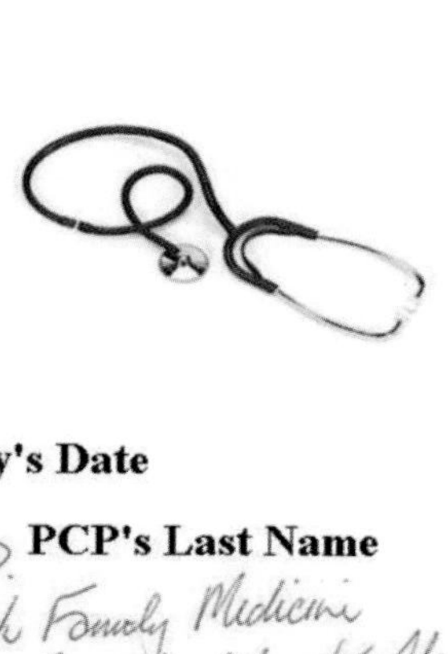

Suburban Medical Group

101 Elm Street
Sherman, TX 77521

PH: (214) 674-2000
FX: (214) 674-2100

Today's Date

Jon D. **PCP's Last Name**
Clark Family Medicine
1200 E. Woodhurst St.
Waterford, MO 65804

Re: **Your Patient's Name**

Dear Dr. **PCP's Last Name,**

Thank you for allowing me to participate in this pt's care. If you have any questions or observations for me, please do not hesitate to call.

Below please find a copy of the recent examination

Sincerely,

J D Smith MD

Source Document 9 Patient Lab Results

TEST PERFORMED AT:
Lab Corp
4380 Federal Dr. Suite 100
Marsdon, MO 65803

PATIENT:
Your Patient's Name
DOB: 10/08/1989
Gender: F

Ordering Physician: John O. Smith MD
Accnt No: 444051
Lab Specimen: No N321850003

Test Name	In Range	Out Of Range	Reference Range
Strep Screen	Normal		Normal

Test Date: 08/05/2011

Source Document 10 Telephone Call Message

Suburban Medical Group
PH: (214) 674-2000
FX: (214) 674-2100

Telephone Call Message

To: Demo

Date: Today's Date Time: 10:35 (A.M.) P.M.

From:

Phone Number: 417-881-3968

- [x] Telephoned
- [ ] Returned Your Call
- [ ] Please Call
- [ ] Will Call Again
- [x] Please Rush Request
- [ ] Special Attention

Message:
Pt called and requested letter regarding her recent lab work results.
She needs to show her employer that the strep results were negative.

Name: User Demo Signed: [signature]

Source Document 11 Letter to Patient

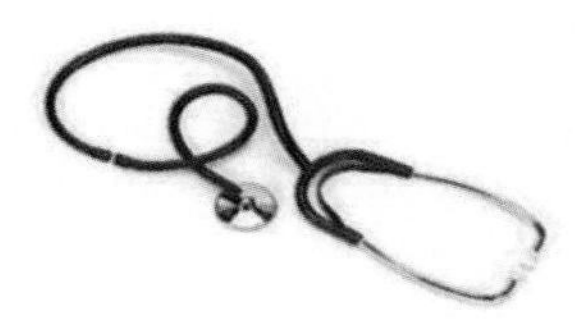

Suburban Medical Group

101 Elm Street
Sherman, TX 77521

PH: (214) 674-2000
FX: (214) 674-2100

Today's Date

Your Patient's Name

78 Richards St
Loganlea, MO 65807

Re: Lab Results from Recent Visit

Dear Ms. **Patient's Last Name,**

Please find enclosed lab results from our recent visit. Included is a basic explanation of the lab results.

If you have any questions regarding these results, please call the office + schedule an appointment to meet with me.

Thank you for allowing me to be your physician. Stay well.

Sincerely,
John D. Smith, MD

glossary

A

Addendum An addendum is a notation added to an office visit note after it has been permanently signed and locked to supplement the information in the original encounter note.

Ambulatory This term means the ability to walk or to move from one place to another. In the medical sense it is used to distinguish walking patients from bedridden patients, as in inpatient hospitals or skilled nursing facilities.

American Medical Association (AMA) The American Medical Association is a national association founded in 1847. Its purpose is to promote the art and science of medicine in order to improve professional and public health concerns in America's healthcare system.

American Recovery and Reinvestment Act (ARRA) ARRA is commonly referred to as the *stimulus package* or the *Recovery Act*. This legislation, which Congress enacted in 2009, was intended to create jobs and promote investment and consumer spending during the late-2000s recession.

Analyte See *Lab analyte*

Application server provider (ASP) An ASP enables access to an EHR via the Internet; the EHR software and database are housed and maintained by a separate company in a remote location.

Appointment schedule The appointment calendar or schedule—known officially in SpringCharts as *Office Calendar*—displays past, current, and future patient appointment schedules and time blocks for activities. Multiple appointment schedules can be created within an EHR program to display patient appointments for different medical providers and other resources. Appointment schedules can show a variety of appointment length slots.

Archive In electronic terms, an archive is a long-term storage folder or device that contains records and information of groups of patients no longer used but important to keep for future reference.

Attending physician An attending physician is the individual who has final responsibility, legally and otherwise, for patient healthcare, even when many of the medical decisions are being made by subordinates such as physician assistants, nurse practitioners, medical interns, and so on.

B

Best practice guidelines Best practice guidelines are methods that have consistently shown superior results and are used as a benchmark or standard until improvements are discovered or developed.

Body mass index (BMI) BMI is a measure of body fat based on height and weight that applies to adult men and women. BMI is the measurement of choice for studying obesity. It is calculated by a mathematical formula that divides a person's weight in kilograms by height in meters squared ($BMI = kg/m^2$).

C

Care plans (or **practice guidelines**) Care plans are specific documents that guide all individuals who are involved in a patient's care, outlining the appropriate treatment that will ensure the optimal outcome. A caregiver unfamiliar with the patient should be able to find all of the information needed to care for the patient in these documents.

Care tree The care tree is a portion of the patient's electronic chart that lists categories in which encounters (progress notes), tests, excuse notes, letters, reports, and other current records are stored.

Category preferences The Category Preferences table on the SpringCharts server enables the clinic administrator to create customized lists of medical data. The lists are displayed in SpringCharts to enable rapid selection of items with which to build the face sheet and other areas of the program.

Centers for Medicare & Medicaid Services (CMS) CMS, formerly known as the *Health Care Financing Administration* (HCFA), is a federal agency responsible for administering Medicare, Medicaid, the Health Insurance Portability and Accountability Act (HIPAA), and other health-related programs.

Certification Commission for Health Information Technology (CCHIT) The Certification Commission's mission was to accelerate the adoption of health information technology by creating an efficient, credible, and sustainable product certification program. It is now one of several ONC-certifying bodies.

Chart Alert Chart alerts in EHR programs highlight important text that appears in prominent areas of the patient chart or as warning pop-up messages when certain areas of the program are accessed.

Chart evaluation A chart evaluation is a CDS (clinical decision support) tool that defines preventive health criteria and allows providers to search patient charts to ensure the criteria are met, thereby supporting disease management, providing routine preventive services, and ensuring wellness healthcare standards.

Clinical decision support (CDS) CDS is an EHR-integrated system designed to assist physicians and other healthcare professionals with evidence-based decision making concerning patient healthcare by using clinical databases.

Clinical quality measures (CQMs) CQMs are measures of processes, experiences, and outcomes of patient care. They encompass observations or treatment that relate to one or more quality aims for healthcare.

Computer on wheels (COW)/workstation on wheels (WOW) COW or WOW is a computer placed on a mobile desk or stand so it can be moved around an office, unit, or patient room.

Computerized provider order entry (CPOE) The CPOE is the process of communicating a clinician's instructions for patient treatment over a computer network to departments within a hospital or testing facilities outside the patient setting.

Consolidated Health Informatics (CHI) CHI is a federal government initiative that promotes the adoption of health information interoperability standards for health vocabulary and messaging.

Conversion Calculator This type of calculator in SpringCharts converts imperial measurements to metric units and converts metric measurements to imperial units in weight, length, and temperature.

Coordination of care Coordination of care comprises making available all resources to ensure healthcare providers have access to all required information on a patient's conditions and treatments and that the patient receives appropriate healthcare services.

Co-pay A co-pay is an amount paid by a policyholder for each medical office visit or other type of medical service obtained by a patient covered under a health insurance policy (for example, $25 per visit). It must be paid before the insurance company will pay any policy benefit to the healthcare provider.

Current Procedural Terminology (CPT) codes CPT codes are five-digit codes the AMA developed and insurance carriers and managed care companies adopted as the means for identifying common medical procedures.

D

Deductible Most medical insurance policies require the patient to pay an annual deductible–an amount of money the policyholder pays toward medical expenses before the insurance company pays its share—for example, $500 per year.

Demographics Demographics are the statistical data of a person or population. They are typically comprised of address, phone numbers, gender, age, marital status, employment, and education. However, demographics can be very broad to include disabilities, mobility, home ownership, income, and personal preferences.

Diagnosis codes Diagnosis codes are used in healthcare to group and identify diseases, disorders, and symptoms. These codes are also used to track the relative frequency of a particular disease (morbidity) and the causes of death (mortality). Diagnosis codes are officially known as International Classification of Diseases (ICD) codes.

Draw program The Draw program accessed in the *OV* screen enables providers to document injuries, pain locations, skin abnormalities, and so on, on templates of body areas or imported images. The completed drawing remains a permanent part of the OV note.

Drug formulary A drug formulary is a database of approved medications in drug therapy categories that includes information on the medications' preparation, safety, effectiveness, and cost.

E

Electronic health record (EHR) An electronic health record is the most commonly accepted term for software with a full range of functionalities to store, access, and use patient healthcare information.

Electronic medical record (EMR) EMR is a term for medical software that lacks a full range of higher-end functionalities to store, access, and use patient medical information. EMRs are not interoperable.

Eligible professional (EP) To participate in the HITECH Act incentive program for meaningful use (MU) on an ONC-certified EHR program, an EP qualifying under Medicare must be a doctor of either medicine, osteopathy, dental surgery, dental medicine, podiatry, optometry, or chiropractic. Individuals qualifying under the Medicaid program must be a doctor of medicine or osteopathy, nurse practitioner, certified nurse-midwife, dentist, or qualifying physician assistant.

Encounters Encounters is a specific tab in the care tree of the patient's chart that stores many of the documents created from patient encounters.

Encrypting To be transmitted securely, computer data are changed from their original form, making the data unintelligible to unauthorized parties, and then decrypted back into their original form for use by the receiving entity.

End-to-end solution This software industry term suggests the vendor of an application program can provide all the hardware and software components to meet the client's requirement and that no other supplier need be involved.

E-prescribing Electronic prescribing is the use of computerized tools, usually embedded in an EHR program, to create and sign prescriptions for medicines, thereby replacing handwritten prescriptions. Electronic prescriptions are sent to pharmacies over the Internet via a clearinghouse.

Evaluation & Management (E&M) code The Evaluation & Management (E&M) code is a five-digit number used by a physician to report evaluation and management services provided to a patient. The E&M encounter may include documenting a patient's medical history, a physical examination, and medical decision making. For example, a 99213 code indicates an outpatient visit with a limited amount of diagnoses and limited complexity and complications.

E&M Coder The Evaluation & Management Coder is a built-in function of many EHR programs that recommends the appropriate evaluation & management code for office visits. The coder looks for keywords used within the review of systems and physical exams in the office visit note. The *E&M Coder* then uses this information, in conjunction with diagnoses, to determine the most appropriate E&M code level for billing.

F

Face sheet The face sheet portion of the patient's chart contains relatively static patient information, such as allergies, problem list, past medical history (PMHX), and so on.

Family medical history (FMHX) This portion of the patient's face sheet contains health information about a patient's close relatives. Because families have many factors in common, including genes and lifestyles, medical information from three generations of relatives can give clues to a patient's increased risk of developing a particular condition.

G

Graphic user interface (GUI) A GUI (pronounced Goo-ee) is a software program screen that can display icons, subwindows, text fields, and menus designed to standardize and simplify the use of the computer program by allowing a user to type in fields and use a mouse to manipulate text and images.

H

Health information exchange (HIE) HIE is the transmission of healthcare information electronically across organizations within a region, community, or hospital system.

Health information technology (HIT) HIT deals with the storage, retrieval, sharing, and use of electronic healthcare information involving computer hardware and software.

Health Information Technology for Economic and Clinical Health (HITECH) Act The HITECH Act was initiated by Congress in 2009 to stimulate and increase independent physicians' and hospitals' use of electronic health records over a five-year period.

Health Insurance Portability and Accountability Act (HIPAA) Passed by Congress in 1996, this legal act enforces standards for electronic patient health, administrative, and financial data.

Health Level 7 (HL7) Health Level 7 is an international computer language by which various healthcare systems can communicate. HL7 is currently the selected standard for interfacing clinical data between software programs in most institutions.

Healthcare Common Procedure Coding System (HCPCS) codes HCPCS codes are used by HHS's Centers for Medicare & Medicaid Services (CMS) to identify medical supplies such as durable medical equipment and medical procedures. The coding of supplies ensures uniformity for billing and financial reimbursement.

History & physical (H&P) report An H&P report documents the patient's healthcare history, such as past medical history, family medical history, routine medications, problem lists, and so on, as well as the details of the current physical exam. The H&P report is a required document when admitting a patient to a hospital as an inpatient.

I

Imperial units This system of weights and measures conforms to the standards legally established in Great Britain and is still widely used in the United States.

Inpatient An inpatient is a person who is admitted to the hospital and stays overnight or for an indeterminate amount of time, usually several days or weeks.

Institute of Medicine (IOM) This independent, nonprofit organization works outside the government to provide unbiased and authoritative medical advice to decision makers and the public.

InterFax InterFax is one of many subscriber-based online fax services that enable users to fax wherever Internet access is available.

International Classification of Diseases (ICD) codes ICD codes are the international standard diagnostic classification for all medical data concerning the incidence and prevalence of disease in large populations and for other health management purposes.

Interoperability Interoperability is the ability of a software program to send and communicate data from its database to multiple vendors' software programs as well as accept data from other vendors' programs.

Intranet An intranet is a privately maintained computer network that provides secure accessibility to authorized people and enables sharing of software, databases and files.

L

Lab analyte This blood test compound is the subject of its own specific chemical analysis. A lab panel is composed of multiple analytes that undergo analysis.

Letter templates Letter templates allow users to create form letters that can be used as a *Letter to the Patient* or *Letter About the Patient*. Only the body of the letter template and the subject line need to be created; SpringCharts automatically completes the appropriate recipient's name, address, and greeting.

Local area network (LAN) A LAN is a wired and/or wireless connection of computers on a single campus or facility.

M

Mandated reporters A mandated reporter is a professional who has regular contact with children, disabled persons, older adults, and other identified vulnerable individuals. Such a professional is legally required to report any observed or suspected maltreatment or neglect to the appropriate authorities.

Meaningful use (MU) Meaningful use is healthcare providers' use of certified EHR technology in ways that can be measured significantly in quality (e.g., e-prescribing) and in quantity (e.g., set percentage of patients). By demonstrating MU with an ONC-certified EHR program, providers then can receive stimulus money, as set up through the HITECH Act of 2009.

Medicare Improvements for Patients and Providers Act of 2008 (MIPPA) Enacted by Congress in 2008, this 275-page piece of legislation blocked scheduled cuts in Medicare's payments to physicians and increased benefits to low-income beneficiaries and other vulnerable areas of the population.

Medicare Part A This part of the federally funded Medicare insurance program covers hospitals, skilled nursing facilities, home health agencies, and other non-ambulatory services.

Medicare Part B This part of the federally funded Medicare insurance program covers medical providers' supervision, outpatient hospital care, diagnostic tests, ambulance services, and other ambulatory services.

Message Archive The message archive is a storage area in SpringCharts for saved messages. A sent or received message that does not concern a patient can be saved as an archived message, which can be reactivated. Messages regarding patients are saved in the patient's chart.

Metric units This system of weights and measures, based on the metric system, is mandatory in a large number of countries; also known as the International System of Units.

N

National Committee on Vital and Health Statistics (NCVHS) Formed in 1949 and restructured following the passage of HIPAA, the NCVHS is an advocate for uniform health data sets, particularly for underrepresented populations. This advisory committee has responsibility for providing recommendations on health information policy and standards to the Department of Health and Human Services (HHS).

National Guideline Clearinghouse (NGC) NGC is a public healthcare resource created by the HHS in partnership with the American Medical Association (AMA) and the America's Health Insurance Plans (AHIP). Its mission is to provide healthcare professionals with an accessible system for obtaining, disseminating, and implementing detailed information on clinical practice guidelines.

No show This term is used to indicate a patient missed a scheduled appointment without calling in advance to inform the clinic or to reschedule.

Office of the National Coordinator for Health Information Technology (ONC) The ONC was established in 2004 within the Office of the Secretary for HHS for the purpose of serving as a resource for the entire health system, supporting the adoption of HIT, and promoting a nationwide health information exchange.

Office Visit (OV) The acronym OV (for office visit) is used in SpringCharts to designate the graphic user interface (GUI) window in which the encounter note is created and in which the patient's chief complaints, body systems, vital signs, physical exam, diagnoses, and medications, among other things, are reviewed and documented.

Office visit templates These templates allow users to create the majority of an office visit note that includes verbiage common to all patients with the same ailment. When the OV template is selected in the *OV* screen the provider only needs to add limited details for a specific patient.

Order templates These templates store orders commonly used in a medical office. For example, physician order templates can be created for the most common laboratory, imaging, and medical tests and procedures.

Outpatient An outpatient is a person who is not hospitalized for 24 hours or more but may visit a hospital, a medical clinic, or other healthcare facility for diagnosis or treatment.

P

Past medical history (PMHX) This portion of the patient's face sheet contains healthcare information gained by clinicians regarding the patient's major illnesses, previous surgeries/operations, and so on. This information is used to help in formulating a diagnosis and providing medical care.

Patient Instructions Manager The Patient Instructions Manager is a central location in SpringCharts that houses all patient education material. From here patient instructions can be created, modified, and linked to diagnoses, labs, procedures, and medications for flagging in a patient's *OV* screen.

Patient portal Patient portals are online applications designed to allow patients access to and storage of some of their medical records and allow communication with their healthcare providers across the Internet. Some patient portals exist as stand-alone websites, while others are integrated into the healthcare provider's existing website.

Patient status The patient status allows clinical staff to know in general terms what is currently happening with a patient or what needs to be done next. The *Status* is chosen from a drop-down list that the clinic customizes.

Patient Tracker The Patient Tracker function enables all users across the network to see at a glance the current location and status of all patients in the clinic. It records the time each patient enters and leaves the clinic.

Personal digital assistant (PDA) The term PDA was first used in 1992 by Apple Computer CEO John Sculley. These handheld mobile devices function as a personal information manager.

Personal health record (PHR) PHRs allow patients access via the Internet to the medical office's website to store and update personal medical information. A patient can make enquiries of the healthcare provider regarding prescriptions, appointments, and other concerns.

Point of care Point of care is the time and place the healthcare provider gives the patient medical care.

Pop-up text Pop-up text is large groups of predefined text that SpringCharts users can rapidly select to complete office visit notes, letters, reports, messages, and to-do/reminder lists. The program includes 34 static categories and 20 categories of pop-up text that can be customized to suit the needs of each user. Each category has the capacity to hold 60 lines of customized type.

Practice management system (PMS) This type of software program manages, among other things, financial transactions, both charges and payments, and the billing of insurance claims and patient statements.

Pregnancy Estimated Delivery Date (EDD) Calculator The EDD calculator has been programmed to add 280 days (9 months and 7 days) to the first day of the patient's last menstrual period (LMP). Use of the LMP date to establish the due date may overestimate the duration of the pregnancy and can be subject to an error of approximately 2 weeks.

Primary insurance Because long term healthcare can be expensive, individuals and families have the option to purchase health insurance that covers a portion of the incurred medical expense. Typically, a patient will pay a monthly premium for the medical insurance policy from an insurance company which is known as the primary insurance carrier.

Procedure codes Procedure codes are numbers or alphanumeric codes that are used to identify specific health interventions taken by healthcare professionals. The codes ensure the standardization of definitions. Procedure codes are officially known as Current Procedural Terminology (CPT) codes.

Procedure templates A procedure template is text associated with specific procedures documented on the encounter note every time the procedure is used. It ensures the same explanation and discussion are provided for each patient undergoing the same procedure.

Protected health information (PHI) Regulated under HIPAA, PHI includes any information (past, present, or future) about health status, provision of healthcare (including mental health), and payment for healthcare that can be linked to a specific individual.

R

Reference lab The Reference lab is a secured area within SpringCharts accessed only by users who have appropriate security permission to view or process the information. When test results are received electronically from specific lab companies, they are automatically imported into the Reference lab for processing.

Return on investment (ROI) This measure, expressed as a percentage, is the amount earned from a company's total purchase or investment, calculated by dividing the total capital into earnings or financial benefits.

Review of systems (ROS) A review of systems is a structured technique used by providers to gather healthcare history covering the organ systems from a patient. It is therefore a component of the 'subjective' portion of the SOAP note. There are 14 body systems recognized by the CMS.

Rich text format (RTF) The rich text format is a document file format developed by Microsoft for cross-platform document interchange so that most word processors are able to read and write in the RTF format.

Routing slip The routing slip is a form that contains the medical office's most common procedure and diagnosis codes and descriptions. It also contains the patient's name, demographics, and billing information and may or may not include pricing. In a paper environment the physician usually indicates on the routing slip which procedures and diagnoses were used in the office visit. With an EHR program, only the codes and description selected in the office visit print on the routing slip. Some other names for a routing slip are Superbill, encounter form, charge ticket, and fee ticket.

S

Secondary insurance Secondary health insurance is an insurance policy that pays for some of the patient's medical expenses that primary health insurance does not pay, for example, the deductible and co-payments.

Server A server is a main computer designed to provide services to a client, workstation, or desktop computers over a local area network or the Internet. Many network software programs have a server component and workstation component.

SOAP This is an acronym for *Subjective, Objective, Assessment,* and *Plan.* The SOAP note is a convenient format for healthcare providers to document a patient's healthcare evaluation in a typical office visit.

Structured data Structured data is information organized in a format so it is identifiable, storable, retrievable, and analyzable in a computer system. Conversely, unstructured data is unidentifiable and not stored in a database (e.g., free text).

Superbill This form includes the medical office's most common procedure and diagnosis codes with descriptions. It is used to record procedures and diagnoses and for billing purposes. In SpringCharts, the Superbill displays billable codes and other items often overlooked or not available in the OV exam.

Surveillance Reports The main purpose of surveillance reports is to provide information to the federal Centers for Disease Control and Prevention to enable effective monitoring of rates and distribution of disease, detection of outbreaks, monitoring of interventions, and predicting emerging hazards.

T

Tablet A tablet is a portable, hand-held computer that allows users to document directly on the screen with a stylus pen or by touch.

Telehealth services These services use electronic and communication technology to deliver medical information and services over large and small distances through a standard telephone line.

Template This is an electronic document predesigned with a set format and structure. It serves as a model for a letter, fax, report, or note that a user then completes with patient-specific information.

Template manager The template manager in the SpringCharts EHR program allows for the creation, editing, and storage of three template types: office visit notes, orders, and letters.

Test script A test script in software testing is a set of instructions performed on the system to ensure the system functions as expected.

Time clock system Electronic time clock systems replace cumbersome time-tracking paperwork and eliminate manual collection of payroll information. They enable employee work time and attendance to be organized accurately into reports for payroll.

Toolbar The Toolbar displays a lineup of icons that give the user shortcut access to the most commonly used functions of the program.

U

User preferences Choices the user makes in software programs to preset elements of the program, such as the default practice name, physician name, schedule, and various other features displayed when the user logs into the program.

W

Wellness screenings These tests are periodic medical checkups to test for or inoculate against significant diseases. Wellness screenings are preventive services given to patients to prevent medical conditions.

Well patient visit The focus of a well patient visit is regular preventive care. Such healthcare measures include routine immunizations to prevent disease for children and adolescents and screening procedures for early detection and treatment of illness for adults. There is typically no treatment for a specific medical condition during a well person healthcare visit and the CPT and ICD codes reflect a wellness visit.

Wireless connectivity Wireless connectivity is the ability to make and maintain a connection between two or more points in a telecommunications system without using "hard" wires or cables. It allows for viewing of data between computer systems and transfer of data from one computer system to another, using electromagnetic waves.

World Health Organization (WHO) This international organization was established in 1948 for the purposes of coordinating international public health to achieve the highest possible level of global healthcare. It is a specialized agency of the United Nations (UN) and is headquartered in Geneva, Switzerland. The WHO has been responsible for developing and modifying ICD codes since 1948.

notes

Chapter 1 The Electronic Health Record

1. *EHR, Electronic Health Record: HIMSS*. 1999. www.himss.org/ASP/topics_ehr.asp (accessed June 25, 2011).
2. *eHealth Health Connect*. June 20, 2008. www.health.gov.au/healthconnect (accessed June 26, 2011).
3. *HealthConnect: Health Information When You Need It*. June 28, 2008. www.health.gov.au/internet/hconnect/publishing.nsf/Content/home (accessed June 25, 2011).
4. *eHealth Health Connect*, 2008.
5. National Committee on Vital and Health Statistics. *Report to the Secretary of the US Department of Health and Human Services on Uniform Data Standards for Patient Medical Record Information*. Washington, D.C., July 6, 2000.
6. "HIV Surveillance Report: Diagnoses of HIV Infection and AIDS in the United States and Dependent Areas, 2009." *Centers for Disease Control and Prevention*. 2009. www.cdc.gov/hiv/topics/surveillance/basic.htm#hivaidsexposure (accessed October 17, 2011).
7. Ross Koppel. "Google Gave Up on Electronic Personal Health Records, But We Shouldn't." *KevinMD.com*. August 2011. www.kevinmd.com/blog/2011/08/google-gave-electronic-personal-health-records-shouldnt.html (accessed October 17, 2011).
8. Chun-Ju Hsiao, Esther Hing, Thomas C. Socey, and Bill Cai. "Electronic Medical Record/Electronic Health Record Systems of Office-Based Physicians: United States, 2009 and Preliminary 2010 State Estimates." *HIMSS website*. December 2010. www.himss.org/content/files/359-3%20-%20EMR-EHR%20Systems%20of%20Office-based%20US%20Physicians.pdf (accessed October 24, 2011).
9. American Rhetoric—Online Speech Bank" "George W. Bush 2004 State of the Union Address" delivered 20 January 2004. http://www.americanrhetoric.com/speeches/stateoftheunion2004.htm (accessed March 2012).
10. "Bush Proposes Update to Patient Records." *Associated Press*. 2004.
11. B. Obama. "Transcript: Obama's Speech to Congress. Washington, D.C." February 24, 2009. http://www.cbsnews.com/stories/2009/02/24/politcs/main4826494.shtml (accessed June 23, 2010).
12. Families USA Issue Brief. "Congress Delivers Help to People with Medicare: An Overview of the Medicare Improvements for Patients and Providers Act of 2008." *Families USA website*. October 2008. www.familiesusa.org/assets/pdfs/medicare-improvements-act-2008.pdf (accessed October 24, 2011).
13. U.S. Department of Health and Human Services. *"Incentive Program Made Simple."* 2010. www.cms.hhs.gov/EPrescribing (accessed July 13, 2010).
14. SureScripts Progress Report. "The National Progress Report on E-Prescribing and Interoperable Healthcare, Year 2010." *SureScript website*. October 24, 2011. www.surescripts.com/about-e-prescribing/progress-reports/national-progress-reports.aspx# (accessed October 24, 2011).
15. *"EHR Incentive Program." CMS.gov/Centers for Medicare & Medicaid Services*. 2010. www.cms.gov/EHRIncentivePrograms (accessed June 2011).
16. Office of National Coordinator. *"Beacon Community Program."* 2011. http://healthit.hhs.gov/portal/server.pt/community/healthit_hhs_gov__onc_beacon_community_program__improving_health_through_health_it/1805 (accessed June 1, 2011).
17. Stephen Buse. "Benefits for All—More Patients in Less Time." *SpringMedical website*. April 11, 2011. www.springmedical.com/YPracticeYWay.html (accessed October 20, 2011).
18. A. H. Melczer, L. Berkeyheiser, S. Miller, and M. Yeager. "Background on Electronic Health Records for Small Practices." *White Paper: Illinois State Medical Society*. January 2005. www.providersedge.com/ehdocs/ehr_articles/Background_on_EHRs_for_Small_Practices.pdf (accessed August 7, 2007).
19. J. T. Scott, T. G. Rundall, T. M. Vogt, and J. Hsu. "Kaiser Permanente's Experience of Implementing as Electronic Medical Record: A Quantitative Study. BMI, 331, 1313–1316." *The Commonwealth Fund Website, Volume 29*. February 24, 2006. www.commonwealthfund.org. (accessed July 13, 2010).
20. L. Stammer. "Chart Pulling Brought to Its Knees." *Healthcare Informatics Volume 18*, 2001: 107–108.
21. D. Dassenko and T. Slowinski. "Using the CPR to Benefit a Business Office." *Healthcare Financial Management 68*, 1995: 68–70, 72–73.
22. J. Mildon, and T. Cohen. "Drivers in the Electronic Medical Records Market." *Health Management Technology 22*, 2001: 14–16, 18.
23. Melczer et al., 2005.
24. Market research study of group medical practice in the United States: "Office-based physicians and group practices." *SK&A—A Cegedim Company*. 2011. www.skainfo.com (accessed October 24, 2011).

Chapter 2 Standards and Features of Electronic Health Records

1. Certification Commission for Health Information Technology. *About the Certification Commission for Health Information Technology*. Modified 2011. www.cchit.org/about (accessed November 2011).
2. Ibid.
3. The Office of the National Coordinator for Health Information Technology. *About ONC*. Modified November 1, 2011. http://healthit.hhs.gov/portal/server.pt/community/healthit_hhs_gov_onc/1200 (accessed November 2011).
4. CMS.gov. "CMS EHR Meaningful Use Overview." *Centers for Medicare & Medicaid Services*. October 12, 2011. http://www.cms.gov/EHRIncentivePrograms/30_Meaningful_Use.asp (accessed November 2011).
5. Centers for Medicare & Medicaid Services. "Eligible Professional Meaningful Use Table of Contents Core and Menu Set Objectives." *CMS website*. October 7, 2011. www.cms.gov/EHRIncentivePrograms/Downloads/EP-MU-TOC.pdf (accessed November 2011).
6. D. W. Bates, et al. "Effect of Computerized Physician Order Entry and a Team Intervention on Prevention of Serious Medication Errors." 1998. *JAMA* 280 (15): 1311–1316.
7. U.S. Department of the Treasury. "USA PATRIOT Act." *Financial Crimes Enforcement Network*. Modified 2011. www.fincen.gov/statutes_regs/patriot/ (accessed October 2011).
8. P. A. Potter and A. G. Perry. *Fundamentals of Nursing (7th ed.)*. 2009. St. Louis, MO: Mosby.
9. Andrew H. Melczer, et al. "Background on Electronic Health Records for Small Practices." 2008. *Indiana State Medical Society:* 50–60.
10. U.S. Department of Labor, Employment and Training Administration. Used with permission.

Chapter 3 Introduction and Setup

1. The ONC-ATCB 2011/2012 certification does not represent an endorsement by the U.S. Department of Health and Human Services nor does it guarantee the receipt of incentive payments. The ONC certification number assigned to SpringCharts EHR 2011 is IG-2444-11-0037 (issued March 9, 2011).
2. Jack Smyth. *Spring Medical Moves Beyond ONC-ATCB Certification with SpringCharts EHR 2011*. March 15, 2011. www.springmedical.com/pr03112011.html (accessed August 2011).
3. Office of Management and Budget. *Revisions to the Standards for the Classification of Federal Data on Race and Ethnicity*. October 30, 1997. www.whitehouse.gov/omb/fedreg_1997standards/ (accessed August 2011).

index

A

B

C

D

E

F

G

H

N

O